Control of Movement for the Physically Disabled

Springer-Verlag London Ltd.

Dejan Popović and Thomas Sinkjær

Control of Movement for the Physically Disabled

Control for Rehabilitation Technology

With 297 Figures

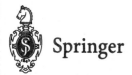
Springer

Dejan B. Popović, PhD
Thomas Sinkjær, PhD, DrMed

Center for Sensory Motor Interaction, Aalborg University, 9220 Aalborg, Denmark

Cover design adapted from the original painting "The Dance", by Djordje Popović, 1976. Used with permission.

ISBN 978-1-4471-1141-2

British Library Cataloguing in Publication Data
Popović, Dejan.
  Control of movement for the physically disabled : control
for rehabilitation technology
  1. Rehabilitation technology 2. Automatic control
  I. Title II. Sinkjær, Thomas
  617'.03
ISBN 978-1-4471-1141-2

Library of Congress Cataloging-in-Publication Data
Popović, Dejan.
  Control of movement for the physically disabled : control for rehabilitation technology /
Dejan Popović and Thomas Sinkjær.
     p. cm.
  Includes bibliographical references and index.
  ISBN 978-1-4471-1141-2   ISBN 978-1-4471-0433-9 (eBook)
  DOI 10.1007/978-1-4471-0433-9
  1. Rehabilitation technology. 2. Orthopedic apparatus. 3. Movement
disorders—Patients—Rehabilitation. I. Sinkjær, Thomas. II. Title
  RM950.P67 2000-06-13
  617'.03—dc21   99-462017

Apart from any fair dealing for the purposes of research or private study, or criticism or review, as permitted under the Copyright, Designs and Patents Act 1988, this publication may only be reproduced, stored or transmitted, in any form or by any means, with the prior permission in writing of the publishers, or in the case of reprographic reproduction in accordance with the terms of licences issued by the Copyright Licensing Agency. Enquiries concerning reproduction outside those terms should be sent to the publishers.

© Springer-Verlag London 2000
Originally published by Springer-Verlag London Berlin Heidelberg in 2000
Softcover reprint of the hardcover 1st edition 2000
The use of registered names, trademarks etc. in this publication does not imply, even in the absence of a specific statement, that such names are exempt from the relevant laws and regulations and therefore free for general use.

The publisher makes no representation, express or implied, with regard to the accuracy of the information contained in this book and cannot accept any legal responsibility or liability for any errors or omissions that may be made.

Typesetting: Camera ready by authors

69/3830-543210 Printed on acid-free paper SPIN 10756734

Foreword

Sensory-motor disability is one of the most debilitating injuries that man can experience following an injury of the neuro-musculo-skeletal system. Humans with motor disability often find themselves totally dependent on other people or devices for even the simplest tasks, which are normally taken for granted. Providing independence and mobility to a person with disability will ultimately improve his/her quality of life. Only full dedication to research and development that integrate the body of knowledge of living systems and technology is likely to allow humans with disability to enjoy the life again.

Medical management and rehabilitation engineering do not reverse paralysis or amputation; there is no cure yet for the pathology and the impairment, but much has been done to improve health and to restore functions. The investigation of new rehabilitation technologies and treatments has received much attention for several years, but the integrated, neuroscience-based research leading to an improved rehabilitation service, being measurable and verifiable, is still in its infancy.

This book follows many years of research and development in the field of motor control and rehabilitation technology for humans with sensory-motor disability. Designing and applying devices for restoring movement were an art for long time, only performed by skilled craftsman and physicians; today, it should be a regular constituent used to improve the life of millions of humans by returning them to every day activities and pleasure. The scientific and technological basis used as the template for writing this book was based on four elements: 1) assessing the difference between the motor performance of able-bodied humans and humans with disability; 2) designing rehabilitation methods aiming to maximize the use of the preserved neuro-musculo-skeletal system; 3) assessing the contribution that this rehabilitation is functioning and improving the quality of life; and 4) revising the rehabilitation accordingly.

The book provides a comprehensive reference material for individuals who study control of movement related to rehabilitation. The book is organized so that it can be used for teaching and assisting at different phases of the research and development of new rehabilitation technologies for restoring movement in humans.

Chapter 1 is a concise review of the basic neuroscience related to movement. The first section of Chapter 1 reviews the structure of the central nervous system; sections two and three the sensory and motor systems involved in the control of movement. The skeletal, muscular, and neural structures of extremities are described in the last two sections of Chapter 1. The organization of movement addressing the posture, walking, reaching, and grasping is detailed in Chapter 2. Chapter 3 summarizes the pathology leading to sensory-motor disorders and introduces methods for classifying and assessing the level of disability.

Chapter 4 gives an extensive review of the state of the art of rehabilitation systems and methods used to restore movement. The first section of Chapter 4 describes the basics of the neuroregeneration methods aiming to cure the disability. This section includes consideration of other surgical techniques aiming to cure neural damages. The Neurorehabilitation section of the chapter presents the methods developed to maximize the function of the preserved neuro-muscular structures by extensive functional therapy and augmented feedback. The Neuroprostheses section covers functional electrical stimulation and orthoses for restoring movement of paralyzed humans, and it includes a review of artificial extremities. The final section of Chapter 4 addresses some problems in the daily use of neuroprostheses (e.g., spasticity, efficiency, and functionality).

Chapter 5 is dealing with the control methods to restore movement. The authors suggest that an assistive system is effective only if it becomes integrated into the preserved neuro-muscular structures and benefits from all available resources. Modeling, identification of model parameters, and control based on those elements form the first section. Hierarchical hybrid control is described in the second section. Rule-base control is singled out as a suitable method for the coordination of movement. Methods for automatic acquiring of the knowledge base for rule-based control and examples of the application of these techniques form the remaining three sections of Chapter 5.

The opinion of authors how the basic, applied medical and engineering research will better serve the rehabilitation of movement is summarized in the Epilogue.

After studying the book, you will find yourself challenged with a controversy. On one side, you will find the extraordinary advances in understanding the control movements and the dramatic technological development, especially in microelectronics, micromachining, new biocompatible materials, and over all computer hardware and software. In contrast, there is a very slow acceptance of rehabilitation technology that uses some of the listed advances to restore motor functions. Why is the field of rehabilitation of sensory-motor functions developing relatively slow in the presence of both advanced technology and know-how? The most likely answer is that the future requires experts who are able to integrate the novel advances in technology and neuroscience into innovative ideas and solutions. It is the authors' wishes that the book will provoke you, the reader, being one of the individuals who will make the difference in assuring that the motor rehabilitation technology follows the success of other medical devices such as the heart pacemakers and cochlear prostheses.

Originally, both authors received engineering degrees, however, they have spent long periods of their professional carriers working with clinicians; they dedicated their work to the biomedical field, specifically to neuroscience. After teaching several courses and supervising many graduate students in both Europe and North America, it became apparent that a reference book, which can be used as a textbook, will facilitate this process and speed up the start of the research of young people. There is no other book that comprehensively presents the results from research and available rehabilitation technology. The book covers the state of the art of artificial extremities; external skeleton based orthoses and neural prostheses. The selection of the material for the book follows the research of the authors, yet it is not limited to techniques and methods developed by the authors; it gives a broad prospective of the field and should serve as a runway for the future research.

Without any reservations, the authors hope that the book provides a solid foundation to conquer some enigmas in the rehabilitation technology.

We wish to acknowledge our colleagues from Center for Sensory-Motor Interaction (SMI), Aalborg University, for providing material for the book and feedback after reading chapters or sections during the production of the book. Among them special thanks to Dr. Zlatko Matjačić who carefully read most of the material and made excellent suggestions, and Drs. Ken Yoshida, Ronald Riso, Johannes Jan Struijk, Francisco Sepulveda, and Morten Haugland. This book includes material that has been contributed by many of the graduate students who worked for obtaining their degrees in several laboratories and institutions, with which the authors have been working or collaborating during the last 20 years.

The greatest help in this project came from Dr. Mirjana Popović from the Institute for Medical Research, Belgrade, who read most of the book, provided many comments and suggestions, and assisted in many phases of the work.

We also express our special thanks to Ms. Susanne Nielsen from SMI, Aalborg, who edited carefully most of the material in the book.

Finally, we would like to acknowledge the Danish National Research Foundation, which partly supported the writing of the book.

May 2000   Dejan Popovic
                                                      Thomas Sinkjær

Table of Contents

1. Organs and Tissues for Human Movement   1

  1.1 Neuroanatomical Basis for Control of Movement   2
    1.1.1 The Central Nervous System   4
    1.1.2 The Functional Systems of the Brain   12
    1.1.3 The Morphology and Physiology of the Neuron   14
    1.1.4 The Membrane Theory of Excitation and Contraction   16
  1.2 Sensory Systems for Control of Movement   18
    1.2.1 Hierarchical and Parallel Organization of Somatic Sensors   18
    1.2.2 Frequency and Population Codes   21
    1.2.3 Dermatomes   23
    1.2.4 Cutaneous Mechanoreceptors   24
    1.2.5 Muscle Receptors   26
  1.3 Skeletal Muscles – Natural Actuators for Movement   28
    1.3.1 Structure of Skeletal Muscle   29
    1.3.2 Nerve Supply of Muscles   31
    1.3.3 Microscopic Structure of a Myofibril   31
    1.3.4 Neuromuscular Junction   33
    1.3.5 The Nature of Contraction   34
    1.3.6 Sliding Filament Theory of Muscular Contraction   35
    1.3.7 Muscle Function   43
    1.3.8 Tendons and Ligaments   45
  1.4 Skeleto-Muscular Structure of Extremities   46
    1.4.1 The Leg   46
    1.4.2 The Upper Limb – Arm and Hand   57

2. Mechanisms for Natural Control of Movement   69

  2.1 Organization and Mechanisms for Control of Movement   69
    2.1.1 Hierarchical Organization of the Motor Systems   71
    2.1.2 Parallel Organization of Motor Control Channels   74
    2.1.3 Afferent Fibers and Motor Neurons   75
    2.1.4 Interneurons and Propriospinal Neurons   76
    2.1.5 Neuronal Pathways   77
  2.2 Mechanisms for Control of Posture   78
    2.2.1 Biomechanical Principles of Standing   80
    2.2.2 Postural Adjustments for Focal Movement   83
    2.2.3 Sensors for Control of Posture   84
    2.2.4 Central Neural Mechanisms for Control of Posture   86

2.3 Mechanisms for Control of Walking — 87
   2.3.1 The Development of Walking — 88
   2.3.2 Bipedal Walking — 89
   2.3.3 Role of Various Neural Mechanisms in Walking — 91
   2.3.4 Central Pattern Generator: A Mechanism for the Control of Walking — 92
   2.3.5 The Role of Peripheral Input in Generation of Normal Walking Patterns — 95
   2.3.6 Effects of Sensory Feedback — 95
   2.3.7 Motor Programs for Walking — 96
   2.3.8 Motor Program in Humans with Paraplegia — 97
   2.3.9 Biomechanics of Bipedal Walking — 98
2.4 Control of Goal-directed Movement — 99
   2.4.1 The Development of Reaching and Grasping — 100
   2.4.2 Mechanisms for Control of Reaching and Grasping — 100
   2.4.3 Motor Planning — 101
   2.4.4 Visual Guidance in Goal-directed Movement — 105
   2.4.5 Precision of Positioning of the Hand — 106
   2.4.6 The Planning Space and Frames of Reference — 107
   2.4.7 Redundancy and Synergies — 109
   2.4.8 Redundancy and Motor Equivalence — 111
   2.4.9 The Equilibrium Point Hypothesis — 111
   2.4.10 The Muscle Patterns Underlying Movement — 114
   2.4.11 Optimization Theory — 115
   2.4.12 Motor Execution — 118
   2.4.13 Reaching Movement — 119
   2.4.14 Grasping — 120
   2.4.15 Coordination of Reaching and Grasping — 123

3. Pathology of Sensory-Motor Systems and Assessment of Disability — 125

3.1 Pathology of Sensory-Motor Systems — 125
   3.1.1 Cerebro-Vascular Infarction (Stroke) — 125
   3.1.2 Diseases of Transmitter Metabolism — 129
   3.1.3 Spinal Cord Injuries — 130
   3.1.4 Injury of the Neuron — 135
   3.1.5 Diseases of the Motor Unit — 138
   3.1.6 Neurogenic and Myophatic Diseases — 138
   3.1.7 Peripheral Neuropathies — 139
   3.1.8 Myopathies — 140
   3.1.9 Muscle Atrophy — 141
   3.1.10 Fatigue in Paralyzed Muscles — 143
   3.1.11 Spasticity — 144
   3.1.12 The Amputation — 145
3.2 Assessment Methods of Sensory-Motor Disorders — 146
   3.2.1 Standards for Classifying the Sensory-Motor Disability — 146
   3.2.2 The Functional Independence Measure (FIM) — 149
   3.2.3 The Quadriplegia Index of Function (QIF) — 149
   3.2.4 Muscle Assessment — 150

3.3 Movement Analysis ... 152
   3.3.1 Instrumentation for Data Capturing – Geometry ... 152
   3.3.2 Gait Events Data Capturing Systems ... 156
   3.3.3 Instrumentation for Recording Contact Forces ... 156
   3.3.4 Energetics of Walking ... 158
   3.3.5 Capturing Muscle Activity – EMG ... 159
   3.3.6 Measurable Characteristics of Walking ... 160

4. Restoring Movement: State of the Art ... 171

4.1 Neuroregeneration ... 171
   4.1.1 Techniques to regenerate CNS Structures ... 174
   4.1.2 Surgery to Provide Muscle Innervation - Grafting Peripheral Nerves ... 177
   4.1.3 Surgery to Provide Muscle for Movement - Tendon Transfer ... 180
4.2 Neurorehabilitation ... 185
   4.2.1 Neurorehabilitation of Walking ... 189
   4.2.2 Neurorehabilitation of Standing ... 194
   4.2.3 Upper Extremity Augmented Feedback ... 198
   4.2.4 Electrical Therapy ... 199
4.3 Neuroprostheses ... 205
   4.3.1 Functional Electrical Stimulation (FES) Principles ... 206
   4.3.2 Instrumentation for FES ... 212
   4.3.3 Neuroprostheses for Restoring Grasping and Reaching ... 250
   4.3.4 Neuroprostheses for Restoring Standing and Walking ... 259
   4.3.5 Orthoses - External Skeleton Neuroprostheses ... 268
   4.3.6 Hybrid Assistive Systems ... 277
   4.3.7 Issues Impeding the Effective Use of Neuroprostheses ... 281
4.4 Artificial Legs ... 290
   4.4.1 The Lower Limb Prosthesis ... 290
   4.4.2 Transfemoral Prosthesis ... 291
   4.4.3 Transtibial Prosthesis ... 300
   4.4.4 Hip-Disarticulation and Hemipelvectomy Prostheses ... 301
   4.4.5 Preparatory Prostheses ... 301
4.5 Artificial Hands and Arms ... 302
   4.5.1 Transhumeral Prosthesis ... 302
   4.5.2 Artificial Hand ... 304
   4.5.3 Activity Specific Artificial "Hand" ... 306
   4.5.4 Passive Arm-hand Prosthesis ... 307
   4.5.5 Body Powered Prosthesis ... 308
   4.5.6 Electrically Powered Prosthesis ... 310
   4.5.7 Hybrid Prosthesis ... 312
   4.5.8 Artificial Extremities – Summary ... 313

5. External Control of Movement — 317

5.1 Overview of Control Systems for Movement — 318
   5.1.1 Modeling of the Musculoskeletal System — 323
   5.1.2 Modeling of the Musculotendonal Systems — 327
   5.1.3 Identification of Model Parameters — 330
   5.1.4 Control Methods for Movement of a Single Joint — 335

5.2 Hybrid Hierarchical Control Systems — 350
   5.2.1 Nonanalytical Methods for Coordination of Movement — 353
   5.2.2 Rule-Based Control Systems — 354
   5.2.3 Methods and Tools to Define Rules for RBC — 355
   5.2.4 Machine Learning for Determining of the Rules for RBC — 360

5.3 Control Methods to Restore Standing — 364

5.4 Controlling Neuroprostheses for Walking — 371
   5.4.1 Analytical Methods to Control Walking — 371
   5.4.2 Nonanalytical Techniques to Determine Walking Synergies — 374
   5.4.3 Hierarchical Hybrid Control of Walking — 387

5.5 Controlling Neuroprostheses for Grasping and Reaching — 391
   5.5.1 Control Methods to Restore Grasping — 391
   5.5.2 Control Methods to Restore Elbow and Wrist Movement — 400

6. Epilogue — 409

References — 413

Abbreviations — 473

Index — 475

1. Organs and Tissues for Human Movement

> "The skeletal muscles are the motor machinery for all the life of the animal which the older physiologists were wont to call the "life of external relation." Of the importance of that life of external relation the moralist has written that even in man the crown of life is an action, not a thought. Should we demur to this distinction, we can still endorse the old adage that to move things is all that mankind can do, and that for such the sole executant is muscle, whether in whispering a syllable or in felling a forest."
>
> Charles Sherrington
> Kinacre Lecture, Cambridge, England, 1924

The question of which mechanisms are controlled and how the nervous system control the movement this has been investigated extensively and discussed at practically every stage of the history of motor control studies [e.g., Bernstein 1967; Granit, 1970; Arbib, 1980; Stein, 1982; Latash, 1993]. One important reason for controversies is the difference in understanding the word control. Human can control virtually any variable characterizing voluntary movement: joint angle (position), joint torque (force), movement speed, and accuracy. A systematic search for the "independently controlled" variables is connected to the classic work of Norbert Wiener [1948]; however, the pioneering, yet very well defined conclusions come from Bernstein [1967]. He was the first to address the motor control system as a "black box" with a virtually unknown internal structure that must control an effector apparatus of multiple links and degrees of freedom [Latash, 1993]. His experimental studies were based on mapping of input and output variables of the motor system. The conclusions are the following:

1) the control system is a hierarchical structure with several levels;

2) feedback loops connect the lower levels with the higher ones in order to tune the descending (efferent) commands;

3) time delays in the feedback loops require combining feedback and predictive, open-loop modes of control; and

4) the number of degrees of freedom in a motor system is always excessive, and the process of control can be regarded as overcoming the ambiguity caused by redundant degrees of freedom.

The hierarchical scheme should not be considered a reflection of actual organization of the central nervous system controlling movement. It is rather a simplified model (Figure 1.1) that appears helpful for understanding some phenomena that are of interest for controlling artificial extremities and neuroprostheses. The upper level in the scheme is associated with production of a "voluntary central motor command," in most cases a combination of conscious and unconscious decision. There is an interface that "translates smart and experienced" commands to the lower level, which now distributes control signals to the appropriate actuators controlling a single or more joints. The actuators receive proprioceptive information from the afferent sources, combine it with information from the descending sources and generate relevant controls to drive actuators. There is a constant exchange of information between lower and upper levels of control.

The engineering methods include two phases: defining the problem and solving of the defined problem. Controlling movement seems as an already defined problem: identify structures that are involved in movement, and find the relationship between them. Solving the problem is a much more difficult task, since there are no engineering methods that are fully suitable for interfacing natural control mechanisms. A general scheme, which seems to be promising, that authors are advocating relies on learned lessons from motor control studies and integrating those with modern computing and other technological advancements.

In order to be able to design artificial control it is essential to understand the richness of biological mechanisms and tissues that are involved in movement. As it will be presented the hierarchical, yet with many parallel pathways, self-organized natural control system that relies on extreme redundancy of both the sensory and motor systems is what automatic control is aiming at in the field of rehabilitation technology.

1.1 Neuroanatomical Basis for Control of Movement

Human motor performance appears to be remarkably flexible and easy. Yet, the underlying neuronal operations are only vaguely understood, even for well studied movements [Jeannerod, 1988]. Given the flexibility and the large number of degrees of freedom in the motor system, one might wonder what happens for simple motor tasks such as grasping a nearby small object. An object in the same position can be grasped in various ways by different combinations of joint angles in wrist, elbow, and shoulder, and by using different grasps (e.g., palmar, pinch). Is the same motor task realized by movement that are chosen randomly from the available repertoire, or is there a consistent reproducible patterns of behavior?

If the latter, can we then understand the constraints that are imposed in order to reproduce the same motor behavior every time when we repeat the same motor task [Bernstein, 1967]? The spectrum of functional motions, which a human can master during his lifetime, is impressive. Most of these movements are learned in early childhood, but the repertoire is increased on a daily basis if so required. As far as is known at present, this is possible because each functional motion relies upon perceptuo-motor coordination that involves three major components: the intake of sensory information, the internal coding of this information in a format that is adequate for driving a motor action, and the generation of movement itself. The last statement supports several interesting findings about the organization of the motor control with respect to the activity of neural cells within the premotor and motor cortex [e.g., Georgopoulos et al., 1982, 1993].

Since the work of Evarts [1966] it has been possible to monitor the activity of cells in the motor cortex of exhibiting monkeys. Initially, studies were restricted to simple movements about a joint, but Georgopoulos and his colleagues have extended these studies to reaching movements in two and three dimensional space [Georgopoulos *et al.*, 1983b]. Many of these findings were confirmed and expanded at later date [Schwartz *et al.*, 1988]. These results suggest that the motor cortex is concerned with the general planning of the direction of movement, rather than the details of the load or the muscles that will have to be activated to produce a desired end point.

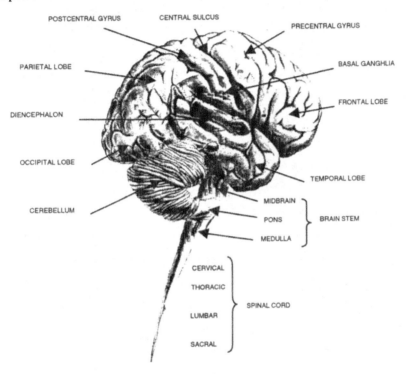

Fig. 1.1: The major division of the central nervous system. The top portion is a cerebral hemisphere. The six parts are: cerebral hemispheres, diencephalon, midbrain, pons, medulla and spinal cord.

Clearly, these signals must be transformed to produce the right movements under various conditions, but the mechanisms underlying these transformations remain unknown. Some aspects must arise from the pattern of anatomical connections from the motor cortex to the spinal cord and others from the variety of input that impinges on the motor neurons from sensory pathways and from other brain centers involved in the control of movement. Nonetheless, the generality of the signals available at the level of the motor cortex is intriguing. If one could record chronically from a number of cells in the human motor cortex, this technique might be used to control a prosthesis or for functional electrical stimulation of paralyzed muscles.

In this chapter we present the organization of both the nervous and muscular systems that is necessary for understanding of the complexity of controlling rehabilitation systems that restore movement.

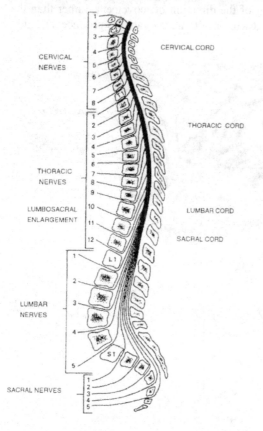

Fig. 1.2: Lateral view of the spinal cord and its location in the spinal canal.

A relatively simple set of functional and organizational principles governs the architecture of the nervous system, although that is in itself complex. These principles provide a foundation for understanding the control of movement. A review of the parts of the central nervous system considering their functional relevance to movement is given in this section.

1.1.1 The Central Nervous System

The brain and spinal cord are organized along the long axis of the human. The long axis of the nervous system bends at the juncture between the brain stem and the region just above it, the diencephalon (Figure 1.1). The central nervous system consists of six main regions: the spinal cord, medula oblongata, the pons, the midbrain, the diencephalon and the cerebral hemispheres.

The spinal cord, the most caudal part of the central nervous system receives information from the skin, joints, and muscles in the trunk and limbs, and it is the final station for issuing commands for movement. In the spinal cord (Figure 1.2) there is an orderly arrangement of motor and sensory nuclei, controlling the limbs and trunk. In addition to nuclei, the spinal cord contains afferent pathways for sensory information to flow to the brain and efferent pathways for commands necessary for motor control to descend from the brain to motor neurons. Afferent pathways carry information to the central nervous system; efferent pathways carry commands out of the central nervous system. The spinal cord also receives sensory information from the internal organs and controls many autonomic functions. The spinal cord has several functions: 1) it is a relay for sensory information; 2) it carries both ascending afferent pathways and descending motor tracts that serve the trunk and limbs; and 3) it contains the interneurons and motorneurons that control the movements of the trunk and the limbs.

A transverse section of the spinal cord shows that it is organized into a butterfly-shaped central gray area, where the cell bodies of spinal neurons are located, and a surrounding region of the white matter that contains afferent and efferent axons, most of which are myelinated (Figure 1.3).

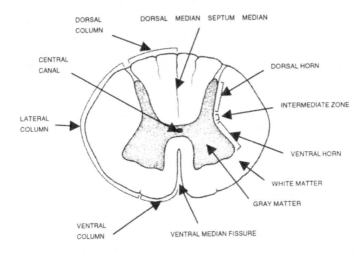

Fig. 1.3: The cross-sectional view of the spinal cord. The gray matter is divided into the dorsal and ventral horns, which are concerned respectively with receiving sensory and sending motor output of the cord.

The gray matter is divided into a dorsal horn, an intermediate zone, and a ventral horn (Figure 1.3). Each of these zones can be subdivided into nuclei. Six nuclei are particularly important: 1) the marginal zone, which is located in the outermost region of the dorsal horn and serves as an important relay for pain and temperature sense; 2) the substantia gelatinosa of the dorsal horn, which integrates afferent information from unmyelinated afferent fibers; 3) the nucleus proprius, which is located in the base of the dorsal horn and integrates sensory information with information that descends from the brain; 4) Clarke's nucleus, or cell column, which lies in the intermediate zone and relays information about limb position and movement to the cerebellum; 5) the intermediolateral nucleus, or cell column, which is located in the intermediate zone and contains autonomic preganglionic neurons; and 6) the motor nuclei of the ventral horn, which contain motorneurons that innervate the skeletal muscles.

The white matter is divided into three bilaterally paired columns, or funiculi: 1) the dorsal columns, which lie medial to the dorsal horns, contain axons that relay somatic sensory information to the medulla; 2) the lateral columns, which lie lateral to the spinal gray matter, contain axons descending from the brain that control sensory, motor, and autonomic functions as well as somatic sensory pathways ascending to the brain; and 3) the ventral columns, which lie medial to the ventral horns, contain axons of the motor neurons that control the axial muscles of the body.

In addition to the major ascending (sensory) and descending (motor) tracts that make up these columns, the spinal cord contains pathways for the axons of propriospinal neurons that connect different regions of the spinal cord.

Dorsal root fibers, whose cell bodies are in the dorsal root ganglia, enter the spinal cord at its dorsolateral margin. The largest cells have large myelinated axons that are up to 20 μm in diameter, and these fibers enter the spinal cord medially. The smallest cells have small unmyelinated axons less than 1 μm in diameter, which enter the spinal cord more laterally. After entering the spinal cord, the dorsal root fibers branch to ascend and descend in the white matter and arborize in the gray matter. Some ascending branches project to the medulla. The axons from large and small cells, carrying information from different somatic modalities, have different distributions.

There are two major ascending systems for somatic sensation: the dorsal column-medial lemniscal system, and the anterolateral system. These systems relay afferent information to the brain for three purposes: perception, arousal, and motor control. The dorsal columns relay information about somatic stimuli to the medulla. This tract runs ipsilaterally in the spinal cord. It originates both from the ascending axons of large-diameter primary afferent fibers and from the axons of neurons in the dorsal horn. The axons of the dorsal columns ascend to the caudal medulla where they synapse on the cells of the dorsal column nuclei. From there, by means of the medial lemniscus, a brain stem pathway, information is relayed first to the contralateral thalamus and then to the anterior parietal lobe. The dorsal column-medial lemniscal system mediates tactile sensation, including vibration sense, and proprioception from the contralateral side of the body. Proprioceptive information from the contralateral arm ascends in the dorsal column, whereas information from the contralateral leg ascends in the dorsal part of the lateral column, a region termed the dorsolateral funiculus.

The anterolateral system carries information chiefly about pain and temperature. It originates from cells in the dorsal horn. These cells send their axons to the contralateral side of the spinal cord and ascend in the anterolateral portion of the lateral column. In addition to pain and temperature, this ascending system also relays some tactile information. Parallel pathways are advantageous for two reasons: they add subtlety and richness to a perceptual experience by allowing the same information to be handled in different ways, and they offer a measure of insurance. If one pathway is damaged, the others can provide residual perceptual capability.

The proprioceptive information from the limbs is used at least in two ways. First, it mediates reflex responses through a local circuit in the spinal cord. Some of this information is relayed through the spinocerebellar pathways to the cerebellum, which modulates the actions of reflexes and voluntary movement. Proprioceptive information projects to the cerebral cortex where it is used for the perception of limb position. The distinction between the information carried by the spinocerebellar tracts and that carried by the dorsal columns and the anterolateral system is important because it illustrates that not all afferents or ascending information gives rise to sensation. It is therefore useful to distinguish afferent pathways, which carry information into the nervous system that does not enter consciousness, but contributes to movement from sensory pathways, which carry information that contributes to conscious perception.

The dorsal columns are primarily composed of the central branches of dorsal root ganglion cells (primary afferent fibers), which ascend to the caudal medulla without synapsing. It has recently been shown, however, that about 15 percent of the fibers in the dorsal columns are actually ascending axons of dorsal horn neurons, and therefore are second-order cells.

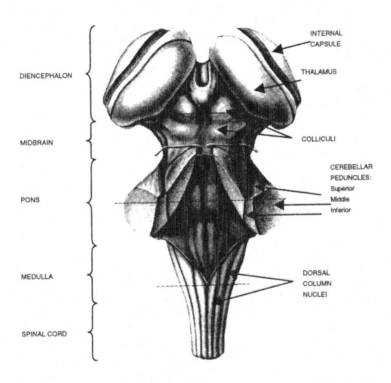

Fig. 1.4: Dorsal view of the brain stem with the cerebellum and cerebral hemispheres removed.

The spinal cord continues as the brain stem, which comprises the next three main divisions of the central nervous system (Figure 1.4): the medulla oblongata, the pons, and the midbrain. *The medulla oblongata* contains ascending and descending fiber tracts and a number of cranial nerve nuclei. It is easily distinguished from other parts of the brain stem at the point where the descending tracts cross and continue to the spinal cord on the contralateral side of the body (called decussation of the pyramids). The medulla houses the most caudal portion of the reticular formation, which, at this level, exerts inhibitory influences on spinal cord neurons.

The pons, which lies above the medulla, contains a massive set of neurons that relay information from the cerebral hemispheres to the cerebellum. The cerebellum is not part of the brain stem, but because of its position behind to the pons, it is commonly grouped together with the pons. The cerebellum is important for determining the timing sequence and the pattern of muscles activated during movement. Evidence suggests that it may also play a role in reflex modification and motor learning.

In another nomenclature the term metencephalon is used to describe the system consisting of the pons and part of the reticular formation. The cerebellum and vestibular apparatus are usually associated with the metencephalon because of location, although they are not considered to be a part of this subdivision.

The pons, like the midbrain, contains ascending and descending tracts and a large mass of transverse fibers on its ventral aspect. The literal meaning of the word pons is "bridge," which implies its function: it interconnects the two sides of the cerebellum and brain stem as well as the fibers connecting the cortex with the spinal cord. Also, several cranial nuclei are located in the pons, notably the main motor nucleus of the fifth nerve and the nucleus of the seventh nerve.

That portion of the reticular formation located at metencephalon level is concerned with facilitation and inhibition of lower spinal cord neurons.

The cerebellum is often dubbed "the great motor coordination center." It overlies the pons and presents a convoluted appearance with numerous fissures. Its specialty as a center for sensory-motor coordination is noted by the many afferent and efferent fibers associated with it. Sensory input is received from the vestibular system, spinal fibers, auditory and visual systems, reticular formation, and various regions of the cerebral cortex. In turn, it sends efferent fibers to the thalamus, reticular formation, and other parts of the brain stem. The cerebellum is often subdivided anatomically, and this type of organization appears to have some functional significance.

An extremely important aspect of the cerebellum is its extensive connections with many parts of the brain stem and cerebral cortex. It is involved in a large number of circles or loops, projects to many parts of the brain including the cerebral cortex, and is importantly involved in the descending tracts to the spinal cord.

The midbrain lies above the pons and is important in the control of eye movement. The midbrain also contains an essential relay in the auditory pathway and several structures critically involved in motor control of skeletal muscles.

Like the spinal cord, the three divisions of the brain stem contain motor and sensory nuclei, but most of these are related to structures in the head and neck, rather than in the limbs or trunk. In addition to the afferent and efferent systems that innervate the skin and the skeletal muscles, the brain stem contains systems that innervate blood vessels and glands in the head, neck, and viscera of the body.

The two pairs of relay nuclei, which subserve the visual and auditory systems, easily identify the dorsal portion of the midbrain (the tectum). The ventral portion of the midbrain (tegmentum) contains nuclei for the third and fourth cranial nerves, all of the ascending and descending tracts mentioned earlier in the section concerned with internal capsule, and a portion of the reticular formation. Two important centers are also located here: the substantia nigra and the red nucleus [Thompson, 1967]. The function of the substantia nigra is controversial, yet it is the major center for excitation of the gamma loop associated with the neuromuscular spindle. Its importance is recognized because it activates the gamma efferent system even before the alpha motorneurons to muscles are activated, and provides the background muscular tone so that discrete and highly coordinated movements can be performed. The red nucleus is primarily concerned with gross body movement especially as the body deviates from the standing upright posture.

Neural structures unique to the brain stem mediate some of the special senses, for example, hearing and taste. Each level of the brain stem also contains fiber tracts that descend from the higher levels of the brain to regulate activity in the brain stem and spinal cord, and tracts that relay sensory input from the spinal cord to the cerebral cortex.

Many of the neurons in the brain stem are grouped into orderly clusters with specific afferent and efferent fiber systems and reasonably well-delineated functions. The brain stem also contains clusters of neurons lying among the bundles (fascicles) of the crossing fibers and outside the discrete nuclear groups. These neurons constitute the reticular formation. Many reticular neurons have axons that spread widely in both directions, up and down the brain stem. As we shall see in later chapters, they also have a unique functional role in the regulation of overall levels of brain activity and the modification of spinal reflexes. Other reticular neurons have a more conventional pattern of either ascending or descending projections.

The diencephalon consists of the thalamus and the hypothalamus. The thalamus processes and relays most of the information coming from the lower regions of the central nervous system en route to the cerebral cortex. The hypothalamus helps in integrating the autonomic nervous system and regulating hormonal secretion. The thalamus serves many important functions other than the ones related to motor control. Along with the subthalamus, substantia nigra, and red nucleus, the thalamus operates in close cooperation with the basal ganglia to exert influences on motor activity. Also, impulses from the cerebellum are transmitted back to the motor cortex via a specialized nucleus of the thalamus, the ventral lateral nucleus. The subthalamic nuclei are importantly involved in the total circuitry that provides the background discharge necessary for the success of fine coordinated movements.

The basal ganglia are composed of the caudate nucleus, putamen, globus pallidus, amygdaloid nucleus, and claustrum. The latter two are not directly concerned with motor function and will not be discussed. Numerous pathways exist between the motor cortex and the caudate nucleus and putamen (collectively labeled the striate body); the latter sends numerous fibers to the globus pallidus, which communicates back to the motor area of the cortex via the thalamus. These circular pathways operate as a kind of feedback loop or servo-control mechanism [Guyton, 1991]. The functions of the basal ganglia are generally associated with the extrapyramidal system, one of the systems by which the cortex communicates with the final common pathways to muscle. If the cortex was destroyed, discrete movements of the body, especially the hands, would be impossible, but gross movements of a subconscious nature would still be possible; *i.e.*, walking and controlling equilibrium.

It is important to recognize the basal ganglia function as a total system. Therefore, assigning specific functions to each portion will not completely describe the physiology of the system. As a whole, the basal ganglia are generally recognized as centers capable of inhibiting muscle tone throughout the body [Noback and Demarest, 1981]. The striate body seems to initiate and regulate gross movements performed unconsciously. The globus pallidus is usually ascribed the ability to provide background muscle tone for movements that are initiated either by the striate body or by the cortex. Thus, the basal ganglia, together with other centers, modulate motor activities through circuits that feed back to the cortex.

The reticular formation is a vast network of neurons and nuclei, which anatomically is located throughout most of the brain stem. A portion of it is located in the diencephalon. It exerts powerful influences on phasic and tonic motor activities. That portion of the reticular formation located in the diencephalon is generally ascribed the ability to exert facilitatory influences on spinal motor discharge. Thus, flexor and extensor reflexes decerebrate rigidity, and responses evoked from the motor cortex are facilitated. An appreciation of some of the facilitatory and inhibitory influences initiated in the diencephalon structures can be attributed the reticular formation and some of the cerebellar and vestibular nuclei.

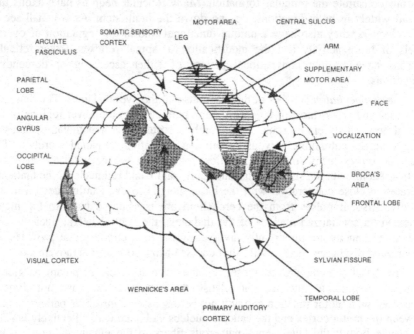

Fig. 1.5: The lateral view of the cerebral cortex of the left hemisphere.

The internal capsule is a massive bundle of nerve fibers, which links the cerebral cortex with other portions of the central nervous system. If the reader can imagine the diencephalon as a structure shaped something like a fist and inserted upward "inside" the cerebral cortex, it is easier to understand that the major routes to and from the cortex travel through the diencephalon. Ascending fibers projecting from subcortical nuclei to the cerebral cortex and descending fibers projecting from the cerebral cortex to lower centers of the brain and spinal cord are massed together and include both sensory and motor pathways. Generally, the internal capsule is divided into anterior and posterior limbs, each of which has distinct pathways associated with them. For example, the corticospinal tract (cerebral cortex to spinal cord) passes downward through the rostral portion of the posterior limb of the internal capsule and the brain stem, crossing to the opposite side at the medulla. The caudal half of the posterior limb of the capsule contains various projections from the many pathways of the thalamus to the cortex [Noback and Demarest, 1981]. The anterior portion of the capsule includes mostly the many fibers, which connect the several portions of the brain stem with each other and with portions of the cortex. Overall, the internal capsule, elaborated at the diencephalon level, can be thought of as the great "elevator" system of the human body because it represents the only means by which nervous system impulses may descend from or ascend to the cerebral cortex.

The cerebral hemispheres consist of the cerebral cortex and the basal ganglia. Collectively termed the cerebrum, these structures are concerned with perceptual, cognitive, and higher motor functions. Some of these complex functions and other specific behavioral functions have now been localized to specific regions of the cerebral cortex.

The cerebral cortex is thrown into infoldings called fissures and sulci. The most prominent fissure separates the brain along the midline into two fairly symmetrical hemispheres (Figure 1.5), each artfully divided into four lobes named for the overlying bones of the skull: frontal, parietal, temporal, and occipital. The central sulcus separates the frontal lobe from the parietal lobe. The parietal lobe is separated from the occipital lobe by the parietal-occipital sulcus (medial aspect of the hemisphere). The Sylvian fissure or lateral fissure separates the temporal lobe.

Large regions of the cerebral cortex are committed to movement and sensation (Figure 1.5). Areas that are directly committed are called primary, secondary, and tertiary sensory or motor areas. For example, the primary motor cortex, which lies within the precentral gyrus, contains neurons that project directly to the spinal cord. The primary sensory areas (the visual, auditory, somatic sensory and gustatory areas) receive information from peripheral receptors with only a few synapses interposed. The primary visual cortex is located at the back of the occipital lobe on its medial aspect. The primary auditory cortex lies in the temporal lobe, where it makes up a portion of the lower bank of the lateral sulcus. The primary somatic sensory cortex lies on the postcentral gyrus.

Surrounding the primary areas are higher order (secondary and tertiary) sensory and motor areas. These areas process more complex aspects of a single sensory modality or motor function than the primary areas. The purpose of the higher order sensory areas is to achieve greater analysis and integration of information coming from the primary sensory areas. In contrast, the flow of information from the motor areas is in the opposite direction. Higher order motor areas distill complex information about a potential motor act and relay it to the primary motor cortex, which is the site from which voluntary movement is initiated. The posterior parietal lobe, called the posterior parietal cortex, is transitional between sensory and motor functions.

Three other large regions of cortex, called association areas, lie outside the primary, secondary, and tertiary areas and function mainly to integrate diverse information for purposeful action. These three regions (the parietal-temporal-occipital association cortex, the prefrontal association cortex, and the limbic association cortex) are all involved in the control of the three major functional systems of the brain: sensory reception, motor control, and motivation.

1.1.2 The Functional Systems of the Brain

There are four principles that govern the functional systems of the brain:

1. The major system in the brain is composed of several distinct pathways in parallel. The sensory, motor, and motivational systems have subdivisions that perform subtasks. The sensory systems have separate divisions for each of the senses, and each of these divisions has components. The motor systems also consist of several pathways that run from the highest centers of the brain to the spinal cord. The pyramidal tract, a pathway that descends from the cerebral cortex to the spinal cord, mediates the performance of accurate voluntary movements of the hand. Other motor pathways control overall body posture and regulate spinal reflexes.

2. Each pathway contains synaptic relays. The multiple sensory, motor, and motivational pathways of the central nervous system are all interrupted by synaptic relays. These relays are not simply one-to-one connections between presynaptic and postsynaptic neurons, but a complex convergence of neurons. At these sites the sensory input, motor output, or motivational component are modified by processing that occurs within the relay nucleus itself as well as by input from other parts of the brain that converge on the relay nucleus. Two types of relay nuclei are particularly important: projection (or principal) cells that constitute the output from that nucleus. These axons leave the nucleus to synapse upon other nuclei or the cortex; and local interneurons that remain confined to the area around the cell body. Almost all of the sensory information that reaches the cerebral cortex does so after first having been processed by a relay nucleus in the thalamus.

3. Each pathway is topographically organized. The most striking feature of the sensory pathways is that the peripheral receptor surface (e.g., the retina, skin receptor) is represented in an organized way within a particular pathway. There is a somatotopic map, a map of the body surface, in the cerebral cortex. This map is also highly distorted in favor of regions that are particularly important for somatic sensitivity, such as the fingertips and the lips, whose representation occupies a relatively large cortical area.

The motor map, like the sensory maps, is distorted and reflects the fineness of control of the individual muscles. These central sensory and motor maps are clinically important; knowledge of them permits the neurologist to localize lesions in the central nervous system with precision because damage to a particular subdivision of a pathway will produce specific deficits in restricted aspects of motor or sensory function.

4. Most pathways are crossed. The bilaterally symmetrical neural pathways cross the midline; hence, the sensory and motor events on one side of the body are interpreted and controlled by the cerebral hemisphere on the opposite side. Furthermore, the pathways cross at different anatomical levels in different systems. In the somatic sensory system, crossing usually occurs soon after the first synapse is established by a primary afferent fiber. As a result, somatic sensation is processed on the contralateral side of the brain. The direct cortical motor pathway to the spinal cord crosses at the level of the medulla, and consequently the cerebral hemisphere on each side regulates the activity of muscles on the opposite side of the body.

All parts of the brain and nervous system are linked together in an elaborate network of pathways. Descending pathways are the means of communication from the cerebral cortex to the spinal cord, terminating on lower motorneurons. They are functionally divided into two systems: the corticospinal system (also called the pyramidal system) and the extrapyramidal. Other descending efferent projections are used to communicate with other parts of the brain and are named for the parts with which the fibers interconnect.

The corticospinal system (pyramidal system) includes roughly 60 percent of the fibers, which arise from the motor cortex (sensory fibers comprising the remainder) and descend through the internal capsule, crossing over at the medulla level and continuing down into the lateral white columns of the spinal cord. These pathways supply the motor nerves of the contralateral side of the body. The corticospinal system is often regarded as a very fast system because one synapse exists in the circuit between the motor cortex and the effector at the juncture with the alpha motorneuron. The sensory fibers project to the dorsal horn of the spinal cord for the purpose of modifying information, which is entering from the periphery.

The extrapyramidal system is the second means of communication from the motor cortex (as well as other cortical areas) to the final common pathway to muscle. The communication takes place via a series of "side trips" which involve other parts of the brain so that they can modify the signal, which finally arrives at the spinal cord level. None of these pass through the pyramids in the medulla; they can travel ipsilaterally or contralaterally. These pathways are also named according to the parts of the central nervous system with which they communicate. Thus, the names rubrospinal, vestibulospinal, reticulospinal, and tectospinal immediately convey to the reader the fact that the fibers originate in the red nucleus, vestibular nuclei, reticular formation, and the roof (tectum) of the midbrain, respectively, and all terminate at the spinal cord level.

The rubrospinal pathway, which originates in the red nucleus of the midbrain, descends in the lateral white column and innervates the distal muscles. The vestibulospinal pathway, which originates in the lateral vestibular nucleus, descends in the ventral white column of the spinal cord. The reticulospinal pathway, which originates in the reticular formation at the pons level, descends in both the ventral and lateral white columns of the spinal cord. Both the vestibulospinal and reticulospinal pathways terminate on proximally located musculature. The tectospinal pathway, which originates in the tectum of the midbrain, descends in the ventral white column and innervates the "neck" muscles.

The vestibulospinal pathways are divided into medial and lateral tracts. Vestibular nuclei located in the upper medulla and lower portion of the pons travel in the medial vestibulospinal tract, project to the spinal cord, and end in the cervical and thoracic level of the cord. The labyrinthine response, which corrects head position with respect to gravity, is mediated by the vestibular nerve, which feeds into this tract and modifies neck and upper-extremity muscle activity.

Lateral vestibular nuclei are somatotopically organized and influence postural mechanisms. They project down to the spinal cord via the lateral vestibulospinal tract and are generally known to facilitate extensors and inhibit flexors in order to maintain the upright position.

The reticulospinal are not somatotopically organized. They are divided into medial and lateral reticulospinal tracts: the medial is often called a reticulo-facilitatory tract because it facilitates extensor reflexes and inhibits flexor responses;

the lateral, the reticulo-inhibitory tract, is involved with inhibiting stretch reflexes in extensor muscles and facilitating flexor responses.

The medial reticulospinal tract assists the lateral vestibulospinal tract with problems of balance, although the vestibular pathways are more substantially involved. Both of the reticulospinal tracts act on the alpha and gamma motorneurons for the purpose of modifying and coordinating reflexes at the spinal cord level.

Ascending pathways are the means of communication from the spinal cord to the many brain centers, *i.e.*, sensory information. They can be divided into two functional units: those which contribute to conscious awareness, and those which may not reach the cerebral cortex, but play an important role in coordination. Most of the ascending pathways travel via the thalamus, especially those concerned with conscious perception; the "unconscious" pathways terminate in the cerebellum.

Proprioceptive pathways carry set of information from the muscle spindles and the Golgi tendon organ via two neurons, which travel ipsilaterally. The first order neuron terminates in the cord for lower extremities and in the medulla for the upper extremities. The second order neuron enters the cerebellum via the inferior cerebellar peduncles and terminates there.

The ventral spinocerebral tract, which also carries information from the neuromuscular spindle and the Golgi tendon organ, makes the first order neuron ascend ipsilaterally to the medulla. The second-order neuron crosses to the contralateral side and enters the cerebellum via the superior cerebellar peduncles. Some fibers may recross to the original ipsilateral side.

Ascending pathways subserving other functions include the spinotectal, which is associated with head and eye movement; the spino-olivary, which is presumed to be associated with movement; and the spinovestibular, which is concerned with postural reflex mechanisms.

1.1.3 The Morphology and Physiology of the Neuron

The nervous system is composed of two types of cells: neurons and glial cells. The neuron is the functional unit of the nervous system. Each neuron possesses in miniature the integrative capacity of the entire nervous system.

There are many more glial cells than neurons in the central nervous system. Glial cells are generally divided into macroglia (astrocytes, alogodendrocytes, and ependeryma cells) and microglia (phagocytic cells). Glial cells are typically small and do not generate active electrical signals. These cells are supporting elements that provide firmness and structure for the brain. Some glial cells are scavengers that remove debris after neuronal death. Certain classes of glial cells guide the migration of neurons, and some possibly have nutritive functions. The role of glial cells is essential in eventual regeneration of central nervous system, as described in section 4.1.

Neurons are usually greatly elongated cells with axon diameters ranging from 0.5 μm in small unmyelinated fibers to 22 μm in the largest myelinated fibers. Some axons exceed one meter in length. The diameters of cell bodies range from 10 to 50 μm. The neurons are specialized to receive, conduct, and transmit excitation.

A generalized neural cell or neuron consists of four morphologically and physiologically distinct portions: a receiving pole, a terminal transmitting pole, an

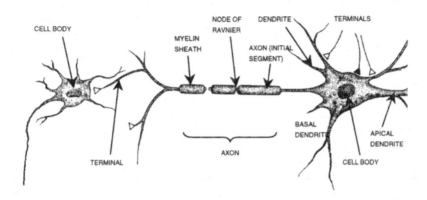

Fig. 1.6: The sketch of a typical neuron.

intervening conducting segment, and a cell body or soma (Figure 1.6). Each is specialized for its particular role in the function of the cell. The neurons possess two types of protoplasmic processes extending outward from the nucleated soma: dendrites and axons. The processes vary in length and in the amount and extent of their branching. The dendrites are usually multiple, short, and highly branched. The space occupied by their three-dimensional spread is often extensive. They constitute the receiving pole of the cell. The axons are usually single, long, and although one or more collateral branches may occur, relatively unbranched except at their ends. The axon is responsible for both conduction of excitation and its transmission to other cells.

An axon generates action potentials (nerve impulses) and conducts them from the receiving portion of the cell to the transmitting region. It is a delicate cylinder of neural cytoplasm with a limiting membrane, the axolemma. It varies in length and in diameter in different types of neurons. Axons are enclosed in a cellular sheath of lipid material, the myelin sheath, which serves to electrically insulate individual axons from one another and from adjacent neural components. The myelin sheath is formed by concentric wrappings of membranous processes from sheath cells, called oligodendrocytes within the central nervous system and Schwann cells in the peripheral nervous system. Small axons, which are invested by only a single layer of sheath cell process, are called "unmyelinated" fibers. Large axons are enclosed in increasingly more numerous sheathing layers formed by more and more windings of sheath cell processes. As the folds become tightly packed together, most of the cytoplasm is squeezed out so that the sheath is ultimately composed of spiral layers of lipid rich cellular membrane. The myelin sheath of the larger axons is segmented rather than continuous, and a single sheath cell encloses each segment. The length of the segments and the thickness of the myelin are quite consistent for neurons of a given caliber, large axons having longer segments (1 to 2 mm long) and thicker sheaths. The diameter of myelineated fibers usually ranges from 1 to 20 μm. The segments are separated by short unmyelinated gaps, so-called Ranvier nodes. Collateral branches, when present, arise at nodal gaps and exit from the parent axon at approximately right angles.

Nerve impulses are generated in the initial segment of the axon, which is unmyelineated even in myelineated fibers. The axon ends usually divide distally into a spray of terminals, which lose the myelin sheath and end in naked tips.

The cell body or soma of the neuron is the metabolic center of the cell, which is under control of its single nucleus, proteins, and other metabolically important substances. The materials are moved from the cell body into and along the neuronal processes. There are three channels for axoplasmic transport: the endoplasmic reticulum; the microtubules, and the neurofilaments. When severed from the nucleated portion of the cell, a nerve process will soon degenerate because it is no longer supplied with essential materials, and a new process will grow out from the cut stump, which is still attached to the cell body.

Mitochondria are present in axons, especially at the nodal areas, and are numerous in the cell body and in both the receiving and transmitting portions of the neuron, being abundant in the latter. Ribosomes are mostly restricted to the cell body. Minute and unique neurofilaments are distributed throughout the cytoplasm. Normally, the excitation is conducted only from the receiving to the transmitting pole of the cell. This polarity results from nerve cells stimulated at the receiving end. An axon that is stimulated at a point along its length is capable of conduction in both directions. Conduction of impulses in a direction opposite to the normal is referred to as antidromic excitation; for conduction in the normal direction, the descriptor is orthodromic.

Neurons may be classified as either receptor neurons or synaptic neurons based on the type of input, which they receive. Receptor neurons receive and transduce environmental energy such as light, sound, heat, or chemical or electrical energy. They are specialized to react to specific types of stimuli, and their dendritic portions are appropriately modified in structure. Synaptic neurons receive information from other neurons by means of synaptic transmission. Their dendritic geometry may be extensive and complex.

1.1.4 The Membrane Theory of Excitation and Contraction

The essential function of a nerve cell is to transmit excitation to other cells, and it responds by releasing a chemical transmitter substance at its synaptic terminal. A number of different kinds of stimuli may excite neurons. The normal stimulus for synaptic neurons is the action upon their membranes of chemical transmitters released by other neurons. Stimulation of receptor neurons is normally provided by chemical, thermal, mechanical, and electromagnetic energies. In a few instances, rare among the vertebrates, a neuron is stimulated by direct electronic stimulation from another neuron.

Some Characteristics of Nerve Conduction

Refractory Periods. As the action potential travels along the fiber surface, it consists of a wave of negativity followed by an area of gradually recovering positivity. While an area is in its reversed (active) state, it is absolutely refractory and cannot be re-stimulated. During recovery, the membrane is relatively refractory; a state which lasts many times longer than the absolute refractory period. Intense or sustained stimuli may restimulate the original site during repolarization.

Afterpotentials. During the relative refractory period both the amplitude and velocity of the spike are altered, reflecting changed conditions in the fiber. In some neurons the latter portion of the downward course of the spike is considerably less rapid than its rise, showing a marked concavity before reaching its initial level. This is the negative after potential because it indicates a delay in return to the resting potential and a prolongation of some slight depolarization (hence negative). During this period of 12 to 80 ms, the membrane is hyperexcitable or super normal and hence more easily restimulated. The recovery may continue into a hyperpolarized state, the positive afterpotential, which persists for a much longer time, up to 1 full second, during which the membrane is subnormal in excitability.

Frequency of Impulses. Neurons normally carry trains of impulses. In general, natural stimuli are of sufficient duration to reactivate the membrane after the absolute refractory period. A single electric shock may produce a single action potential, but only because its duration does not outlast the refractory period of the fiber. The stronger the stimulus, the earlier it will re-excite, and the shorter will be the time span between impulses, hence, the greater the frequency.

Because each action potential is followed by an absolute refractory period, action potentials cannot summate, but remain separate and discrete. The neurons do not conduct impulses at rates as high as the absolute refractory periods would suggest. Cognizance must also be taken of the characteristics of the relative refractory period. A fiber with a spike duration of 0.4 ms might be expected to conduct impulses at a frequency of 2500 per second, but its upper limit will be closer to 1000 per second. Conduction frequencies rarely approximate their possible maxima. Motorneurons usually conduct at frequencies of 20 to 40, rarely as high as 50, impulses per second, although, at the start of a maximum contraction, rates greater than 100 Hz have been recorded. Upper-limit frequencies for sensory neurons normally lie between 100 and 200 impulses per second although auditory neurons may conduct between 800 and 1000 impulses per second. Information is conveyed by the presence or absence of an action potential, as well as by the frequency of action potentials.

Velocity of Conduction. Velocity of conduction depends not only on myelination but also, more importantly, on the diameter of the fiber. It can be fairly accurately said that the conduction velocity is proportional to the diameter of the axon, and is in the range of 50 meters per second. The largest motor and sensory nerve fibers, with diameters near 20 µm, have conduction velocities up to 120 m/s. In small unmyelinated fibers, the velocities range from 0.7 to 2 m/s. Large fibers not only conduct more rapidly than small fibers, but characteristically have lower stimulus thresholds and larger spikes with shorter duration.

Classification of Nerve Fibers. As a result of the classic experiments of Erlanger and Gasser in 1937, nerve fibers are classified into three major groups, A, B, and C on the basis of conduction velocities. Group C contains the unmyelinated postganglionic fibers and group B the small myelinated preganglionic fibers of the autonomic nervous system. Group A includes the large, rapidly conducting myelinated somatic fibers. Group A has been further divided into four subgroups: alpha (α), beta (β), gamma (γ), and delta (δ) based on the velocity and diameter. The fastest fibers are those with the largest diameters. Sensory nerve fibers have been separately classified by Lloyd [1943] according to diameter into groups I, II, III, and IV, with corresponding velocities. These do not correspond exactly in size and velocity to the subgroupings of the Erlanger-Gasser class, but among afferents from the skin and muscles, group I approximates Aα, and group II approximates Aβ and Aγ. In order to avoid confusion, use of the alphabetical designations is restricted to efferent fibers and the numerical designations to afferent fibers.

1.2 Sensory Systems for Control of Movement

Sensory receptors are highly specialized neural structures that are receiving information about the external world. Various natural stimuli that impinge upon our bodies are transformed into neurally relevant signals at these neural structures. Sensory information is coming from the environment and from within our bodies (e.g., blood vessels, the actions of skeletal muscles). To distinguish the systems that convey signals from these different sources, the sensory systems are divided into three categories: exteroceptive, proprioceptive, and interoceptive.

Exteroceptive sensors are sensitive to external stimuli and include vision, audition, skin sensation, and some chemical senses. *Proprioceptive sensors* provide information about the relative position of body segments to one another and about the position of the body in space. *Interoceptive sensors* are concerned with internal bodily events such as blood pressure and the concentration of glucose in the blood. Unlike exteroceptive and proprioceptive stimuli, of which we are typically aware, interoceptive signals do not often reach consciousness.

The somatic sensory system receives and processes stimuli that impinge on the body surface or originate from within the deeper tissues and viscera. The somatic sensory system serves all three classes of stimulus reception. We may view the somatic sensory system as comprising several different perceptual modalities, or subclasses, each related to different stimuli. There are four major modalities: 1) tactile sensations, elicited by mechanical stimulation applied to the body surface; 2) proprioceptive sensations, elicited by mechanical displacements of the muscles and joints; 3) thermal sensations, including separate cold and warm senses; and 4) pain sensations, elicited by noxious stimuli.

1.2.1 Hierarchical and Parallel Organization of Somatic Sensors

The organization of a pathway for perception of somatic stimuli is schematically illustrated in Figure 1.7. The first neuron in the chain of events leading from the periphery to the central nervous system is the receptor neuron, which, in this example, is a dorsal root ganglion cell. Receptor neurons convert or encode natural stimuli into neural events. Only the distal portion of the peripheral axonal branch of the dorsal root ganglion cell is specialized to encode stimulus energy. The remaining portion of the axon is specialized to conduct information, encoded in the form of action potentials, to the central nervous system. A receptor neuron encodes stimulus information from a restricted region of the receptive surface. This region, called the neuron's receptive field, is the area of the skin within which a stimulus excites the receptor.

Receptor neurons in the somatic sensory system converge onto second-order neurons in the central nervous system. The second-order neurons also have a receptive field because they receive input from receptor neurons. The second-order neurons, which may be located in the spinal cord or the medulla, project to third order neurons in the thalamus. The neurons in the thalamus project in turn to the parietal lobe of the cerebral cortex.

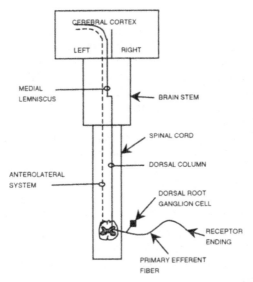

Fig. 1.7: The hierarchical and parallel organization of sensory system in two ascending parallel pathways: dashed and full line. See text for details.

Most modalities are subserved by more than one serially organized pathway. The dorsal column medial lenmiscal pathway and the anterolateral pathway mediate reflex functions. The parallel organization of sensory systems is important clinically because when one pathway is damaged, the remaining pathway can mediate residual sensory capabilities.

Sensory capacity reflects both the stimulus intensity necessary to elicit a perception and the precision with which the site of stimulation can be recognized. Different parts of the body vary greatly from one another in their sensory capacities. For example, the fingertips are very sensitive. When they move over a surface, their afferent fibers convey detailed sensory information about that surface to the central nervous system. In contrast, the skin over the elbow is limited to only the crudest discriminations.

Psychophysical investigation allows us to explore the performance of the neural machinery. Three observations will be discussed here: sensory threshold, evaluation of stimulus intensity, and two-point discrimination.

Sensory Thresholds for Perception

The absolute sensory threshold is the lowest stimulus intensity that a subject can detect. The threshold is determined statistically. If a subject is given several series of stimuli of different intensifies; the intensity at which the stimulus is first detected in each series (*i.e.*, the threshold) will differ slightly. Moreover, if a subject receives a series of stimuli, whose intensity is close to the average threshold, the subject typically fails to detect a certain proportion of stimuli. The threshold should therefore be defined as the stimulus intensity detected in 50 percent of the trials.

Stimulus Intensity

Not only is the somatic sensory system remarkably sensitive in detecting when stimuli occur, but it also provides information about the magnitude of the stimulus. This is important for our ability to discriminate between stimuli and to estimate stimulus intensity. The capacity to distinguish stimuli that differ only in magnitude depends on how large the stimuli are. Consider the discrimination of two weights. One can perceive a 5 N weight as different from a 10 N weight, but it is very difficult to distinguish between a 45 and a 50 N weight. Yet both sets differ by only 5 N [Weber, 1846], who developed a quantitative relationship between stimulus intensity and discrimination, now known as Weber's law. This law states that $\Delta S = K \times S$, where ΔS is the minimal intensity difference that can be perceived relative to a reference stimulus S (*i.e.*, background), and K is a constant. Thus, as the intensity of the reference stimulus increases, the difference in magnitude necessary to perceive a second stimulus as different from the reference stimulus also increases.

Fechner introduced the relationship between stimulus intensity and the intensity of the sensation experienced: $I = K \log S/S_0$, where I is the subjectively experienced intensity, S_0 is the threshold, S is the suprathreshold stimulus used in the estimation of stimulus magnitude, and K is a constant. Later experiments suggested the polynomial relation between the intensity and sensation: $I = K(S-S_0)^n$. This is important because natural stimuli vary greatly in intensity. The sensation is also sensitive to the discharge rate of primary afferent fibers.

Spatial Discrimination

Weber's early work on somatic sensation highlighted two attributes of the awareness of the spatial aspects of sensory experience: the ability to localize the site of stimulation and the ability to distinguish two closely spaced stimuli. The capacity to resolve two stimuli is quantified by measuring the distance between the stimuli, a measurement that Weber called the two-point threshold. The two-point threshold is 1 mm at the fingertip and increases markedly for more proximal parts of the body. The palm has, for instance, a two-point threshold of 10 mm; the arm, 20 mm. As the two-point threshold increases from the fingertip to the arm, there is a corresponding decrease in the accuracy with which we are able to localize the site of stimulation. Insight into the neural mechanisms for fine spatial discriminations on the finger tips has come from the work of Vallbo and Johansson [1984], who have systematically evaluated the receptive fields of mechanoreceptors that innervate the glabrous, or hairless, skin of the human hand. Vallbo found that the density of receptor innervation is four times greater on the fingertips than on the palm. The greater detail in the fine-grain resolution of the receptive sheet is reflected in a greater spatial sensory capacity.

Characteristics of the Stimulus

Sensory transduction is the first step in the extraction of stimulus features in the periphery. The unmyelinated ending of a single afferent fiber forms one kind of receptor. Here we consider the process by which the receptive portion of an afferent fiber converts natural stimulus energy into neural activity. This is the process of stimulus transduction. To activate a receptor, a stimulus must have a suitable intensity (greater than threshold) as well as a suitable quality. The dimensions of the receptive field typically exceed the regions of tissue directly innervated, since stimulus energy can be transmitted through body tissue.

The key to understand sensory transduction lies in the analysis of the receptor (or generator) potential, which is a local depolarizing potential that propagates only by electronic means and is therefore restricted to the receptive membrane. An opening of cation channels selective for Na^+ and K^+, similar to those that produce the excitatory postsynaptic potential produces the potential. When the amplitude of the receptor potential reaches the threshold of the trigger zone, an action potential is generated. The trigger zone is located on the myelinated portion of the axon. Because the trigger zone is close to the receptive membrane, the potential across this region reflects the sum of the receptor potential and action potentials. Farther from the receptive membrane and trigger zone, only action potentials are recorded. Suprathreshold stimuli lead to receptor potentials with faster rates of rise and greater amplitude. These receptor potentials evoke trains of action potentials at progressively higher frequencies.

1.2.2 Frequency and Population Codes

Stronger stimuli evoke larger receptor potentials, which cause not only a greater number of action potentials, but also action potentials at higher frequencies. The relationship between discharge frequency and stimulus intensity resembles the relationship between a subject's estimate of the magnitude of a stimulus and its intensity.

Stronger stimuli also activate a correspondingly greater number of receptors so that stimulus intensity is also encoded in the size of the responding population; therefore the term "population code" is used to describe the activity of the ensemble of responding receptors. As the stimulus intensity becomes greater, it is encoded in two ways: the conduction of a greater number of action potentials by each afferent fiber and the activation of more fibers.

Receptor Adaptation and Feature Extraction

An important feature of all somatic receptors is that they adapt. The receptor potential invariably decreases in amplitude in response to a maintained and constant stimulus, but it may do so either slowly or fast. An example of a slowly adapting receptor is the muscle spindle receptor, which is located within muscle and is sensitive to stretch. An example of a fast adapting receptor is the Pacinian corpuscle, which is located in subcutaneous tissue and is sensitive to vibration. The Pacinian corpuscle responds only transiently at stimulus onset and sometimes also at the end of a step change in stimulus position.

Adaptation often results from characteristic properties of the excitable membrane of the sensory neuron. However, in the case of the Pacinian corpuscle, adaptation depends on the nonneural accessory structure that surrounds the central unmyelinated axon. This accessory structure consists of concentric layers of connective tissue surrounding an afferent nerve fiber terminal. A steady stimulus applied to the outermost layer deforms the inner unmyelinated axon, but there is transverse slippage between the layers of the accessory structure so that the effective stimulus reaching the axon decreases with time. As a result, the accessory structure filters steady or slow components of mechanical stimuli, and the receptor responds only to rapid changes in pressure. It was shown that after removal of the connective tissue accessory structure transforms the Pacinian corpuscle from a fast adapting receptor into a slowly adapting one.

Fast adaptation in the Pacinian corpuscle is an example of a simple form of feature extraction - the selective detection by sensory neurons of only certain features of a stimulus. With a steady and maintained stimulus, stimulus onset and offset uniquely define the duration. Any intervening neural discharges are redundant and carry no additional information.

To investigate the composition of afferent fibers in peripheral nerves it is essential that the efferent fibers are eliminated. The simplest way to accomplish this is to remove the efferent fibers from the peripheral nerve in experimental animals by cutting both the ventral roots and the nerve trunks that contain the postganglionic motor supply. To ensure that the motor fibers distal to the transaction degenerate, a period of recovery must be allowed.

The conduction velocity of a fiber has important functional significance. The faster a fiber conducts action potentials, the quicker the central nervous system receives the information. Consider that in an average adult a stimulus delivered to a fingertip activates receptors that are located about 1 m from the spinal cord. An Aβ fiber, conducting at 50 m/s, conveys its information to the central nervous system in 20 ms. In contrast, a C fiber, conducting at the rate of 0.5 m/s, takes 2 s or more to convey the information, it carries to the central nervous system. If the stimulus is noxious and carried only by the C fibers, damage to the fingertip can begin long before the central nervous system receives the information. Time delays also occur in the central processing of a stimulus, which further increase the possibility of damage.

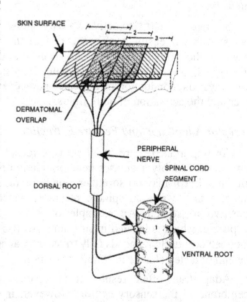

A peripheral nerve innervating the skin contains tens of thousands of axons, which may be subdivided into 20 fiber types based on the site of termination and function. Of these, eight fiber types are efferent and 12 afferent. The efferents consist of one extrafusal motor, two intrafusal motor, and five sympathetic fiber types. The 12 afferent fiber types are grouped into three classes, each containing four types: 1) cutaneous mechano-receptors, which are sensitive to skin deformations of various kinds; 2) proprioceptors, which are

Fig. 1.8: Sketch of dorsal roots innervating the skin. There is no clear border between dermatomes.

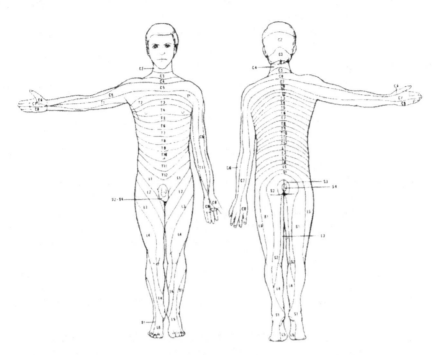

Fig. 1.9: The dermatomes of each spinal segment are located on particular regions of the body: S- sacral; L - lumbar; T - thoracic; and C - cervical.

sensitive to joint angle and muscle force and length; and 3) small diameter myelinated and unmyelinated axons, which are sensitive to thermal and nociceptive stimuli.

1.2.3 Dermatomes

Information from the periphery is brought into the central nervous system by afferent nerve fibers that run together with efferent fibers in peripheral nerves. As the peripheral nerves approach the spinal cord, they join together into spinal nerves. The afferent fibers in the spinal nerves separate from the efferent fibers and enter the spinal cord as the dorsal roots. Each dorsal root innervates a restricted peripheral region called a dermatome (Figure 1.8). At various points, called plexuses, located between the spinal cord and the periphery, the afferent fibers are regrouped so that each spinal nerve receives afferents from several peripheral nerves. As a result of this mixing of fibers, the area innervated by an individual dorsal root is less well defined than the area innervated by a single peripheral nerve. In fact, the areas innervated by adjacent dorsal roots overlap a good deal (Figure 1.8). Therefore, sectioning of the distal portion of peripheral cutaneous nerve results in a circumscribed area of sensory loss in the skin. In contrast, damage to a spinal nerve or a dorsal root often results only in a modest sensory deficit.

Dermatomes are arranged in a highly ordered way on the body surface (Figure 1.9). It has been possible to map the distribution along the body surface of the dermatomes for all of the spinal segments by studying the sensibility and responsiveness that remain after injury to dorsal roots.

The segmental organization of the dorsal roots is preserved in the various ascending systems. This shows that there is an orderly topographic arrangement between adjacent regions of the receptive sheet and all of the sites in the nervous system that receives sensory projections. This ordered mapping of the body surface onto central neural structures is called somatotopy.

1.2.4 Cutaneous Mechanoreceptors

The preceding specification of the sensory afferents and their response properties is a specification of the first stage of sensory coding, the encoding stage. However, it does not specify the relationship between our sensory capacity and the neural activity in these afferents. In some cases, the relationship is relatively simple. For example, the only afferents activated by small, continuous indentation of a fingertip are SAI afferents, and therefore the ongoing mechanical sensation must depend solely on activity in these afferents. Then, the question to be answered is: How does the sense of cutaneous indentation relate to the activity in these afferents? In most other cases, for example texture perception, the responses evoked by the relevant stimuli are very complex, and it is not possible to infer the basis of sensory capacity from a simple description of the encoding properties of single afferent fibers.

The standard method used to infer the neural mechanisms underlying human sensory capacity is the one pioneered by Mountcastle in his studies of vibratory sensation [Talbot *et al.*, 1968; Mountcastle *et al.*, 1972]. In that design, psychophysical studies of a particular aspect of perceptual behavior are followed by neuro-physiological studies using identical stimuli and stimulus conditions. The object of the neurophysiological studies is to reconstruct the population responses to all of the stimuli in order "to inquire which quantitative aspects of the neural response tally with psychophysical measurements" [Mountcastle *et al.*, 1963].

Combined psychophysical and neurophysiological studies have produced a rather neat picture of the neural mechanisms underlying tactile sensory function: the (slowly adapting I (SAI) system is responsible for form and texture perception, the fast adapting (FA) system is responsible for motion detection and perception, and the PC system is responsible for vibratory sensation. The role of the slowly adapting II (SAII) system is less clear because it has not been subjected to the same kind of combined analyses, as have the other afferent systems. By SAI system, we mean the primary slowly adapting type 1 afferent population and all of the central mechanisms that convey its signals to memory and perception. Similar definitions hold for the FA, SAII, and Pacinian (PC) systems. We do not mean to imply that there is no central convergence, *i.e.*, no overlap between the systems.

The psychophysics of tactile form perception and the evidence linking form perception to the SAI system, which has been reviewed recently", is as follows. The human ability to recognize complex patterns like Braille or embossed letters is essentially the same with or without horizontal scanning movements and whether the patterns are scanned actively or presented passively [Loomis, 1985]. The psychophysical results show that humans first begin to resolve spatial periods of 1 mm and reach threshold performance at a spatial period of 2 mm [van Boven and Johnson, 1994]. This corresponds exactly with the predicted limits based on spacing of SAI afferents at the finger pad and the response properties of SAI afferents, which resolve the spatial structure of gratings with 0.5 mm groove and bar widths. The psychometric function relating performance to the element size (gap, bar, dot size) is identical for gratings and more complex stimuli such as embossed letters and Braille characters. The SAI system appears to allow resolution of spatial frequencies up to 5 cycles/cm.

The only exception to the claim that the SAI system is responsible for form perception relates to the perception of microscopic surface structure. Katz [1989] demonstrated that finely etched glass is easily distinguished from smooth glass and surmised that the irregularities were too fine to be detected by the "spatial sense". LaMotte and Srinivasan [1991] showed that an etched pattern only 0.1 µm high could be detected based on responses of PC afferents [Johansson and LaMotte, 1983; LaMotte and Whitehouse, 1986]. Thus, it appears that the FA and PC afferents but not the SAI afferents transduce microscopic surface structure, which is easily detected.

Texture Perception. Tactile perception of texture has at least three perceptual dimensions and two of them are "smooth-rough" and "soft-hard" [Hollins *et al.*, 1993]. Both of these dimensions are based on measures extracted from the SAI spatial neural image evoked by textured stimuli [Johnson and Hsiao, 1992]. Combined psychophysical and neurophysiological studies, using identical textured surfaces have shown that roughness perception is not based on some measure of mean impulse rate or on some temporal measure of the afferent discharge in any of the afferent populations.

PC System. It is well known that Pacinian afferents are responsible for the detection of sinusoidal vibrations with frequencies exceeding 60 Hz [Talbot *et al.*, 1968]. While that fact alone does not suggest an obvious role for Pacinian corpuscles in ordinary tactile perception, the observation that textured surfaces can be differentiated effectively through a rigid probe by scanning the probe across she surfaces does suggest an important role for PCs. The basis for this discrimination is vibration induced in the probe; Katz [1989] demonstrated that this ability is diminished by any mechanism that attenuates vibrations transmitted through the probe or from the probe to the skin. Although a detailed study of the frequencies and amplitudes of such vibrations is needed, the primary candidate for the transduction of this vibratory information is the PC system because of its sensitivity to transmitted vibration. In experiments involving microneurography in humans, when an object was lifted from a platform and returned to it, there were abrupt mechanical transients that activated PCs vigorously, but affected SAIs and FAs minimally.

FA system. A puzzle emerging from the finding that SAI afferents are responsible for fine (but not microscopic) form perception is why the FA afferents should have the highest innervation density [Johansson and Vallbo, 1979; Darian-Smith and Kenins, 1980]. One of the earliest results of carefully combined psychophysical and neurophysiological study was that FA afferents are responsible for the detection of vibratory stimuli in the frequency range from 2 to approximately 60 Hz. However, that function does not seem to be the reason for the high innervation density. A more compelling reason is the recent discovery that FA afferents are responsible for the detection of motion on the surface of the skin [Srinivasan *et al.*, 1990]. A particularly important form of motion detection for motor control is the detection of overt or incipient slip. Johansson and Westling [1987] showed that subjects detect the coefficient of friction of a surface without overt horizontal movement between the skin and the surface, and that the FA afferents provide a signal inversely related to the coefficient of friction. High innervation density provides redundant sampling, which ensures that local slip is detected, and provides amplification of the signal. Considering that a typical FA afferent receptive field area is 10-15 mm^2, then any local slip, no matter how confined, is monitored by at least 10-15 afferents. These properties of the FA system identify it as the best candidate among the cutaneous afferents to provide signals for control of neuroprostheses for grasp and release.

Nociceptors

The receptors that respond selectively to damaging stimuli are called nociceptors. They are connected to axons belonging to two fiber classes: AS and C. There are three main types of nociceptors: 1) mechanical nociceptors are activated only by strong mechanical stimulation and most effectively by sharp objects. No response is evoked in this type of nociceptor when a blunt probe is pressed firmly into the skin, but a pinprick or pinch causes a brisk response; 2) heat nociceptors respond when the receptive field is heated to temperatures above 45 degrees Celsius, the heat pain threshold in humans; 3) polymodal nociceptors respond equally to all kinds of noxious stimuli (e.g., mechanical, heat, and chemical). Morphologically, nociceptors are bare nerve endings. It is not known, however, whether nociceptors respond directly to the noxious stimulus or indirectly by means of one or more chemical intermediaries released from the traumatized tissue. There are two different types of pain: fast and slow. Fast pain is an abrupt and sharp sensation that is carried by AS fibers. Slow pain, which comes from C fibers, is a sickening, burning sensation, which follows fast pain. Both types of pain can be felt in succession when, for example, the fingernails pinch the web between the fingers hard and quickly.

1.2.5 Muscles Receptors

Muscles and joints contain a variety of receptors. Some inform the central nervous system about the length of the muscle, others detect its tension, and still others respond to pressure or to noxious stimuli. Among these different receptors, two have been most thoroughly studied and have important and specific actions on motorneurons. These are the muscle spindles and the Golgi tendon organs. Although both of these receptors discharge when the muscle is stretched, differences in their anatomical arrangement within the muscle are reflected in differences in the information they convey to the central nervous system. Muscle spindles, arranged in parallel with the muscle fibers, provide information about the length of the muscle. Golgi tendon organs are arranged in series with the muscle fibers and inform the nervous system of the tension exerted by the muscle on its tendinous insertion to the bone (Figure 1.10).

Muscle Spindles. Mammalian muscle spindles are receptors that are distributed throughout the fleshy parts of skeletal muscle. Each spindle, which consists of an encapsulated group of fine specialized muscle fibers, is tapered at each end and expanded at its center in a fluid-filled capsule. Within this capsule the terminal branches of afferent fibers entwine the muscular elements.

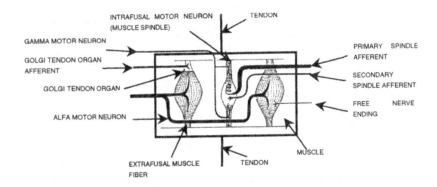

Fig. 1.10: The muscle spindles (intrafusal fibers) are in parallel with the extrafusal fibers; the Golgi tendon organs are in series. The intrafusal fibers attach actually to the extrafusal fibers, not to the tendons.

The small muscle fibers within the spindle are called intrafusal fibers; they do not contribute to the overall tension of the muscle, but regulate the excitability of the spindle afferents by mechanically deforming the receptors. Intrafusal fibers are innervated by small motor cells of the ventral horn called gamma motorneurons (Figure 1.10). The large skeletal muscle fibers that do develop substantial muscle tension are called extrafusal fibers and are innervated by the large alpha motorneurons in the ventral horn.

Muscle spindles contain two types of intrafusal muscle fibers called nuclear bag fibers and nuclear chain fibers after the arrangement of nuclei in their equatorial region (Figure 1.11). The bag fibers have nuclei clustered in twos or threes; the chain fibers have nuclei in single file and are shorter and more slender than the bag fibers. The bag and chain fibers also differ in the kind of contraction they exhibit: bag fibers produce slow contractions, whereas chain fibers produce fast (or twitch) contractions.

There are two types of afferent terminals in muscle spindles: primary and secondary. The primary and secondary endings differ in several ways. The most important difference is their relationship to the two types of intrafusal fibers. Primary endings innervate every single intrafusal fiber within a spindle. Secondary endings lie almost exclusively on nuclear chain fibers.

The Golgi tendon organ is a slender capsule approximately 1 mm long and 0.1 mm in diameter. Each organ is in series with about 15-20 extrafusal

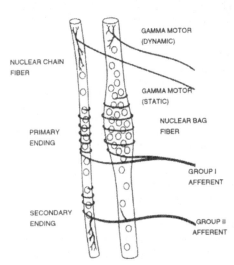

Fig. 1.11: Nuclear bag and nuclear chain intrafusal fibers within a muscle spindle.

skeletal muscle fibers that enter the capsule through a tight-fitting collar. The muscle fibers terminate in musculotendinous junctions after entering the capsule and give rise to collagen fiber bundles that become braided and run the length of the capsule. An afferent fiber enters the capsule in the middle and branches many times so that the axons of the afferent fiber become twisted within the braids of the collagen fiber bundles. When the skeletal muscle fibers contract, they cause the collagen bundles to straighten, causing compression of the afferent fibers and thereby, their firing. Thus, the organization of the collagen fiber bundles gives them an advantage in sensitivity to small changes in muscle tension. The afferent fiber responds to multiple motor units and so can register the effects of recruitment.

Muscle stretch receptors convey information about muscle length, tension, and velocity of stretch. Matthews [1933], who found that when the muscle is stretched, the afferent fibers from either the tendon organ or the spindle would increase their rate of discharge, first analyzed the relationship between muscle spindles and Golgi tendon organs. In contrast, when the muscle was made to contract actively while still stretched, then the tendon organ farther increased its discharge, but the spindle discharge decreased or ceased altogether. He explained this difference by the anatomical difference: the spindle organs are arranged in parallel with the extrafusal muscle fibers, whereas the Golgi tendon organs are arranged in series with the extrafusal fibers.

Loading of the muscle activates both the tendon organ and the muscle spindle receptors. Contraction further stretches the tendon organ. However, active contraction of the extrafusal muscle fibers makes the intrafusal fibers go slack, unloading the spindle so that it is no longer stretched.

The primary and secondary afferents in the muscle spindles respond quite differently when a muscle is stretched. Both fiber types respond to static (steady-state) stretch, but they respond differently to the dynamic phase of stretch. Primary endings are very sensitive to the dynamic phase of stretch, whereas the secondary endings are not. Thus the secondary endings are mainly sensitive to the length of the muscle, whereas the primary endings are sensitive both to the length of the muscle and to the rate of change in length. The dynamic sensitivity of the primary endings is largely due to the mechanical properties of the nuclear bag fibers.

There are two types of *gamma motorneurons*. One type innervates nuclear bag fibers (gamma dynamic or γ_d); the other type innervates nuclear chain fibers (gamma static or γ_s). The reason for the names dynamic and static is that these gamma motorneurons regulate the sensitivity of the spindle afferents either to dynamic or to static phases of stretch. An important role of the gamma system is to allow the spindle to maintain its high sensitivity over a wide range of muscle lengths during reflex and voluntary contractions.

1.3 Skeletal Muscles - Natural Actuators for Movement

The motor system of the human comprises three interrelated anatomical systems: the skeletal system, the muscle system, which supplies the power to move the skeleton; and the nervous system, which directs and regulates the activity of the muscles. Man has about 330 pairs of skeletal muscles of many shapes and sizes that are situated across more than 300 joints, being attached at two or more points to bones via tendons. Movement is produced by a shortening and broadening of the muscle, which brings the muscle ends closer to each other, ultimately changing the joint across which it acts.

The muscles differ in shape according to their functions. Some are long and slender for speed and range of movement (e.g., Biceps Brachii m.); others are sheet-like to form supporting walls (e.g., Oblique Abdominal m.); and some are multiple-headed to distribute and vary movement (e.g., the Deltoid m.).

Muscle has four well-developed characteristic properties: contractility, irritability, distensibility, and elasticity.

The most distinguishing characteristic of muscle is *contractility*. By contractility, reference is made to the capacity of muscle to produce force between its ends. Relaxation is the opposite of contraction. It is entirely passive; the giving up of force. Both relaxation and contraction progress from zero to maximal values over a finite time. Neither is instantaneous.

Irritability is the ability of muscle tissue to respond to stimulation. The muscle is the second most highly irritable tissue in the human body, being exceeded in this capacity only by neural tissue.

The muscles are *distensible*; thus, they can be lengthened or stretched by an external force. The stretching force can be the pull of an antagonistic muscle, of gravity, or of a force exerted by an opponent. Distensibility is a reversible process and the muscle suffers no harm so long as it is not stretched in excess of its physiological limits.

Unless a muscle has been over stretched, it will recoil from a distended length owing to *elasticity*. Distensibility and elasticity oppose each other, yet they assure that contractions will be smooth and that the muscle is not injured by a sudden strong change in either stretch or contraction.

1.3.1 Structure of Skeletal Muscle

It is necessary to consider the structure of the skeletal muscle before discussing its functions, because structure and function are interdependent and inseparable. The presentation starts with the macroscopic structure, *i.e.*, the muscle as a discrete organ; followed by important elements of the ultrastructure of the contractile machinery of the fibers, the myofibrils.

A *skeletal muscle* is composed of two types of structural components: active contractile elements and inert compliant materials. The contractile elements are contained within the muscle fibers. Each muscle is composed of many muscle fibers, a medium-sized muscle containing approximately 1 million. The fibers vary in length from a few millimeters to more than 40 cm, and their width is between 1 µm to 150 µm.

The fibers run with their long axes parallel to the length of the muscle (e.g., Sartorius m.), or they are arranged in the form of a spindle, so-called fusiform muscles (e.g., Gastrocnemius m.), or they have fan-shaped form (e.g., Adductor Magnus m.) as shown schematically in Figure 1.12. Finally, they can belong to a group of so-called pennate muscles. Pennate muscles are characterized by an arrangement of short fibers in a feather-like pattern. This type of muscle may be single or double pennate as in the forearm muscles, or the fibers may be arranged between multiple tendons as in the Gluteus Maximus m. The arrangement of the fibers is related to the function of the muscle concerned. Fast-acting muscles generally have parallel fibers, while those designed for strength are more often pennate. In general, individual muscle fibers run from tendon to tendon of the muscle.

About 85 percent of the mass of a muscle consists of the muscle fibers, while the remaining 15 percent is composed largely of connective tissues, which contain variable proportions of collagen, reticular, and elastic fibers. The distensibility and elasticity of muscles assure that the force of the muscle is transmitted smoothly to the load, and that an elongated muscle will recover its original length after being stretched. The connective tissues provide an arrangement of simple, spring-like elements (elastic components of the muscle), and which exist both in series and in parallel with the contractile elements.

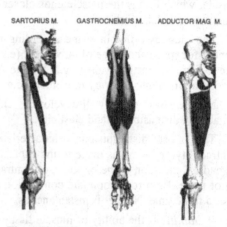

Fig. 1.12: Different types of skeletal muscles: parallel (right), fusiform (middle), and fan-type (right) fibers.

A connective tissue sheath, the epimysium, surrounds the muscle and sends septa (the perimysia) into the muscle to envelop bundles (fascicles) of muscle fibers. Larger bundles may be subdivided into several smaller bundles. From the perimysia delicate strands of fine connective tissue (the endomysia) pass inward to invest individual fibers.

The total number of fibers and hence the cross-section area of a muscle are related to its strength requirements, but the bundle size reflects the general function of the muscle. Muscles whose function it is to produce small movement increments, such as those required in manipulation, are composed of small bundles, whereas those concerned with powerful gross movements contain larger fascicles. As a result, the proportion of connective tissue is greater in the muscles, which are capable of finely graded movements.

The connective tissues of the muscle blend with the collagen bundles of the tendon, forming a strong and intimate union, the myotendinous junction. The connective tissues of the muscle and tendon are continuous. They act together as a buffer system against the possibility of too-rapid development of contractile force in the muscle.

Fascia and tendons act to harness the pull of the muscle fibers to the bony levers. When a relaxed muscle is stretched passively or when it actively contracts, the initial force developed is due to the elasticity of the connective tissues. In order to do work on a load, a muscle must first stretch out the elastic components until their force is appropriate to the load before any shortening of the muscle becomes apparent. Until then, there is effectively no load on the contractile elements. Once muscle force and load are in equilibrium, further expenditure of energy may be used to lift the load and perform external work.

The muscle obtains a rich blood supply from branches of neighboring arteries. The arteries and veins travel in the epimysium, while arterioles and venules course in the perimysia and capillaries run longitudinally in the endomysia between individual muscle fibers. Frequent transverse linkages between capillaries of adjacent fibers provide an abundant circulatory network. Capillary anastomoses are especially well developed in the neighborhood of motor end plates. In some instances, dilated cross-connecting vessels appear and are thought to act as reservoirs from which the muscle fibers may draw oxygen during sustained contraction, at which time the capillary flow may be significantly reduced by compression of the supply vessels.

1.3.2 Nerve Supply of Muscles

Nerves enter the muscle near the main arterial branch and divide to distribute both motor and sensory fibers to the muscle bundles. Motor fibers fall into two categories: large fibers (alpha subdivision of Group A) and smaller fibers (gamma subdivision of Group A). Each large alpha motorneuron, with its cell body lying in the ventral horn of the spinal cord, supplies a number of muscle fibers by successive bifurcation of its axis cylinder. One motorneuron and all of the muscle fibers that are innervated with the axon terminals constitute a motor unit. The number of muscle fibers per motor unit varies considerably with both the size of the muscle and the type of its function. Small muscles and muscles concerned with fine gradations of contraction have necessarily smaller motor units than larger bulky muscles whose job is the maintenance of strong contraction. For example, motor units in the extraocular muscles of the eye consist of about five muscle fibers per motor unit, while those of the gastrocnemius may have as many as 2000 fibers activated by one motorneuron. The size of the motor unit is related to the size of the muscle fascicles. A specific motor unit tends to be distributed among several fascicles in a limited area of the muscle.

The smaller gamma motorneurons innervate the muscle spindles, providing a means of central regulation of muscle contraction over an indirect pathway known as the gamma loop. Sensory nerve fibers are also of two general sizes: large Group I neurons whose sensory terminals lie in the muscle receptors (spindles and tendon organs) and smaller Group III fibers, which subserve the sense of muscle pain.

1.3.3 Microscopic Structure of a Myofibril

The muscle fiber is a syncytial mass of sarcoplasm, cylindrical in form with a bluntly tapered end and surrounded by a specialized membrane, the sarcolemma. The sarcolemma is a unit membrane about 0.01 μm thick. A number of nuclei lie peripherally just under the sarcolemma, and numerous myofibrils, each about 1 μm diameter, lie longitudinally embedded in the sarcoplasm. The myofibrils are the contractile elements of the muscle. There are about one thousand in each muscle fiber.

Viewed under the ordinary light microscope, the muscle fiber has a distinct cross-striated appearance of alternate dark and light areas appearing in a regular and repeating pattern. High magnification shows the striping to be a property of the myofibrils, which are oriented in register with dark regions adjacent to dark regions and light to light so that the pattern appears to extend across the whole fiber. Dark areas are known as A bands because of their anisotropic (doubly refracting) effect upon polarized light. Each appears to be somewhat lighter in its mid-region, the H zone, which is crossed by a darker line, the M line. The light regions are known as I bands because of their more nearly isotropic effect. Each I band is clearly bisected by a dark line, the Z disc or line. The region from one Z disc to the next constitutes a sarcomere. A sarcomere is both the structural and functional unit of the myofibril.

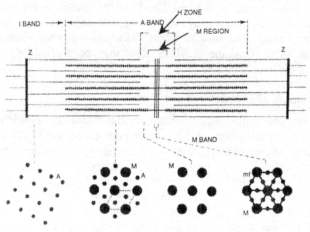

Fig. 1.13: The banding pattern of striated muscles results from alternating A- and I- bands, which are composed of thick and thin filaments. Transverse sections (bottom) at various locations along the myofibrils indicate spatial relationship of the filaments.

Each myofibril is composed of two types of filaments: one thick and short, and another thin and long. These are seen to lie longitudinally in a very definite parallel orientation (Figure 1.13). Each thick filament extends the length of the A band, while a thin filament passes from each Z line through the I band and into the adjacent A band as far as the edge of the H zone. Therefore, the denser outer portions of the A band are produced by the overlapping of thick and thin filaments for part of their lengths. The central H zone region is less dense because it contains only thick and no thin filaments. The I band is least dense because it contains only thin filaments. The H zone is not homogeneous, but shows variations in its density. Across its center is the dense region of the M line, on either side of which there appears a narrow region whose density is lower than that of the rest of the H zone. The lightest portion, known as the pseudo-H zone, maintains a constant width regardless of stretch or contraction, indicating that it is a structural feature of the thick filaments and not just another reflection of overlap.

The relation of filaments to fiber banding is clearly demonstrated by cross-sections through these areas. If sections are taken through the denser part of the A band, the thin filaments are found surrounded by thick filaments in an orderly hexagonal array; if through the H zone of the A band, only thick filaments are present, the thin ones being absent; if through the I band, only thin filaments are present. Thus, the cross-striations of the muscle fiber seen with the light microscope are found to be due to a repeating pattern of varying filament densities along each myofibril with the patterns of adjacent fibrils in register.

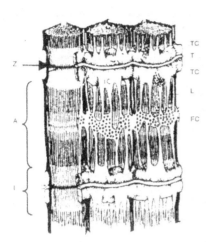

Fig. 1.14: Diagram illustrating the organization of myofibrils, internal membranes, and thick and thin filaments of skeletal muscle. The transverse tubule (T) and two adjacent terminal cisternae from the three-part triad structure involved in excitation-contraction coupling. The sarcoplasmatic reticulum consists of a fenestrated collar (FC), longitudinal tubules (L), intermediated cisternae (IC), and terminal cisternae (TC).

Chemical analysis of the fibrils shows them to be composed of about 20 percent protein, the rest being a watery suspension of salts and other metabolically important substances. About 80 percent of the protein consists of actin and myosin in a ratio of about 1:3. Actin is a low-viscosity protein, while myosin is more viscous. During contraction these two proteins combine to form a complex, actomyosin, which is the contractile material *per se* of the muscle fiber. Smaller amounts of two other proteins, tropomyosin and troponin, are also present.

The endoplasmic reticulum of the muscle fiber displays certain distinctive characteristics, which have merited the use of the term *sarcoplasmic reticulum* in reference to it. First, instead of being distributed throughout the cytoplasm, the membrane-limited tubules and cisterns form lace-like sleeves around the myofibrils in a distinct pattern, which is repeated in a definite phase relationship to the striation bands of each sarcomere. Secondly, there is a special arrangement of reticular elements in characteristic groups of three, known as triads, consisting of two cisterns separated by a transversely oriented tubule, the *T tubule* (Figure 1.14). The triads are found at the same site in muscle tissue of any given species. The T tubules are now known to be distinct from the sarcoplasmic reticulum, although they are functionally associated with it. The T system, as it is called, communicates with the sarcolemma or perhaps represents invaginations of it. The content of the tubules is continuous with the extracellular fluids and contains sodium in significant amounts. The cisterns of the sarcoplasmic reticulum contain a high concentration of calcium.

1.3.4 Neuromuscular Junction

As a terminal axon approaches a muscle fiber, its myelin sheath narrows and finally ceases a short distance before the end plate. It has been firmly established that there is no continuity of nerve and muscle protoplasms. The nerve axon does not penetrate the sarcolemma; its arborizations lie on the surface of the muscle fiber. Axon terminals may lie under the endomysium, but do not penetrate the sarcolemma. The neuromuscular junction is formed by axolemma and differentiated sarcolemma in apposition to each other. The structure of the muscle fiber in the junctional region is highly specialized. The sarcolemma is profusely folded into troughs and grooves, presenting a spiny or laminated appearance. The muscle portion of the neuromuscular junction has been called the subneural apparatus. Many muscle fiber nuclei are seen in the vicinity of the junction, accompanied by an abundance of mitochondria. Most authorities believe that the gap between the nerve terminus and the sarcoplasm is a specialized barrier across which excitation must be transmitted by chemical means.

1.3.5 The Nature of Contraction

Muscle may be excited and caused to contract by natural or artificial means. Normally, excitation is accomplished only by the nervous system: nerve impulses arriving at the neuromuscular junction cause the release of a transmitter substance, which diffuses across the junction and chemically excites the muscle fiber. However, whether induced naturally or artificially, the generation and conduction of action potentials in the sarcolemma of the muscle fiber evidence excitation. Action potentials travel along the fiber membrane at a speed of 1 to 3 m/s and initiate the events that lead to shortening of the contractile elements of the myofibrils and the consequent production of force in the muscle.

Muscular contraction requires the expenditure of energy obtained from chemical reactions coupled to a contractile mechanism which uses the energy to generate force and produce external work. Some facts regarding the processes involved are well established; others still controversial. In brief, the source of energy for muscular contraction is the high-energy-producing molecule, adenosine triposphate (ATP). In addition, other chemical substances are essential for muscular contraction. Among them are Ca^{++} and Mg^{++} and actin and myosin combined to form actomyosin. The ATP supply is generally maintained through the metabolism of glucose that is available in the blood stream. Glucose is supplied from storage in the liver in the form of glycogen. There is also an on-the-spot supply of glycogen in muscle cells. Glucose metabolism is accomplished in two ways, anaerobically by glycolysis in the sarcoplasm and aerobically in the mitochondria via the Krebs cycle and electron transport system.

A supplementary and rapid means of supplying ATP in muscle involves creatine phosphate. When vigorous muscular activity persists, wherein the oxygen supply is insufficient to meet the aerobic needs, glycolysis takes over and a condition of oxygen debt is reached and may be tolerated for a short period of time. Eventually the system must be balanced through the oxidative process.

Only about 40 percent of the energy resident in glucose is captured as ATP-stored energy, and of the chemical energy released from the ATP during contraction only about 30 percent can be converted into external work. This metabolically useful energy may be called the available energy. The rest dissipates as heat and represents energy wasted as a result of the inefficiency of the chemical and physical processes.

For almost three decades the work of Hill [1938] dominated thinking with regard to the *heat production* associated with muscular activity. Although some of the recent literature has raised questions concerning some points, it is still reasonable to divide the heat released by an active muscle into two major portions: the initial heat, which appears during the contraction, and the recovery heat, which appears after relaxation. The ratio of initial to recovery heat is the same for twitch and tetanus, whether isotonic or isometric.

The initial heat may be further divided into activation heat, shortening heat, and relaxation heat. Activation heat is produced upon stimulation and is associated with the appearance of the active state. It is probably related to the breakdown of ATP to initiate contraction and perhaps also to the thermal effects of the release and movement of calcium. It is the basal heat production, appearing whether the muscle shortens or not. It is independent of muscle length and force. In tetanic contraction *activation heat* is sometimes called the maintenance heat.

Shortening heat is produced when the muscle is permitted to shorten. It is absent in isometric contraction. Authorities seem to agree that the amount of shortening heat is proportional to the distance shortened and that the rate of its production is a linear function of the velocity of shortening. There is some disagreement as to whether or not it is also load-dependent.

As force subsides, a portion of the initial heat can be identified as *relaxation heat*. It may reflect the release of the energy, which was stored in the elastic components during the development of tendon.

Recovery heat constitutes a larger fraction of the total heat than the initial heat does. It is produced more slowly and over a relatively long period of time following contraction. It represents heat loss during the reconstitution of ATP by interaction with creatine phosphate and by cellular respiration, and during the resynthesis of glucose and glycogen from lactic acid. It can be subdivided into an anaerobic portion related to glycolysis and a larger aerobic portion, which varies with the amount of energy expended (work done), and which reflects the oxidative reactions of the Krebs cycle and electron transport system.

1.3.6 Sliding Filament Theory of Muscular Contraction

From electron micrography it has been concluded that in a stretched muscle the sarcomeres are longer than in a resting muscle, however the A bands are unchanged. Therefore, stretching has not lengthened the thick myosin filaments. The length of the thin actin filaments is also unchanged, as shown by the constancy of the distance from the H zone of one sarcomere through the Z line to the H zone of the next sarcomere. The H zones, however, have increased, and the I bands have lengthened. Apparently the extent of overlap of the two types of filaments has decreased while each filament has maintained its own integrity.

In a moderately contracted muscle, filaments and hence A bands still retain their original lengths, but changes are found in other parts of the striation pattern. Sarcomeres are shorter, and H zones and I bands have diminished. The area of overlapping of thick and thin filaments has increased (Figure 1.13).

Electron-microscopic evidence has led to the theory that the band pattern changes described above are due to the sliding of the filaments past one another, and that contraction is produced by the creeping of the thin actin filaments along the thick myosin filaments, the motion being mediated by chemical interactions between the filaments (gliding filament theory). This theory has been supported by experimental evidence of many kinds, and most physiologists now accept it.

Interactions of actin and myosin have a so-called "ratchet style". The myosin bridges oscillate back and forth, shifting their attachments from site to site along the actin filaments. The orientation of molecules in the myosin filaments suggests that bridge action exert forces that are directionally oriented toward the center of the sarcomere.

As the actin filaments advance farther into the A bands, the H zones will be reduced in size. The maximal number of bridges will be able to attach when the tips of the actin filaments have reached the outer borders of the pseudo-H zones. As further contraction advances the filaments first to the M line and then beyond it, actin filaments from the two opposite sides of the sarcomere will meet and then pass by, producing a double overlap of thin with thick filaments (Figure 1.13). In strong contractions extreme double overlapping will cause the H zone to be replaced by an area which is denser than the outer areas of the A bands, where only single overlap occurs. Electron micrographs of cross-sections taken through the sarcomere midregion show, under such conditions, twice as many thin filaments as are otherwise present. Even in maximally shortened muscle, however, the pseudo-H zones are still distinguishable, remaining constant in location and dimensions and lighter than adjacent portions of the double overlap regions.

The shortening of sarcomeres adds up to produce shortening of myofibrils, which in turn adds up to produce shortening of the muscle fiber; therefore the contractile force of the muscle represents a summation of the short-range forces acting at multiple bridges between the myosin and actin filaments. Each cycle of a bridge contributes its small part to the production or maintenance of force. Action of the bridges cannot be synchronous. While some are pulling, others must be just attaching and still others detaching to shift to a new site of attachment. The peak force at any moment reflects the average number of bridges that are active at that moment.

Relaxation

Muscular relaxation is completely passive. It is basically a cessation of force production and may or may not be associated with lengthening of the previously shortened muscle. Muscle fibers are incapable of lengthening themselves actively. If gross lengthening occurs, a force outside the muscle itself, such as gravity, contraction of antagonists, or of a load brings it about. However, as the bridges detach at relaxation, the internal elastic force, which has been built up within the fibrils during contraction, is released. Recoil of the elastic components then restores the fibrils to their uncontracted lengths. The passive lengthening of the fibrils will be concomitant with the slipping of the actin filaments away from the centers of the sarcomeres.

Contractile Force

The force developed by a contracting muscle is influenced by a number of factors such as the characteristics of the stimulus, the length of the muscle both at the time of stimulation and during the contraction, and the speed at which the muscle is contracting.

Most of what has been learned about muscle has been derived from studies using stimulation by electrical pulses. Although it is an artificial stimulus, electricity has distinct advantages for experimental purposes because it is controllable and reproducible. The intensity, form (time course of rise to and duration of peak intensity), and frequency of pulses can be arbitrarily selected and varied as desired.

Measurable responses of the muscle can be correlated with the quantified stimulus characteristics. Interestingly, new therapeutic locomotor aids are available using controlled electrical stimuli applied to the motor nerve or muscle when regular nerve function is disrupted.

In isolated preparation a muscle may be stimulated directly by pulses applied to the muscle tissue or indirectly by pulses applied to its motor nerve fibers. The response of the whole muscle, of a single motor unit, or of one muscle fiber may be studied under controlled conditions.

When a single pulse is applied directly to a motorneuron, the corresponding muscle fiber will respond in an all-or-none fashion. Increasing the intensity of the pulse will not increase the magnitude of the fiber's response. It is important to mention here that the all-or-none response of the muscle fiber is determined by the all-or-none character of its excitation and not by any all-or-none limitations inherent in the contractile mechanism itself.

When a single adequate pulse is applied to a whole muscle, the muscle will respond with a quick contraction, followed immediately by relaxation. Such a response is called a twitch. Its magnitude will vary with the number of muscle fibers, which respond to the stimulus, and this will vary directly with the intensity of the pulse up to a finite maximal intensity.

The twitch is an indication of force development by the muscle. After a short latent period, the force becomes evident and rises in a hyperbolic manner to a peak (the contraction period). It then declines over a slightly longer time course to zero (the relaxation period).

The time course of the development of overt force in the twitch is influenced by the interaction of the contractile components of the muscle fibrils with the elastic components of the muscle.

The time course of the force generated is studied by the techniques of quick stretch and quick release. Because of the elastic components and the viscosity of muscle tissue, the externally measured force exerted in a twitch is less than the full capability of the contractile material, that is, less than the intensity of the active state. The viscoelastic effect may be counteracted and the full force characteristics of the contractile elements registered by employing quick stretch or quick release. If, coincident with stimulation, the muscle is given a short, quick stretch which pulls out the elastic elements just slightly beyond what their effective excursion would be. The muscle is relieved of the necessity of stretching out the elastic components, and its full force is revealed. By this means the onset, rise time, and duration of the peak intensity of the active state can be determined.

The time course of the decay of the active state is studied by the method of quick release, in which the fiber is stimulated to contract isometrically until its full active state has been developed. Then it is suddenly released to a slightly shorter length. Force falls immediately, but is quickly redeveloped at a rate exceeding that in a normal twitch. The peak level, however, is lower. By varying the time of release and plotting redeveloped force against time, a curve reflecting the decline of the active state is obtained.

A single electrical pulse must have a certain minimal intensity to be effective. This minimal level is an inverse measure of the irritability of the tissue; the smaller the minimal intensity, the greater the irritability. The minimal effective intensity is designated the threshold or minimal stimulus. These terms refer to the weakest stimulus, which will evoke a barely perceptible response. Subthreshold and subliminal refer to a stimulus of inadequate intensity. As the intensity of the single pulse is increased above the minimum, the contractile force in the muscle increases progressively as a result of the activation of more and more muscle fibers. Finally, an intensity is reached evoking the maximal response of which the muscle is capable. Presumably all fibers are then active. Further increase in intensity will not be accompanied by further increase in contraction. The weakest stimulus intensity, which will evoke maximal contraction of a muscle, is called the maximal stimulus.

A weak, but adequate pulse with a rapid rate of rise from zero to its preset intensity will evoke a stronger contraction than a pulse of the same intensity with a slower rise. A minimal rate is required even for an intense stimulus. If intensity rises too gradually, there will be no response at all; the stimulus is then ineffectual. For any stimulus of adequate intensity, the more abruptly it is applied the greater will be the response it evokes within the limits of the muscle's capacity. The greater the intensity, the less rapidly it needs rise to produce a given level of response.

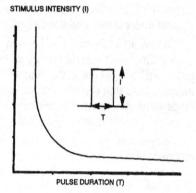

Fig. 1.15: Intensity-duration curve. The upper limb of the curve indicates that a very strong stimulus must be applied for at least a minimal duration, and a minimal pulse intensity is required to activate muscle (lower limb).

For a stimulus of adequate intensity and rise rate, the duration of its peak intensity will influence its effectiveness. Within limits, the longer its duration, the greater will be the response of the muscle. Exclusive limits are found at both extremes: the duration can be so short that no response will occur in spite of the fact that the same intensity and abruptness would be sufficient with longer duration, or the duration can be so long that the response decreases until it ceases altogether. The latter is a common experience in the laboratory when direct current is used to stimulate the tissue. The muscle responds at the closing of the circuit, but ceases to respond as current flow continues at the constant (peak) level. The duration of the peak intensity has exceeded the response capabilities of the tissue. The relationship of intensity and duration of single current pulses in the production of a barely perceptible contraction is presented in the intensity-duration curve (Figure 1.15).

If a stimulus of constant intensity and duration is applied at various rates of rise, effectiveness will be directly related to the rate. The more abruptly the stimulus is applied, the greater the response of the muscle will be. As the rate decreases, the response will diminish until ultimately, regardless of intensity, the stimulus becomes ineffectual. The decreased effectiveness of a constant intensity at long duration and/or low rate of rise are designated adaptation or accommodation. Many tissues besides muscle adapt to a gradual or persistent stimulus.

If an adequate stimulus is applied to a muscle fiber repeatedly at a rate rapid enough for each succeeding stimulus to reactivate the contractile elements before the previous force has completely subsided, successive responses summate, each building upon the previous one until a maximal level is achieved. If stimulation is continued, the contraction peak is maintained at this level. Such a response is known as tetanus or tetanic contraction. Ultimately, fatigue will cause the peak level to decline progressively. When stimulation ceases, contraction terminates, and the fiber relaxes, the force subsiding quickly to zero. If the repetitive stimulation is too prolonged, however, contracture will result, and relaxation will be very much slowed as compared with normal. Unlike rigor, contracture is reversible.

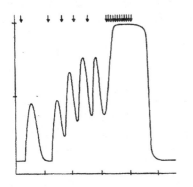

Fig. 1.16: The effect of the frequency of stimulation on the force developed in isometric conditions. First stimulus is a twitch (0.3 Hz), followed by 5 Hz and 50 Hz stimulation.

The frequency of stimulation, usually expressed as number of pulses per second or Hertz, determines both the shape and the magnitude of a tetanic contraction traced on a myograph by an excised muscle. When pulses are delivered with a time span (period) which places successive stimuli during the relaxation phase of the preceding response, the contraction approaches a tremor and a scalloped tracing results. This is incomplete tetanus. With a time span (period) which is short enough to allow for restimulation during the contraction phase, the tracing is smooth.

The force developed in response to repetitive pulses is greater than that evoked by a single pulse of the same magnitude (Figure 1.16). The tetanus to twitch ratio varies with different muscles and may even reach five. To explain the greater force developed in a tetanic contraction, it has been postulated that in a twitch the short duration of the active state allows too few bridge movements to permit the contractile material to shorten enough to stretch out the elastic components fully before the active state begins to subside. Hence the full capacity for force production cannot be realized. Repetitive stimulation, however, by maintaining the active state, permits continuation of bridge activity. The stretching of the elastic components is completed, and full force is developed.

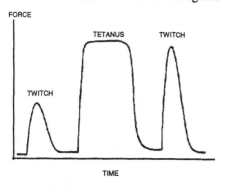

Fig. 1.17: Diagram demonstrating post-tetanic potentiation. Following a fused tetanus, isometric twitch force is greater then the same twitch response developed prior to tetanus.

In many muscles, if twitch responses to single pulses are recorded before and immediately after a period of tetanic stimulation, the postetanic twitch shows an increase in magnitude and a steeper rise of force than the pre-tetanic control. This phenome-non is known as post-tetanic potentiation (Figure 1.17). The effect occurs whether its motor nerve stimulates the muscle directly or indirectly. Potentiation is maximal shortly after the repetitive stimulation and then decays exponentially at a rate, which is dependent on both the frequency of pulses and the number delivered in the train. Short trains produce potentiation without any alteration of the twitch duration, but longer trains result in lengthening of the contraction time and of the half-relaxation time (the time required for force to drop to 50 percent of its peak value).

Muscle Length

The most obvious property of the muscle is its capacity to develop force against resistance. The length of the muscle at the time of activation markedly affects its ability to develop force and to perform external work. When a muscle contracts, the contractile material itself shortens, but whether the whole muscle shortens or not depends on the relation of the internal force developed by the muscle to the external force exerted by the resistance or load.

Three types of muscle contraction are distinguished according to the length change, induced by the relationship of internal and external forces: isometric, isotonic, and eccentric contraction.

If the internal force generated by the contractile components does not exceed the external force of the resistance and if no change of muscle length occurs during the contraction, the contraction is *isometric*. The available energy expended by the muscle and the force produced against the resistance may be considered to be in equilibrium. No contraction in the body is purely isometric because at the fibril level the contractile components do shorten. Stretching of the elastic components, as discussed above under active state, offsets their shortening. By current usage, an isometric contraction is one in which the external length of the muscle remains unchanged.

If the constant internal force produced by the muscle exceeds the external force of the resistance and the muscle shortens, producing movement, the contraction is *concentric*. Energy utilization is greater than that required for producing force that will balance the load; the extra energy is used to shorten the muscle. During concentric contraction, the muscle works against the load. A muscle can develop greater force in isometric than in concentric contraction because none of the available energy is expended in shortening. In concentric contraction the greatest load that the muscle can lift is about 80 percent of its maximal isometric force.

If an external force, greater than the internal force, is placed on an already shortened muscle and the muscle is allowed to lengthen while continuing to maintain force, the contraction is called *eccentric*. The energy expended by the muscle is less than the force exerted on the load, but the muscle acts as a brake controlling the movement of the load. In eccentric contraction a muscle can sustain greater force than it can develop in isometric contraction at any given equivalent static length. During an eccentric contraction the work is done by the load on the muscle. Eccentric contractions are very common. Every movement in the direction of gravity is controlled by an eccentric contraction (e.g., bending forward, placing any object down onto a surface). Electromyograms (which reflect the electrical activity of the muscle and hence provide insights regarding muscle contractions) show not only that anatomically antagonistic muscles are actively controlling the eccentric movement, but also that the electrical activity in these muscles is less than when the same muscles are contracting concentrically to do the same amount of positive work with the same load over the same distance and at the same speed.

Muscle Force vs. Length Relationship

The initial length of a muscle, *i.e.*, its length at the time of stimulation, influences the magnitude of its contractile response to a given stimulus. A stretched muscle contracts more forcefully than when it is unstretched at the time of activation. This is true whether the contraction is isometric, isotonic, or eccentric. Within physiological limits, the greater the initial length, the greater the force capability of the muscle will be. Parallel-fibered muscles exert maximal total force at lengths only slightly greater than rest length. Muscles with other fiber arrangements have maxima at somewhat greater relative stretch. In general, optimal length is close to the maximal body length of the muscle, *i.e.*, the greatest length that the muscle can attain in the normal living body. This is about 1.2 to 1.3 times the rest length of the muscle. Force capability is less at short and long lengths. Therefore, a muscle can exert the greatest force or sustain the heaviest load when the body position is such as to bring it to its optimal length. In isotonic contractions the increased force and longer length permit greater shortening; hence, more work can be done or, alternatively, the same work can be done at lower energy cost. The diminished energy cost of eccentric contraction is in part due to this stretch response, but other factors are also involved, as evidenced by the capacity to produce greater force than with either isometric contraction or isotonic contraction at most equivalent lengths.

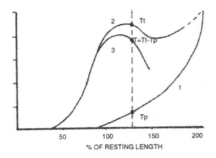

Fig. 1.18: Force *vs.* length curve for isolated muscle: 1) passive elastic tension; 2) total force; and 3) force calculated by subtracting of passive force from total force.

The relationship of force to muscle length may be presented graphically in the form of a force-length curve, in which force in an isolated muscle are plotted against a series of muscle lengths from less than to greater than the resting length (Figure 1.18). Both the passive elastic force (Curve 1) exerted by the elastic components in the passively stretched muscle and the total force (Curve 2) exerted by the actively contracting muscle are plotted.

Maximal contractile force is developed when sarcomere lengths are such that maximal single overlap of actin and myosin filaments exists. At greater lengths the number of cross-links diminishes as overlap decreases, and at shorter lengths double overlap results in reduced force as a result of the antagonistic action of bridges.

Speed of Contraction

Most isolated unloaded muscles normally shorten by about 50 percent or less of their rest length. The absolute amount by which any muscle can shorten depends upon the length and arrangement of its fibers, the greatest shortening occurring in the long parallel-fiber muscles such as the biceps and sartorius. In intact muscle, the structure of joints, the resistance of antagonists, and any load, which opposes the muscle, further limit shortening. The intrinsic shortening speed of a muscle reflects the rate of shortening at the sarcomere level. It is limited by the rate at which bridges can attach, move, and detach and by the rates of the chemical reactions involved. With muscle attachments severed, shortening speed of the contractile material is maximal but no force is developed. A muscle can produce force only when shortening against resistance, and the amount of force developed is equal to the load.

When shortening against resistance, speed varies inversely with the load. Therefore in isotonic contraction the less the resistance, the more nearly maximal is the rate of shortening. This may be explained as follows: the active state arises abruptly upon stimulation and persists for a relatively fixed period of time; the less resistance, which is met by the contractile material, the more readily the bridges function and the greater the distance of shortening accomplished during the persistence of the active state.

When a muscle is required to shorten more rapidly against the same load, less force is produced than when it shortens more slowly. This may be due to the fact that fewer links are formed between actin and myosin in the shorter time available and that the bridges, which do form, are detached more quickly. Consequently at higher speeds fewer bridges will be attached at any given moment, and less force is produced.

Force vs. Velocity of Shortening Relationship

The velocity at which a muscle shortens is influenced by the force that it must produce to move the load. In concentric contraction the relationship is evidenced by the decrease in velocity as the load is increased. Shortening velocity is maximal with zero load and reflects the intrinsic shortening speed of the contractile material. Velocity reaches zero with a load just too great for the muscle to lift; contraction is then isometric and maximal force can be produced. When more muscle fibers are activated than are needed to overcome the load, the excess force is converted into increasing velocity and therefore greater distance of movement. A commonly experienced example is the exaggerated movement, which occurs when one lifts a light object anticipated to be much heavier.

In eccentric contraction, values for shortening velocity become negative, and the muscle's ability to sustain force increases with increased speed of lengthening, but not to the extent which might be expected from extrapolation of the shortening curve (Figure 1.19).

Winter [1990] developed an instructive three-dimensional plot to demonstrate the relationship among force, length, and velocity. If force is a

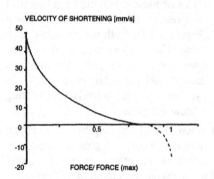

Fig. 1.19: Relationship among the normalized muscle force and velocity of contraction. Negative velocity relates to eccentric contraction, while the positive to active contraction.

function of both length and velocity, "the resultant curve is actually a surface, which represents only the maximal contraction condition." The more usual contractions would be at fractions of this maximum, and surface plots would be required for each level of contraction.

Slow and Fast Muscle Fibers

Although the previous discussion has considered striated muscle in general, there is abundant evidence that there are two types of skeletal muscle, distinguishable by speed of contraction and endurance. Over a hundred years ago Ranvier observed that some muscles of the rabbit were redder in color and that those muscles contracted in a slower and more sustained manner than did the paler muscles of the same animals.

Since then the designations of red and white muscles have become synonymous with slow and fast contraction, respectively. In addition to a slower contraction/relaxation cycle, red muscles have lower thresholds, tetanize at lower frequencies, fatigue less rapidly, and are more sensitive to stretch than the faster white muscles. As might be expected, individual muscle fibers reflect these differences in contractile behavior. Investigations by a number of workers have revealed histological and biochemical differences which distinguish the two types of muscle fibers and which correlate with the physiological differences between fast (white) and slow (red) muscles.

Most human striated muscles contain both types of fibers, but in differing proportions, which determine the color of each muscle. Some show a characteristic arrangement or zonation of the fiber types within the muscle; in others the two types are randomly distributed. In such muscles as the gastrocnemius, tibialis anterior, and flexor digitorum longus, fast fibers predominate, although slow fibers may also be present. In many mammals the soleus muscle appears to consist entirely of slow fibers. The preponderantly slow-fibered muscles are the antigravity muscles, adapted for continuous body support. Their sensitivity to stretch results in a continuously mild (tonic) activity even at rest. The predominantly fast-fibered muscles are phasic muscles, which produce quick postural changes and fine skilled movements. At rest they are electrically silent.

1.3.7 Muscle Function

Motor skill and all forms of movement result from the interaction of muscular force, gravity, and any other external forces, which impinge on skeletal levers. The muscles rarely act singly; rather, groups of muscles interact in many ways so that the desired movement is accomplished. This interaction may take many different forms so that a muscle may serve in a number of different capacities, depending on the movement. Whenever a muscle causes movement by shortening, it is functioning as a mover or agonist. If the observed muscle makes the major contribution to the movement, that muscle is named as the prime mover. Other muscles crossing the same joint on the same aspect, but which are smaller or which are shown electromyographically to make a lesser contribution to the movement under consideration, are identified as secondary or assistant movers or agonists. The muscles whose action are opposite to and so may oppose that of a prime mover are called antagonists. This does not mean that an antagonist, as the name implies, always exerts force against the prime mover; electromyography has demonstrated conclusively an absence of electrical activity in opposing muscles.

Synergy

Synergic action has been defined as cooperative action of two or more muscles in the production of a desired movement. A synergist, then, may be regarded as a muscle which cooperates with the prime mover so as to enhance the movement. Synergic interaction may take many forms and variations as discussed below. Two muscles acting together to produce a movement, which neither could produce alone, may be classed as conjoint synergists. Dorsiflexion of the foot at the ankle is an example. The movement is produced by the combined action of the tibialis anterior and the extensor digitorum longus. The tibialis anterior alone would produce a combination of dorsiflexion and inversion, while shortening of the extensor digitorum longus alone would produce toe extension, dorsiflexion, and eversion. Acting together, the muscles produce a movement of pure dorsiflexion. Another example occurs in lateral deviation of the hand at the wrist; e.g., ulnar deviation results from the simultaneous action of the flexor carpi ulnaris and the extensor carpi ulnaris.

The *sine qua non* of an effective coordinate movement involves greater stabilization of the more proximal joints so that the distal segments move effectively. The greater the amount of force to be exerted by the open end of a kinematic chain (whether it is the peripheral end of an upper or of a lower extremity), the greater is the amount of stabilizing force that is needed at the proximal links.

When a joint is voluntarily fixed rather than stabilized, there is, in addition to immobilization, a rigidity or stiffness resulting from the strong isometric contraction of all muscles crossing that joint. These muscles will forcefully resist all external efforts to move that joint. As fixation can be very tiring, it is seldom used and rarely useful. From the above discussion one should recognize the difference between stabilization and fixation of joints. As stated, fixation denotes a rigidity or stiffness in opposition to all movement, whereas stabilization implies only firmness. Economy of movement involves the use of minimal stabilizing synergy and no fixation of joints.

Multiarticular Muscles

A muscle crossing two or more joints has certain characteristics, capabilities, and limitations when compared with those muscles which cross only one joint. When a muscle crosses more than one joint, it creates force moments at each of the joints crossed whenever it generates force. The moments of force it exerts at any given instant depend on two factors: the instantaneous length of the moment arm at each joint and the corresponding amount of force that the muscle is exerting. The joint with the longest moment arm, and hence with the greatest moment of force, is normally the one at which the multiactuator muscle will produce or regulate the most action. The Hamstring muscles are specific; the moment arm at the hip is at least 50 percent longer than the one at the knee, and electromyography has repeatedly demonstrated that activity such as slow hip flexion as in toe touching is controlled by eccentric contraction of these muscles and that, when the action is reversed, they return the body to the upright posture without the assistance from the Gluteus Maximus m.

1.3.8 Tendons and Ligaments

Tendons and ligaments are composed of fibrous connective tissues. They contribute to a movement by transmitting the tension. Unlike muscles, tendons and ligaments are passive tissues. Tendons transmit forces from muscle to bone, whereas ligaments join bones to bones. Both tendons and ligaments contain relatively few cells, and their extracellular matrices are made up of a small number of components. These components are combined in different proportions to give mechanical properties appropriate to the function of the particular tendon or ligament.

The constituents of tendons are the gel-like ground substance, collagen, and elastic fibrils. A weak gel, known as "ground substance," which consists largely of water, surrounds the fibrils of the extracellular matrix. Tendons and ligaments typically contain about 60-70 percent of water, most of which is associated with the ground substance [Elliott, 1965; Nachemson and Evans, 1968]. Water is attracted to the ground substance because it contains glycosaminoglycans [Maroudas, 1975]. Collagen fibrils are able to reinforce the weak ground substance because of their much greater stiffness and strength in tension [Minns et al., 1973; Hukins, 1982]. Each fibril is like a rope in which linear molecules are packed together with their axes parallel, within a few degrees, to the fibril axis.

The function of collagen fibrils must withstand axial tension. They are like any rope weak in compression and flexion [Hukins, 1982]. Whenever a fibril is pulled, its length increases. This length increase, which is normally expressed as a fraction of the original length and is then termed "strain" leads to a restoring force in the fibril that balances the applied force. This behavior is rather like a loaded spring, which stretches to enable it to bear the load but returns to its relaxed length on removing the load. Similarly, collagen fibrils are able to reinforce a tissue if they are oriented so that an applied force tends to stretch them [Hukins, 1984].

The function of the tendon is to transmit the force generated by a contracting muscle to the correct point of application on a bone and to manipulate a joint. The tendons are often preferable to direct attachment of the muscle to the bone because of various functional requirements. Muscles have a low tensile strength, defined as load-at-fracture per unit cross-sectional area. The muscle is located further away and a tendon makes attachment (e.g., flexor digitorum profundus and flexor digitorum superficialis flex the last and metacarpal phalanx of fingers being remote in the forearm). The tendons are strong, so even if they are thin and stiff they are able to transmit the force. The tendons are elastic and they store some of the energy.

The size of the tendon (cross sectional area) is directly related to the elastic properties. The forces transmitted by tendons can be very high. Tendons can be relatively elongated of up to about 4 percent [Haut and Little, 1972]. Beyond this strain a tendon does not return to its original length when the applied stress is removed. A tendon will break at strains of 10 percent [Haut and Little, 1972]. The initial stages of tendon extension involve straightening the crimp of the collagen fibrils described previously. When the crimp is removed, all the collagen fibrils are highly aligned along the direction of the tendon, so the tendon becomes much stiffer. The advantage of a material with this form of stress-strain relationship is that it also confers a measure of protection to the material. The area under the stress-strain curve gives the energy stored in the stretched tendon.

Ligaments have a role similar to tendons; to transmit tension, but they connect two bony tissues. Ligaments differ greatly from tendons in composition [Hukins, 1984]. The range of structures and compositions is understandable when it is realized that the function of a ligament is very dependent on its position in the body; the medial collateral ligament in the knee, operates at strains of about 2 percent, whereas the ligamentum flavum of the human spine operates at strains of up to 60 percent [Nachemson and Evans, 1968]. A ligament contains a high proportion of elastin (about 60-70 percent of the dry weight), which enables it to withstand these high strains without fracture [Minns et al., 1973].

If the stress applied to a tendon or ligament is sufficiently high, the tissue will be damaged. When a tissue is stretched, work is done on it and most of that work is stored as energy of deformation in the tissue. Because tendon and ligaments are viscoelastic, causing fluid flow of the ground substance as previously described, this dissipates some of the energy, but the rest is stored in the stretched tissue. This stored energy can be used to disrupt structure within the material and thereby cause damage.

1.4 Skeleto-Muscular Structure of Extremities

1.4.1 The Leg

The human leg is a biomechanical structure involving many bones, joints and muscles. The leg can be divided into three main parts: the foot, the shank and the thigh. These three "segments" connect at the ankle joint, the knee joint and the hip joint (thigh to body contact). A diagram of the skeleton is shown in (Figure 1.20).

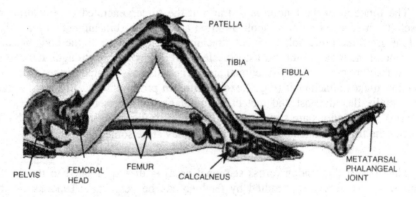

Fig. 1.20: Sketch of the skeleton of the leg.

The Hip Bone

The bony pelvis consists of the two hipbones, the sacrum and the coccyx. The hip bone consists of three parts, the pubis, the ilium and the ischium which synostose in the acetabular fossa (Figure 1.21). The two hip bones are joined at the symphysis pubis by a fibrous cartilage with a hyaline cartilage covering, the interpubic disk. Within the disk a small nonsynovial cavity may be present. The auricular surface of the hip bone and the auricular surface of the sacrum form the articulation. Both are covered by fibrous cartilage. A very taut joint capsule encloses the almost immobile joint.

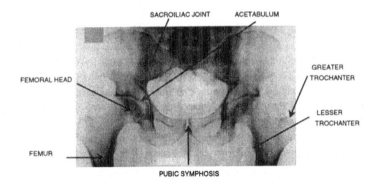

Fig. 1.21: Xerogram of the pelvis and hip joints.

The Hip Joint

The articular surfaces of the hip joint are formed by the lunate surface of the acetabulum and the femoral head (Figure 1.21). The lunate surface of the joint cavity presents a section of a hollow sphere and is extended beyond the equator by the acetabular lip (fibrocartilaginous material).

The lunate surface and the lip cover two thirds of the femoral head. The bony socket is incomplete and closed inferiorly by the transverse acetabular ligament. The joint capsule is attached to the hip bone outside the acetabular lip, so that the latter projects freely into the capsular space. The capsular attachment at the circumference of the head of the femur lies at about the same distance from the cartilaginous rim of the head of the femur so the extracapsular part of the neck is shorter in front than at the back. Several ligaments provide firm mechanical constraints and limit the range of movement. Muscle tone also restricts joint movement, most noticeably when the extended limb is elevated anteriorly.

Movements of the hip joint include flexion (anteversion) and extension (retroversion), abduction and adduction, and circumduction and rotation. Flexion and extension occur about a transverse axis through the head of the femur. With the knee bent, the thigh may be raised against the abdomen. This movement of flexion is much greater than that of extension, which can only be executed slightly beyond the vertical. Abduction and adduction occur about an anterior-posterior axis through the femoral head. Rotation of the femur occurs around a (vertical) axis through the head of the femur and the medial femoral condyle. With the leg extended, a rotation of about 60 degrees is possible.

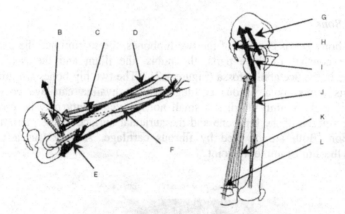

Fig. 1.22: Muscles contributing to the flexion (left panel) and extension (right panel) at the hip joint. B) Illipsoas m; C)The Tensor Fascia Latae m; D) Rectus Femoris m; E) Adductor Brevis m, Adductor Longus m. and Gracilis m; F) Sartorius m; G) Gluteus Minimus m; H) The Piriformis m; I) Gluteus Maximus m; J) The Adductor Magnus m; K) Semimembranosus m; L) Semitendonosus m.

Circumduction is a compound movement in which the leg describes the surface of an irregular cone, the apex of which lies in the head of the femur.

There are many muscles contributing to movement at the hip joint (Figures 1.22, 1.23 and 1.24):

Femur flexion – Psoas m, Iliacus m, Rectus Femoris m;

Femur extension – Gluteus Maximus m, Biceps Femoris m, Semimembranosus m, Semitendinosus m;

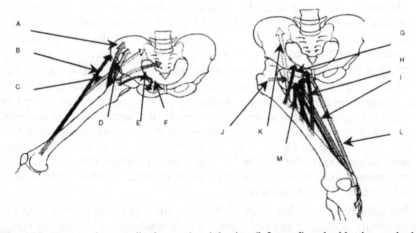

Fig. 1.23: The muscles contributing to the abduction (left panel) and adduction at the hip joint (right panel). A) Gluteus Medius m; B) The Tensor Fascia Latae m; C) Gluteus Maximus m. (with the attachment to the Tensor Fascia Latae; D) Gluteus Minimus m; E) The Piriformis m; F) Obturator Internus m; G) Pectineus m; H) Adductor Longus m; I) Semitendonosus m; J) Quadratus Femoris m; K) Gluteus Maximus; L) Gracilis m; M) Adductor Minimus m.

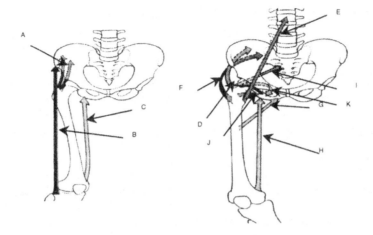

Fig. 1.24: Muscles controlling the hip joint: medial rotation (left panel) and lateral rotation (right panel). A) Gluteus Medius m. and Gluteus Maximus m; B) The Tensor Fascia Latae m; C) Adductor Magnus; D) Gluteus Minimus m. and m; E) Illipsoas m; F) Gluteus Maximus m; H) Gracilis m; G) Pectineus m; I) Piriformis m; J) Quadratus Femoris m; K) Obturator Internus m.

Femur adduction – Adductor Brevis m, Adductor Longus m, Adductor Magnus m, Gracilis m;

Femur abduction – Tensor Fascia Latae m Gluteus Maximus m, Gluteus Medius m, Gluteus Minimus m;

Femur medial rotation – Gluteus Medius m, Gluteus Minimus m;

Femur lateral rotation – Gluteus Medius m, Inferior Gemellus m, Obturator Externus m, Sartorius m.

The Thigh

The thigh bone, or femur, is the largest tubular bone of the body and comprises a shaft with a neck and two ends, proximal and distal. An angle is formed between the shaft and neck, the angle of inclination. The shaft exhibits three surfaces: anterior, lateral, and medial. The transition of the neck into the shaft is marked at the anterior surface by the intertrochanteric line and at the posterior surface by the intertrochanteric crest. At the boundary between the middle and proximal third of the intertrochanteric crest is a rounded elevation, the quadrate tubercle. Directly below the greater trochanter is a pit-like depression, the trochanteric fossa.

The angle formed between the neck and the shaft of the femur is called the collodiaphysial angle or, more correctly the neck-shaft angle, *i.e.*, the angle of inclination. In the newborn it is about 150 degrees, decreasing throughout life to about 120 degrees. The angle of inclination influences the relation of the femoral shaft with respect to the weight-bearing line of the leg.

The weight-bearing line of the leg lies along a line from the middle of the femoral head through the middle of the knee joint to the middle of the calcaneus. The plane, which passes through the lower surface of the femoral condyles, is at right angles to this vertical line. This produces an angle between the axis of the shaft of the femur and the weight-bearing line. This angle is to the angle of inclination and is important in relation to the correct position of the lower limb.

The Patella

The patella is the largest sesamoid bone of the human body. It is triangular in shape with its base facing proximally and its tip, the apex patellae facing distally. It has two surfaces, one toward the joint with the femur and the other directed anteriorly. These two surfaces join at a lateral (thinner) and a medial (thicker) margin. The anterior surface may be divided into three parts and incorporates the tendon of the quadriceps femoris muscle. In the upper third there is a coarse, flattened, rough surface, which often has exostoses and serves largely for the attachment of the tendon of the quadriceps muscle. The middle third is characterized by numerous vascular canaliculi while the lower third includes the apex, which serves as the origin of the patellar ligament. The inner surface may be divided into an articular surface covering about three-quarters and a distal surface with vascular canaliculi. This is filled by fatty tissue, the infrapatelar adipose body.

The Knee Joint

The knee joint is the largest joint in the human body (Figure 1.25). It is a hinge joint, a special type of mobile trochoginglymus. Its flexion combines rolling and gliding movements. In the flexed position some rotation is possible. The articular bodies of the knee joint consist of the femoral and the tibial condyles. The incongruence of these joint surfaces is compensated by a relatively thick cartilaginous covering and by the menisci. In addition to the tibia and femur, the patella also forms part of the knee joint.

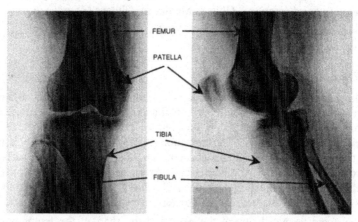

Fig. 1.25: Xerogram of the knee joint: anteroposterior view (left panel), lateral view (right panel).

The knee joint is surrounded with several ligaments: patellar ligament being the continuation of the quadriceps tendon; the tibial collateral, fibular collateral, oblique poplietal, arcuate poplietal, anterior cruciate, posterior cruciate ligaments and several retinaculum structures.

The menisci consist of connective tissue with extensive collagen fiber material, infiltrated with cartilage-like cells. The collagen fibers run in two principal directions. The strong fibers follow the shape of the menisci between their attachments, while weaker fibers pass radially to an imaginary midpoint and interlace between the longitudinally running fibers. The medial meniscus is semicircular in shape and is fused with the tibial collateral ligament. The medial meniscus is wider posteriorly than anteriorly. Its attachment makes it far less mobile than the lateral meniscus. External rotation of the lower leg causes the greatest displacement and pulling stress on it. Internal rotation relaxes it. The lateral meniscus is almost circular; its points of attachment lie close together, and it is of uniform width. It is more mobile than the medial meniscus, as it does not fuse with the fibular collateral ligament, and therefore the different movements less stress it. From its posterior horn arise one or two ligaments.

The joint space itself has a complicated structure. Anteriorly, in the exposed joint, there is a wide fatty pad, the intra-patellar fat pad, inserted between the synovial and fibrous membranes.

Movement at the Knee Joint

The knee may be flexed and extended about an almost transverse axis, and in the flexed position rotation is possible about the axis of the lower leg. In the extended knee both collateral ligaments and the anterior part of the anterior cruciate ligament are taut. During extension the femoral condyles glide into the almost extreme position in which the lateral tibial collateral ligament is completely unfolded. During the last 10 degrees of movement before complete extension there is an obligatory terminal rotation of about 5 degrees. This is caused by stretching of the anterior cruciate ligament and is permitted by the shape of the medial femoral condyle. Both lateral ligaments become taut and at the same time there is a slight unwinding of the cruciate ligaments. Final rotation of the non-weight-bearing active leg is produced by lateral rotation of the tibia, and in the standing leg by medial rotation of the thigh. In the position of extreme extension the collateral and cruciate

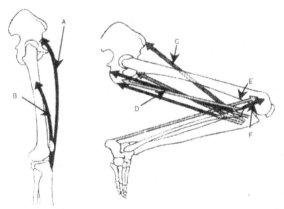

Fig. 1.26: Muscles contributing to extension (left) and flexion (right) at the knee joint: A) Rectus Femoris m; B) Vasti m; C) Sartorius m; D) Semitendinosus m, Biceps Femoris m, Gracilis m, and Semimembranosus m; E) Gastrocnemius m; F) Poplioteus m.

ligaments are tensed. Normal extension is to 180 degrees, although in children and adolescents the leg may be overextended by about degrees.

The extent of medial rotation of the leg is less than of lateral rotation. During medial rotation of the tibia on the femur, the cruciate ligament is twisted around each other and so prevents any appreciable medial rotation. In the same way, the dorsal fibers of the tibial collateral ligament are tensed at extreme medial rotation. During lateral rotation, the cruciate ligaments become unwound. The tibial collateral ligament primarily determines the limit of lateral rotation; its maximal extent is 45 to 60 degrees. During rotation, the femur and menisci move over the tibia, and during flexion and extension the femur rolls and glides on the menisci, so that the knee should be considered as a polycentric (mobile) joint.

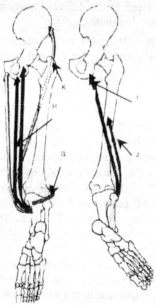

Fig. 1.27: Posterior view of the muscles contributing to the lower leg medial rotation (left panel), and lateral rotation (right panel). G) Popliteus m; H) Semimembranosus m, Semitendonosus m. and Gracilis m; K) Sartorius m; I) Biceps Femoris Long Head m; J) Biceps Femoris Short Head m. The knee joint is flexed at both panels.

There are several muscles controlling the movement at the knee joint (Figures 1.26 and 1.27). Based on the functioning the muscles can be clustered into the following groups:

Tibia extension – Rectus Femoris m, Vastus Lateralis m, Vastus Medialis m, Vastus Intermedius m;

Tibia flexion – Sartorius m, Biceps Femoris m, Semimembranosus m, Semitendonosus m, Plantaris m;

Medial rotation of tibia – Gracilis m, Semimembranosus m, Semitendonosus m, Popliteus m;

Lateral rotation of tibia – Biceps Femoris m.

The Lower Leg - Shank

The bones of the lower leg are the tibia and fibula. The tibia is the stronger bone, which alone provides the connection between the femur and the bones of the ankle and foot. The tibia has a somewhat triangular shaft at proximal and distal ends. At the proximal end lie the medial and lateral condyles. The fibula corresponds approximately in length to the tibia, but is a slimmer and therefore more flexible bone.

The tibiofibular joint is an almost immobile synovial joint (amphiarthrosis) between the head of the fibula and the fibular articular surface of the lateral tibial condyle. It possesses a tease capsule, which is reinforced by the anterior and posterior ligaments of the head of the fibula.

It is also known as the compensation joint because, during maximal forward dorsiflexion in the ankle (talocrural) joint, there is expansion of the malleolar mortise, and this results in a compensatory movement in the tibiofibular joint. In addition to the synovial joint between the leg bones, the interosseous membrane of the leg, as a fibrous joint, fixes the two bones.

The fibers in the interosseous membrane run inferiorly from the tibia to the fibula and are very tense.

The Foot

The skeleton of the foot may be divided into the tarsus, the metatarsus and the digits (Figure 1.28). The tarsus consists of seven bones, the talus, calcaneus, navicular, cuboid and the three cuneiform bones. The metatarsus consists of five metatarsals, and the digits are formed by the phalanges. The talus transmits the weight of the entire body to the foot. The head of the talus carries the navicular articular surface for articulation with the navicular bone. The calcaneus is the largest tarsal bone. The Achilles tendon is inserted into the roughened area on the tuber calcanei. The navicular bone articulates with the talus and with the three cuneiform bones.

The cuneiform bones differ from each other in size and position in the skeleton of the foot, the medial being the largest and the intermediate the smallest. All three cuneiform bones have articular surfaces proximally for articulation with the navicular. Distally and directed toward the digits are articulations for the metatarsals. The five metatarsals are long bones and are dorsally convex. The metatarsal connects to the bones of the digits, *i.e.,* phalanges. The second to fifth digits each have a proximal, middle and distal phalanx, while the first digit has only two phalanges. Each phalanx has a base, a shaft and a head. The distal phalanx has a distal tuberosity. There are small grooves on the proximal and middle phalanges.

Joints of the Foot - The Ankle

The joints of the foot include the upper ankle joint, or talocrural joint, and the lower ankle joint, or subtalar and talocalcanconavicular joints, in addition to the cuneonavicular, calcancocuboid, cuncocuboid and intercuncifom articulations (Figure 1.28). The tarsonietatarsal joints are articulations between the tarsal and metatarsal bones. Articular connections between the bases of the metatarsals are the intermetatarsal joints and those between the metatarsals and the phalanges of the foot are the metatarsophalangeal joints, and interphalangeal articulations of the foot.

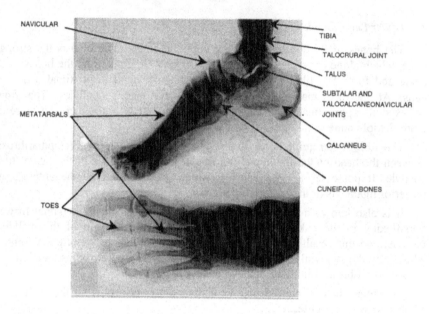

Fig. 1.28: Xerogram of the foot: lateral view (top panel), anteroposterior view (bottom panel).

The Ankle Joint

The malleolar morthe and the superior surface of the talar trochlea along with its medial and lateral malicolar surfaces form the articular surfaces of the talocrural joint. The tibia and fibula form a mortise or "clasp" for the roll of the talus. The joint surface of the fibula extends further distally than the tibia. The joint capsule is attached to the margins of the cartilaginous layer of the articular surfaces. The joint cavity contains anterior and posterior synovial folds. Many ligaments provide the necessary stability, yet flexibility. Both plantar and dorsiflexion are possible. In plantar flexion, as the trochlea of the talus is narrower posteriorly, which leaves more free play in the mortise, slight side-to-side movement is possible. The ankle joint is a hinge joint with a transverse axes, beginning just beneath the tip of the medial malleolus and running through the thickest part of the lateral malleolus. The range of movement between dorsal and plantar flexion is up to 70 degrees.

The *subtalar joint* forms the posterior part and the *talocalcanconavicular joint* forms the anterior part of the joint (Figure 1.28). The talus and the calcaneus form the articular surfaces of the subtalar joint. The capsule is loose and thin and is strengthened by the medial and lateral talocalcaeneal ligaments. The talocalcanconavicular joint is made up of three bones. In addition to the joint surfaces of the talus, calcaneus and the navicular, there is an additional articular surface covered by cartilage on the plantar calcanconavicular ligament. In summary, the ankle joint permits hinge movement while the subtalar and the talocaleanconavicular joints permit two other degrees of freedom: inversion/eversion, and medial/lateral rotation.

There are several muscles contributing to movement at the ankle joint (Figure 1.29). These muscles can be clustered to the following groups:

Plantar flexion - Peroneus Brevis m, Peroneus Longus m, Flexor Digitorum Longus m, Triceps Surae (Gastrocnemius m, Plantaris m, Soleus m), Tibialis Posterior m;

Dorsiflexion – Tibialis Anterior m, Extensor Digitorum Longus m, Extensor Hallucis Longus m, Peroneus Tertius m;

Inversion - Triceps Surae m, Tibialis Posterior m, Flexor Hallucis Longus m, Flexor Digitorum Longus m, Tibialis Anterior m;

Eversion – Peroneus Tertius m, Peroneus Brevis m, Peroneus Longus m., Extensor Digitorum Longus m.

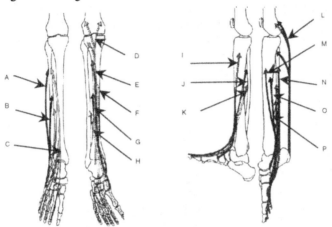

Fig. 1.29: Muscles contributing to ankle movement: eversion (left), inversion (middle left), dorsiflexion (middle right), plantar flexion (right). A) Peroneus Longus m; B) Peroneus Brevis m; C) Extensor Digitorum Longus m. and Peroneus Tertius m; D) Triceps Surae m; E) Tibialis Anterior m; F) Flexor Digitorum Longus m; G) Tibialis Posterior m; H) Flexor Hallucis Longus m; I) Tibialis Anterior m; J) Extensor Digitorum Longus m; K) Extensor Hallucis Longus m; L) Triceps Surae m; M) Flexor Digitorum Longus m; N) Peroneus Longus m; O) Tibialis Posterior m; P) Peroneus Brevis m.

Joints of the Digits

The metatarsophalangeal joints and the interphalangeal joints of the foot may be divided into the proximal and the middle and distal joints. The proximal metatarsophalangeal joints are ball-and-socket joints, although collateral ligaments restrict their mobility. The middle and distal joints are pure hinge joints.

Many muscles play role in movement of toes (Figure 1.29):

Big toe extension – Extensor Hallucis Longus m.

Big Toe flexion – Abductor Hallucis m, Flexor Hallucis Longus m.

Toes extension - Extensor Digitorum Longus m, Extensor Digitotrum Brevis m;

Toes flexion – Flexor Digitorum Longus m, Flexor Digitorum Brevis m, Quadratus Plantae m, Lubricalis m, Flexor Digiti Minimi Brevis m.

Abducting toes – Abductor Digiti Minimi m, Abductor Ossis Metatarsi Quinti, Dorsal Interossei m;

Adducting toes - Plantar Interossei m.

The Plantar Arch

The plantar arch is normally in a position of supporting the weight of the body. The bony points of support of the arch on a level ground surface are the calcaneal tuberosity, the head of the first metatarsal and the head of the fifth metatarsal. Thus, the supporting surface is in the form of a triangle. If a footprint is examined, a somewhat larger supporting surface is found, which is produced by the soft tissues. The line of transmission of the weight of the body runs from the tibia to the calcaneus and to the midfoot and forefoot. The transmission of pressure to the arch in both directions tends to flatten its curvature, and the ligaments and the plantar muscles oppose this.

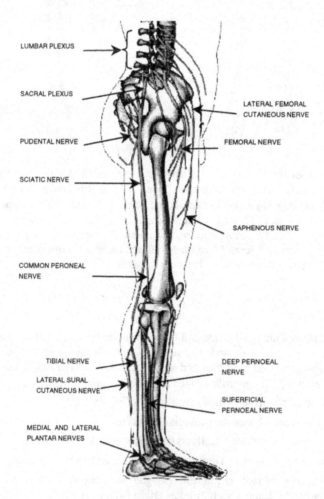

Fig. 1.30: Schematic diagram of the nerves of the leg (right side, lateral aspect).

Peripheral Nerves of the Leg

The peripheral nerves of leg are connected to the spinal cord at several lumbar and sacral segments. Both sensory and motor nerve come into the vertebral column through lumbar plexus (T12-L3), sacral plexus (L4-S3) and pudental plexus (S2-S4) as shown in Figure 1.30. The main nerves for movement are sciatic nerve that divides into common peroneal and tibial nerve. Common peroneal nerve divides into superficial and deep branches. All these nerves are mixed; they contain both sensory and motor neurons.

1.4.2 The Upper-Limb - Arm and Hand

The upper-limb is a complex neuro-musculo-skeletal system that has been developed through evolution specifically to serve for goal-directed movements, and which allows humans to operate differently from all other living species. Here, some anatomical elements relevant for farther elaboration are presented.

The upper limb is attached to the shoulder girdle (Figure 1.31). The scapulae and the clavicles form the shoulder girdle. Connections with the trunk are made through a continuous fibrous (costoclavicular) ligament and discontinuous synovial joints (sternoclavicular articulation). In the same way, the parts of the shoulder girdle are connected to each other by continuous fibrous (coracoclavicular ligament) and discontinuous synovial joints (acromio-clavicular articulation).

Sternoclavicular joint has an articular disk, which divides the space of the joint cavity in two. The socket is a shallow concave indentation in the sternum, and the sternal end of the clavicle forms the head. The incongruity is adjusted by the cartilage-like fibrous tissue, which covers both articular facets. The articular disk is fixed cranially to the clavicle and caudally to the sternum. The capsule is slack and thick and is strengthened by the anterior and posterior sternoclavicular ligaments. The interclavicular ligament interconnects the clavicles. The sternoclavicular joint functions as a ball-and-socket type and has three degrees of freedom.

Acromnoclavicular joint consists of two opposing, almost flat joint surfaces covered by cartilage-like fibrous tissue. The capsule has a strengthening ligament on its superior surface, the acromnoclavicular ligament. The coracoclavicular ligament extends between the coracoid process and the clavicle.

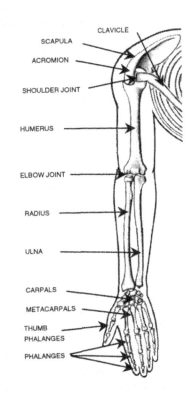

Fig. 1.31: Sketch of the upper extremity connected to the shoulder girdle.

The Shoulder Joint

The bony socket, the glenoid cavity, of the ball-and-socket shoulder joint is much smaller than the head of the humerus (Figure 1.32). A fibro-cartilaginous lip, the glenoidal lip, enlarges the socket. The socket is perpendicular to the plane of the scapula, and the position of the scapula determines the attitude of the entire joint.

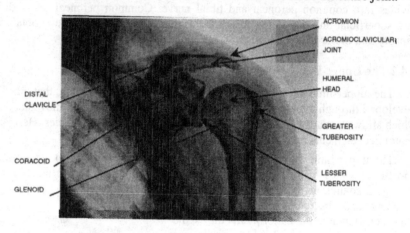

Fig. 1.32: Xerogram of the shoulder joint.

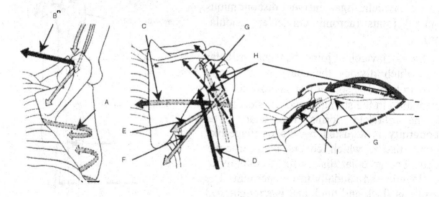

Fig. 1.33: The muscles contributing to the shoulder elevation (left), adduction (middle) and abduction (right). A) The Seratus Anterior m; B) Trapezius m; C) Pectoralis Major m; D) Triceps Brachii m; E) Teres Major m; F) Latissimus Dorsi m; G) Biceps Brachii m; H) Deltoid m; I) Supraspinatus m.

There are no strong ligaments and the shoulder joint is maintained by the action of the enveloping muscles. It is known as a "muscle-dependent joint." The shoulder joint has three degrees of freedom of movement. Abduction and adduction refer to movements away from the position of rest of the head of the humerus in the scapular plane. Purely lateral abduction always produces retroversion and slight rotation, while abduction from the scapular plane is anteriorly directed. Flexion (anteversion) is forward lifting of the arm. Because of rotary components associated with these other movements, a compound movement, called circumduction occurs in which the

1 Organs and Tissues for Human Movement   59

arm traces the surface of a cone. Abduction is always associated with movement of the scapula; excessive associated scapular movement occurs with abduction of more than 90 degrees, because then the coraroacromial ligament restricts the movement of the joint.

Muscles Acting at the Shoulder Joint

Many muscles are acting at the shoulder joint (Figure 1.33). Most of the muscles have several function, *i.e.,* they contribute to spatial movement. These muscles can be clustered in the following groups:

Upperarm abduction – Deltoid m, Supraspinatus m;

Hymerus adduction - Coracobrachialis m, Triceps Brachii (long head) m, Latissimus Dorsi m, Pectoralis Major m, Teres Major m;

Upperarm flexion - Coracobrachialis m, Pectoralis Major m, Deltoid m;

Upperarm extension - Triceps Brachii (long head) m, Latissimus Dorsi m, Teres Major m;

Upperarm medial rotation – Latissimus Dorsi m, Pectoralis Major m, Deltoid m, Teres Major m, Subscapularis m;

Upperarm lateral rotation – Teres Minor m, Infraspinatus m.

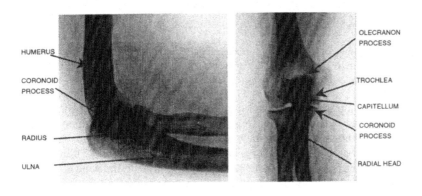

Fig. 1.34: Xerogram of the elbow joint: lateral view (left) and anteroposterior view (right).

The Upperarm - Humerus

The bones of the upper limb are the humerus, the radius and ulna, the carpal and metacarpal bones and the phalanges.

The humerus articulates with the scapula and the radius and ulna. It consists of the body and upper (proximal) and lower (distal) ends. The head of the humerus, adjoining the anatomic neck forms the proximal end. On the anterolateral surface of the proximal end lies the greater tubercle, and medially is the lesser tubercle. Between these tubercles begins the intertubercular sulcus, which is bounded distally by the crests of the lesser and greater tubercles. The sulcus for the radial nerve lies on the posterior surface of the body. The distal end of the humerus bears on its medial side the large medial epicondyle and on the lateral side the smaller lateral epicondyle.

The humerus is twisted at its proximal end, *i.e.*, the head is posteriorly rotated at about 20 degrees in relation to the shaft.

The Elbow Joint

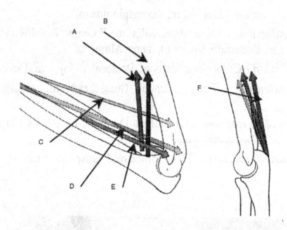

Fig. 1.35: The muscles contributing to the elbow flexion (left) and extension (right). A) Biceps Brachii m; B) Brachialis m; C) Brachioradialis m; D) Extensor Carpi Radialis m; E) Pronator Teres m; F) Triceps Brachii m.

The elbow joint is a compound joint with the three articulating surfaces of the bones within the joint capsule (Figure 1.34). It consists of three joints, the humeroradial, humeroulnar and proximal radioulnar joints. Bone and ligament secure it. The trochlea of the humerus and the trochlear notch of the ulna into which it fits provide bony stability. Ligamentous stability is due to the annular ligament of the radius and the collateral ligaments.

The thin, lax joint capsule encloses the joint surfaces. In order to prevent pinching of the capsule between these surfaces during movement of the joint, fibers from the brachialis and triceps brachii muscles act as articular muscles and radiate into the capsule in order to tense it. The very strong collateral ligaments are embedded in the sides of the joint capsule. The ulnar collateral ligament arises from the medial epicondyle of the humerus and usually possesses two strong fiber bundles, an anterior one, which is directed to the coronoid process, and a posterior one, which extends to the lateral margin of the olecranon.

Because of the interaction of these three joints in any flexed or extended position, a simultaneous rotation of the radius around the ulna is possible. The following movements are possible: flexion, extension, supination and pronation.

The "angle of excursion," *i.e.*, the anteriorly measured angle between the upper arm and forearm at maximal extension is insignificantly greater in females (180

1 Organs and Tissues for Human Movement   61

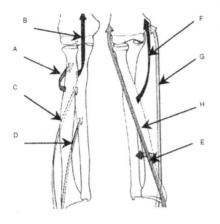

Fig. 1.36: The muscles contributing to the forearm supination (left) and pronation (right). A) Supinator m; B) Biceps Brachii m; C) Abductor Pollicis Longus m; D) Extensor Pollicis Longus m; E) Pronator Quadratus m; F) Pronator Teres m; G) Flexor Carpi Radialis m; H) Extensor Carpi Radialis m.

degrees) than in males (175 degrees). Hyper-extension is possible in children. At maximal flexion the upper arm and forearm forms an angle of about 35 degrees (soft tissue restraint).

The Muscles at the Elbow Joint

Muscles contributing to the movement in elbow are (Figures 1.35 and 1.36):

Forearm supination - Biceps Brachii m, Extensor Carpi Radialis Longus m, Supinator m;

Forearm pronation - Pronator Teres m, Pronator Quadratus m, Brachioradialis m;

Forearm flexion - Brachialis m, Biceps Brachii m, Brachioradialis m, Abductor Pollicis Longus m;

Forearm extension - Triceps Brachii m, Anconeus m.

The Forearm

In the forearm (antebrachium), the shorter bone, radius lies laterally, the longer bone ulna, medially (Figure 1.37). The *radius* comprises a shaft or body and a proximal and a distal ends. The proximal extremity contains the head with its articular fovea, which continues, into the articular circumference. Medially, at the

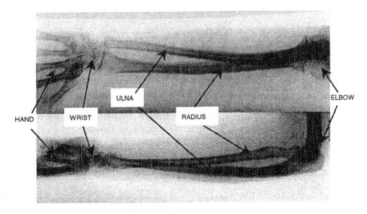

Fig. 1.37: Xerogram of the forearm: anteroposterior view (top) and lateral view (bottom).

transition between the neck of the radius and its shaft, lies the radial tuberosity. At the distal end of the radius is the styloid process and medial to it, the ulnar notch. The carpal articular surface is directed distally. Dorsally are found various distinctly developed grooves in which course the tendons of the long extensors.

The *ulna* possesses a shaft and a proximal and distal extremity. The proximal end exhibits a book-shaped, curved process, the olecranon, which has a roughened surface. In front is the trochlear notch, which extends up to the coronoid process. The radial notch lies laterally and articulates with the articular circumference of the radial head.

The Wrist Joint and the Hand

The head of the ulna and the ulnar notch of the radius form the distal radioulnar joint, a pivot joint (Figure 1.38). Between the radius and the styloid process of the ulna lies an articular disk, which separates the distal radioulnar from the radiocarpal joint. The capsule is lax and extends from the inferior recessus sacciformis up to the shaft of the ulna. The proximal and distal radioulnar joints are necessarily combined joints to permit pronation and supination.

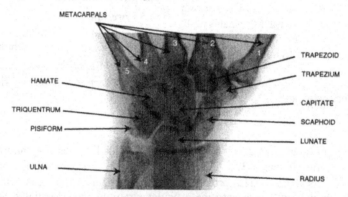

Fig. 1.38: Xerogram of the wrist joint including part of the hand (carpal bones).

The carpus consists of eight carpal bones arranged in two rows of four (Figure 1.38). In the proximal row from lateral to medial are the scaphoid, lunate, triquetrum and, superimposed on it, the pisiform. In the distal row from the lateral to the medial side are: the trapezium, the trapezoid, the capitate and the hamate. Each carpal bone has several facets for articulation with the neighboring bones.

Both rows of bones together, *i.e.*, the entire carpus, form an arch, which is convex proximally, and concave distally. The palmar surface of the carpus is also concave and is spanned by the flexor retinaculum, which forms the osteofibrous carpal tunnel. It stretches from the scaphoid and trapezium to the hamate, triquetrum and pisiform. Projections on these named bones are palpable through the skin.

The five metacarpals of the hand each have a head, a shaft and a base. On all of these there are articular facets at one end (base) for articulation with the carpals and at the other (head) for the phalanges. The palmar surface is slightly concave and the dorsal surface slightly convex. The dorsal surface exhibits a characteristic triangular configuration toward the head.

1 Organs and Tissues for Human Movement   63

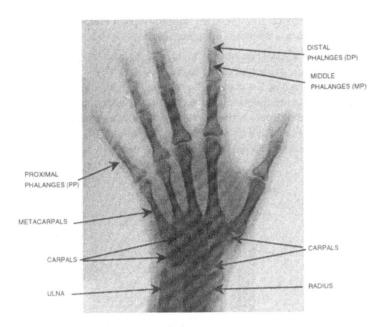

Fig. 1.39 Xerogram of the hand (posteroanterior view).

The proximal articular facet of the first metacarpal is saddle-shaped; the second metacarpal has a notched base proximally for articulation with the carpus, and on the medial side with the third metacarpal. On the dorso-radial side of the base of the third metacarpal is a styloid process and radially an articular facet for the second metacarpal. Proximally, for junction with the carpus, there is one articular facet, and on the ulnar side there are two articular facets for articulation with the fourth

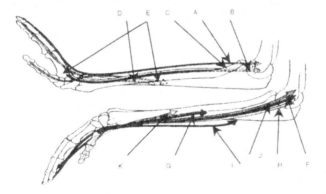

Fig. 1.40: The muscles contributing to the dorsiflexion (up) and palmar flexion (bottom) - wrist movement. A) Extensor Digitorum m; B) Extensor Carpi Radialis Longus m; C) Extensor Carpi Radialis Brevis m; D) Extensor Indicis m; E) Extensor Pollicis Longus m; F) Flexor Digitorum Superficialis m; G) Flexor Digitorum Profundus m; H) Flexor Carpi Ulnaris m; I) Abductor Pollicis Longus m; J) Flex. Carpi Radialis m; K) Extensor Indicis m.

metacarpal. The fourth metacarpal has two articular facets radially but only one on its ulnar side for articulation with the fifth metacarpal.

The bones of the digits (Figure 1.39). Each digit consists of more than one bone, namely a proximal, a medial, and a distal phalanx. The sole exception is the thumb, which has only two phalanges. Each proximal phalanx has a flattened palmar surface, dorsally and transversally it is convex and has roughened sharpened borders for the attachment of the fibrous tendon sheaths of the flexor muscles. It has a shaft, a distal phalangeal head (also called a "trochlea"), and aproximal base. The base has a transverse oval socket, an articular facet for the metacarpals.

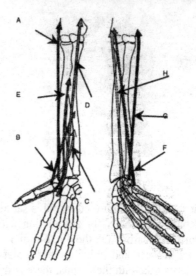

Fig. 1.41: The muscles contributing to the radial abduction (left) and ulnar abduction (bottom) - wrist movement. A) Extensor Carpi Radialis Longus m; B) Abductor Pollicis Longus m; C) Extensor Pollicis Longus m; D) Flexor Carpi Radialis m; E) Flexor Pollicis Longus m; F) Extensor Carpi Ulnaris m; G) Extensor Digitorum m; H) Extensor Digiti Minimi m.

The radiocarpal or wrist joint is an ellipsoid joint formed on one side by the radius and the articular disk and on the other by the proximal row of carpal bones. Not all the carpal bones of the proximal row are in continual contact with the socket-shaped articular facet of the radius and the disk. The triquetrum, only makes close contact with the disk during ulnar abduction and loses contact on radial abduction. The capsule of the radiocarpal joint is lax, dorsally relatively thin, and is reinforced by numerous ligaments. The joint space is unbranched and sometimes contains synovial folds. Often the wrist joint is in continuity with the midcarpal joint.

The midcarpal joint is formed by the proximal and distal row of carpal bones and has an S-shaped joint space. Each row of carpal bones can be considered as a single articular body, and they interlock with each other. Although there is a certain limited degree of mobility between members of the proximal row of carpal bones, this is not true of the distal row because they are joined one to another, as well as to the metacarpal bones by strong ligaments.

Four groups of ligaments can be distinguished around the wrist joint. These include the ulnar collateral ligament, the radial collateral ligament, the palmar radiocarpal ligament, the dorsal radiocarpal ligament, and the palmar ulnocarpal ligament.

Starting from the midposition it is possible to distinguish marginal movements of radial deviation (abduction) and ulnar deviation (adduction) from movement in the plane of the hand, *i.e.*, flexion (volar flexion) and extension (dorsiflexion) as well as intermediate or combined movement.

The carpometacarpal ioint of the thumb is a saddle joint, which allows abduction and adduction of the thumb, as well as opposition, reposition and circumduction. The metacarpophalangeal joints are ball-and-socket joints in shape with lax capsules. The articulation is between the head of the metacarpal and the base of the first phalanx. Restriction of movement is caused by the collateral ligaments, whose origin is dorsal to the axis of motion of the joint of the beads of the metacarpals. The greater the movement, the tighter the ligaments become. In flexion, movements of abduction are almost impossible. The joints may be rotated passively by up to 50 degrees. The joints between the bones of the fingers, the interphalangeal joints of the hand, are hinge joints, which may be flexed and extended. They, too, have collateral (5) and palmar ligaments.

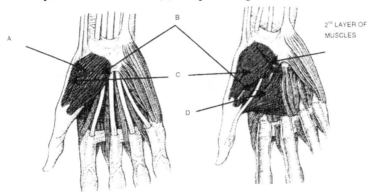

Fig. 1.42: Thenar muscles. A) Abductor pollicis Brevis m; B) Flexor Pollicis Brevis m; C) Opponens Pollicis m; D) Adductor Pollicis m. Other muscles in the hand are not shown (metacarpus muscles - Palmar Interossei m, Dorsal Interossei m; palmar aponeurisis muscles - Palmaris Brevis m; hypothenar muscles - Abductor Digiti Minimi m, Flexor Digiti Minimi Brevis m, Opponens Digiti Minimi m.)

The Muscles at the Wrist Joint and Hand (Figures 1.40, 1.41 and 1.42)

Hand flexion - Flexor Carpi Radialis m, Palmaris Longus m, Flexor Carpi Ulnaris m, Flexor Digitorum Superficialis m, Flexor Digitorum Profundus m;

Hand extension - Extensor Carpi Radialis Longus m, Extensor Carpi Radialis Brevis m, Extensor Digitorum m, Extensor Carpi Ulnaris m;

Hand radial deviation - Flexor Carpi Radialis m, Extensor Carpi Radialis Longus m, Extensor Carpi Radialis Brevis m, Abductor Pollicis Longus m, Extensor Pollicis Brevis m;

Hand ulnar deviation - Flexor Carpi Ulnaris m, Extensor Carpi Ulnaris m;

Fingers flexion (proximal and middle phalanges) - Flexor digitorum Superficialis m, Flexor Digiti Minimi Brevis m, Palmar Interossei m, Dorsal Interossei m, Lumbircals m;

Fingers flexion (distal phalanges) - Flexor Digitorum Profundus m;

Fingers extension - Extensor Digitorum m, Extensor Digit Minimi m, Extensor Indicis m;

Abduction of fingers - Extensor Digitorum m, Extensor Digit Minimi m, Abductor Digiti Minimi m, Dorsal Interossei m.;

Adduction of fingers - Extensor Indicis m, Palmar Interossei m;

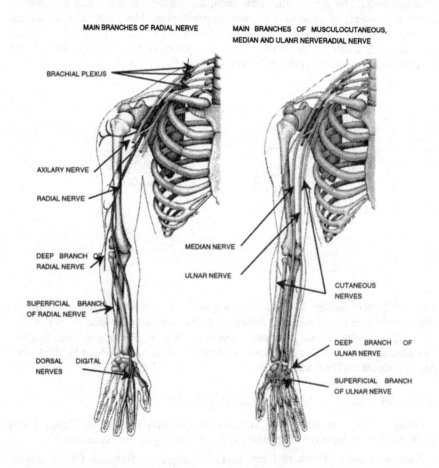

Fig. 1.43: The schematic drawing of main branches of radial nerve (left), and median and ulnar nerve (right). Only some nerves are shown for simplicity.

Thumb flexion (distal phalanx) - Flexor Pollicis Longus m, Abductor Pollicis Brevis m, Flexor Pollicis Brevis m;

Thumb extensor - Abductor Pollicis Longus m, Extensor Pollicis Brevis m, Extensor Pollicis Longus m;

Thumb abduction - Abductor Pollicis Brevis m, Abductor Pollicis Longus m;

Thumb adduction - Adductor Pollicis m;

Thumb opposition - Opponens Pollicis and Opponens Digiti Minimi m.

Peripheral Nerves of Upper Extremities

The upper extremities connect to the spinal cord at the cervical level, and the connection is called brachial plexus. Brachial plexus spans over four vertebral segments (C4-C7) and it branches to lateral, posterior and medial cords (Figure 1.43). The medial cord branches to axillary and radial nerve. The lateral cord includes the median nerve and the posterior cord the ulnar nerve. Radial, median and ulnar nerves are all mixed nerves containing both sensory and motor nerves.

2. Mechanisms for Natural Control of Movement

> "One of the major challenges facing clinical neurobiologists is how to exploit the untapped reserves of coordinated movement contained in the spinal cord circuits of patients with a functionally isolated spinal cord."
>
> Robert Burke [1981]

This chapter presents the anatomy and organization of cyclic and goal-directed movement of humans. Diagrammatic representation and condensed description cannot do full justice to the complex relation involved. The illustrations do not attempt to show all details of movement, but only to describe the richness of movement that extremities support.

2.1 Organization and Mechanisms for Control of Movement

The skeleto-motor system provides the structure and drives to move the body and limbs relative to the surroundings and to maintain the posture in space. The entire behavioral repertoire is made up of movement and postural adjustments performed to achieve certain goals. How do the motor systems achieve this action? In contrast to the sensory systems, which use physical energy and transform it into neural information, the motor systems act on the environment by transforming neural information and metabolic energy into movement. Changes in external events or in our internal environment, signaled by our sensory systems, set up commands that are transmitted to the skeletal muscles by nerve impulses. The muscles translate this neural information into a command that transforms chemical into mechanical energy by generating a contractile force.

The control of movement and posture is achieved solely by adjusting the degree of contraction of skeletal muscles, however, this control requires that the motor systems are provided with a continuous flow of information about events from the periphery. Exteroceptors provide the motor systems with information about the spatial coordinates of the objects. Proprioceptors relay information about the position of the body vs. the vertical, the angles of the joints, the length and tension of muscles, etc. Through proprioceptors, the motor systems gain access to information about the condition of the peripheral motor plant, the muscles and joints that have to be moved. The motor systems need information about the consequences of their actions. Both exteroceptors and proprioceptors provide this information, which can then be used to calibrate the next series of motor commands. Thus, motor mechanisms are intimately related to and functionally dependent upon sensory information.

The control of movement and posture and its regulation and updating by afferent information have to be examined having in mind all the constraints imposed on the motor system by the muscles and bones that are to be moved. The motor systems are organized hierarchically, being the consequence of self-organization through evolution.

Our motor systems may produce either a change in muscle length and a resultant change in joint angles, as when we reach for an object, or merely a change in tension, as when we tighten our grasp on an object already within our reach. To accomplish these different goals, the motor systems must take into account the limitations on movement imposed by the physical characteristics of the musculo-skeletal system. Three constraints are especially important.

Muscles contract and relax slowly. Changes in muscle tension do not represent a simple one-to-one transformation of the firing patterns of motor neurons. The muscle filter the information contained in the temporal pattern of the spike train produced by motorneurons. Because of this filtering action, muscles faithfully reproduce only those signals that vary slowly. The ability of the muscular force to follow those fluctuations is greatly diminished if the signals fluctuate rapidly. This indicates that it is necessary to alternate contraction in opposing muscle in order to produce fast change of the force.

Muscles have spring-like properties; thus, within limits, the tension exerted by muscles varies in proportion to length. Neural input is changing the muscles' resting length and stiffness. The actual change of muscle length depends on the neural drive and also on both initial lengths of the muscle and external loads. The mechanisms localized in spinal segments could be responsible for compensating for some of the more complex properties of muscle; hence, eliminate the needs for "accurate" control of muscle contractions by the higher structure of CNS. The complex properties of muscles and the loads to which they are ultimately attached also require that the motor systems calibrate their commands based on previous experience. Therefore, learning is the key for the skilled motor performance.

A somewhat different constrain is that typically, the motor systems need to control many muscles acting at the same joint simultaneously with muscles acting at different joints. Reaching while standing is an example of using many muscles to achieve a task. Bringing a segment of the hand to a desired position requires contraction of a group of muscles acting as prime movers (agonist muscles), yet antagonist muscles, which oppose the actions, must be controlled. For example, the antagonists may need to relax so that movement can take place with the least expenditure of energy, or they may need to contract late in the trajectory to decelerate the moving limb. In postural control, some muscles contract in order to fix the angle of proximal joints, while others prevent the loss of balance. When one is in an upright position and lift his/her arm, the muscles of the legs contract before those of the arm; this prevents us from falling over when our center of gravity shifts suddenly. Finally, besides compensating for the inevitable changes in the center of gravity that occur when we move our limbs, or merely when we breathe, the motor systems also have to keep many bones aligned end to end to maintain the posture.

Our motor systems permit a large number of adjustments in both posture and movement. As pointed out by Bernstein [1967], the principal task of motor integration is to select one or more options from the large number of possibilities, so-called degrees of freedom, that are available. The motor systems of the brain and spinal cord reduce this wide array of choices to manageable proportions primarily by means of a hierarchy of several interconnected components.

2.1.1 Hierarchical Organization of the Motor Systems

It has been noticed that the motor systems are organized hierarchically [Jackson, 1932]. Different motor behaviors could be classified on a continuum that ranges from the most automatic behavior (e.g., reflex) to the least automated behavior. Many automatic responses are organized at the level of the spinal cord, whereas the less automatic behaviors are organized by successively higher centers. This indicated that the motor systems consist of separate neural circuits that are linked. These neural circuits are located in four distinct areas: 1) the spinal cord; 2) the brainstem and the reticular formation; 3) the motor cortex; and 4) the premotor cortical areas (Figure 2.1).

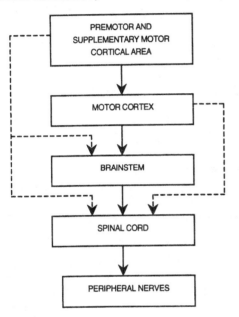

Fig. 2.1: The hierarchical and parallel organization of the motor system.

The lowest part of the motor hierarchy is the spinal cord. It is responsible for organizing the most automatic and stereotyped responses to stimuli. These automatic behaviors are known as reflexes (e.g., phasic behavioral responses such as the knee jerk or the withdrawal of the leg when touching a sharp obstacle on the ground). In the spinal cord, sensory inputs are initially distributed either directly to the motor neurons innervating different muscles or indirectly to motor neurons through interneurons. The spinal cord also contains a center or region, the so-called "central pattern generator" (CPG), which plays a major role in alternating, cyclic movement (e.g., walking). The existence of the CPG, described in next section of this chapter, has been documented in mammals, and evidence suggests the existence of one in humans [e.g., Calancie et al., 1994].

Although motor neurons are the final common pathway for motor actions, many of these actions are coordinated at the level of interneurons. For example, networks of spinal interneurons organize the reflex withdrawal from a noxious stimulus, or the alternating activity in flexors and extensors during locomotion. Indeed, simple descending commands can produce surprisingly complex effects by acting on these interneurons.

In order to move a limb in a desired direction, descending connections from the brain can activate the relevant motor neurons, yet a simple descending command acts simultaneously on motor neurons innervating the agonist muscles and on interneurons that inhibit the antagonists. The reciprocal control of two groups of muscles receives a simple command signal, much as Ia afferents act both on the motor neurons to agonistic muscles and on the motor neurons to their antagonists.

As said, locomotion relies on networks of interneurons within the spinal cord that control alternating activity in flexor and extensor motor neurons. The existence of this circuitry at a low level in the motor hierarchy allows execution of highly complex sequences of muscle contractions required for walking by sending only simple commands.

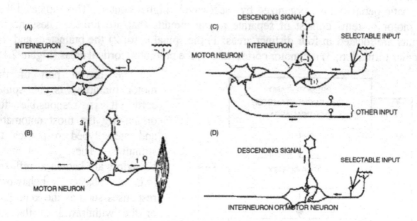

Fig. 2.2: Combinations of neuronal connections: (A) Collaterals of a single neuron synapse on several target neurons; (B) Activity of a single neuron is the summation of afferent input (1), interneurons (2), and descending fibers (3); (C) An inhibitory command preventing peripheral input from acting on a motor neuron; (D) Descending command controlling afferent input by acting on presynaptic terminals.

A given descending pathway exerts control on the final motor response by acting either through interneurons or on motor neurons directly. Descending pathways can engage spinal interneurons to enhance or suppress specific reflexes. These interneurons can act at the terminals of afferent fibers, thereby enabling or preventing peripheral input from affecting motor output. Primary afferent fibers can be inhibited presynaptically by the afferent information. Higher centers can preselect which of several possible responses will follow a certain stimulus at a given moment using the mechanisms in the spinal cord. This decreases substantially the information processing required, and even more importantly eliminates the need for a decision during the interval between stimulus and response.

The activity of both the spinal motor neurons and the interneurons reflects the sum of the several inputs impinging upon them: inputs from the periphery, from supraspinal regions, and from other interneurons or motor neurons (Figure 2.2). The convergence of peripheral and descending synapses on spinal neurons allows the flexibility instrumental in the central nervous system's affecting of motor neuron activity. The subthreshold depolarization of motoneurons by descending pathways facilitates the excitatory action of concurrent peripheral input. The strength of a reflex can be increased in this way. Descending inhibitory influences on motoneurons also decrease the reflex strength. In addition, interneurons and motoneurons branches (collaterals), that diverge and connect with other neurons, allow individual motor neurons and interneurons to effect the activity of other neurons. All motoneurons and interneurons receive converging inputs from many different sources. The neuron's activity reflects the sum of excitatory and inhibitory influences (postsynaptic potentials) prevailing on it at the same time.

The next, higher level from the spinal cord is the brainstem. It contains neuronal systems that are necessary for integrating motor commands descending from higher levels as well as for processing information that ascends from the spinal cord and is conveyed from the special senses. The brainstem motor systems are essential in processing two categories of afferent input: the ones related to cranial nerve nuclei and others that are essential for postural adjustments. This pathway is very important for control of the posture required muscular adjustments. The importance of the brainstem motor systems is also illustrated by the fact that all descending motor pathways to the spinal cord, except the corticospinal tract, originate in the brainstem.

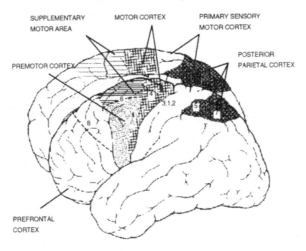

Fig. 2.3: The cortical regions (Broadman's areas) within the human brain. Areas 4 and 6 are the most important for central motor programs.

The motor and premotor cortices are the top two levels in the motor hierarchy [Brodmann, 1909]. The Brodmann's Area 4 of the motor cortex (third level) is the node upon which the cortical organization converges, and from which most descending motor commands requiring cortical processing are sent to the brainstem and other subcortical structures including the spinal cord. The corticospinal system mediates the commands. After being mediated, the command signals control segmental neurons in the spinal cord.

The premotor cortical regions in Brodmann's Area 6 (Figure 2.3) play important role in planing the movement. These areas are closely connected by corticocortical association fibers to the prefrontal and posterior parietal cortices. The premotor areas are responsible for identifying targets in space, for choosing a course of action, and for programming movement. These premotor areas act primarily on the motor cortex but also exert some influence on lower order brainstem and spinal systems.

Three features of the hierarchy of motor structures are particularly important. Different components of the motor systems contain somatotopic maps. The areas that influence adjacent body parts can be found adjacent to each other can be found in these maps. This somatotopic organization is also preserved in the most interconnections at different levels (e.g., the regions of motor cortex controlling the arm receive input from

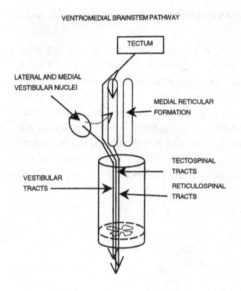

Fig. 2.4: Ventromedial brainstem pathway, one of the brainstem motor pathways controlling different groups of motor neurons, *i.e.,* muscles. See text for explanation.

premotor arm areas and influence corresponding arm-control areas of the descending brainstem pathways). A hierarchical level receives information from the periphery, so that sensory input can modify the action of descending commands. Finally, a feature of the organization of the motor systems is the capacity of higher levels to control the information that reaches them, allowing or suppressing the transmission of the afferent volleys through sensory relays.

The cerebellum and basal ganglia play important roles in controlling movement. The cerebellum adjusts the actions of both the brainstem motor structures and the motor cortex by comparing descending control signals responsible for the intended motor response with sensory signals resulting from the consequences of motor action. Based on this comparison, the cerebellum is able to update and control movement when the movement deviates from its intended trajectory. The basal ganglia are not as well understood. They receive inputs from all cortical areas and focus their actions principally on premotor areas of the cerebral cortex. Diseases of the basal ganglia produce a unique set of motor abnormalities consisting of involuntary movement and disturbances in posture.

2.1.2 Parallel Organization of Motor Control Channels

The brainstem and the motor and premotor cortical areas are organized hierarchically, but there are connections (channels) allowing them to also work in parallel. They can act independently on the final common pathway (Figure 2.4). For example, the corticospinal projection controls brainstem by descending pathways and also controls spinal interneurons and motor neurons. This parallel organization allows commands from higher levels either to modify or to supersede lower order reflex behavior (Figure 2.5). The combination of parallel and hierarchical control results in an overlap of different elements of the motor systems. The overlap allows motor commands to be divided into separate components, each making a specific contribution to motor behavior. This is also important in the recovery of function after local lesions.

The principles of hierarchical and parallel organization explain most of the functional interrelationships between various components of both sensory and motor systems. Sensory receptors carry information into the spinal cord by primary afferent fibers. These axons act on segmental interneurons and motor neurons. The spinal cord is mediating these reflex-type activities.

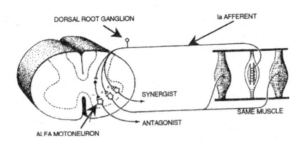

Fig. 2.5: The schema of organization of the myotatic reflex. Note the inhibitory interneuron (black) going to antagonist and monosynaptic excitatory mechanism to the same muscle.

The neuronal networks of each segment connect to those of other segments through propriospinal neurons. Ascending pathways convey information to motor centers of the brainstem and to the cerebral cortex. Both the brainstem and cortical centers project back to the segmental networks and thereby are able to control reflex activity as well as produce voluntary movement. The output of these supraspinal centers is influenced and ultimately integrated by the cerebellum and basal ganglia. Note that the receptors in muscle sense the displacement of muscles and limbs and influence the output from spinal segments or higher levels.

2.1.3 Afferent Fibers and Motor Neurons

On entering the spinal cord, the axons of the dorsal root ganglion cells send terminal branches to all laminae of the dorsal horn except lamina II (Figure 2.6). Some fibers continue within the intermediate zone, and a few of them reach the groups of motor neuron cell bodies in the ventral horn. In the ventral horn, the afferent fibers bifurcate and travel in rostral and caudal directions, sending off terminals at various segmental levels. The motor neurons lie in the ventral horn. Those innervating a single muscle are collectively called a motor neuron pool. The motor neuron pools are segregated into longitudinal columns extending through two to four spinal segments.

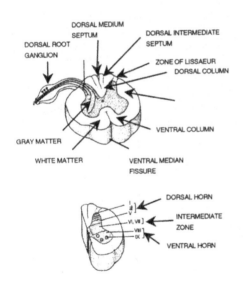

Fig. 2.6: The white matter of the spinal cord is divided into columns, and the gray matter is divided into horns. The Roman numbers show laminae divided in three major divisions.

Two groups or divisions of motor neuron pools can be distinguished in the ventral horn. One group is located in the medial part of the ventral horn; the other, much larger group lies more laterally. These motor neurons connect to muscles according to a strict functional rule: the motor neurons located medially project to axial muscles; those located more laterally project to limb muscles (Figure 2.6). The motor neurons of the lateral division innervate the muscles of the arms and legs. Within the lateral group, the most medial motor neuron pools tend to innervate the muscles of the shoulder and pelvic girdles, while motor neurons located more laterally project to distal muscles of the extremities and digits. In addition to the proximal-distal rule, there is a flexor-extensor rule: motor neurons innervating extensor muscles tend to lie ventral to those innervating flexors.

2.1.4 Interneurons and Propriospinal Neurons

Between the dorsal horn and the motor neuron pools lies the intermediate zone of the spinal cord. This zone contains interneurons that direct the impulse traffic according to their connections. The lateral parts of the intermediate zone project ipsilaterally to the dorsolateral motor neuron groups that innervate distal limb muscles. The medial regions of the intermediate zone project bilaterally to the medial motor neuron groups that innervate the axial muscles on both sides of the body.

Many of the interneurons in the intermediate zone have axons that course up and down the white matter of the spinal cord and terminate in homologous regions several segments away. These interconnecting interneurons, known as propriospinal neurons, send axons in the lateral columns that extend only a few segments (Figure 2.7). Those in the ventral and ventromedial columns are longer and may extend the entire length of the spinal cord. This pattern of organization allows the axial muscles, which are innervated from many segments, to be activated in concert for appropriate postural adjustment. In contrast, distal limb muscles tend to be used independently.

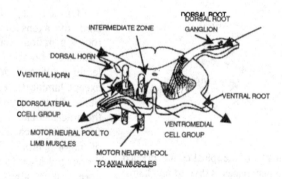

Fig. 2.7: Input-output organization of spinal segments and interconnections between segments.

In addition to an overall topographic organization, the interneurons also make precise connections. Many of these interneurons receive characteristic connections from descending pathways. These descending pathways terminate either on neurons in the dorsal horn and intermediate zone or directly on the motor neurons.

2.1.5 Neuronal Pathways

The brainstem contains many groups of neurons whose axons form pathways projecting to the spinal gray matter. Different pathways could be subdivided into two distinct groups [Kuypers, 1981] according to the location of their terminations in the spinal cord. The first group, the ventromedial pathways, terminates in the ventromedial part of the spinal gray matter; thus affects motor neurons innervating proximal muscles. The second group, the dorsolateral pathways, terminates in the dorsolateral part of the spinal gray matter and influences motor neurons controlling the distal muscles of the extremities. The difference in termination corresponds to a systematic difference in the functional roles of these two sets of descending systems. The ventromedial pathways are important in maintaining balance and in postural fixation. The dorsolateral pathways play a crucial role in steering the extremities and in the fine control required for manipulating objects with the fingers and hand. The different usage to which we put proximal and distal muscles are reflected in differences in the fine organization of the connections of the ventromedial and dorsolateral systems.

The *ventromedial group* of pathways descends in the ipsilateral ventral columns of the spinal cord and terminates predominantly on medial motor neurons that innervate axial and girdle muscles. The pathways also end on interneurons, including long propriospinal neurons in the ventromedial part of the intermediate zone.

The ventromedial pathways are characterized by the divergent distribution of their terminals. Many axons in the ventromedial pathways terminate bilaterally in the spinal cord. In addition, they send collaterals to different segmental levels. Thus, about one-half of the axons that reach the-lumbar cord also has collaterals in the cervical gray matter. Moreover, the long propriospinal neurons controlled by this system also have many axons spreading widely up and down the spinal cord.

The ventromedial system has three major components: 1) the lateral and medial vestibulospinal tracts originate in the lateral and medial vestibular nuclei and carry information for the reflex control of equilibrium from the vestibular labyrinthof the inner ear; 2) the tectospinal tract originates in the tectum of the midbrain, a structure that is important for the coordinated control of head and eye movement directed toward visual targets; and 3) the reticulospinal tract originates in the reticular formation of the medulla and the pons. The reticular formation is an area of the medulla and pons composed mainly of interneurons and their processes and can best be considered as a rostral extension of the spinal intermediate zone into the brainstem.

The *dorsolateral group* of pathways descends in the lateral quadrant of the spinal cord. It terminates in the lateral portion of the intermediate zone and among the dorsolateral groups of motor neurons innervating more distal limb muscles. In contrast to the ventromedial pathways, in which individual fibers send off large numbers of collaterals at different levels, the dorsolateral pathways terminate on a small number of spinal segments.

The dorsolateral brainstem system is primarily composed of rubrospinal fibers that originate in the magnocellular portion of the red nucleus in the midbrain. Rubrospinal fibers cross the midline ventral to the red nucleus and descend in the ventrolateral quadrant of the medulla. The magnocellular portion of the red nucleus also gives rise to rubrobulbar fibers, which project both to the cranial nerve nuclei controlling facial muscles and to nuclei with a sensory function: the sensory trigeminal nucleus and the dorsal column nuclei (the cunaete and gracile nuclei).

The cerebral cortex sends command signals that are conveyed to the motor neurons by two main routes: the corticobulbar and corticospinal tracts. The corticobulbar tract controls the motor neurons innervating cranial nerve nuclei, and the corticospinal tract controls the motor neurons innervating the spinal segments. The two systems act directly on the motor neurons. These two systems also act on the descending brainstem pathways, mainly the reticulospinal and rubrospinal tracts. Moreover, like the descending brainstem pathways, the corticospinal tract has both ventromedial and dorsolateral subdivisions that influence axial and distal muscles, respectively.

Strictly speaking, the corticobulbar fibers originate in the cortex and terminate in the medulla. In practice, however, the term is often used to include cortical fibers that terminate either in cranial nerve nuclei or in other brainstem nuclei, such as the nuclei giving rise to descending pathways, dorsal column nuclei, and nuclei projecting to the cerebellum). The corticospinal fibers originate in the cortex and terminate in the spinal cord, in the medulla; the corticospinal fibers form the medullary pyramids. The term pyramidal tract is therefore often used synonymously with corticospinal tract. However, because many fibers leave the medullary pyramids to innervate brainstem nuclei, the terms corticospinal and pyramidal are not strictly synonymous.

All regions of the cortex are ultimately capable of influencing both the motor and premotor cortices through their corticocortical connections. These pathways take the form of bundles of axons in the white matter that links the different regions of cortex with each other.

An additional source of corticocortical inputs comes from the corpus callosum, which relays information from one hemisphere to the other. Callosal fibers interconnect homologous areas of both the sensory and motor cortices. The regions that receive information from or project to the distal regions of the limbs do not receive callosal connections. These regions (the hand and foot areas of the somatic sensory and motor cortices of the two hemispheres) are thus functionally disconnected from one another.

2.2 Mechanisms for Control of Posture

There are multiple definitions of posture. Posture is the genetically defined position of body segments, characteristic for each species. This view is supported by the classical works by Sherrington [1906] and Magnus [1924] showing that the body orientation with respect to gravity is determined by a set of complete sensory-motor processes defining the orientation of the body segments and stabilizing this orientation against external disturbances. Posture can also be defined based on anatomical and functional backgrounds [Kuypers, 1981]. Axial and proximal body segments and their corresponding musculature serve as a support for the distal segments such as the hands for reaching and grasping. Bouisset *et al.* [1992] proposed a concept of posturo-kinetic capacity, meaning that posture is a capacity of the supporting segments to anticipate the disturbing effect on posture and balance provoked by ongoing movement. An interesting concept is to oppose posture to movement. In this view, posture means that the position of one or several segments is fixed with respect to other body segments or with respect to space; this position is stabilized against external disturbances. By contrast, movement means that a new position is controlled by the central nervous system.

With respect of defining posture two functions emerge [Massion, 1998]. A first function is an antigravity function. This function includes first the building up of the body segment configuration against gravity. A related function is the static and dynamic support provided by skeletal segments in contact with the support base to the moving segments. A second function is that of interface for perception and action between the environment and the body. The orientation with respect to space of given segments such as head or trunk serves as reference frame for the perception of the body movements with respect to space and for balance control. They also serve as a reference frame for the calculation of the target position in space and for the calculation of the trajectories for reaching the targets.

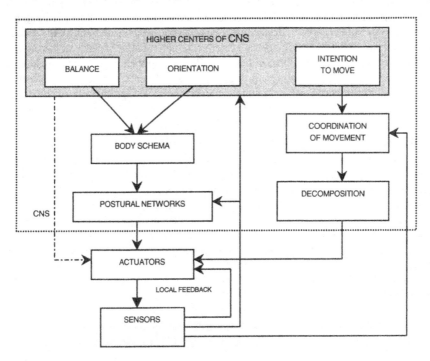

Fig. 2.8: Central organization of postural control. The schematic diagram summarizes the main components involved in postural and movement control. There are two references: body segment orientation and equilibrium control. The schema shows various feedback commands involving different sensory sources (e.g., vision, labyrinth, proprioception, cutaneous sensors, and gravitoreceptors). Body schema is an internal representation of the organization of the body.

The coordination needed for posture is better understood when referring to the hierarchical model of posture (Figure 2.8) which includes both the inborn reactions and those built up by learning [Gurfinkel and Levik, 1991]. They claim that in the postural domain two levels of control can be identified. The first level is a level of representation or postural body schema, and a second level is a level of implementation in terms of kinematics and force. Actually, this schema is not different from the concept of internal models proposed by Bernstein [1967] for the organization of movement. The level of representation can be documented by a set of observations made by artificial or biased sensory inputs, such as a moving visual scene [Lestienne et al., 1977], or galvanic stimulation of the labyrinth [Lund and Broberg, 1983].

Two main hypotheses have been formulated. According to one, a single controller does exist, acting on the various joints and achieving the various goals and task constraints. This hypothesis has been put forward by Bernstein [1967], and Aruin and Latash [1995]. According to others, two or several parallel controls exist, one for the main task [Massion, 1992], the others for the associated task constraints such as balance and body segment orientation, these multiple controls being coordinated.

Sensory-motor organization for postural orientation includes neural mechanisms for active control of joint stiffness and global variables such as trunk and head alignment. Biomechanical models of posture suggest that much of the coordination and control of posture emerges from biomechanical constraints inherent in the musculo-skeletal system and that the nervous system takes advantage of these constraints. The control of dynamic equilibrium has a reflex component (automatic response to disturbances), yet it is anticipatory postural adjustments that are instrumental in voluntary, focal movement. Postural coordination is significantly influenced by previous experience, practice, and training. The relative roles of the somatosensory, vestibular, and visual inputs for postural orientation and equilibrium can change, depending on the task and on the particular environmental context.

Orienting the body to environmental variables (e.g., vertical line), and aligning various body parts is termed postural orientation. The orientation of the trunk may be one of the most important controlled variables, since this will determine the positioning of the limbs relative to the objects with which we may wish to interact. Body posture can be oriented to a variety of reference frames depending on the task and behavioral goals. The frame of reference can be visual, based on external cues in the surrounding environment; somatosensory, based on information from contact with external objects; or vestibular, based on gravitoinertial forces. Alternatively, the frame of reference may be an internal representation of body orientation to the environment, such as an estimated reference position from memory.

2.2.1 Biomechanical Principles of Standing

During quiet standing, the gravity, ground reaction forces and inertial forces produced by swaying are in equilibrium. The center of mass (CoM) is the point at the body where the resultant gravity force acts. The projection of the CoM to the base of support is called the center of gravity (CoG). The point of origin of the ground reaction force, the point through the resultant ground reaction forces passes, is named the center of pressure (CoP). Maintaining posture is a process of continuos swaying of the body around the position of labile stability. Since the human body contains many segments that move relative to each other, CoM constantly changes its position; therefore CoG is constantly moving in the plane of feet. The central nervous system has constantly to adjust the relative position of segments to prevent falling, that is to control many muscles according to ensure dynamic equilibrium.

The support while standing on both legs is the region bounded by the feet, a quadrangle bounded by the heels and toes (Figure 2.9). When the body is in contact with objects (e.g., parallel bars, walker, crutches, or cane), the support base extends to include all support points. During walking the support region is very small, being only part of one foot at some phases of the gait cycle. During standing the projection of the CoM lies within the base of support, yet while walking it is never within this zone. The actual movement of the CoP and CoM for an able bodied subjects is presented in Figure 2.10. Walking is only dynamically stable; precise control continually prevents the fall of inherently unstable system. Very slow walking, called ambulating with hand supports belongs to postural problem.

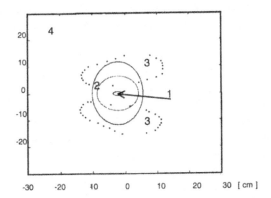

Fig. 2.9: Zones of preference for the center of pressure (CoP): 1) high preference; 2) low preference; 3) undesirable preference; and 4) unstable. Adapted from Popović MR et al. 1999, with permission.

Stability in standing is a function of many factors. The standing quadruped is stable because the four contact points determine the base of support; it is relatively large (e.g., standing or ambulating with the walker or crutches). In contrast, the base of support is small in a standing bipedal human. For the purpose of biomechanical analysis the body can be modeled as a multijoint multiactuator inverted pendulum. The control of stability of a multi-body, inverted pendulum is very difficult, even if the torque at the base is unconstrained. However, the torque that a human generates at the surface is limited because of the feet. The position of CoM is relatively high - somewhere at the trunk region, being on average about one meter above the ground. The frequently used models use only one or two segments. The single body inverted pendulum studies consider only the ankle joints for control of posture, while in the three-link models (Figure 2.11) the ankle and hip joints are studied [Winter, 1992].

Postural adjustments for maintaining orientation and equilibrium arise from neural programs that are formulated and implemented by complex sensory-motor control processes. The concept of a motor program has developed from accumulated evidence that postural adjustments are not merely the sum of simple reflexes, but arise from a complex sensory-motor control system. The motor program represents the dynamic reordering of the many postural variables that are controlled, into a hierarchical structure. For any part of the program, one or more postural goals, such as trunk orientation, gaze fixation, or energy expenditure may take precedence over another set of goals, but this ordering will change depending on the task and context. Many variables are controlled dynamically in the performance of postural adjustments from the relatively simple variables of muscle length or force to the more global variables of body segment orientation or position of the CoM. Current studies of postural control attempt to determine which variables are controlled and how that control is achieved. There may be simple programs available to the postural control system for a given task, whether it is a postural adjustment to an unexpected disturbance or a voluntary movement. The neural program applies constrains to the musculo-skeletal system by setting the hierarchical order of controlled variables, in order to achieve one particular solution for the postural task.

The nervous system commands the contraction and relaxation of muscles throughout the body (Figure 2.12). Forces developed by the muscles are transformed to joint torque. The joint torque displaces the body segments in order to restore postural

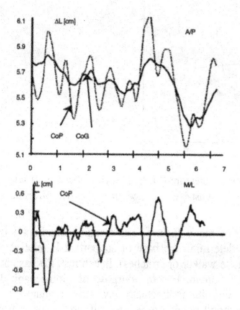

Fig. 2.10: Displacement of the center of gravity and center of pressure in anteroposterior (A/P) and mediolateral (M/L) directions during standing. Adapted from Winter *et al.* 1996, with permission.

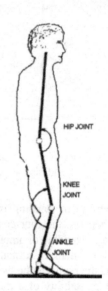

Fig. 2.11: The sketch of a three-link model used for biomechanical analysis of standing

orientation, and the friction force from the support surface moves the CoM to a new equilibrium position. Here, one should notice that the redundancy of both the skeletal system and the actuators provides an infinite number of trajectories. However, analyses of quiet standing in able-bodied human shows that some postures are preferred to others, and that the preference is based on the task and environmental constraints. Recordings from muscles show reproducibility from one human to another. Analysis of joint trajectories and torque in the phase space shows high correlation between neighboring joint movement. This behavior is termed synergy. The synergies are not fixed; they depend on many factors such as the initial conditions and environmental constraints. Similar behavior found in electromyography recordings is called a muscle synergy, consisting of the spatial and temporal patterns of activation and relaxation of muscles.

Biomechanical analyses provide important results in the control of the posture (e.g., effects of cocontraction). Cocontraction results in an increased stiffness of joints. Controlling a series of loose joints (ankle, knee, hip), which should support the trunk, neck, head, and arms against gravity in an erect position, is comparable with the automatic control of a bicycle chain or rope in the vertical position, while regulating a series of stiff joints to be translated into the control of an inverted pendulum.

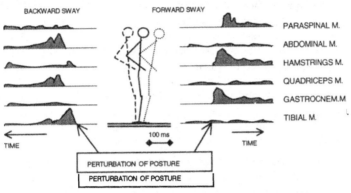

Fig. 2.12: Postural response to a moderate perturbation of a movable platform in anteroposterior direction. Muscle activity of main movers is showing the complexity of responses in first 300 ms. Adapted from Horak and Nashner, 1986.

2.2.2 Postural Adjustments for Focal Movement

A voluntary focal movement (e.g., pointing movement) produces forces that affect all the segments of the body, therefore the CoM will move. Focal movement does not occur in isolation; it is accompanied by activity in many distant muscles that does not contribute directly to the focal movement itself. Such activity represents an active postural adjustment that either precedes the activation of the prime movers in a voluntary movement, or is simultaneous with the voluntary movement [Horak and Macpherson, 1995]. Experiments involving able-bodied humans picking objects from the desk while walking close to it showed that the reaching movement of the arm is the latest in a series of events, preceded by the lowering of the CoM and postural movement of the legs and the trunk [MacKenzie and Iberall, 1994]. Through learning and adaptation, the nervous system anticipates the mechanical effects of a voluntary movement and adjusts the amplitude and timing of the accompanying postural component in order to minimize the disturbance to balance.

If the reaction time for the focal movement changes, the latency of the anticipatory postural activity does too so that the temporal relations are maintained between postural activity and focal activity [Belecki *et al.*, 1967]. Furthermore, the latency for activation of a muscle is shorter when that muscle serves a preparatory postural role than when it acts as a prime mover. The spatial pattern of EMG activity in the postural adjustment that accompanies voluntary movement is specific to the movement being performed, and is not merely a generalized co-contraction [Horak and Macpherson, 1995]. For example, the activity of the muscles in the two legs is asymmetric for a single arm raise, but symmetric when both arms are raised together because of the differences in the reaction forces related to the arm lift [Belecki *et al.*, 1967; Bouiset and Zattara, 1981].

2.2.3 Sensors for Control of Posture

There are many common features in the sensory control of postural orientation and of dynamic equilibrium. Both use sensory information from multiple channels, including somatosensory (cutaneous and proprioceptive), vestibular, and visual. These sensory systems do not operate as independent, parallel channels that sum together at some point to result in a motor output. Multiple sensory inputs are integrated and resolved by the postural control system to provide a coherent interpretation of the body's orientation and dynamic equilibrium. This information is then compared with an internal model of the body and any resulting error signal is used to generate motor commands in order to maintain the required postural variables at the desired level. This process occurs at the subconscious, involuntary level, producing automatic adjustments with short latencies.

The information coded by each sensory modality is unique, and each class of receptor operates optimally within a specific range of frequency and amplitude of body motion. Nevertheless, there is enough redundancy of sensory information to maintain balance in certain environments when information from one or more sensory channels is not available. Multiple channels of input are necessary in order to resolve ambiguities about postural orientation and body motion. Because the sensory receptors are part of the body itself, the interpretation of the afferent information within the reference frame of the surrounding world may not be singular; thus, leading to ambiguity.

Dynamic weighting of sensory inputs may be necessary to optimize the control of the postural stability. As mentioned previously, the main controlled variable for dynamic equilibrium may be the position and orientation of the trunk in space. How information about the trunk is derived from sensory inputs is task and context-dependent. When the support surface is stable and firmly contacted, then proprioceptive and cutaneous information from the legs and feet may give the most reliable information about the trunk relative to the environment. In contrast, when the surface is unstable or contacted for only brief periods such as during rapid locomotion, then the combination of vestibular and neck proprioceptive information may provide the most veridical information about trunk orientation and velocity. Vestibular inputs detect acceleration of the head in a gravitoinertial reference frame, whereas the neck proprioceptors provide information about the head relative to the trunk. Thus, the combination of vestibular and neck inputs allows the system to derive trunk position and velocity relative to the environment.

An example of the relative dependence of postural control on visual, vestibular, and somatosensory information comes from a study by Nashner and colleagues [Black et al., 1988; Nashner et al., 1982]. They measured postural sway during erect stance while systematically manipulating one type of sensory information at a time: visual information by either eye closure or by stabilizing the visual surround with respect to body sway at the hip, called "sway referencing"; and somatosensory information by "sway referencing" the tilt of the support surface and, therefore, ankle joint angle. The role of vestibular input was examined by studying patients with various types of vestibular deficits. In the sway-referenced conditions, sensory information is not rendered absent, but is "inaccurate" as a postural orientation reference.

Somatosensory afferents, which include mechanoreceptors in the skin, pressure receptors in deep tissues, muscle spindles, Golgi tendon organs, and joint receptors, provide critical information about postural orientation and equilibrium. New studies of postural orientation in unusual gravitoinertial environments suggest that somatosensory information alone may be sufficient for maintaining body orientation in stance. In order to remain standing in a large room that is rotating at constant velocity, the subjects must orient to the tilted force field, which is the summation of gravitational and angular inertial vectors [Fisk *et al.*, 1993].

The vestibular receptors in the semicircular canals and macular otoliths are sensitive to angular and linear acceleration of the head, respectively [Fitzpatrick *et al.*, 1996]. The otolith signal gives a combination of all the linear accelerations acting on the head, including the constant acceleration due to gravity. Thus, the otoliths are stimulated as the head tilts with respect to gravity, such as during body sway. Otolith signals alone are probably not responsible for our sense of verticality [Mittelstaedt, 1983].

The semicircular canals, as angular accelerometers, are sensitive to higher frequencies of head motions than the otoliths. The anterior and posterior canals, which detect pitch (rotation about the interaural axis) and roll (rotation about the nasooccipital axis) are important for detecting rapid postural sway, which occurs with rapid hip flexion or extension, but not for detecting low frequency sway such as in quiet stance [Nashner, 1972; Nashner *et al.*, 1989].

Vestibular afferents are responsible for triggering the response to sudden, unexpected falling. In contrast, vestibular inputs are not required for the triggering of postural responses to movements of the support surface, especially when the subject is in contact with a stable, large surface [Allum *et al.*, 1993; Diener and Dichgans, 1985; Horak *et al.*, 1990].

Several lines of physiological and psychophysical evidence indicate that the continuous drift of textured images over the retina excites a visual subsystem distinct from that which signals stimulus location and stationary features of the visual array.

The two modes of transcoding spatial relationships are provided by these two distinct, yet complementary visual subsystems. Static vision, that detects stable spatial features, is specially tuned for coding, object shape, pattern, contour, and relative position in a configuration space. It includes the foveal and parafoveal regions up to 10-15 degrees eccentricity (central retina). Dynamic vision detects the continuous motion of a stimulus and image drift on the retina. It is tuned for velocity coding and direction selectivity. It predominates in the peripheral retina. The former has high spatial acuity whereas the latter manifests higher temporal acuity. Psychophysical studies of visual function are confirming the duality of neural mechanisms subserving the perception of movement: one mechanism infers motion from the successive positions of a moving object and the other perceives directly the movement of the moving target signal [Paillard, 1999].

Behavioral, psychophysical, and neurophysiological data lead in the direction of a potential interaction between two analyzing systems for visual motion detection. This may explain the dominant role of positional cues in central vision over fast continuous movement detection and the prevalence of movement cues over stable patterned cues in peripheral vision [Paillard *et al.*, 1981]. This kind of reciprocal inhibition, observed at the behavioral level, may intervene at different levels in the central processing of visual information. It could explain why structures, receiving anatomically identified fibers from both systems, may nevertheless react separately to one or the other, according to the priority of access gated by the actual visual context, notwithstanding the possible role in this gating of specific reafferent information derived from self-motion.

Selective use of visual information as proprioceptive cues for controlling body movements has been reported. Two kinds of proprioceptive visual cues have been distinguished: those provided by vision of a moving body segment in relation to other body parts and those supplied by changes in the visual array related to displacement of the head in space.

The parallel computation of position and movement cues in two separate channels and networks allowing a somewhat redundant description of space relationships. Theoretically, both descriptions may be complete and self-sufficient. In one channel, immobile and stationary features can be inferred from the null velocity signal, and the final position of a movement can be derived from the integral of its velocity. Velocity signals conveyed by the dynamic channel are the essential descriptors of what may be called a "movement space." In the second channel, motion information can be derived from the discrete successive changes of stimulus position, thereby primarily defining a "relative position space." Thus, information about position is available directly from the static channel and indirectly from the integral of velocity provided by the kinetic channel. Conversely, velocity, which is directly coded in the movement channel, can also be indirectly evaluated by the position channel as a derivative of the extent of location change with respect to time. Two main descriptions of space relationships are available for the brain, therefore. One is based on the coding of relative distance between stable points of the visual array, and the other is based on the velocity and direction coding of moving features, being probably the more primitive from an evolutionary viewpoint.

2.2.4 Central Neural Mechanisms for Control of Posture

Current evidence suggests that spinal cord circuits alone are not capable of producing the organized equilibrium responses characteristic of intact mammals [Pratt et al., 1994]. The vestibular nuclear complex in the medulla and pons is an important center for the integration of vestibular, somatosensory, and visual information that plays a large part in the control of postural orientation and equilibrium [Wilson and Melvil-Jones, 1979]. Vestibulospinal pathways from this region, as well as reticulospinal pathways from the adjacent reticular formation, terminate on both motoneurons and interneurons that influence neck, axial, and limb musculature [Wilson and Peterson, 1981]. The extent to which these and other descending tracts from the brain stem structures influence and shape programs for postural orientation and equilibrium is not known.

The basal ganglia play an important role in postural alignment and control of stability [Alexander and Crutcher, 1990; Hallet, 1993]. They appear critical for adapting postural strategies to changes in initial conditions and environmental support. Normally, the strategy for postural equilibrium changes rapidly when subjects stand on a different support configuration or support themselves with their hands, trunk, or by sitting.

The cerebellum plays several different roles in the control of posture involving sensory-motor integration [Babinski, 1896]. Lesions in different regions of the cerebellum produce very different effects on postural control [Holmes, 1939]. Lesion of the vestibulo-cerebellum results in impaired vertical orientation of humans who slowly drift away from upright posture, even with eyes open [Diener et al., 1983a and b]. The most profound deficits in dynamic postural control occur with damage to the anterior lobe of the cerebellum, which receives somatosensory inputs from throughout the body and projects to the spinal cord via the red nucleus and reticular formation [Allum and Honneger, 1993; Carpenter *et al.*, 1999; Diener and Dichgans, 1985].

Subjects with lesions restricted to the cerebellum invariably show normal latencies of automatic postural responses evoked by unexpected perturbations of the support surface, suggesting that the initiation of these responses is independent of the cerebellum. In fact, the entire pattern of agonistic and antagonist activation throughout the body in response to external postural perturbations is preserved in cerebellar patients, suggesting that the postural synergy is not selected or triggered by the cerebellum [Horak and Diener, 1994]. In contrast, the duration and amplitude of automatic postural responses are much larger than normal in subjects with anterior lobe disorders and may contribute to their large trunkal tremor and gait ataxia.

Although the motor areas of the cerebral cortex are involved in the preparation of voluntary movement, their role in postural mechanisms and, in particular, in response to unexpected perturbations of stance is a point of discussion [Massion, 1992]. The latency of the postural response to an unexpected perturbation is long enough to involve a loop through the sensory-motor cortex, and this fact has been invoked as evidence of the participation of the cortex in such responses. A medium-latency response to unexpected perturbations has been referred to as a "transcortical reflex" [Evarts, 1976]. However, latency alone does not provide sufficient proof of the involvement of the cortex. Studies have also demonstrated that the medium-latency responses can arise even from the isolated spinal cord, perhaps through reverberating loops within spinal interneuronal circuits [Eklund *et al.*, 1982a and b].

Cortical involvement is most important in the anticipatory postural adjustments that accompany voluntary movement. The extent to which these postural adjustments share the same mechanisms and processes as those elicited by unexpected perturbations is not known. Anticipatory postural adjustments may be either an integral and inseparable part of motor planning for voluntary movement, or a distinct process, organized in a parallel fashion and utilizing different circuits and mechanisms.

2.3 Mechanisms for Control of Walking

Walking is amongst the most highly automated movements of humans. The cycle to cycle repetition of all elements comprising walking is characteristic for each particular subject when walking [Bernstein, 1967, Cavagna and Margaria, 1966, Patla, 1991; Cappozzo *et al.*, 1978]. Locomotion displays an extremely widespread synergy incorporating the whole musculature and the entire moving skeleton and bringing into focus a large number of areas and conduction pathways of the central nervous system. Walking belongs to the category of extremely ancient movements. It is phylogenetically older than the cortical hemispheres and has undoubtedly affected the development of the central nervous system in the same manner as have the distance receptors mentioned by Sherrington [1900, 1910].

The bipedal locomotion of humans is an unusually stable structure, although the mechanical structure is far from the favorable. All basic details of normal walking may be found in each and every able-bodied subject. Individual differences between subjects do not depend on the differences in the structure of walking, nor on the assembly of elements encountered, but only in the rhythms and amplitudes of the ratios between these elements.

2.3.1 The Development of Walking

Human and animal walking develop through maturation and experience. The capacity to walk is genetically available. Human newborns exhibit stepping movements when held beneath the shoulders, provided their feet can touch the ground [André-Thomas and Autgarden, 1966]. The development of walking follows a number of milestones: t baby first lifts its head, then supports its body on its arms, next turns over, then sits up, then creeps, next walks with assistance, and finally walks alone.

Disappearing Reflexes. The development of walking comes as a consequence of several reflexes that come into play. In addition, some reflexes present in infancy disappear [Easton, 1972]. The disappearance of reflexes accompanies neurological changes, which allow for mature walking behavior. Babies show a variety of reflex behaviors. The startle reflex (arms and legs move symmetrically, first outward, then upward, then inward, the hands open and clench, as do the legs); the tonic neck reflex (an asymmetrical pose adopted by newborns, the baby's head and arm extend to one side and on the opposite side, the arm and leg flex); the righting reflex (the attempts to keep the head erect); the Babinski reflex (involuntary response to stimulation of the bottom of the feet); the crawling reflex (alternating pattern of extensions and flexion of the arms and legs); and the stepping reflex (alternate lifting and planting the two feet in succession when held so the feet come in contact with a solid surface) are all disappearing with maturing.

The stepping reflex disappears by around 4 weeks of age, only to reappear several months later in a different form. Why does stepping disappear and then reappear in human infants can be explained by development of supraspinal control and cognitive functions [Thelen, 1983]. He attributed the reemergence of stepping to physical changes. Infants can kick throughout the beginning of the life, yet they can not walk. This may be attributed to the inability to maintain bipedal posture and balance during the first year of life [Thelen et al., 1981].

Although physical factors may account for the re-emergence of stepping around one year of age, not all developmental phenomena in motor control can be explained so easily. The reflexes discussed earlier, for example, disappear under normal conditions, presumably because of neurological changes. Researchers concerned with these changes have suggested that they are organized on the basis of several major principles:

1) During development, nerve fibers in the central nervous system undergo myelination, the process by which axons are coated with the fatty substance that allows for speeded neural transmission. Once this coating has formed, finer coordination becomes possible [Yakolev and Lecours, 1967].

2) Cortical centers come to take over functions that were previously performed by subcortical centers, or they inhibit those subcortical centers [McGraw, 1943]. This explains why reflexes seen in young infants, such as the tonic neck reflex and the grasp reflex, are supplanted by other, more flexible behaviors. The same explanation holds also for the postures adopted during sleep in able-bodied adults being similar to those exhibited by babies (during sleep the inhibitory influences of the higher brain centers are temporarily suspended).

3) The neural maturation proceeds in a distinct cephalic-caudal (head-to-tail) and proximal-distal direction [Woollacott *et al.*, 1987].

2.3.2 Bipedal Walking

As described in Section 2.2 the posture is the state of equilibrium in which the net torque and force generated by gravity and muscles are zero, and only minimal sway exists around the quasi-stable inverted pendulum position. Walking occurs once the equilibrium ceases to exist because of the change of internal forces caused by muscle activity. The change of internal forces will cause the center of gravity to move out of the stability zone, and the body will start falling. Human walking starts, therefore, after the redistribution of internal forces allowing gravity to take over. The falling is prevented by bringing the contralateral leg in front of the body, hence, providing new support position. Once the contralateral leg supports the body weight and the ipsilateral leg pushes the body up and forward due to the momentum the body will move in the direction of progression, and ultimately come directly above the supporting leg. This new inverted pendulum position is transitional; momentum and gravity will again bring the body into the falling pattern. Cyclic repetition of the described events is defined as bipedal locomotion or walking.

The major requirements for successful locomotion are: 1) production of a locomotor rhythm to ensure support to the body against gravity; 2) production of muscle forces hat will result with the friction force required for propelling it to the intended direction; 3) dynamic equilibrium of the moving body; and 4) adaptation of these movements to meet the environmental demands and the tasks selected by the individual.

Walking is achieved through the repetition of a well-defined movements; thus, the emphasis in the research to date has often been on identifying principles and mechanisms that govern the generation of the basic rhythm. However, walking is not only a simple repetition of movements The movements of the leg while walking could be also classified as goal directed movements (e.g., ballet dancing), but after many repetitions it became automatic. The walking is result of a planned action where and how to move. Walking over uneven terrain, changing the pace and other activities require the action of higher centers of the central nervous system. This view does not contradict the ideas that there is a center at the spinal cord, called central pattern generator, that plays an important role in generating the necessary rhythm, once the decisions are made.

Functional movements in humans follows the cognitive decision: the task and a plan how to achieve the task. Walking is a function that follows the decision to transfer from one point to another in space maintaining the vertical posture. The first element in planning of locomotion in able-bodies subjects is a visual cue. Walking is possible without visual cues (e.g., walking in dark room, blind people); nut it is based on anticipation of no obstacles and good performance requires knowing the environment and excessive training. Natural environments rarely afford an even and uncluttered terrain for walking. A hallmark of successful and safe walking is the ability to adapt the basic gait patterns to meet the environmental demands [Patla *et al.*, 1985]. The visual system allows a human to make the anticipatory adjustment to the walking pattern necessary for overcoming environmental constraints. This can be easily seen when analyzing walking in environments with obstacles [Berger *et al.*, 1984; Patla *et al.*, 1991]. They found that reactions are mediated through proprioceptive and vestibular sensory channels. Patla with his colleagues [Corlett, 1985; Patla *et al.*, 1991; Bélanger and Patla, 1984] showed that the walking adaptations are not simple variations of the basic walking pattern; they are complex functional reorganization of the normal walking pattern. If humans are walking over a terrain with obstacles, which are appearing as perturbations, they select different strategies (Figure 2.13) depending on the size of the obstacle, and on the timing of perturbations with respect to the period of the gait cycle.

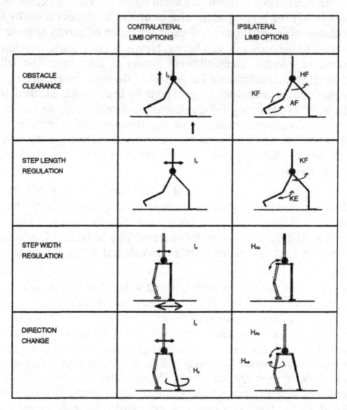

Fig. 2.13: A schematic diagram showing the contra- and ipsi-lateral options for implementing various avoidance strategies: HF - hip flexion, KF - knee flexion, AF - ankle flexion, KE - knee extension, $I_{x,y,z}$ - impulse in the direction of x, y, a-axis respectively, H - torque impulse around y-axis, abduction, and lateral femoral rotation, Ab - abduction, rot – rotation. Adapted from Patla, 1991, with permission.

In Chapter 1 the involvement of different sensory systems and motor systems was presented to stress that the repetitive behavior is a preferred manner of moving, and that this preference is task and motivation dependent. The richness of plausible options that one have while will walking be described by using an example when obstacles appear in the visual field of able-bodied subjects while walking. During a single step that is presented in Figure 2.13, the contralateral leg is supporting the body (stance), while the ipsilateral leg is swinging for the major part. Once an obstacle appears in front of the walking subject, he/she should avoid it and continue to walk. Therefore, he/she is forced to change the walking pattern. The change primarily involves the ipsilateral leg trajectory and a subsequent placement of the foot. There are several options that the subject can select, and four of them are shown: obstacle clearing, step length regulation, step width regulation, and direction of walk change. All options involve the ipsilateral, the contralateral, or both legs. The most "difficult" option that the subject can select is to change the direction of walking because it involves much larger forces to override inertia. Once more, this example is included to draw the readers' attention to the fact that the analysis of walking must be comprehensive, otherwise the results may be leading to wrong conclusions.

2.3.3 Role of Various Neural Mechanisms in Walking

Identifying the roles of various neural substrates in the control of locomotor is important when trying to restore walking of a human with disability. The only way to test some hypotheses is from animal experiments. Animal walking is in principle quadrupedal; thus, findings are sometimes difficult to transfer to bipedal walking. The three methods most frequently used for studying neuro-muscular mechanisms are the spinal, decerebrate, and decorticate preparations. Depending on the level of spinal transaction, one can either observe the locomotor ability of all four limbs or just the hind limbs; the latter being more commonly investigated. The spinal preparation needs an external stimulus, electrical or pharmacological, to produce locomotion. The decerebrate preparation can also be done at different levels. Depending on which nuclei are left intact, spontaneous locomotion may be possible although generally an external stimulus is needed to elicit locomotion. A decerebrate preparation leaves the brain stem, cerebellum, and the spinal cord intact. In contrast, the decorticate preparation also spares the basal ganglia with only the cortex removed. These preparations do not require an external stimulus to produce locomotion.

In the spinal preparation one can study how the spinal cord can produce reasonably complex and "normal" muscle activation patterns in response to an unpatterned stimulus. These patterns of muscular activation are not restricted to muscles within a limb. The spinal cord can provide appropriate interlimb coordination in addition to the intralimb coordination. It is also able to functionally modulate reflex responses [Forssberg, 1979 a and b] and carry out other stereotypic tasks concurrently [Carter and Smith, 1986a and b]. The modulation of reflex responses indicates that the spinal cord produces not only the appropriate patterns for the effector system, but also suitably primes the sensory system so that the reflex responses are compatible with the movement pattern. The ability to carry out other stereotypic tasks concurrently suggests that the spinal cord is not "fully used" for locomotion; reserves can be applied for other tasks.

In a decerebrate preparation, locomotion can be reliably induced and sustained by a simple pattern of stimulus to well defined regions [Shik *et al.*, 1966; Grillner and Dubuc, 1988]. The cerebellum is essential for the fine coordination of the locomotor patterns by virtue of the afferent information it receives and the influence it has on various descending pathways. Weight support and active propulsion are the added features compared to the spinal preparation. Decerebrate preparations are all limited to treadmill walking being very different from the previously described preparation since the propelling forces are not required. Experiments indicate that the added supraspinal drive is adequate for active propulsion and weight support. Decerebrate preparations do not have adequate equilibrium control.

The evidence for the sufficiency of basal ganglia and other caudal structures to provide range of locomotor abilities was tested in a decorticate preparation. Armstrong [1988] and Drew [1988] showed that the cortex, normally quiescent during unperturbed normal locomotion, is active when the animal is required to walk over uneven terrain. Therefore, it is possible to conclude that cortical structures play an important role in the expression of skilled locomotor behavior.

The demonstration that a simple unpatterned input to the spinal cord can produce complex rhythmic activation patterns led to the principle of central pattern generator (CPG) for the control of locomotion [Delcomyn, 1980; Grillner, 1985; Shik and Orlovsky, 1976]. The input plays no role in the generation of basic rhythm (Figure 2.14). The CPG has a dual role in controlling the activity of individual muscles. The first role is time keeping, periodically repeating the activation to the appropriate muscles. The second and more important role pertains to the production of specific forms of activation for each muscle. Oscillators have been proposed as models for these central pattern generators. The two roles for CPGs can thus be thought of in terms of time keeping and information storage function for oscillators [Patla, 1986].

This model for the control of basic locomotor rhythm is attractive because it narrows the locus of study to identifying neuronal organization at the spinal level that can produce the appropriate activation profiles. The time keeping of the locomotor rhythm unlike the heart rhythm relies not on pacemaker neurons, but rather appears to be an emergent property of neuronal networks. Understanding and deciphering these neural networks offers an unique opportunity to determine how the nervous system encodes and generates complex rhythmic movements.

The fact that supraspinal input, which is complex and patterned, can modify not only the timing of the rhythm, but also the activation profiles of specific muscles [Armstrong, 1988; Drew, 1988] suggests that the model is not necessarily appropriate for locomotor control. The input is not merely utilized to release stored patterns, but is also used to alter the motor patterns. This has led to researchers re-examining the validity of the earlier concept of a CPG [Pearson, 1995; Pearson and Gordon, 1999]. Therefore, the locomotor control model should emphasize information transformation, requiring not only the study of neuronal organization at the spinal level, but also characterization of the inputs, and subsequent transformations to predict the observed output patterns. Perhaps analytical models of complex input transformation play an important guiding role in empirical research.

2.3.4 Central Pattern Generator: A Mechanism for the Control of Walking

A central pattern generator (CPG) is a neuronal network capable of generating a rhythmic pattern of motor activity in the absence of phasic sensory input from peripheral receptors. CPGs have been identified and analyzed in more than 50 rhythmic motor systems, including those controlling such diverse behaviors as walking, swimming, feeding, respiration and flying. Although the centrally generated pattern is sometimes very similar to the normal pattern, there are often some significant differences. Sensory information from peripheral receptors and signals from other regions of the central nervous system usually modify the basic pattern produced by a CPG.

The generation of rhythmic motor activity by CPGs depends on three factors: the cellular properties of individual nerve cells within the network, 2) the properties of the synaptic junctions between neurons and 3) the interconnections between neurons.

Most CPGs produce a complex temporal pattern of activation of different groups of motor neurons. Sometimes the pattern can be divided into a number of distinct phases. The sequencing of motor patterns is regulated by a number of mechanisms. The simplest mechanism is mutual inhibition; interneurons fire out of phase with each other, in most cases reciprocal due to their inhibitory connections.

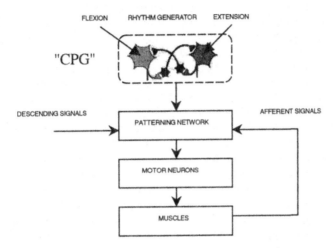

Fig. 2.14: The motor program for walking comprising descending signals, rhythm generator and feedback.

Normal walking is automatic, however it is not stereotyped. Able-bodied humans adjust their stepping patters to variations in the terrain, possible loading, and certainly to unexpected events. Three important types of sensory information are used to regulate stepping somatosensory input from receptors of muscles and skin; input from the vestibular apparatus for adjusting posture and balance, and visual input. This is not to say that other input are not used (e.g., auditory system).

The somatosensory sensors comprise proprioceptors and exteroceptors. One of the proofs that proprioception regulates the stepping pattern comes from experiments with spinalized cats. Spinalized cat adjusts the stepping to the velocity of the treadmill, and even reacts to unexpected events such as obstacles (e.g., "foot in hole" experiments by Prochazka and coworkers [Hiebert et al., 1994]). Some studies show that manipulating hip can generate locomotor like moving pattern [Calancie et al., 1994]. Golgi tendon organs provide a measure of the load carried by the leg. The excitatory action of the Golgi tendon organs on extensor motor neurons during walking is opposite to their inhibitory action when locomotor activity is not being generated. The functional consequence of this reflex reversal is that the swing phase will not be initiated until the leg is unloaded and the forces exerted by extensor are low.

Proprioceptive feedback from muscle spindles and Golgi tendon organs contributes significantly to the generation of burst activity in extensor motor neurons, being necessary for CPG to operate. A monosynaptic pathway from Ia fibers, a disynaptic pathway from Ia and Ib fibers and a polysynaptic pathway from Ia and Ib fibers certainly contribute in transmission from extensor sensory fibers to extensor motor neurons. Exteroceptors in the skin have a powerful influence on the central pattern generator for walking. They detect obstacles in order to adjust the stepping to avoid them. This behavior can be classified as reflexive, however, it also can be attributed to modulation of CPG regulated activity.

As said, CPG gives the basic rhythm for stepping, and it is located within the spinal cord. The leg movements within a step can also be considered as a goal-directed movements, however, is became highly automated due to the number of previous repetitions. Motor cortex, cerebellum and various sites within the brain stem play essential role in mediating the neuronal network in spinal cord. This has been documented from recordings of the neuronal activity in different regions within the higher CNS structures. Rhythmic activity was found that is in phase with the rhythm of stepping; thus it is involved in the locomotion. Supraspinal control can be divided in several functional systems: system for control of the rhythm of CPG, systems for responding to sensory input (feedback) and systems responding to the visual input (planning and feedback). Decisions to initiate walking and control its speed are generated within the brain stem, following commands from motor cortex and feedback [Shik et al., 1966]. The information is transmitted to CPG via reticulospinal pathway. Fine regulation and precise stepping are controlled form the motor cortex. The cerebellum fine-tunes the walking pattern by regulating the timing and intensity of descending signals. The cerebellum receives information about both the actual stepping movement and the state of spinal rhythm generated network via ventral and dorsal spinocerebellar tracts. The cerebellum might be the center where the planned and actual movement are compared, and corrective measures decided [Houk, 1979]. The cerebellum influences all the vestibular nuclei, red nucleus and nuclei in the medullary reticular formation.

All information presented heavily rely on animal experiments. Analyzing movement of newborn suggest similar locomotor behaviors to be available: rhythmic stepping when baby is held erect and moved over a horizontal surface, reciprocal movements of legs when manipulating legs. This strongly suggests that some of the basic neuronal circuits for locomotion are inherited. These neuronal networks are located bellow the brain stem since stepping was seen in anencephalic infants [Pearson and Gordon, 1999]. These basic circuits are suppressed, that is brought under supraspinal control during the development of bipedal walking. The suppression may come from the development of reticulospinal pathways and regions activating reticulospinal neurons, but also as a result of maturation of descending systems originating form the motor cortex and brain stem nuclei modulated by the cerebellum. Recent experiments with humans after spinal cord injury receiving tonic stimulation of the spinal cord at T12 level and resulting with locomotor like behavior strongly support that human walking relies on the same principles as walking of quadrupeds: intrinsic oscillatory networks are activated and modulate by other brain structures and by afferent input. Human walking, however, requires descending commands from higher centers to cope with the problem of balance and intrinsic biomechanical instability of the bipedal posture.

The other aspect of the proposed model that has not been adequately addressed is the nature of the output patterns from the spinal circuit. Often it is implied that these can be mapped directly to the muscle activation patterns quantified by the full-wave rectified electromyographic signals. There are two problems with this assumption. First, if we accept this, the number of output patterns would be large and imply that the nervous system controls each muscle independently. This is highly unlikely. Secondly, such an assumption ignores the contribution of the rich spinal neural connections between muscles to the complexity of activation patterns. The spinal cord must be able to utilize the rich neural and anatomical complexity in the effector system to simplify the control signals.

2.3.5 The Role of Peripheral Input in Generation of Normal Walking Patterns

In many studies, the results are confined to the analysis of sub-systems of components and behaviors. Researchers often pay little attention to the properties of the sensors and actuators actually available, assuming that these should and can be converted to simple state variables, such as end-effector position, joint angles, velocity, and force by computational processes known as coordinate transformations [Soechting and Flanders, 1992]. We suggest that one have to consider both the control plant and the controller in order to define relationships that might be expected among the brain, spinal cord, and sensory-motor apparatus. All levels in a human work synergistically in the performance of most behaviors. Three levels of the sensory-motor hierarchy must be considered. At the bottom is the musculo-skeletal plant itself, whose many sensors and actuators have complex intrinsic properties, which are determined both by their physical form and by their postural deployment and activation by the central nervous system. The medium level comprising the motor program that incorporates the CPG is at the lower part of the central nervous system. This is a primitive, but powerful machine for rapid, tactical responses to a wide range of input. These first two are the "lower levels". At the top is the upper part of the central nervous system.

2.3.6 Effects of Sensory Feedback

One way to assess the role of sensory input is selectively to abolish it, for example by transecting the sensory nerves entering the CNS and then to look for deficits in the motor performance. This has been carried out in numerous different ways in animals ranging from insects, lobsters, and crabs to amphibia, reptiles, birds, fish, and mammals, including humans [e.g., Grillner, 1975; Sanes et al., 1990; Sainburg et al., 1993]. In nearly all cases, purposeful or rhythmic motor action persisted after deafferentation, but accuracy and adaptability were diminished.

Though deafferentation experiments seem simple enough in principle, the results have been varied and confusing, engendering much controversy and debate. The full capability of a deafferented limb is only expressed if the contralateral limb is also deafferented or bound [Taub et al., 1975a and b]. Even the remnants of sensory input may suffice for reasonable control, especially of simple movements [Sainburg et al., 1993]. New motor strategies to circumvent deficits are always developed, making the impairments less obvious [Cole and Sedgwick, 1992]. Deficits are prominent when tasks are complex [Gordon et al., 1994a and b], yet they may be missed if testing in relatively simple tasks [Bizzi et al., 1978].

The following conclusions regarding deafferentation with respect to walking are now fairly secure: 1) the ability to move is preserved after deafferentation, and voluntary force production may be fairly normal. The movements are, however, generally uncoordinated and inaccurate, especially when visual guidance is absent [e.g., Nathan et al., 1986; Ghez et al., 1990]; 2) walking is feasible after deafferentation, but it is irregular. In humans who have lost limb proprioception, gait is severely impaired [Cole and Sedgwick, 1992]; and 3) the control of tasks involving simultaneous changes in several variables, coordination of several limb segments, or adaptation to changes in the external environment is impaired [Gordon et al., 1994a and b].

The question is how well the motor program works if proprioception is diminished, modified, or absent. Grillner and colleagues acknowledged that after deafferentation the locomotor rhythm was more fragile and labile [Grillner and Zangger, 1975, 1984].

In certain specific cases, movements in an intact animal can be attributed fairly clearly to central programming [Zill, 1985a and b; Delcomyn, 1991a and b]. In rapid ballistic movements in humans, sensory feedback is too delayed to play a significant role [Desmedt and Godaux, 1979a and b]. Human subjects plan in advance the force of certain movements, based on visual judgement and prior memory [Gordon et al., 1994 b]. Although the neural activity involved in this planning has been recorded in several different ways [Ashe et al., 1993], even the simple co-contraction strategy, which humans use to stiffen limbs when learning novel tasks [Bernstein, 1967], is not fully explained.

Grillner [1975] suggested that in locomotion, reflexes are "prepared to operate, but are without any effect so long as the movement proceeds according to the set central program". It is clear that afferent input can play a decisive and overriding role in modulating centrally generated activity. The hind limbs of spinal cats walking on a split-belt treadmill separately adapt their speed to that of their corresponding belt because of the sensory activity elicited by foot contact with the belt [Forssberg and Svartengren, 1983]. Obstruction of hip movements [Andersson and Grillner, 1981] or loading of extensor muscles [Duysens and Pearson 1980; Pearson and Duysens, 1976] can completely suppress rhythmicity in a leg, while the other legs continue to be rhythmically active. In the absence of sensory feedback, obstacles or inclines are not compensated for, and if the animal is not otherwise supported, it falls [Giuliani and Smith, 1987]. The relative role of different sensory systems, specifically the role of Ia, Ib and II afferents is described in detail in Sinkjær et al. [2000].

2.3.7 Motor Programs for Walking

The evolution from quadrupedal to bipedal walking freed the "forelimbs" for tasks other than locomotion and had a tremendous impact on control. For one, the base of support has been reduced and coupled with this, the placement of a large proportion of body mass constituting the head, arms, and trunk (approximately 66 percent of body mass) high above the ground (center of mass being approximately 65 percent of the body height) over two narrow structures, the limbs, imposes stringent balance constraints. During normal human walk, the center of mass is outside the base of support for approximately 80 percent of the stride representing an unstable condition defined purely from a static perspective. In quadrupeds, a tripodal support is ensured at all times by having three limbs on the ground. The body center of mass probably never falls outside this base of support. If this is the case, then equilibrium control of the moving body during walking is greatly simplified in four legged animals. The balance control in bipedal walking is in contrast very complicated, almost critical. This probably explains why humans require far greater time than any other animal to develop independent walking ability. Greater supraspinal involvement in the control and expression of locomotor behavior in humans would be expected.

The functional modulation of muscle afferent feedback has also been demonstrated in humans [Capaday and Stein, 1986; Sinkjær et al., 1996a and b].

Although not as clear cut, the role of various neural substrates in the control of locomotion can be inferred from studying patients with specific pathologies. The constraints on *in vivo* experiments in humans are balanced by other benefits that are realized when working with subjects where two-way communication is possible, and instructions can be used creatively in experiments to provide insights into the inner workings of the nervous system. Besides developing experimental paradigms suitable for human subjects, researchers studying human movement in general have examined the observable output patterns far more creatively and rigorously to provide different perspectives on the control issue.

One way to understand what is being controlled is to determine the variant and invariant features in the motor output patterns relying in the CPG (Figure 2.13). The premise being that the invariant features in the motor output patterns can be stored and retrieved when needed, while the variant features are the result of modulation of the basic patterns. The name given to the stored invariant features could be "motor program", but the concept of CPG providing the rhythm, and mediation by both peripheral input and central commands remain the same. How the invariant features are determined from the motor pattern, and what constitutes the control patterns have and will be the points of future debate. Analysis of individual patterns, whether they are muscle activity, joint torque, joint powers, or ground reaction forces, does not imply that the nervous system controls them independently.

2.3.8 Motor Program in Humans with Paraplegia

Until recently it was thought that stepping movements could not occur in accidentally spinalized humans as supraspinal circuits are more dominant than spinal circuits in humans [Forssberg *et al.*, 1980a]. However, involuntary stepping movements have been observed in humans after spinal cord injury, indicating that a spinal motor program generator also exists in humans [Forssberg *et al.*, 1980b; Kuhn, 1950]. An improved effect of locomotor rhythm may be achieved by the induction of spinal reflexes and by pharmacological means: stimulation of cutaneous afferents [Calancie *et al.*, 1994] or of load receptors within the leg extensor muscles [Wernig *et al.*, 1995] can evoke functional complex leg muscle EMG patterns in able-bodied subjects. Spinally generated EMG patterns and their close interaction with the locomotor pattern generator can be assumed on the basis of the onset latencies of their appearance and their modulation during the step cycle [Duysens *et al.*, 1977].

In subjects with paraplegia, supraspinal activation of spinal locomotor centers is absent even though the locomotor apparatus is intact. The following two specific elements have been confirmed: 1) coordinated stepping movements can be elicited by treadmill stimulation and training when the body is partially unloaded. By this approach, subjects with incomplete paraplegia have been shown to gain the stepping ability. Determining the ability to perform stepping movements is instrumental in this method. This ability includes the possible restriction by the level of the lesion, whether or not the lesion is complete or partial, the frequency and duration of the artificial stimulation, the influence of the feedback and the extent to which the body weight is supported; and 2) spinal reflex mechanisms can be released in order to activate and control additional spinal locomotor rhythms. This can be achieved by unilateral electrical stimulation of cutaneous nerves and/or of extensor muscles (which contain load receptors).

These reflex mechanisms are known to generate complex patterns of leg muscle activation (within bilateral, distal, and proximal muscles) at a spinal level. Results from experiments involving humans with complete spinal cord injury (paraplegia) at high thoracic level [Pinter and Dimitrijević, 1999] suggest that the phasic, epidural, single channel electrical stimulation to the posterior structures at L2 level in some subjects leads to generation of alternate, locomotion-like movement of the leg (Figure 2.15). By varying stimulation parameters, it is possible to change the amplitude of joint rotations, as well as the rhythm of movements within limits. Stimulation below or above the L2 level resulted with tonic or rhythmic (symmetric) EMG responses. In the case, that there is any peripheral input coming from lower legs (e.g., force acting at the soles, which would be the case in standing), the locomotor rhythm would be suppressed. There is as yet no definitive answer to why and how the peripheral input suppresses this locomotor behavior. The later finding follows the results of treadmill induced stepping [Wernig *et al.*, 1995; Dietz *et al.*, 1994; Dietz, 1992; Barbeau and Rossignol, 1994] in which a harness was used to partially support the body weight and provide vertical posture of paraplegics.

For the purposes of simplifying the problem we suggest that the CNS can autonomously generate detailed patterns of muscle activity that can form the substrate of complex movements, yet these patterns must be under direct feedback control to provide functional walking.

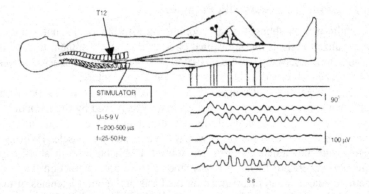

Fig. 2.15: Schematics of the experiment by Pinter and Dimitrijević showing the existence of CPG in humans with paraplegia. The traces show about 30 seconds of locomotor-like movement (angles in the hip and knee joints, and EMG activities from hip and knee flexor and extensor muscles). Adapted from Pinter and Dimitrijević, 1999, with permission.

2.3.9 Biomechanics of Bipedal Walking

In addition to studying the neurophysiology of walking it is of interest to understand the mechanics behind it. The first most important element is to grasp how complex analysis is required to use the tools of mechanics comprehensively. In Chapter 1 the skeleto-muscular structure of the systems available for walking are described.

The important element for understanding bipedal walking it to grasp that the organism should constantly benefit from gravity. Using this methodology, human walking can be described in the following way: The body rotates about the supporting foot, as an inverted, multilink pendulum. This rotation moves the center of mass in the direction of movement (e.g., forward, sideways, and backwards). The other, not loaded leg swings (like pendulum) and contacts the ground in front of the moving body, preventing the fall. During the swing phase of the leg the body rotates (if imagined as a single body) about a point above the head [Jonić et al., 2000]. When the swinging leg contacts the ground, the "inverted pendulum" motion will be repeated [Basmajian, 1976; McGeer, 1993; McMahon, 1984; Mochon and McMahon, 1980]. This hypothesis of ballistic walking has been partly confirmed by using the EMG recordings from the leg muscles. The muscles show very little activity in the swing leg during walking at normal speed, except at the beginning and the end of the swing phase. The muscles are active during the double support period, when the initial conditions on the angles and velocities of each of the limb segments are being established. Thereafter, all the muscles turn off and allow the leg to swing through like a jointed pendulum.

Coordinated movements of all body segments are required to achieve the walking. Simultaneous control of "external" and "internal" forces is essential. External forces like gravity and friction force are existing, but the interplay of internal forces change their effects (e.g., friction force changes its direction based as the consequence of muscle contractions (e.g., bending back or for in hips while standing, changing direction of walking). One should not forget that *sine qua non* condition for walking is the ability to maintain vertical posture on one or two legs under different environmental conditions that include perturbations.

2.4 Control of Goal-directed Movement

Goal-directed movement is a complex sequence of kinematic events, which can be divided into different phases. Reaching, grasping, pointing, fitting, throwing, drawing, handwriting, keyboarding, tracking, object manipulating and catching are different modalities of goal-directed movements. Although the listed movements are different they all share very similar characteristics: high level of coordination at joints of the arm and hand, and use of the same command system.

One of the earliest systematic studies of arm and hand movements [Woodwort, 1899] described goal-directed movements as being two-phased. After the goal is identified, and the decision to move is generated at the cortical level, an initial, ungoverned movement occurs, followed by a final, controlled adjustment. The limb is transported quickly towards the target location in the initial phase, and the current control phase subsequently corrects any error made along the way, using sensory feedback to reach the target accurately. Jeannerod [1981, 1988] suggested two phases in prehensile movements: an initial, faster arm movement during which the hand and fingers preshape, and slower arm movement beginning after maximum aperture, during which the fingers enclose to make contact with object. He argued that the arm (reaching) is controlled separately from the hand (prehension and grasp). MacKenzie and Iberall [1994] described three components of prehension: planning phase, movement before contact and movement after contact. The planning process involves three aspects: perceiving task-specific object properties, selecting a grasp strategy and planning a hand location and orientation.

2.4.1 The Development of Reaching and Grasping

In order to grasp the complexity of the control of reaching and grasping one can analyze the development of goal-directed movements in newborn and young children. The newborn can automatically take hold of an object placed in its palm (reaction known as the grasp reflex). This grasp is powerful enough to support an infant's weight. This behavior usually disappears at about 6 months of age. As the "grasping reflex" is disappearing, a defined task dependent grasp is being developed. The development of the grasping can be observed in babies after they are 3 months old. The grasp is developing in average for about four years, and the full dexterity is reached only at about 10 years of age. The development of control of grasping is related strictly to self-organization, that is heuristics and learning from examples. The learning is taking place constantly in all daily activities (e.g., playing with toys).

Reaching to an object of interest develops gradually over a period of several months after birth. At an early phase infants preprogram their reaches in the correct general direction. Young infants can reach with rough accuracy for objects placed in different radial position, but their estimate of distance is typically wrong. The direction gets better when they are about 5 months of age. By the end of this period, infants are so skilled at preprogramming the direction of their reaching movements that they can direct their hands to the future positions of moving objects, effectively catching the objects while moving [von Hofsten, 1980]. Other studies are somewhat controversial; suggesting that directional learning takes longer time.

Judgement of the distance to an object is developed at a slower pace. Some studies suggest that infants first develop the perception on what us within and out of reach [Bower, 1972; von Hofsten, 1979]. It is a general belief that infants start to "understand" the distance at the age of 5 months [White *et al.*, 1964]. Reaching skills require training of 12 to 16 months on average.

Control requires both the sensory and motor systems, as described in previous sections; hence, these systems have to be developed and perfected before an organized activity such as grasping takes place. A rudimentary form of eye-hand coordination is present in the neonate and it is on this background that visual reaching is established. However, it has to be developed in the context of a task, and integrated in the overall anticipation of movement. The sensory and motor systems must reach the level of maturity and integrate before they can contribute to complex movements.

In summary, a human needs to develop visual cues, *i.e.*, the understanding of distance and object shape with respect to his grasping apparatus to allow the nervous system to learn movement. Learning relies on heuristics, and it becomes a skill after trial and error episodes. It takes many months of practicing and learning by examples to build a database within the motor cortex, which then is capable of producing voluntary movements of all kinds. The central nervous system allows relearning and learning of new skills throughout the life.

2.4.2 Mechanisms for Control of Reaching and Grasping

Goal-directed movement is a planned change of arm and hand segments positions, ultimately leading to a task. Goal-directed movement depends on a balance of initial programming and subsequent correction. Initial programming is based partly on visual perception of an objects, and partly on proprioception (e.g., a visual cue is used to decide whether to pick up the object with one or two hands, and what type of grasp to use). The accuracy of visual perception determines the initial programming. This can be documented easily seen in sports when a human has to respond functionally to objects coming towards him quickly (e.g., receiving a service in tennis). If the perception is accurate and timely, will the correct response follow. The differences in manipulating object depend on the task to be accomplished (e.g., tossing or gently placing an object in a container [Marteniuk et al., 1987], feeling the texture of an object or evaluating its temperature [Klatzky and Lederman, 1987]).

Despite many controversies, motor control theories have agreed about the generation of goal-directed movement. Generating movement requires the nervous system to solve the following three problems: multi-modal sensory integration or sensory intake; complex transformations between different spatial and intrinsic coordinate systems, and motor commands adequate to attain the aim (resolving problems associated with movement dynamics).

The question of essential importance for a study of motor systems, that is both theoretical and neurophysiological, and is as yet unresolved, is which variables are controlled by the brain. Joint torque, angular position, angular velocity, joint stiffness, and muscle stiffness have all been suggested as possible variables controlled directly by the brain [Feldman, 1986; Bizzi et al., 1984]. Answers to this question and better understanding of the control schemes employed by the nervous system in the execution of desired motor plans are of fundamental significance when dealing with motor adaptation.

Over the past decade there have been a number of experiments, which suggest that in planning movement the nervous system has considerable information about the physical world with which it interacts, and about the kinematics and dynamics of the motor systems in control. What remains unclear is the influence of these factors on neural control. For example, how precisely the nervous system accounts for workspace-dependent changes in order to produce movement? Does the nervous system maintain an exact representation of geometry, which it adjusts with changes in workspace position, or can the nervous system use a simplified approximation of musculo-skeletal geometry when planning movement? One way to explore the neural representation of factors such as geometry and mechanics is to use detailed models of motor systems to assess the consequences of possible simplifications in neural encoding. Assumptions about the details of neural encoding can be implemented in models and tested (e.g., movement amplitudes, movement errors).

This section brings only general ideas on the organization of control of goal-directed movement, although the neural mechanisms are still, to a large extent unknown, an adequate language of motor control science has not yet been accepted as standard [Gelfand and Latash, 1998] and construction of a global model for movement control is still underway [Desmurget et al., 1998].

2.4.3 Motor Planning

There is no doubt that the anticipation of the next movement is instrumental for the successful performance. If one is catching a falling object, and he/she knows that the object is heavy, the posture before catching will be adjusted to compensate for the expected load [Bennett et al., 1994]. There is general agreement that the initial events of motor planning occur in the premotor cortical areas, retrieving a kind of a motor program [Jeannerod et al., 1995], or memory trace of specific examples [Wilberg and Guay, 1985]. It is also established that this initiation of computational process ultimately produces the descending corticospinal commands. Traditional view separates a planning phase from subsequent execution phase [Kandel et al., 1999]. In contrast, Morasso and Sanguinetti [1997] speculate that motor planning in the motor and premotor areas, could not proceed without the detailed geometric information provided by the body-schema in the posterior parietal areas; such areas must be updated with the ongoing plan in order to maintain a coherent sensory-motor representation and this implies a closed loop or bi-directional interaction between precentral and post-central areas.

The neuronal events subserving the aimed movement at the level of the spinal cord are largely unknown as yet, although it is expected that the appropriate motoneuronal pools are excited and/or inhibited when the reaching movement is implemented. These pools could be addressed directly at their segments by supraspinal signals, but the possibility exists that this action is indirect, via propriospinal neuronal networks. A population of propriospinal neurons at the C3-C4 level has been identified that receives monosynaptic, convergent input from almost all the major descending motor tracts and, in turn, excites monosynaptically or inhibits disinaptically motoneurons innervating forelimb muscles [Illert et al., 1978]. Surgical interruption of the projection from these propriospinal neurons to the segmental forelimb pools resulted in a severe impairment of reaching but not of grasping [Alstermark et al., 1981]. They also suggested that the precise aiming in the normal target-reaching movement depends exclusively or very largely on the C3-C4 propriospinal neurons and that the segmental neuronal circuitry alone cannot substitute for them appropriately. The findings about this propriospinal system indicate that it may subserve the synergistic activation of the motoneuronal pools involved in reaching. Moreover, the rich convergence of these neurons suggests that several supraspinal systems possess a direct access to the reaching synergy for its on-line modification, if needed, according to changes in the environment or in the behavioral goal.

Features of virtually all movements are represented in the primary motor cortex. The movement feature most extensively studied is direction. Murphy and his colleagues [1982] recorded the activity of cells in the motor cortex during forward reaching by monkeys. They concluded that the production of any movement engages a complex population of precentral neurons, such that any one neuron may behave similarly for different movements. It further implied that the unique trajectory of the movement is represented at the level of the neuronal population and not of the single neuron. This problem was investigated by Georgopoulos et al. [1982, 1983a], who studied neuronal discharge in relation to the direction of 2-D aimed movement in the motor and posterior parietal (area 5) cortex [Kalaska et al., 1983] of behaving monkeys. The discharge of single cells was broadly tuned to the direction of the 2-D movement, frequently in a sinusoidal fashion. In 3-D space studies, it was observed that the discharge of motor cortical cells is indeed tuned to the 3-D movement direction [Georgopoulos et al., 1988]. Although motor cortical cells possess a *preferred direction*, their broad tuning suggests that the coding of movement direction may be, instead, a function of a neuronal population. Indeed, this was found to be the case, given certain assumptions ("*vector hypothesis*"), Georgopoulos et al. [1983c, 1984]. Briefly, the relations between the direction of movement and the population discharge were formulated within a spatial vector context, in which a population "vector" is derived on the basis of the preferred direction and the change in activity of individual constituent cells. Experimental results showed a good correspondence between the direction of the population vector and the direction of the upcoming movement [Georgopoulos et al., 1993].

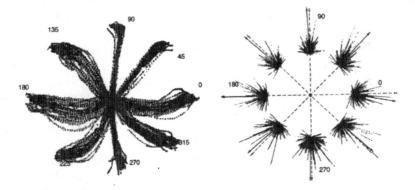

Fig. 2.16: Trajectories of 30 movement (the numbers show degrees) to eight targets positioned at 0, 45, 90, 135, 180, 225, 270, and 315 degrees made by monkey (left), and the corresponding population vectors recorded in the motor cortex (full line) slightly biased from actual directions (dashed lines). Modified from Georgopoulos et al, 1982, with permission.

Georgopoulos found that cells in primary motor cortex (M1) responded to movement in a characteristic way. More than 80 percent of the cells were tuned so that the strength of their activation in different directions could be fitted well by a cosine function of the form, $r = b + k\cos(\theta - \theta_0)$ where r is the firing rate, b and k are constants, θ is the angular direction of movement, and θ_0 is the direction of movement for which the cell would fire maximally. Thus, each cell becomes characterized, fundamentally, by a single parameter, which is called its preferred direction. Once each cell is described by its preferred direction, Georgopoulos calculated a quantity, which he named the population vector:

$$\vec{P}(\vec{M}) = \sum_{i=1}^{N} w_i(\vec{M})\vec{C}_i$$

The preferred direction of each cell (the $\vec{C}$ in the equation above) is taken as a unit vector, and multiplied by the activity $w_i(M)$ of the cell during movement in some direction. The cells within the primary motor cortex fire with lower frequency when the movement is in the opposite direction and high frequency when it is in the preferred direction; hence, the vector sum points *always* in the direction of the movement as illustrated in Figure 2.16.

The nature of the representation of reaching movement in M1 (zone in the primary motor cortex) is under continues study. The covariation of motor cortex activity with the hand path is well documented [Sanger, 1996; Georgopoulos et al., 1982, 1988; Schwartz et al., 1988; Kalaska et al., 1989] and studies are extended to movement sequences [Kettner et al., 1996a and b]. It is also well established that motor cortex cell activity varies as a function of output forces [Taira et al., 1996]. These studies support a primary role for motor cortex in processing directional information about movement [Georgopoulos, 1992, 1995]. There is evidence specific to muscle centered information in M1. Scott [1997] reported preliminary evidence of parallel trends in the variation of onset times and magnitude of activity as a function of arm movement direction between groups of shoulder and elbow muscles, and functionally corresponding groups of M1 cells. Bennett and Lemon [1996] identified corticomotoneuronal cells that made direct monosynaptic connections to spinal motoneurons innervating more than one muscle. Both studies indicate that MI can provide specific information about the coordinated patterns of muscle activity required for multi-articular movements.

The mathematical analysis by Mussa-Ivaldi [1988] showed that cells relating to movement direction in muscle length space (*i.e.*, cells coding muscle shortening velocities) will necessarily have cosine-shaped tuning curves when analyzed with respect to the spatial direction of movement. This property is evident in neural network models by Burnod *et al.* [1992] and Bullock *et al.* [1993]. Cosine-shaped tuning curves are not built into the model cells but instead arise as a result of learning the mapping between spatial directions and joint rotations.

Schieber and Hibbard [1993] have shown that single motor cortical neurons do not discharge specifically for a particular flexion-extension finger movements but instead are active with movements of different fingers, which suggested that control of any finger movement utilizes a distributed population of neurons. Using these data, Georgopoulos and colleagues [1999] applied the neuronal population vector analysis [Georgopoulos *et al.*, 1982] to determine whether single cells are tuned in an abstract, three-dimensional (3D) instructed finger and wrist movement space with hand-like geometry and whether the neuronal population encodes specific finger movements. Authors found that the activity of 75 percent of motor cortical neurons related to finger movements was tuned in this space. Moreover, the population vector computed in this space predicted well the instructed finger movement. Thus, although single neurons may be related to several disparate finger movements, and neurons related to different finger movements are intermingled throughout the hand area of the motor cortex; the neuronal population activity does specify particular finger movements.

Using probability theory, Sanger [1996] proposed an alternative to the population vector method for estimating the population signals. Cell activity is expressed as a probability density function that is proportional to the cell's tuning curve for movement in different spatial directions. The population signal is then defined as the product of the tuning curves for all cells active for a given movement.

The discussion above referred to the neural coding of spatial attributes of the aimed movement. Unfortunately, there is no knowledge of abstract characteristics of the aimed movement, e.g., its accuracy or its visual guidance. It is remarkable, however, that studies in brain areas related to motor control of the arm have not revealed invariance relating to the endpoint of the aimed movement; instead, a clear relationship to movement direction has been observed [Georgopoulos *et al.*, 1982, 1983b; Kalaska *et al.*, 1983]. Indeed, when monkeys made movements from several points on a circle to the same final endpoint, neuronal discharge in the motor and parietal cortex was related to the movement direction but not to the final position of the hand [Georgopoulos *et al.*, 1985]. These results indicate that, if the endpoint control hypothesis [Polit and Bizzi, 1979] is correct, the motor and parietal areas are involved after the process that specifies the endpoint.

Other areas of CNS were studied in regard to different aspects of aimed movement. Several researchers studied complex spikes discharged from Purkinje cells of the cerebellum and proposed their contribution to the initiation of arm movement [Bauswein *et al.*, 1983; Mano *et al.*, 1986, 1989; Simpson *et al.*, 1996], or to the gradual improvement of motor skills [Simpson *et al.*, 1996]. Kitazawa and colleagues

[1998] used information theory to show that the complex spikes convey multiple types of information; spikes occurring at the beginning of the reach movement encode the absolute destination of the reach, and the complex spikes occurring at the end of the short-lasting movement encode relative errors. This is consistent with the idea that Purkinje cells contribute both to the generation of movement and to its gradual, long-term improvement.

An essential property of movement coordination is the ability to compensate for the interaction torque arising during a reaching movement, and recent data have shown that the cerebellum is involved in this compensation [Bastian *et al.*, 1996]. Detailed analysis performed by Schweighofer and his colleagues [1998] suggests that the cerebellum form part of the inverse model of the arm: motor cortex is an approximate inverse model and the cerebellum is the locus of the part of the inverse dynamics specifically involved in compensating for the interaction torque. The authors developed a novel computational model of the cerebellum and tested the validity of this hypothesis.

Recent studies provided further support for the hypothesis that spatial representation of arm position, target locations, and potential motor actions are expressed in the neuronal activity in parietal cortex [Kalaska *et al.*, 1997]. In contrast, precentral cortical activity expresses processes involved in the selection and execution of motor actions more strongly.

2.4.4 Visual Guidance in Goal-directed Movement

The visual information is used to identify a target and its location in space, and also for corrections of ongoing movement. Preparation for a movement toward a visual target happens in posterior parietal cortex. Goal-directed movement for a seen object usually benefits from visual feedback. This observation raises the question of how visual guidance is used in the control of reaches and grasps. There are at least three aspects of this problem: 1) visual localization of the target in extra-personal space and suitable coding of that information for use by the arm motor system; 2) visual monitoring of the hand before and during its movement through space; and 3) visual adjustment of the final position of the hand to touch, grasp, or retrieve successfully the object of interest [Georgopoulos, 1986].

Goodale [1996] advocates the hypothesis that the visual system is modular, with a fundamental division between systems dedicated to perception and to more cognitive functions and those concerned with visuomotor behavior. In this scheme, key functions of the parietal cortex are to extract information about the structure of the external world, such as the spatial location, distance, physical dimensions, and spatial orientation of objects, and to perform some of the associated visuomotor transformations that are required to organize successful visually guided movement.

It has been shown unequivocally that reaching is more accurate in the presence than in the absence of vision of the arm just before [Prablanc *et al.*, 1979b] and during the movement [Conti and Beaubaton, 1976; Prablanc *et al.*, 1979 a and b]. Since this improvement was observed even for movement that were completed within 200 ms, it was proposed [Paillard, 1982] that visual cues from arm motion are being processed at higher speeds than the timing assumed necessary (190-260 ms) to utilize external visual feedback [Keele and Posner, 1968].

Two visual systems have been identified that process information related to arm/hand movements during reaching [Paillard, 1982; Jeannerod and Biguer, 1982]. Their contribution to the visual guidance of movement and the cues they use have been studied in experiments that allowed separate control of target and hand vision through a colored filter in normal and split-brain monkeys [Beaubaton et al., 1978]. In other experiments, continuous or stroboscopic illumination was used to dissociate position cues from motion cues during the course of prismatic adaptation in human subjects [Paillard et al., 1981]. It was found that one system utilizes central vision and it is facilitated by the presence of a foveated target, and analyzes positional (displacement) cues, for it is unaffected under conditions of stroboscopic. Presumably, this system subserves the accurate placement of the hand on the target near the end of the reaching movements. The other system employs peripheral vision and analyzes motion cues, as evidenced by its impairment under conditions of stroboscopic illumination. More importantly, the motion cues that seem to be meaningful to this system are those arising from the motion of the arm when actively moved by the subject but not when passively moved by the experimenter. These findings are consistent with earlier results that suggested that the development of visually guided reaching depends on "self-produced movements with its concurrent visual feedback" [Held and Hein, 1963].

2.4.5 Precision of Positioning of the Hand

The nervous system can learn to achieve desired levels of accuracy by adjusting control signals to accommodate factors such as changing musculo-skeletal geometry, and dynamics. For example, when an object is grasped and lifted with fingers, the grip force varies directly in an anticipation of the load force as determined by mass and acceleration of the object [Flanagan and Wing, 1993, 1997a and b]. This suggests that the nervous system may utilize knowledge about dynamics when planning movement. Additionally, Ghilardi with coworkers [1995] show that subjects can be trained to make accurate reaching movements in areas in which before training, they produce errors. Interestingly however, they note that after training, movement initiated from locations that were previously error free showed new biases. However, the possible sources of these biases are unknown and could include different factors.

It is difficult to distinguish between different sources of position errors. Wolpert et al. [1994] has demonstrated that distortion in visual perception of extra-personal space can contribute to inaccuracies in the production of multi-joint arm movements. Gordon et al. [1994a and b] have shown that direction-dependent errors in reaching tasks are related to direction-dependent differences in total limb inertia, and they suggest that subjects may not fully compensate for workspace-dependent differences in limb dynamics. Soechting and Flanders [1989] suggested that movement errors may result from approximations in sensory-motor transformations. Specifically, the nervous system may use an approximation to the transformation between extrinsic coordinates (the location of the hand in 3D space) and intrinsic coordinates (joint configurations of the arm). Moreover, the relative distribution of muscle spindles in one and two joint muscles may affect the positioning accuracy of the limb [Scott and Loeb, 1994].

Fitts' law. Fitts [1954] analyzed the relationship between the precision of aiming and time to perform the task. He studied the effect of the distance to the centers of targets and their width (size). The experimental results have been fitted with the following equation:

$$T = a + b\log_2(\frac{2A}{W})$$

where T denotes movement time, A the distance to the centers of targets, and W the size of the targets. The second term is called the index of difficulty. This law was confirmed later in several experiments (e.g., moving a joystick [Jagacinski *et al.*, 1980], transferring pegs over a distance to be inserted into a hole [Annet *et al.*, 1958]). This behavior can be explained by thinking of a movement as a sequence of component movements, being iteratively corrected [Jagacinski *et al.*, 1980]. The alternative explanation assumes that Fitts' law reflects the initial ballistic phase being followed by the feedback phase (corrective movement). Tomović *et al.* [1995] suggested that an aiming movement is composed of a sequence of straight-line movement, the following being corrected by the visual feedback. This assumption follows the idea of mapping of the visual and motor cortex, and matching of the fields during the execution of movements.

2.4.6 The Planning Space and Frames of Reference

The central neuronal processes that control eye and arm movement aimed at visual targets are often described as a sequence of sensory-motor co-ordinate transformations between a signal of spatial location and pattern of muscle activity [Kalaska and Crammond, 1992; Soechting and Flanders, 1995]. The most commonly encountered view in the motor control literature postulates that the nervous system controls the spatial characteristics of the movement directly, rather than the joint angle characteristics. Morasso [1981] documented that for pointing movements humans tend to move the hand following a straight line that connects the initial and target position with bell-shaped spatial velocity profiles, Figure. 2.17 left panels. Morasso's key study of kinematic properties of planar arm movements provided some of the strongest experimental support for spatial planning. These characteristics of the hand trajectory appeared to be invariant across different regions of the workspace. In contrast, the temporal patterns of joint angles did not follow straight lines in joint space, often exhibited single-peak velocity profiles, and double-peaked accelerations, Figure 2.17 right panels.

Although the results of Morasso [1981] are usually taken as strong evidence for spatial planning, several investigators have pointed out that end-point trajectories are not completely straight but instead gently curved in many parts of workspace, particularly in the sagittal plane [Hollerbach *et al.*, 1986]. This might be evidence for joint space trajectory planning, but the curvature seen in this movement is insufficient to support simple joint space interpolation, which would lead to much larger curvature. To account for this, Hollerbach *et al.*, [1986] proposed a modification to joint space interpolation, which they termed "staggered joint interpolation", in which different joints begin moving at different times in order to produce straighter trajectories. However, this model cannot account for the reversals seen in the study of Morasso [1981]. Hollerbach and Atkeson [1987] proposed a way to directly control joint, which also yields straight-line hand paths. The method is to vary the onset times for the motions of the joints. This method coming from mechanics of systems of rigid bodies is certainly applicable for control of manipulation robots. Another experiment that tried to prove that movement is joint space planned [Soechting and Lacquaniti, 1981] was a simple act of pointing to a target. The analysis of movement in vertical plane shows that peak angular velocities are synchronous, and that the joints equaled the ratio of the radial distances that they cover. Such regularities have been attributed to planning in the joint space.

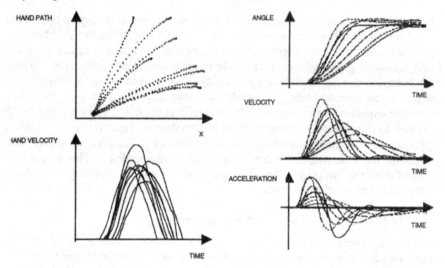

Fig. 2.17: What is controlled by nervous system – spatial (left) or joint angle (right) characteristics? Hand trajectory (left, top) and bell-shaped velocity profile (left bottom) for eight movements in different directions and with different amplitudes. Joint angles, (right, top), joint angular velocity (right, middle), and accelerations (right, bottom) for eight joint rotations performed with different speeds.

According to a model based on minimization of the torque change along the trajectory proposed by Uno et al. [1989], curvatures are an inherent side effect of a control strategy, which controls joints instead of hand trajectories. Although this model provides one possible explanation for much of the curvature seen in reaches, a study by Wolpert et al,. [1995] showed that increasing the perceived curvature of movement through altered visual feedback caused subjects to change their movement to produce visually straighter hand paths, at odds with non-spatial planning models such as torque change model. In order to explain the curvature of human reaches under the assumption of spatial trajectory planning Wolpert et al. [1994] demonstrated that some of the curvature of hand trajectories could be attributed to perceptual distortion; i.e., in some parts of the workspace, a curved reach appears straighter than it usually is. However, perceptual distortion alone did not appear to be sufficient to account fully for the curvature of reaches in this study.

Flash [1987] suggested that curvature arises as the result of interactions between the viscoelastic properties of muscles and the inertial properties of the arm following a straight-line "equilibrium trajectory".

In the experiments where humans have been instructed to draw curved lines [Abend et al., 1982] results suggest that the curved path is composed of a series of straight - line segments. Popović M and Popović [1994] showed high correlation between the joint co-ordinates for a given orientation of movement, suggesting that movement is planned in external coordinates, and that the synergy between joint co-ordinates is the key issue for control of goal-directed movement. This result follows studies of Bernstein [1967] who concluded that the natural control of movement is achieved by planning of the movement of the most distal segment in the external reference frame, and controlling the most proximal segment. The intersegmental control follows "memorized and learned" synergies. This explanation finds support in many experiments, but the best prove is the development of reaching and grasping in infants previously described.

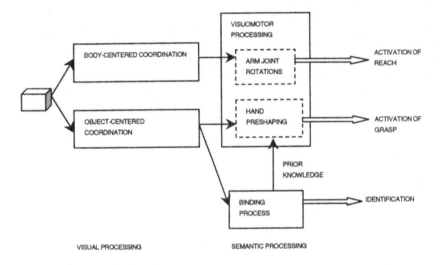

Fig. 2.18: Extrinsic and intrinsic object properties are processed in body-centred and object-centred co-ordinates, respectively. Activation of reach and grasp are thought to rely on separate, parallel processes, both pertaining to the dorsal visual pathway and to the posterior parietal areas. Semantic processing, in spite of using the same object primitives as visuomotor processing, is thought to occur in the ventral visual pathway and can improve visuomotor performance using connections between the two pathways [Jeannerod, 1993].

Description of events depends on the frame of reference that has been adopted. During the action of grasping, several systems of coordinates for describing the same object coexist [Jeannerod, 1993] as shown in Figure 2.18. In this example, a viewer-centered system is used for generating movements at the proximal joints and performing the reach. An object-centered system is used for generating movement with the distal motor apparatus and performing the grasp. The fact that the representations for "what and how" both operate in object-centered coordinates, in spite of their very different behavioral implications, suggests that the coordinate system is defined early in the processing of the object attributes, that is, before the object information is distributed to the semantic and pragmatic representations, respectively.

2.4.7 Redundancy and Synergies

The method used by nature to resolve problem of *redundancy* and increase the efficiency of movement comes from the dependencies between components of the motor system. These dependencies could be understood as *constraints* and they ultimately decrease the number of variables to be controlled. This type of constraints has been used frequently in machines.

The mechanical linkage having N joints is considered as a system with N degrees of freedom (DoFs). This is to say that the position of the final member of the linkage should be adjusted by a larger number of variables, all N degrees of freedom. The position of a rigid body is determined with six independent variables; minimal number of hinge joints to be controlled is N = 6. If N > 6, the system is called redundant, and then constraints must be introduced between the joint trajectories in order to make the system deterministic. Each constraint reduces the number of DoFs at least by one. Natural control uses task dependent constraints in order to reduce the number of variables that have to be controlled voluntarily to the lowest possible by forcing other variables to follow the memorized schemes. This method was named *synergistic control*, first analyzed and described by Bernstein [1967]. According to the particular motor task, the neuromuscular system develops and modifies synergies.

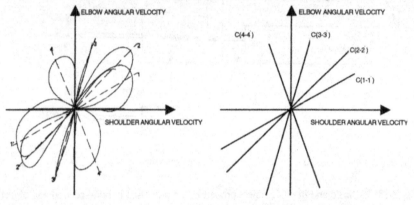

Fig. 2.19: Complex relationship between shoulder and elbow joint angular velocities for four different reaching movements with return (left) is simplified with scaling coefficient-C (right) according to linear synergy. Note that 1-1', 2-2', 3-3', 4-4' are for four different movements directions. Adapted from Popović M, 1995.

Bernstein suggested that the problem of motor redundancy is solved using flexible relations (synergies) among control variables directed at *individual elements*. These were further developed in *structural units* [Gelfand et al., 1971]. For any task, elements of the system for movement production are assembled into task-specific structural units (synergies). Structural units and their corresponding synergies can be formed at different levels of the central nervous system. For example, reflexes among muscles crossing different joints of a limb can be viewed as elements of synergies decreasing the system redundancy. Synergy can be found between individual muscles. An example of *anatomic synergists* is that of the Biceps Brachii and Brachioradialis m. acting together to flex the elbow. Another example is of using *coordinative synergies* [Popović M and Popović, 1994, 2000; Popović M, 1995; Popović M et al., 1999] to reduce the dimensionality of the control vector from two to one in reaching. Based on experimental study of humans in self-paced planar point-to-point movement, the authors found synergy between shoulder and elbow joint angular velocities expressed by scaling parameter (Figure 2.19). The choice of scaling is predictable based on initial and target hand positions relative to the shoulder. This inherent ratio as a kind of "biological signature" is imposed to the arm motion during reaching. This velocity space synergy does not mean that the problem is reduced to kinematics, and that the dynamics is taken out of considerations; it only provides proof about the high correlation that can be seen effectively in the "velocity" information, which is "measured" by somato-sensory system.

2.4.8 Redundancy and Motor Equivalence

Bernstein [1967] postulated the main problem of control of voluntary movement as the elimination of redundant degrees of freedom (DoFs). Originally, it had been expressed with respect to the discrepancy between the number of apparent kinematic DOFs of the body and the number of dimensions of the external space. However, this problem can emerge at virtually any level of analysis of the system for movement production. In particular, if the task is to generate a certain level of force (torque) at the effector's endpoint, then the large number of muscles that can contribute to force are contracting (Bernstein problem). The redundancy leads to an undetermined mechanical problem: an infinite number of combinations of muscle forces can produce the same total force output. Since Bernstein's original work, the question of how a large number of muscles bring a required common output has received considerable attention [Crowninshield and Brand 1981a and b; Dul *et al.*, 1984; Zatsiorsky *et al.*, 1984; Latash, 1996; Prilutsky *et al.*, 1996].

Attempts to find theoretical solutions for problems of motor redundancy have involved mathematical modeling, in particular optimization [e.g., Nelson, 1983; Seif-Naragfhi and Winters, 1990]. This method is based on many simplifying assumptions and morphometric data that are only roughly estimated. The outcome of the modeling is very difficult to verify. Direct measurement of the tendon forces and a search for regularities in their behavior was proposed [Gregor and Abelew, 1994], but is not yet practical for human subjects.

Motor equivalent behavior can be understood as the ability to use redundant degrees of freedom to compensate for temporary constraints on the effectors while producing movement trajectories to targets. Motor equivalence is seen in a variety of human behaviors, including handwriting and reaching, but also in a variety of species. Motor equivalence is no doubt the evolutionary result of its utility: animals capable of using different motor means to carry out a task under different environmental conditions have a tremendous advantage over those that cannot. There are some advantages of having the ability to perform a task in many ways (e.g., such as avoiding obstacles). The essence of motor equivalence is the ability to transform one type of sensory information into another. This is not present at birth. Transformations must be adapted (calibrated) in different circumstances like growth or handicap. This property has important implication for biological movement control. It suggests how a person can easily overcome constraints on the effectors.

2.4.9 The Equilibrium Point Hypothesis

Feldman [1966] suggested that the control is organized directly in terms of commands to individual muscles making movement arise from shifts in the equilibrium position (EP) of the limb. The hypothesis implies that the brain does not compute all the forces required to move a limb from one place to another, but simply launches the limb, depending on reflexes and the intrinsic elasticity of the muscles to get it to its destination. Theory holds that this is possible because intrinsic springiness makes opposing muscles seek an equilibrium, or balance, whenever the brain perturbs the system by setting the limb in motion.

The EP is a consequence of the interaction of the central neural commands (muscle λs), reflex mechanisms, muscle properties, and external loads. Feldman's λ-model implies that by changing the values of λs over time, the nervous system can shift the system from one posture to another. As the λs change value, forces develop in each muscle in proportion to the difference between the muscle's current length and its threshold length (λ). These forces then drive the system towards a new equilibrium position. In this way, the model proposes that the nervous system may produce

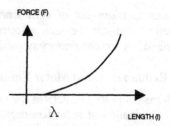

Fig. 2.20: Feldman's λ-model. Force-length characteristic curve represents monoparametric control of a single muscle.

movement by specifying appropriate time-varying sequences of λs. Many experiments have confirmed the principle that the nervous system is adjusting the muscle length and tension of agonistic and antagonistic muscles to be in dynamic equilibrium.

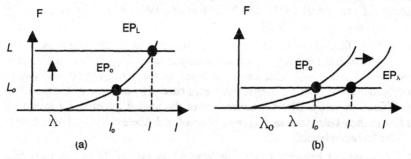

Fig. 2.21: Changes in muscle length from l_o to l can be induced by change in (a) load characteristic from L_o to L; (b) central motor command from λ_o to λ, or both.

λ-model is illustrated on force-length diagram, Figure 2.20. Changes in muscle length and/or force can be induced by a change in central motor command, load characteristics, or both. Figure 2.21 illustrates a change in muscle length, from l_0 to l. According to this theory, equilibrium point EP_0 than shifts to a new position EP_L or EP_λ as a result from change in load (L_0 to L, Figure 2.21a) or a change in central command (λ_0 to λ, Figure 2.21b), or both.

Goal-directed movement generally requires coordinated motion of several joints of the arm and hand. A pair of antagonistic muscles-flexor and extensor controls a joint. Their central control can be described with a pair of λ values on torque-angle diagram, Figure 2.22. A muscle is active when its length exceeds the threshold λ. That is, the flexor is active to the right of λ_f, and the extensor is active to the left of λ_e. The activation of the antagonist leads to development of torque directed against the agonist muscle torque and/or movement in a joint in the opposite direction. That is why the curve for antagonist is mirrored in regard to angular axis so it corresponds to negative values of torque. Behavior of the joint is defined by the algebraic sum of the two λ characteristics and the load characteristic [Feldman, 1979].

Neurophysiological data have provided some evidence to support the equilibrium trajectory control hypothesis; the characteristics of the force fields elicited by micro-stimulating the spinal gray matter in frogs during either posture or coordinated multijoint leg movements were found to be converging fields characterized by single equilibrium point [Bizzi et al., 1992], although many investigators argue against it.

The equilibrium point hypothesis, and λ-model was refined to suggest that, rather than choosing just end-points, a series of moving equilibrium points - a virtual trajectory – is chosen to produce the desired trajectory, leading to the so-called virtual trajectory control hypothesis [Bizzi et al., 1984]. In contrast to this theory, some other models support the idea that the nervous system uses a control space in which control variables are specified for each kinematic degree of freedom separately [Ostry and Munhall, 1994; Sergio and Ostry, 1995].

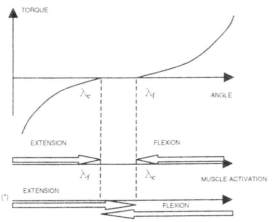

Fig. 2.22: The characteristics of muscle couples when either one is active, or both are inactive. (*) shows the case when the zones of activation overlap, *i.e.*, both muscles are active simultaneously.

Major criticism about equilibrium hypothesis [e.g., Enoka, 1983; Gielen and Houk, 1984; Atkeson, 1989] is based on the fact that the experimental basis of the λ-model included only static experiments, being unable to account for the experimentally observed EMG patterns during voluntary movement. That led to further development of λ-model [Feldman et al., 1990a and b].

Gomi and Kawato reported in 1996 that equilibrium point hypothesis is not valid. By tracking a moving arm and measuring its stiffness along the way with their apparatus [Gomi and Kawato, 1996] evidence has been provided that the brain *de facto* controls constantly a movement, does all the "calculations" required to assess which and when to activate muscles. Gomi and Kawato's experiment focused on a variant of the equilibrium point hypothesis that implies that the brain picks the endpoint for a movement and then specifies the trajectory the arm will follow by triggering a sequence of muscle contractions that ensure it reaches that final position.

This finding is in accordance with earlier challenge to the equilibrium point hypothesis posed by Lackner and DiZio [1995]. Lackner and DiZio [1995] used a round rotating room and subjects were placed in the center of this room. Subjects lost the ability to tell whether the room is spinning or not; they could not rely on sensory clues to correct their movement for external forces. If the equilibrium point hypothesis is valid, subjects should be able to touch a target whether or not the room is spinning. However, when subjects tried this task while rotating, they were very inaccurate. After several tries their accuracy improved, but then when the room stopped rotating, the subjects missed the target again.

2.4.10 The Muscle Patterns Underlying Movement

The first detailed EMG analysis [Wachholder and Altenburger, 1926] of agonist and antagonist muscle activity in humans during flexion-extension movements of the arm showed a so-called triphasic pattern. The triphasic pattern is a strict alteration between agonist and antagonist EMG activity: the initiation of a distinct burst of activity in the agonist is followed by a distinct burst of activity in the antagonist. After a brief silent period in the agonist, activity returns in the form of second burst (Figure 2.23).

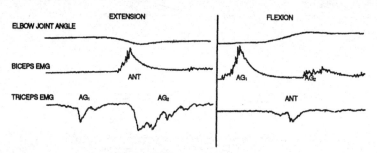

Fig. 2.23: The triphasic EMG activity patterns of the agonist and antagonist muscles in two opposite elbow rotations: extension (left) and flexion (right). AG_1 and AG_2 are agonist bursts and ANT is the antagonist burst of activity.

Another consistent finding was that the bursts of activity of the agonist muscle tended to increase in duration when the movement amplitude increased, although the burst of the antagonist decreased. Since then, the triphasic EMG pattern of simple voluntary movements has been amply confirmed [e.g., Hallet et al., 1975]. The main concern remains about the origin of the muscle bursts. The first, or initiating burst of the agonist muscle AG_1 is of central origin. The amplitude and duration of AG_1 are directly dependent on movement amplitude: the larger the movement, the greater the amplitude and the longer the duration of the burst. Amplitude of AG_1 also reflects the force of the movement [Gordon and Ghez, 1984]. AG_1 duration seems to be constant (around 70 ms) for movements of small amplitude (up to 20 degrees) [Hallet and Marsden, 1979], and increases sharply (up to 200 ms) for larger movements [Brown and Cooke, 1984]. The duration of AG_1 may only increase with movement duration for simple movements (e.g., flexion-extension); the duration of AG_1 increases with amplitude beyond certain range [Lestienne, 1979]. The origin of other two bursts of the triphasic EMG: the antagonist (ANT) and second agonist (AG_2) are less easily determined. The fact that ANT is not a stereotyped phenomenon, and can be influenced by the subject's strategy is a strong indication that this component belongs to the program of accurate movement, the function being to decelerate and stop the movement at the target, and to produce linear trajectories.

The EMG patterns underlying the performance of aimed movement differ according to the movement path and dynamics. The existence of a consistent relationship between muscle activation patterns and the kinematic (or kinetic) variables of movement (Figure 2.23), indicates which of these variables are important in planning appropriate motor output [Soechting, 1989].

For example, forward reaching movement involve primarily activation of the anterior deltoid to implement the protraction at the shoulder, and various degrees of activation of the Biceps to brake the action of gravity on the extending forearm [Soechting and Lacquaniti, 1981; Murphy *et al.*, 1982]. The extension may even be produced by gravity, depending on the height of the target; accordingly, the magnitude of activation of the Biceps will vary widely [Soechting and Lacquaniti, 1981]. These patterns of muscle activation pertain to forward reaching movement made at [Soechting and Lacquaniti, 1981] or near [Murphy *et al.*, 1982] the sagittal plane. When the initial position of the hand and the location of the target require aimed movement in different directions, the muscles involved and the patterns of their activation are much more complicated.

An EMG analysis of movements (monkeys moving their hand in eight different directions in a plane) showed that at least ten muscles acting on the shoulder joint and girdle had been active [Georgopoulos *et al.*, 1984]. The magnitude of EMG activation was correlated significantly among several muscles, a finding that suggests that the movements employed muscle synergies. These synergies differed in an orderly fashion with the direction of movement.

The complexity of the muscle patterns of activation underlying aimed and other multijoint movements arises from several factors. Firstly, these movements are implemented by the concomitant contraction of several muscles, so a population of muscles has to be considered rather than an agonist-antagonist pair, as is usually the case for movement around joints possessing a single degree of freedom (e.g., elbow). Secondly, the exact contribution of each of these muscles to the torque generated at each joint in the course of the movement is often difficult to measure because the direction along which a muscle will exert its mechanical action may change during the movement. Thirdly, a complete analysis of the muscular patterns of activity contributing to these movements has to take into account the temporal differences between the evolving contractions of the participating muscles, for such differences may affect the movement trajectory.

2.4.11 Optimization Theory

Recent observations have indicated that human reaching movements are characterized by certain stereotypical kinematic features such as straight hand paths and bell-shaped velocity profiles [Kelso *et al.*, 1979; Morasso, 1981; Hollerbach and Flash, 1982; Abend *et al.*, 1982]; thus, suggesting that the generated trajectories are not selected at random, but rather in a preferred way according to some general criteria or organizing principles. In particular, it was argued that the characteristic behavior seen in reaching movements may reflect the tendency of the motor system to select particular motor behavior that maximize or minimize certain objective functions which represent the desired global features of the behavior [Hogan, 1984].

Humans, therefore, do not use the full repertoire of possible trajectories but produce movements with certain invariant properties, suggesting a tendency to select one trajectory from the many available. One way to select a unique trajectory is to place additional constraints on the task, thereby, reducing its effective degrees of freedom. Thus, engineering answer to the question why and how humans, when performing the same tasks select more or less the same strategy is to apply optimization methods. In optimal control a *cost function* is chosen in order to evaluate quantitatively the performance of the system under control [Bryson and Ho, 1975]. The cost function is usually defined as the integral of an instantaneous cost over a certain time interval, and the aim is to minimize the value of this cost function.

In applying optimal control theory to explain the invariance seen in human trajectory formation, the task is to select the cost function that produces the observed trajectory. Several cost functions have been suggested in literature, and they all follow experimental results in analyzing characteristic functional movements.

Early studies of trajectory formation considered cost functions such as *minimum energy*, *minimum torque* and *minimum acceleration* [Nelson, 1983]. A cost function C_E (2.1) can be associated with the energy,

$$C_E = \frac{1}{2A}\int_0^T a^2(t)dt \qquad (2.1)$$

where $a(t)$ is acceleration, A is maximal acceleration, and T is movement time. This cost function is based on the assumption that the input power requirement for muscles is proportional to the square of the muscle force output [Hatze and Buys, 1977] and that muscle force is proportional to acceleration (purely inertial system).

This optimization produces bell-shaped velocity profile and demonstrates an increase in peak velocity with decrease in movement time.

The *minimum jerk* model was originally proposed by Hogan [1984] for one-joint and by Flash and Hogan [1995] for multi-joint movements and it can be described by (2.2). For planar movement the cost function C_J is defined by

$$C_J = \frac{1}{2}\int_0^T \left(\left(\frac{d^3x}{dt^3}\right)^2 + \left(\frac{d^3y}{dt^3}\right)^2 \right) dt \qquad (2.2)$$

using T - the duration of the movement and (x,y) - the hand's position at time t.

Harris and Wolpert [1998] proposed a principle of *maximum precision*. They argue that the motor system is constantly calibrating itself to improve performance, and it is much easier to compute the endpoint error than the degree of smoothness. This unifying theory of eye and arm movements is based on the assumption that the neural control signals are corrupted by noise in which presence, the shape of a trajectory is selected to minimize the variance of the final eye or arm position.

Hasan [1986] proposed *minimum effort* model. He suggested that the cost function is the integrated "effort" of movement, the product of muscle stiffness and the square of the derivative of the equilibrium point position. This definition of effort is in good agreement with the model of position and torque perception suggested by Feldman and Latash [1982], that has been based on the equilibrium-point hypothesis. The cost function C_C (2.3) comprises: k - joint stiffness (assumed constant), r - equilibrium position, and T - movement time.

$$C_C = \int_0^T k\left(\frac{dr}{dt}\right)^2 dt \qquad (2.3)$$

An approach reassembling the minimum jerk model has been suggested by Uno *et al.* [1989] in a form of *minimum joint torque-change*. For a planar two-joint arm movements, the cost function C_T is of the form (2.4) where T is the duration of the movement and τ_1 and τ_2 are the shoulder and elbow torque respectively at time t. Unlike minimum jerk, this cost function is not amenable to analytic solution but can be solved by iterative algorithms. Minimum torque change, like minimum jerk, predicts bell-shaped velocity profiles, but also predicts that the form of the trajectories should vary across the arm's workspace.

$$C_T = \frac{1}{2}\int_0^T \left(\left(\frac{d^3\tau_1}{dt^3} \right)^2 + \left(\frac{d^3\tau_2}{dt^3} \right)^2 \right) dt \quad (2.4)$$

Alternative criteria further included the minimum rate of change of muscle-tensions [Dornay *et al.*, 1996], the minimum work [Soechting *et al.*, 1995] or the minimum rate of change of motor-command [Kawato, 1996]. This optimization cost function may also include multiple variables that are relevant for the function (e.g., weighted sum of squares of muscle activity, shortest path, minimum time, minimum effort, minimum jerk, minimum energy consumption, minimum fatigue, and minimum curvature).

At present, only two cost functions account for the most of the multi-joint experimental movement data. These two competing theories reflect the majority understanding of how motor computations are organized. The first one is the minimum jerk cost function [Hogan, 1984], which is based solely on kinematic variables, *i.e.*, the rate of change of hand acceleration, and assumes that a major objective of the motor system is to maximize the smoothness of the movement expressed in terms of spatial coordinates. The minimum jerk model takes no account of the arm's dynamics, thus the velocity profile of the predicted trajectories are invariant under rotation and translation of start and end points of the movement. Moreover the velocity profiles scale linearly with distance and duration. Once the trajectory is determined in Cartesian space, other processes must be invoked to translate the desired hand trajectory into joint coordinates and finally into motor torque. This model ignores non-kinematic factors in the selection and production of reaching movements and is consistent with a theory that neural computations to produce movement are hierarchically organized and are executed by proceeding from the abstract (*i.e.*, move hand to the target) to the particular (*i.e.*, activate that set of motoneurons in this manner). Nevertheless, a somewhat troubling aspect of this theory is that it seems to imply that, at least at the higher levels of the postulated hierarchy, the brain does not take any dynamic considerations into account such as the energy required, the loads on the limb segments or the force and fatigue limitations of its peripheral neuromuscular system.

To circumvent this problem, an alternative model based on the minimization of the rate of change of joint torque was formulated by Uno *et al.* [1989]. Authors proposed an optimization model, based on a dynamic objective function implying that the brain does consider dynamic factors in selecting and producing human-like behavior. It is also consistent with the theory that neural computations to produce movement are executed in parallel, taking all relevant factors, dynamics as well as kinematics into account simultaneously [Alexander *et al.*, 1992]. Uno with collaborators [1989] showed that there is a reasonably good correspondence between the predictions of the minimum torque change model and actual hand trajectories. They also showed that the minimum torque change model predicts the curved trajectories seen when subjects are instructed to make movement while a spring is attached to their hand, a finding which they argued is inconsistent with the minimum jerk model. However, two recent studies on the effects of dynamic environments on movement have shown that, over the course of several practice trials, subjects adapt their movement, resulting in a straightening of the hand paths [Shadmehr and Mussa-Ivaldi, 1994].

Addressing the question, which one of the above hypothetical cost functions better reflects the control strategies employed by the nervous system during the generation of reaching movement researchers inquire into the nature of motor organization. In particular, optimization theory provides us with a useful mathematical framework for concisely formulating and testing specific hypotheses concerning what aspects of performance are considered important by the motor control system. Even though, human may select the preferred strategy not necessarily being optimal with respect to any of the mentioned variables. In addition, we must have in mind that optimization method requires for all cost functions, movement time to be known in advance [Latash, 1993].

2.4.12 Motor Execution

Realization of motor plan is the motor act. For motor execution and for realization of desired motion plans several alternative schemes exist. One, based on the minimum torque-change model [Uno *et al*., 1989] assumes that the tree factors involved in motor act, namely, trajectory planning, coordinate transformations and generation of motor commands to the muscles are simultaneously solved each time the system is presented with a new motor task or when the external conditions (e.g., loads) undergo particular changes.

An alternative view is that the arm trajectory generation processes involve at least two different hierarchical levels [Hogan and Flash, 1987; Flash, 1990]. Higher levels of the motor system are mainly concerned with the kinematic aspects of trajectory formation. *i.e.*, with the setting up of ideal motion plans, while lower level deal more with dynamic aspects of motor execution. To deal with the later problem, it was suggested that the motor system does not necessarily directly derive and code the time histories of joint torque needed to realize the desired motions but may take, instead, advantage of the viscoelastic properties of neurally activated muscles, thus avoiding some of the complexities associated with the explicit solution of the inverse dynamic problem.

Additional experimental studies have shown that the mechanical behavior of a two-joint arm can be characterized as being spring-like, whereby it was shown that small perturbations displacing the hand from its equilibrium position, give rise to elastic restoring forces that can be derived from a potential field [Mussa-Ivaldi *et al*., 1985; Bizzi *et al*., 1992; Shadhmer *et al*., 1993]. The stiffness field of the arm, which describes the dynamic relation between force and displacement, has characterized the mechanical interactions between the limb and the environment. The stiffness field was than experimentally measured and characterized by end - effector (hand) and joint stiffness matrices where the former matrices were graphically represented as stiffness ellipses characterized by their size, shape and orientation. In the case of unconstrained point-to-point reaching movement it was suggested that arm movements are generated by gradually shifting the equilibrium position of the hand from the starting toward the final position. The results based on experimental measurements indicated that the calculated equilibrium trajectories were straighter than the actual movement. Based on that it was than suggested that the execution of reaching movement involve explicit planing of straight hand equilibrium trajectories, which remain invariant under translation, rotation, speed and amplitude scaling.

2.4.13 Reaching Movement

Reaching movement is described as arm manipulation between two points. As a behavioral act, reaching is the result of complex sensory-motor coordination and is performed under behavioral and biomechanical constraints. Reaching is a complicated multijoint movements directed to a defined point in space performed by means of coordinated rotation at the shoulder and elbow joints (Figure 2.24, left, top). These movements are characterized with an initial acceleration phase and a final deceleration phase, resulting with bell-shaped velocity profile (Figure 2.24, left, bottom). Hand, being the arm end-point, normally follows relatively simple, often almost straight, paths in space (Figure 2.24, right).

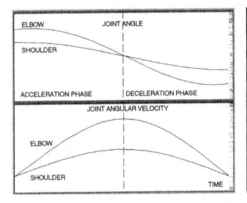
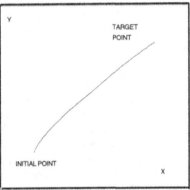

Fig. 2.24: Reaching movement. Joint angles (left, top) and velocities (left, bottom) at the shoulder and elbow joints; hand path from initial to target points (right). Adapted from Popović M, 1995, with permission.

Reaching movement comprises several different activities: pointing - the target position is not defined precisely, yet only the direction of the distal segment of the arm; point to point reaching without grasping - position of both the initial and target positions is known, however the orientation of hand is not relevant, neither the trajectory of the hand between the end points; point to point movement with grasping - complex movement that requires the orientation of the hand that corresponds to the shape of the object to be grasped, in addition to precision in getting to the target with the velocity being about the same as the object to minimize the impact; and tracking - movement along a prescribed trajectory. All of the movement have some specifics, and they require to certain extent different feedback mechanisms in addition to the central program.

Visual guidance of reaching. Much of the research on the control of hand movement has been concerned with the simple task of moving the hand from one position to another, generally as self set speed, yet accurately as possible. This task was studied in detail with both visual feedback and with the eyes closed. It has been shown that when subjects had their eyes closed, mean absolute error remained constant as velocity increased. With the eyes open, mean absolute error decreased with slower movement. This is to prove that proprioception and preprogrammed action works well for the tasks learned, showing a high level of connectivism between activity of actuators, called synergy. The visual feedback adds the corrective mechanism, but it requires time. This lead to the hypothesis that movements have an initial ballistic phase, which when allowed is followed by a feedback-based homing-in phase.

Planning of reaching. The planning of the reaching requires the following: the task, its spatial and temporal characteristics, and dynamics. For example, the desired total movement time can be specified on behavioral grounds for making a slow, intermediate, or fast movement, in relation, of course, to the accuracy desired. The question is also, at which level is the movement planned. It seems that the answer will depend on the instructions given to the subject and on the particular peripheral motor conditions.

Since the motion of the hand will be effected by changes in the angles of joints produced by the action of muscles, it is obvious that planning and/or transformations from one level to the other will take place. The real problem is to identify the level at which a neuron or a neuronal population participates in the generation of the movement. The problem is further complicated by the fact that this relation may change as a function of time. These important questions await rigorous treatment at the theoretical and practical levels.

2.4.14 Grasping

Grasping is a part of the prehension, a process of orienting the hand, opening it so that the object fits comfortably, contacting the object, and forming a firm grip. On the kinetic level, prehension entails applying forces during interaction with an object. Stable grasping requires that the forces are applied by hand surfaces in opposition to other hand surfaces or external objects in order to overcome perturbations. The human hand has a variety of ways to grasp objects firmly.

The selection of the grasp depends on both the function that has to be achieved and the physical constraints of the object and the hand. A fundamental functional constraint is that once the object is grasped it is not to be dropped. The posture used by the hand during the task must be capable of overcoming perturbations and include anticipated forces that may act at the object. There are different prehensile classifications, methods to classify hand postures, developed by researchers from different prospective (e.g., medical, robotics) [McKenzie and Iberall, 1994]. Schlesinger [1919] suggested a taxotomy that was developed to capture the versatility of human hands for designing functionally effective prosthetic hands. The simplest taxotomy includes set of five grasp postures, Figure 2.25. For practical reasons this classification can be further reduced to only three grasps: lateral, palmar and pinch grasps. Analyzing grasping in typical daily activities shows that these three grasps are responsible for almost 95 percent of all functions.

The pattern of finger movements that arises prior to and during grasping reflects the activity of visuomotor mechanisms for detecting the shape of the object and generating appropriate motor commands. The problem is for the motor system of the hand to build an "opposition space", which would take into account both the shape of the object and the biomechanics of the hand [Arbib, 1985; Iberall and MacKenzie, 1990]. Experimental data suggest that there are preferred orientations for the hand opposition space. The hand posture selected during the preshape defines the optimal opposition space for applying the required forces to the object [Iberall et al., 1986]. Using the term opposition authors described three basic directions along which the human hand can apply forces: 1) pad opposition occurring between hand surfaces along a direction parallel to the palm. The surfaces are typically the volar surface of the fingers and thumb near or on the pads (pinch grasp); 2) palm opposition occurring between hand surfaces along a direction perpendicular to the palm (palmar grasp); and 3) side opposition occurring in the direction generally transverse to the palm (lateral grasp). Paulignan *et al.* [1991] showed that the same orientation of the hand was retained during prehension of the same object placed at different positions in the working space, which implies different degrees of rotation of the wrist or the elbow. The kinematic redundancy of the whole arm, and not only its distal segments, are exploited in building appropriate hand configuration for a given object. All these observations suggest the existence of higher order coordination mechanisms that couples the different components of prehension.

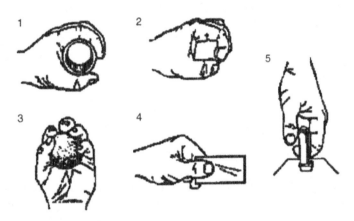

Fig. 2.25: Different patterns of grasping: 1) cylindrical (palmar); 2) tip (pinch); 3) spherical (palmar); 4) lateral (key); and 5) hook.

Forces required to grasp and lift the object are also predetermined during the visual phase of grasping. These forces are calibrated according to visual and cognitive cues. Tactile cues intervene during object loading for adjusting the force level to the real weight and avoiding slippage during manipulation [Johansson and Westling, 1990; Jenmalm *et al.*, 1998]. When an object is gripped and rested in a hand in a pad opposition, a posture involves at least two surfaces. The force system acting on the object is redundant: individual fingers can produce various forces in terms of magnitude and direction insofar as both the net force and moment on the object are zeros. The requirement for equilibrium implies that the normal force developed by the thumb is equal and opposite to the force of the "virtual fingers" – the four fingers combined [MacKenzie and Iberall, 1994]. The grasping hand is a convenient object to study the motor redundancy problem, because all the involved forces can be directly measured and the sharing pattern can be calculated [Zong-Ming Li *et al.*, 1998].

When humans lift and manipulate objects, they apply grip forces that are large enough to prevent the object from slipping but avoid using excessive grip forces that may damage the object or the hand or cause unnecessary muscle fatigue. Grasp stability is achieved by automatically increasing or decreasing grip forces (normal to the grasp surfaces) in parallel with increases or decreases in the load forces (tangential to the grasp surfaces) [Westling and Johansson, 1984].

An important element of understanding grasping is that a stable grasp requires at least three points of contacts that will form three opposition planes, and ensure static equilibrium of the objects, Figure 2.26. The principle of maximizing the contact surface was instrumental for the development of multi-fingered artificial hands as reviewed by Tomović *et al.* [1995].

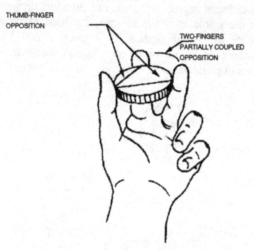

Fig. 2.26: The "tripod" grasp involves three independently controllable fingers, yet the opposition between the thumb and fingers is dominant for safe and stable grasp. Adapted from Cutkosky and Howe, 1990, with permission.

The visual phase of grasping does not imply the use of touch, but it is in direct continuity with the tactile phase and includes preparatory mechanisms for active touch. During the subsequent handling and manipulation, signals for object identification arising from sight and touch are coprocessed [Jeannerod, 1993]. The fingers begin to shape during transportation of the hand at the object location. Preshaping first involves a progressive opening of the grip with straightening of the fingers, followed by a closure of the grip until it matches object size. The point in time where grip size is largest (maximum grip size) is a clearly identifiable landmark which occurs within about 60 to 70 percent of the duration of the reach, that is well before the fingers come in contact with the object [Jeannerod, 1981, 1984; Wing *et al.*, 1986]. The size of aperture during grip formation covaries with object size [Marteniuk *et al.*, 1987, 1990; Gentilucci *et al.*, 1991]. Marteniuk and colleagues [1990] related closure pattern of grip formation to the thumb – finger geometry. Because the index finger is longer than thumb, the finger grip has to open wider than required by object size, in order for the index finger to turn around the object and to achieve the proper orientation of the grip. Indeed, the movement of the index finger contributes the most to grip formation, whereas the position of the thumb with respect to the wrist tends to remain invariant. The extra opening of the grip during preshaping might also represent a safety margin for compensating the effects of the variability of the reach.

2.4.15 Coordination of Reaching and Grasping

A prehensile act requires coordination of its two constituent components, the transport and the grasp components. Transport or reach component brings the hand into the proximity of the object to be grasped. The grasping itself ensures that the object is enclosed. Natural prehension is characterized by the hand opening and closing in tune with the movement of the hand toward the target object. Accordingly, prehension involves the control of both (its reach and its grasp components), as well as their coordination. The issue of how such coordination is achieved and the nature of the coupling of the two components has been a subject of discussion and has inspired a number of experimental investigations [Jeannerod 1981, 1984, 1986, 1994; Arbib 1981, 1985; Zaal *et al.*, 1998]. According to Jeannerod and Arbib, the reach and grasp components evolve independently and are coordinated through central timing mechanism. For instance, Jeannerod [1981, 1984] suggested that the central timing mechanism operates such that peak hand aperture is reached at the moment of peak deceleration. This timing mechanism ensures the temporal alignment of "key moments" in the evolution of the two prehensile components. A number of experiments in which object size, orientation, and/or distance [Gentilucci *et al.*, 1991; Jacobson and Goodale, 1991; Marteniuk *et al.*, 1990; Paulignan *et al.*, 1991] were systematically varied, however, failed to provide evidence for the postulated coincidence of these or other "key moments". In search of other characteristics of the coupling that might then reveal the operation of a central timing mechanism responsible for the control of coordination, Gentilucci *et al.* [1992] noted that the duration of hand closure remained constant over a range of reaching amplitudes. This invariance was found to maintain over conditions in which object location was changed immediately after movement initiation. This led Gentilucci with coworkers [1992] to suggest that the initiation of hand closure (grasp component) was timed based on the time remaining before the hand reached the object (reach component).

The notion of a temporal coordination between reaching and grasping that involved keeping constant the duration of hand closure was included in Hoff and Arbib's update [1993] of Arbib's original model [1981]. The coordination mechanism in the model is based on prior knowledge of the duration of hand closing. Hoff and Arbib argued that hand opening and closing times determine overall movement duration. The duration of the transport component is lengthened accordingly. Importantly, Hoff and Arbib did not suggest that closing times should be equal for movements performed under different condition as if reaches to grasp differently sized objects.

Rather than focusing on the temporal coupling of reaching and grasping, Haggard and Wing [1991] and Haggard and Richardson [1996] note that spatial relation between these two components are highly stable. They studied the traces of normal and perturbed prehensile movements in a state space with hand position and hand aperture size as dimensions. Unperturbed movements exhibited typical traces in this space. Authors showed that the spatial relation between hand position and hand aperture size is stabilized by the system.

3. Pathology of Sensory-Motor Systems and Assessment of Disability

> "The development of the cerebral cortex, with its distinct cellular, molecular, and functional characteristics, is central to our understanding of human cognitive capacity. Recent advances in development neurobiology have helped us to gain new insights into the formation of the cerebral cortex and the pathogenesis of disorders of higher brain function."
>
> Paško Rakic [1995]

Chapter 3 reviews the pathology leading to sensory-motor disorders. The first section is linked to Chapters 1 and 2 by discussing the changes of the organs and tissues that lead to disability when dysfunctional. The presentation indicates which organs and changes are responsible for lost or deprived sensory and motor functions. The second part of Chapter 3 describes relevant classification and medical assessment of subjects with disabilities based on clinical and functional tests. The chapter ends with the description of instrumentation and methods to assess the biomechanics of movement, being essential to quantify the performance and progress of the eventual rehabilitation treatment. The focus of presentation is on injuries and diseases that could be treated with extensive therapy (neurorehabilitation) and assistive systems (neuroprostheses) described in Chapters 4 and 5.

3.1 Pathology of Sensory-Motor Systems

As shown in the first two chapters, organs and tissues responsible for movement are organized in both hierarchical and parallel ways and they are highly interactive; thus, the injury of any part of the system may have many, very different consequences. Before the review of systems dysfunction is given, the injury of a basic element, the neuron, is described.

3.1.1 Cerebro-Vascular Infarction (Stroke)

There is a large population of humans that suffer from cerebro-vascular infarction caused by changes at blood supply of the brain. Stroke is one of the leading medical problems, mostly at elderly subjects. For example, only in Denmark with the population of about five million people there are more than 70 thousand individuals with stroke.

Blood flow to the brain is highly protected, yet the brain remains highly susceptible to disturbances of the blood supply, as reflected in the high incidence of symptomatic cerebral vascular disease. Diseases of the blood vessels are among the most frequent, serious neurological disorders, ranking third as a cause of death in the adult population in the world. The term stroke, or cerebro-vascular accident, refers to the neurological symptoms and signs, usually focal and acute, which result from diseases involving blood vessels. Strokes are either occlusive (due to closure of a blood vessel) or hemorraghic (due to bleeding from a vessel). Insufficiency of blood supply is termed ischemia; if it is temporary, symptoms and signs may clear with little or no pathological evidence of tissue damage. Ischemia reduces blood supply, thereby deprives tissue from the oxygen, glucose, and prevents the removal of potentially toxic metabolises such as lactic acid. When ischemia is sufficiently severe and prolonged, neurons and other cellular elements die; this condition is called infarction.

Hemorrhage may occur at the brain surface (extraparenchymal). Alternatively, hemorrhage may be intraparenchymal (e.g., from rupture of vessels damaged by long-standing hypertension) causing a blood clot or hematoma within the cerebral hemispheres, in the brainstem, or in the cerebellum. Ischemia or infarction may accompany hemorrhage. The mass effect of an intracerebral hematoma may compromise the blood supply of adjacent brain tissue; or subarachnoid hemorrhage may, by unclear mechanisms, cause reactive vasospasm of cerebral surface vessels, leading to further ischemic brain damage. Infarcted tissue may also become secondarily hemorrhagic.

Although most occlusive strokes are due to atherosclerosis and thrombosis and most hemorrhagic strokes are associated with hypertension or aneurysms, strokes of either type may occur at any age from a legion of causes that include cardiac disease, trauma, infection, neoplasm, blood dyserasia, vascular malformation, immunological disorder, and erogenous toxins. The diagnostic strategies and treatment should vary accordingly.

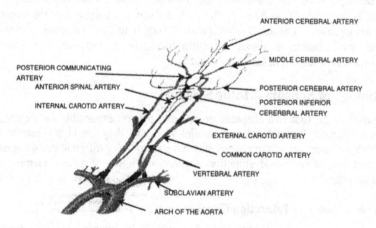

Fig. 3.1: The blood vessels of the brain. Dark areas are common sites of atherosclerosis and occlusion.

Each cerebral hemisphere is supplied by an internal carotid artery, which arises from a common carotid artery beneath the angle of the jaw, enters the cranium through the carotid foramen, traverses the cavernous sinus (giving off the ophthalmic artery), penetrates the dura, and divides into the anterior and middle cerebral arteries (Figures 3.1 and 3.2). The large surface branches of the anterior cerebral artery supply the cortex and white matter of the inferior frontal lobe, the medial surface of the frontal and parietal lobes, and the anterior corpus callosum. Smaller penetrating branches supply the deeper cerebrum and diencephalon, including limbic structures, the head of the caudate, and the anterior limb of the internal capsule. The large surface branches of the middle cerebral artery supply most of the cortex and white matter of the hemisphere's convexity, including the frontal, parietal, temporal, and occipital lobes, and the insula. Smaller penetrating branches supply the deep white matter and diencephalic structures such as the posterior limb of the internal capsule, the putamen, the outer globus pallidus, and the body of the caudate. After the internal carotid artery emerges from the cavernous sinus, it also gives off the anterior choroidal artery, which supplies the anterior hippocampus and, at a caudal level, the posterior limb of the internal capsule.

Each vertebral artery arises from a subclavian artery, enters the cranium through the foramen magnum, and gives off an anterior spinal artery and a posterior inferior cerebellar artery. The vertebral arteries join at the junction of the pons and the medulla to form the basilar artery, which at the level of the pons gives off the anterior inferior cerebellar artery and the internal auditory artery and at the midbrain the superior cerebellar artery. The basilar artery then divides into the two posterior cerebral arteries. The large surface branches of the posterior cerebral arteries supply the inferior temporal and medial occipital lobes and the posterior corpus callosum; the smaller penetrating branches of these arteries supply diencephalic structures, including the thalamus and the subthalamic nuclei, as well as parts of the midbrain.

Interconnections between blood vessels (anastomoses) protect the brain when part of its vascular supply is compromised. The anterior communicating artery connects the two anterior cerebral arteries, and the posterior cerebral arteries are connected to the internal carotid arteries by the posterior communicating arteries.

Middle Cerebral Artery Territory Infarction

Infarction in the territory of the middle cerebral artery (cortex and white matter) causes the most frequently encountered stroke syndrome with contralateral weakness, sensory loss, and visual field cut, and, depending on the hemisphere involved either language disturbance or impaired spatial perception. Weakness and sensory loss affect the face and arm more than the leg because of the somatotopy of the motor and sensory cortex (pre- and postcentral gyri): the face and arm lie on the convexity, whereas the leg resides on the medial surface of the hemisphere. Motor and sensory losses are greatest in the hand, as the more proximal limbs and the trunk tend to have greater representation in both hemispheres. Paraspinal muscles, for example, are hardly ever weak in unilateral cerebral lesions. Similarly, the facial muscles of the forehead and the muscles of the pharynx and jaw are represented bihemispherically and are therefore usually spared. Tongue weakness is variable. If weakness is severe (plegia), the muscle tone is usually decreased initially and is gradually increased over days or weeks to spasticity with hyperactive tendon reflexes. A Babinski sign, reflecting upper motor neuron disturbance, is usually present from the outset. When weakness is mild, or during recovery, there may be clumsiness or slowness of movement out of proportion to loss of strength; such motor disability may resemble Parkinsonian bradykinesia or even cerebellar ataxia.

Acutely, there is often paresis of contralateral conjugate gaze because of damage to the convexity of the cortex anterior to the motor cortex (the frontal eye field). The reason why the gaze palsy persists for only one or two days, although other signs remain severe, is controversial.

Sensory loss tends to involve discriminative and proprioceptive modalities more than affective modalities. Pain and temperature sensation may be impaired or seem altered, but are usually not lost. Joint position sense, however, may be severely disturbed, causing limb ataxia, and there may be loss of two-point discrimination, astercognosis (inability to recognize a held object by tactual sensation), or failure to appreciate a touch stimulus if another is simultaneously delivered to the normal side of the body (extinction).

Visual field impairment (homonymous hemianopsia) is the result of damage to the optic radiation, the deep fiber tracts connecting the thalamic lateral geniculate nucleus to the visual cortex. Destruction of left opercular cortex in human cause aphasia, which may take a variety of forms depending on the degree and distribution of the damage. Frontal opercular lesions tend to produce particular difficulty with speech output and writing with relative preservation of language comprehension, whereas infarction of the posterior superior temporal gyrus tends to cause severe difficulty in comprehending spoken speech and reading. When the damage is widespread, there is severe language disturbance of mixed type (global aphasia). Left-hemisphere convexity damage,

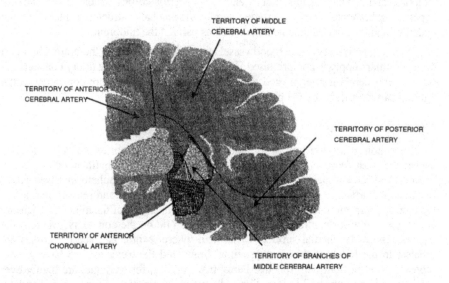

Fig. 3.2: The main blood supply zones within the cerebral cortex.

especially parietal, may also cause motor apraxia, a disturbance of learned motor acts not explained by weakness or incoordination, with the ability to perform the act when the setting is altered.

Right-hemisphere convexity infarction, especially parietal, tends to cause disturbances of spatial perception. There may be difficulty in copying simple pictures or diagrams (constructional apraxia), in interpreting maps or finding one's way about (topographagnosia), or in putting on one's clothes properly (dressing apraxia). Awareness of space and the subject's own body contralateral to the lesion may be particularly affected (hemi-inattention or hemineglect). Subjects may fail to recognize their hemiplegia (anosognosia), left arm (asomatognosia), or any external object to the left of their own midline. Such phenomena may occur independently of visual field defects and in subjects otherwise mentally intact.

Anterior Cerebral Artery Territory Infarction

Infarction in the territory of the anterior cerebral artery causes weakness and sensory loss qualitatively similar to that of convexity lesions, but affects mainly the distal contralateral leg. There may be urinary incontinence, but it is uncertain whether this is due to a lesion of the paracentral lobule (medial hemispheric motor and sensory cortices) or of a more anterior region concerned with the inhibition of bladder emptying. Damage to the supplementary motor cortex may cause speech disturbance, considered aphasic by some and a type of motor inertia by others. Involvement of the anterior corpus callosum may cause apraxia of the left arm (sympathetic apraxia), which is attributed to disconnection of the left (language dominant) hemisphere from the right motor cortex.

Bilateral anterior cerebral artery territory infarction (occurring, for example, when both arteries arise anomalously from a single trunk) may cause a severe behavioral disturbance, with profound apathy, motor inertia, and muteness, attributed variably to destruction of the inferior frontal lobes (orbitofrontal cortex), deeper limbic structures, supplementary motor cortices, or cingulate gyri.

Posterior Cerebral Artery Territory Infarction

This lesion may include, or especially affect, the following structures: the thalamus, causing contralateral hemisensory loss and sometimes spontaneous pain and dysesthesia (thalamic pain syndrome); the subthalamic nucleus, causing contralateral severe proximal chorea (hemiballism); or even the midbrain, with ipsilateral oculomotor palsy and contralateral hemiparesis.

3.1.2 Diseases of Transmitter Metabolism

Diseases of the basal ganglia characteristically produce involuntary movement (dyskinesia), poverty and slowness of movement, and disorders of muscle tone and postural reflexes. These abnormal movements include the following: tremor (rhythmic, involuntary, oscillatory movements of a body part); athetosis (slow, writhing movements of the fingers and hands, and sometimes of the toes and feet, which can also involve the proximal part of the limb); chorea (rapid, flick-like movements of the limbs and facial muscles that may resemble normal restlessness or fidgeting); and ballism (violent, flailing movements primarily involving proximal parts of the limb).

Motor disorders, as described above, fall into two classes of deficits: primary functional deficits (negative signs), which can be attributed to the loss of function subserved by specific neurons; and secondary deficits (positive signs or release phenomena), which may be caused by the malfunction of neurons or the emergence of an abnormal pattern of action in neurons when part of their controlling input (usually their inhibitory input) is destroyed or dysfunctional because of disease. The abnormal movements that occur in basal ganglia disease are thought to fall into the second category. These movements apparently result from abnormal activity in neurons of the basal ganglia caused by removal of inhibitory influences on them.

Parkinson's Disease

Parkinson's disease (paralysis agitans), one of the best characterized diseases of the basal ganglia, is accompanied by a rhythmic tremor at rest, a unique kind of increased muscle tone or rigidity that often has a cogwheel like characteristic, and a slowness in the initiation of movement (akinesia) as well as in the execution of movement (bradykinesia). This slowness is often evident in the way the subject gets up from a bed or chair and in a shuffling gait. The presumptive site of the lesion in Parkinson's disease is the dopaminergic projection from the substantia nigra to the striatum.

The tremor and rigidity of Parkinson's disease have been attributed to a loss of an inhibitory influence within the basal ganglia, leading to an abnormal outflow from the internal segment of the globus pallidus to the ventral anterior and ventral lateral nuclei of the thalamus, and finally to the cortex.

Huntington's Disease

Four features characterize Huntington's disease: (1) heritability, (2) chorea, (3) dementia, and (4) death after 15 or 20 years. This disease has now been shown to affect men and women with equal frequency, about 0.05 percent of the population.

The first signs of the disorder are subtle and may consist of absentmindedness, irritability, and depression, accompanied by fidgeting, clumsiness, or sudden falls. Uncontrolled movement, a prominent feature of the disease, gradually increases, until the subject becomes confined to bed or to a wheelchair. Speech is at first slurred, then incomprehensible, and finally it ceases altogether as facial expressions become distorted and grotesque. Mental functions undergo similar deterioration, and eventually the ability to reason disappears.

Tardive dyskinesia is another clinical disorder that may involve the basal ganglia; involuntary movements, especially manifest it on the face and tongue.

3.1.3 Spinal Cord Injuries

Spinal cord injuries or diseases are a frequent reason of disability and result in total or partial obstruction of flow of both sensory and motor information being instrumental for normal life. Spinal cord injuries are most often caused by trauma, especially following the motor vehicle and sport accidents. The resulting syndrome depends on the extent of direct injury of the cord or compression of the cord by displaced vertebrae or blood clots. In extreme cases trauma may lead to complete or partial transaction of the spinal cord. Knowledge of the anatomy and physiology of the spinal cord helps in recognizing spinal cord disease and localization of the disease to a particular segment or region of the spinal cord. This allows identifying the nature of the disorder.

Lesions of the spinal cord give rise to motor or sensory symptoms that are often related to a particular sensory or motor segmental level of the spinal cord (Figure 3.3, right). Identification of the appropriate level of the motor or sensory loss (called a motor or sensory level) is important for understanding the disability.

When motor roots are involved, or when motor neurons are affected focally, clinical findings may indicate the spinal level of the injury. This clinical evidence would include the typical lower motor neuron signs: weakness, wasting, fasciculation, and loss of tendon reflexes. Because it is clinically difficult to relate the innervation of muscles of the trunk and thorax to specific spinal segments, however, the motor level may not be evident. For instance, a lesion anywhere above the first lumbar segment may cause signs of upper motor neuron disease in the legs. Under these circumstances, sensory abnormalities are more valuable for localizing the lesion.

The characteristic pattern of sensory loss after a transverse spinal cord lesion is loss of cutaneous sensation below the level of the lesion, contralateral to the damaged spinothalamic tract if the lesion is unilateral. The sensory level is often more evident than the motor level. However, sensory loss due to spinal lesions must be differentiated from the pattern of sensory loss caused by lesions of peripheral nerves or isolated nerve roots. In multiple symmetrical peripheral neuropathy (polyneuropathy), there is a glove-and-stocking pattern of impaired perception of pain and temperature. This pattern is attributed to "dying-back" or impaired axonal transport; the parts of the axons most severely affected are those most distant from the sensory neuron cell bodies in the dorsal root ganglia. In injuries of single peripheral nerves, the distribution of sensory loss is more restricted and can be recognized by reference to sensory charts that were originally generated by studies of the long-term effects of traumatic nerve injuries incurred during war.

Nerve root or segmental sensory loss and spinal sensory levels can be identified by the dermatomes typically affected The spinal cord ends at the base of the second lumbar (L2) vertebra. Below this level the spinal canal (Figure 3.3, left) is occupied by the lower nerve roots (the cauda equina).

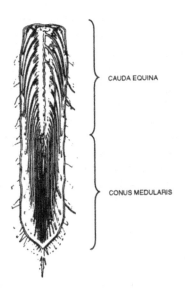
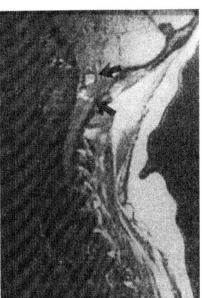

Fig. 3.3: The bottom part of the spinal cord and nerve roots: cauda equina and conus medularis region (left). Magnetic Resonance Image (right) of a spinal cord injury (sagittal view) caused by a vascular disorder; the lesion is located near C1 (indicated with arrows). The functional result of this injury is an incomplete tetraplegia.

A spinal cord lesion (Figure 3.3, right) arises within the spinal cord (intra-axial or intramedullary), or externally (extra-axial or extramedullary). Clinical evidence may give some clues that are helpful in making the distinction. For instance, pain is more common in extra-axial lesions because a compressive lesion (such as a tumor) may affect the dura, posterior nerve roots, or blood vessels that are innervated by sensory neurons mediating pain. In contrast, because there are no pain receptors within the spinal cord and the brain, intra-axial lesions may be painless. Intra-axial lesions may be marked by sacral sparing of sensation or may cause a segmental pattern of sensory loss, as in syringomyelia. The bladder function is affected earlier in intra-axial disorders than it is in extra-axial disease.

The list of terms frequently use in communication between people dealing with rehabilitation technology [Maynard et al., 1997] is the following:

Tetraplegia (preferred to *quadriplegia*). This term refers to impairment or loss of motor and/or sensory function in the cervical segments of the spinal cord due to damage of neural elements within the spinal canal. Tetraplegia results in impairment of function in the arms as well as in the trunk, legs and pelvic organs. It does not include brachial plexus lesions or injury to peripheral nerves outside the neural canal. *Paraplegia.* This term refers to impairment or loss of motor and/or sensory function in the thoracic, lumbar or sacral (but not cervical) segments of the spinal cord, secondary to damage of neural elements within the spinal canal. With paraplegia, arm functioning is spared, but, depending on the level of injury, the trunk, legs and pelvic organs may be involved. The term is used in referring to cauda equina and conus medullaris injuries, but not to lumbosacral plexus lesions or injury to peripheral nerves outside the neural canal.

Quadriparesis and paraparesis terms describe incomplete lesions, where many functions are preserved.

Dermatome refers to the area of the skin innervated by the sensory axons within each segmental nerve (root).

Myotome refers to the collection of muscle fibers innervated by the motor axons within each segmental nerve (root).

Neurological level, sensory level, and motor level. The first of these terms refers to the most caudal segment of the spinal cord with normal sensory and motor function on both sides of the body. Thus, up to four different segments may be identified in determining the neurological level, (*i.e.,* R-sensory, L-sensory, R-motor, L-motor). When the term *sensory level* is used, it refers to the most caudal segment of the spinal cord with normal sensory function on both sides of the body; the Motor level is similarly defined with respect to motor function. *Skeletal level* refers to the level at which, by radiographic examination, the greatest vertebral damage is found.

Sensory and motor scores are numerical summary scores that reflect the degree of neurological impairment associated with the SCI.

Incomplete injury is defined in cases where partial preservation of sensory and/or motor functions is found below the neurological level and includes the lowest sacral segment. Sacral sensation includes sensation at the anal mucocutancous junction as well as deep anal sensation. The test of motor function is the presence of voluntary contraction of the external anal sphincter upon digital examination.

Complete injury is the term used when there is an absence of sensory and motor function in the lowest sacral segment.

Zone of partial preservation (ZPP) refers to those dermatomes and myotomes caudal to the neurological level that remain partially innervated. When some impaired sensory and/or motor function is found below the lowest normal segment, the exact number of segments so affected should be recorded for both sides as the ZPP. The term is used only with complete injuries.

Complete Spinal Cord Transection

The spinal cord may be completely severed acutely in fracture-dislocations of vertebrae or by knife or bullet wounds. Acute transaction of the cord may also result from an inflammatory condition called transverse myelitis or from compression due to a tumor, especially metastatic tumors. In myelitis and tumors, symptoms evolve in days or weeks.

Immediately after traumatic section of the cord, however, there is a loss of all sensation and all voluntary movement below the lesion. Bladder and bowel controls are also lost. If the lesion is above C3, breathing may be affected. Although upper motor neuron signs might be expected, tendon reflexes are usually absent - a condition of spinal shock that persists for several weeks. After a while, the reflex activity returns at the levels below the lesion. Hyperactive reflexes, clonus (rapid and repeated contraction and relaxation of passively stretched muscle), and Babinski signs then appear as signs of damage to the corticospinal tract. The legs become spastic; this condition is often preceded by intermittent hypertonia and flexor spasms that occur spontaneously or may be provoked by cutaneous stimuli. Later, flexor and extensor spasms may alternate, and the ultimately fixed posture may be either flexion or extension of the knees and hips. Bladder and bowel function may become automatic, with emptying in response to moderate filling. Automatic bladder emptying may be retarded by severe distention of the bladder or infection in the acute stage, or by damage to lumbar or sacral cord segments.

Partial Transection

In partial transaction of the spinal cord, some ascending or descending tracts may be spared. In slowly progressing lesions, as in compression by an extramedullary tumor, the same tracts may be affected, but less severely. Partial function is retained, but specific motor and sensory signs can still be recognized.

Hemisection (Brown-Sequard Syndrome)

Because of spinal cord anatomy, hemisection of the right side of the cervical spinal cord (at C4, for example) has four main clinical consequences:

1. Ipsilateral (right) signs of a lesion in the corticospinal tract results with the weakness of the right arm and leg, with more active tendon reflexes in the right arm and leg. In addition, several abnormal reflexes appear. One is the Babinski sign - abnormal extension of the great toe, instead of the normal flexor (downward) plantar reflex in response to a moving stimulus on the lateral border of the sole of the foot. This reflex abnormality reliably indicates a disorder of the corticospinal tract on that side of the spinal cord. Another abnormal reflex is the Hoffmann sign, an abnormal flexor reflex of the thumb and other fingers induced by stretching the flexors of the middle finger by flicking the distal phalanx of that finger. Finally, there may be clonus, which is best detected at the ankle when the examiner abruptly moves the subject's foot upward (stretching the gastrocnemius). Sometimes, clonus is so easily evoked that it occurs vigorously in response to a simple tap on the Achilles tendon or when the subject places the foot on the floor. The reaction can be stopped promptly by passively

moving the foot down or plantar-flexing the foot, relieving the stretched position of the gastrocnemius.

2. *Ipsilateral signs of a posterior column lesion* are indicated by a loss of position sense and vibratory sensation.

3. *Contralateral loss of pain and temperature perception* to the level of C4 follows interruption of the right spinothalamic tract.

4. *Loss of autonomic action* results in Homer's syndrome (miosis, ptosis) on the same side.

Multiple Sclerosis

The two most common nontraumatic disorders of the central nervous system are probably amyotrophic lateral sclerosis and multiple sclerosis. Upper motor neuron signs and proprioceptive sensory loss are almost always present in advanced cases of multiple sclerosis, although there may be no signs referable to a lesion of the spinal cord. Nonetheless, when subjects who have had these signs come to autopsy, there are usually many small lesions throughout the spinal cord. Some combinations of signs are almost diagnostic of multiple sclerosis; for instance, the combination of proprioceptive sensory loss and signs of upper motor neuron disease together with evidence of either cerebellar dysfunction ataxia, tremor of the arms, disorders of eye movement (nystagmus), difficulty in speaking (dysarthria)-or a history or signs of optic neuritis. In addition to signs of disorder elsewhere in the nervous system, there is often a clinical episode of transverse myelitis with corresponding motor and sensory levels.

Syringomyelia

Syringomyelia is a condition defined by the formation of cysts within the spinal cord. The cause is unknown, but the lesion affects the central portion of the cord first and then spreads peripherally. Intramedullary tumors may also cause the same clinical syndrome. The clinical picture of syringomyelia is characterized by two unusual patterns of segmental dysfunction (involving cutaneous sensation and motor neurons) as well as interruption of ascending or descending tracts. Because the lesion starts centrally, the first fibers to be affected are those carrying pain and temperature sensations as they cross in the anterior commissure. This usually causes bilateral loss of cutaneous sensation, restricted to the segments involved and resulting in a "shawl" or "cuirass" pattern, affecting a few cervical or thoracic segments and sparing sensation below. Sometimes the segmental sensory loss is unilateral. The lesion is chronic, and the loss of sensation may lead to painless injuries of the digits or painless burns. Because touch perception is conveyed in posterior columns as well as in spinothalamic tracts, there may be dissociated sensory loss, sparing touch as well as position and vibration sense. If motor neurons in the diseased segment are affected, there are lower motor neuron signs, such as weakness, wasting, and loss of reflexes, in the appropriate area. If the lesion extends laterally, the corticospinal tracts are affected and there may be upper motor neuron signs in the legs.

Friedreich's Ataxia

Friedreich's ataxia is a genetic condition in which the distribution of spinal cord lesions is similar to that of combined system disease. In addition, spinocerebellar tracts are affected. As a result, the first symptoms, occurring in adolescence, are usually unsteadiness or ataxia in walking. There may be spastic weakness of the legs and loss of proprioception. The combination of lesions results in the incongruous appearance of Babinski signs although knee and ankle jerks are lost.

3.1.4 Injury of the Neuron

Cutting an axon interrupts both rapid axonal transport and the slower axoplasmic flow, the two mechanisms that carry materials synthesized in the cell body to the axon terminals [Kelly, 1985]. Therefore, the axon and synaptic terminals degenerate when deprived of their normal metabolic interaction with the cell body. Axonal transport occurs in the retrograde direction along the axon. Retrograde changes are found after axotomy and in some instances they result in death of the neuron, yet in others the neuron survives, but it does not function appropriately. The motor neuron of the spinal cord and the afferent (sensory) neurons of the associated dorsal root ganglia will be used as models for analyzing the consequences of cutting the axon (axotomy).

The sensory information is first encoded by receptors and other afferent neurons, and the series of synaptic interaction that follows leads to the generation of the motor output as described in Chapters 1 and 2. Synapses mediate trophic interactions between neurons; they are instrumental for the normal maintenance of neural cells. Deprived of its synaptic terminals, a neuron may shrink, atrophy, or degenerate. Therefore, when a bundle of axons in the central nervous system is severed, then degenerative changes will be found in the damaged neurons, and also in neurons that receive synapses from the damaged neurons (Figure 3.4). In some injuries, the presynaptic neurons that synapse on the damaged cells are also affected. Such reactions are called transsynaptic or transneuronal because they cross from one neuron to the next via the synapse. These influences can be mild or they can cause degeneration of the affected neurons. Transneuronal changes of various kinds are important in explaining why a lesion at one site in the central nervous system can have effects on sites distant to the lesion, sites that are distributed according to the connections that the lesion interrupts.

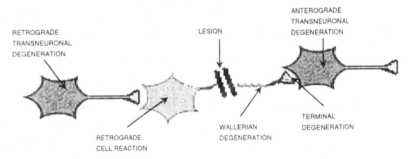

Fig. 3.4: Axotomy can result in degeneration not only in the injured cell, but also in those cells with which is shares synapses.

The zone of trauma is a place where a bundle of axons is cut, either by sectioning of a tract within the central nervous system or by sectioning a peripheral nerve. The part of the axon still connected to the cell body is the proximal segment, and the part isolated from the rest of the cell is the distal segment. The cut ends of both parts of the axon lose axoplasm immediately after injury, but the ends soon become sealed off by fusion of the axon membrane, retract from one another, and begin to swell. Both the proximal and the distal segments swell because fast axonal transport occurs in two directions. The proximal end swells more, however, because newly synthesized neurofilaments, microtubules, and microfilaments, traveling by slow axoplasmic flow, come from the cell body only.

At a zone of trauma in the central nervous system, the axon and myelin sheath undergo rapid local degeneration. Because a lesion usually interrupts blood vessels, macrophages from the general circulation can enter the area and phagocytose axonal debris. Astrocytes and microglia proliferate and act as phagocytes. In the central nervous system, however, the proliferation of fibrous astrocytes leads to the formation of a glial scar around the zone of trauma. Scarring can block the course taken by regenerating axons and establish an effective barrier against the reformation of central connections.

The degeneration spreads in both directions along the axon from the zone of trauma, but only for a short distance in the proximal segment, usually up to the point of origin of the first axon collateral. After few days, a retrograde reaction is seen in the cell body. If the entire cell body dies, then degeneration spreads from the axon hillock down along the remainder of the proximal segment. In the distal segment, outside the zone of trauma, the degeneration first appears in the axon terminal about one day after the occurrence of the lesion. In approximately two weeks, the synapses formed by the distal segment degenerate completely. The process is called terminal degeneration. Degeneration of the distal axon, termed Wallerian degeneration takes place over a period of about two months [Kelly, 1985]. Sometime cells that are prior postsynaptic to the injured neuron may also be affected.

Loss of the Presynaptic Terminal

The axon terminal is very sensitive to interruption of contact with the parent cell body. If cutting a peripheral nerve severs the axon of a motor neuron to a skeletal muscle, degenerative changes begin to occur immediately, at the presynaptic terminals of the motor axon because the maintenance of its integrity is critically dependent on fast axonal transport. Intracellular recordings from muscle fibers few days after the motor axons, which innervate them, are severed show that synaptic transmission fails after the axon is cut. The cells around the synaptic terminal of the motor axon loose differentiation and proliferation ability to form phagocytes that absorb the degenerating terminal. The whole distal axon breaks up into short, beaded segments, which are then phagocytosed by Schwann cells.

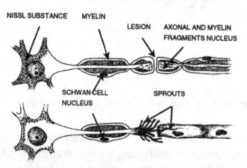

Fig. 3.5: Principles of regeneration of the peripheral neuron. See details in Chapter 4.

About one week after the initial degenerative changes appear in the axon terminal, degeneration begins in the entire distal axon. The myelin sheath draws away from the axon and breaks apart. The axon swells and then becomes beaded. Neurofilaments and neurotubules soon fill the axon. Fragments of the axon and the myelin sheath are absorbed by local phagocytes derived from the glial cell population in the central nervous system or from Schwann cells in the peripheral nervous system. In the central nervous system, macrophages from the general circulation do not absorb the debris produced by Wallerian degeneration, as they do in the zone of trauma.

If the peripherally directed process of a dorsal root ganglion cell is cut, or if a motor axon is cut, then the distal segment of the severed axon will degenerate as described. The connective tissue sheath that surrounds the nerve in which the severed axon ran originally remains intact for longer periods. The proximal segment of a severed axon can regenerate and reconnect to its previous synaptic sites as long as its cell body remains alive. The regenerating axons run along the connective tissue sheath, which acts as a conduit leading the growing axons back to the peripheral target (Figure 3.5). If the centrally directed branches of dorsal root ganglion cells are cut, the glial scar that forms around the degenerating axons in the dorsal aspect of the spinal cord prevents any axons that might regenerate from reaching their central targets.

The cell bodies of different classes of neurons respond to axotomy in two major ways. After an axon is severed, some neurons undergo distinctive regenerative changes as they prepare metabolically for the regrowth of a new axon. For example, cutting the peripheral axon of a dorsal root ganglion cell or a spinal motor neuron causes characteristic changes in the parent neuron within two to three days. The cell body first begins to swell, the nucleus moves to an eccentric position and swells; the endoplasmic reticulum breaks apart and moves to the periphery of the swollen cell body. Peripheral axons will regenerate under relatively simple conditions. If the distal part of the denervated axon (the myelin sheet) is brought in the proximity of the proximal end of the axon that is "alive", the axon will start growing through the sheet at the speed of about 1 mm per day. The survived nucleus will grow if it finds a target (receptors, muscle) at the end of a degenerated axon transformed in the myelin sheet comprising Schwann cells.

At this time, there is very limited confirmation that central axons can regenerate. In normal environment in the spinal canal or the brain, central axons cannot regenerate, yet new cells can be formed. Some evidence suggests that the glial scar is the barrier to the regrowth of central neurons as described in Chapter 4. It is important to recognize the role played by glial cells in normal function as well as in the response to disease or damage of the central nervous system. Two types of glial cells-astrocytes and oligodendrocytes-vastly outnumber neurons. The astrocytes are located predominately in gray matter. In the damaged brain astrocytes phagocytose neuronal debris. The term sclerosis is often used to describe disease states, such as multiple sclerosis, that affect populations of axons in the brain. The term refers to the palpably hard scar of astrocytes that replaces phagocytosed debris resulting from the disease process.

Oligodendrocytes, which form myelin in the central nervous system, predominate in white matter. They have smaller cell bodies and give off fewer processes than astrocytes; each process appears to participate in forming myelin for a single axon. In the central nervous system, each oligodendrocyte contributes to the myelin sheath of several axons by means of its different processes. Damaged neurons receive reduced synaptic inputs, and the evoked excitatory postsynaptic potentials are smaller in amplitude, as if synapses on the cell body and proximal dendrites were removed by encroachment of glial cells.

Transneuronal Degeneration. Two mechanisms have been proposed to explain transneuronal degeneration. The first is that neurons require a certain amount of stimulation to survive. Cutting the axons that provide input to a population of cells could reduce activity below a critical level, and the deafferented cells might atrophy as a consequence of this reduced activity. However, the activity may not be the sole factor. The synaptic terminals release some trophic substance necessary for the normal survival of neurons. Degeneration of the terminals removes this substance and leads eventually to the atrophy of the postsynaptic cell. The two mechanisms could be related if the release of the trophic factor is tied to the level of activity in the presynaptic fiber.

3.1.5 Diseases of the Motor Unit

A mature human skeletal muscle fiber is innervated by only one motor neuron, yet each motor neuron innervates more than one muscle fiber. The synaptic transmission at the nerve-muscle synapse is very effective; thus, every action potential in the motor neuron activates the contraction mechanisms of the muscle fibers innervated by that neuron. The term motor unit refers to the motor neuron in the spinal cord and the population of muscle fibers that it innervates. The motor unit has four functional components: 1) the cell body of the motor neuron, 2) the axon of the motor neuron that runs in the peripheral nerve, 3) the neuromuscular junctions, and 4) the muscle fibers innervated by that neuron.

Most diseases of the motor unit cause weakness and wasting of skeletal muscles. These diseases may differ in other features; however, depending upon which of the four components of the motor unit is primarily affected. A disease can be functionally selective by affecting only the sensory systems or only the motor systems. Motor diseases are regionally selective. They affect only one component of the neuron (e.g., the axon, rather than the cell body). Thus, the distinctions among the different components of the neuron have important clinical implications; reciprocally, clinical observations can provide valuable insights into the functional significance of these components.

The clinical consequences of neurogenic disease are most obvious when a peripheral nerve is cut. The muscles innervated by that nerve are immediately paralyzed and then wasted progressively. Tendon reflexes are lost immediately, as is the sensation in the area innervated by the nerve because the nerve carries sensory as well as motor fibers. In neurogenic diseases, similar effects of denervation appear more slowly, and the muscles gradually become weak and wasted.

In the myopathies, there is dysfunction of muscle without evidence of denervation. The main symptoms are due to weakness of skeletal muscle and often include difficulty in walking or lifting. Less commonly, other muscle symptoms occur, such as inability to relax (myotonia), cramps, pain (myalgia), or the appearance in the urine of the protein that colors the muscle red (myoglobinuria). The muscular dystrophies are a group of myopathies with special characteristics: they are hereditary; all symptoms are due to weakness; the weakness becomes progressively more severe and, histologically, there is evidence of degeneration and regeneration with no storage of abnormal metabolizes.

3.1.6 Neurogenic and Myopathic Diseases

The neurogenic and myopathic diseases are characterized by weakness of muscle, and differential diagnosis is difficult. Neurogenic disorders tend to cause distal limb weakness, while myopathic disorders tend to cause proximal limb weakness. Some signs, however, are restricted to neurogenic diseases. Denervated muscle fibers tend to fire spontaneous motor unit potentials that give rise to spontaneous twitches of the muscle called fasciculation and fibrillation. Fasciculations are visible twitches of the muscle that can be seen as ripples under the skin. They result from the synchronous and involuntary contractions of the muscle fibers innervated by the same motor neuron (a motor unit). Fibrillations, on the other hand, arise from spontaneous activity within single denervated muscle fibers. They are not clinically visible, but can be recognized only by electromyography.

A sign of neurogenic disease is the combination of overactive reflexes (disease of upper motor neurons) in a weak, wasted, and twitching limb (disease of the lower motor neuron). This combination is a diagnosis of amyotrophic lateral sclerosis, a condition that involves both the upper and the lower motor neurons.

Abnormalities can be diagnosed by electromyography (EMG). Attention is given to three measurements: spontaneous activity at rest, the number of motor units under voluntary control, and the duration and amplitude of each motor unit potential.

3.1.7 Peripheral Neuropathies

Because motor and sensory axons run in the same nerves, disorders of peripheral nerves usually cause symptoms of both motor and sensory dysfunction. Some humans with peripheral neuropathy often report abnormal sensory experiences, frequently unpleasant. Similar sensations are recognized by normal individuals after local anesthesia is used for dental work; these sensations are variously called "numbness," "pins-and-needles," or "tingling." When these sensations occur spontaneously without a proximate sensory stimulus, they are called paresthesias. Subjects may be unable to discriminate between hot and cold. Lack of pain perception may lead to painless injuries. Examination of subjects with paresthesias usually reveals impaired perception of cutaneous modalities of sensation (pain and temperature) due to selective loss of the small myelinated fibers that carry these sensations; the sense of touch may or may not be involved. Proprioceptive sensations (position and vibration) may be lost without loss of cutaneous sensation. The sensory disorders are always more prominent distally (the glove-and stocking pattern), presumably because the distal portions of the nerves are most remote from the cell body and therefore more susceptible to disorders that interfere with axonal transport of essential metabolizes and proteins. This concept of dying-back is invoked to explain why both weakness and sensory loss are usually more severe in distal parts of the arms and legs.

The motor disorder of peripheral neuropathy is first manifested by weakness, which may be predominantly proximal in acute cases and is usually distal in chronic cases. Tendon reflexes are usually depressed or lost. Fasciculation is only rarely seen, and atrophy does not ensue unless the weakness has been present for many weeks. Neuropathies may be either acute or chronic. The chronic neuropathies also vary from the mildest manifestations to incapacitating or even fatal conditions, and the list of possible causes seems almost endless.

Neuropathies may be divided in two categories: demyelinating and axonal. The velocity of conduction is slow in axons that have lost myelin. In axonal neuropathies, the myelin sheath is not affected, and conduction velocity is normal. The clinical manifestations may partly be due to disorders of axonal transport. Both axonal and demyelinating neuropathy may lead to two kinds of symptoms, positive or negative. The positive symptoms of peripheral neuropathies consist of paresthesias that are attributed to abnormal impulse activity in the sensory fibers. These paresthesias may arise from spontaneous activity of injured nerve fibers or from electrical cross-talk interactions between abnormal axons. The negative symptoms consist of weakness or paralysis, loss of tendon reflexes, and impaired sensation. Weakness and loss of tendon reflexes result from damage to motor axons. The specific loss of sensation depends on the category of sensory fibers affected. Early in many neuropathies, there is loss of position sense or in the perception of low-frequency vibration, indicating damage to large-diameter fibers. Disordered pain and temperature perception indicates that small-diameter fibers are also affected. Negative symptoms have been studied most thoroughly in demyelinating neuropathy and are attributed to three basic mechanisms: conduction block, slowed conduction, and impaired ability to conduct impulses at higher frequencies.

If an axon that has become demyelinated, as in diabetic neuropathy or an inherited neuropathy, the high resistance, low-capacitance insulation of the myelin sheath is damaged or lost completely. Reflecting the different degrees of demyelination along the axon, the action potentials in the axons of a nerve begin to conduct at slightly different velocities, with the result that the nerve loses the normal synchrony of conduction.

3.1.8 Myopathies

Muscle diseases are conveniently divided into those that are inherited and those that seem to be acquired. The best-known inherited diseases are the muscular dystrophies, which are separated based on clinical and genetic patterns into four major types. Two types can be distinguished that are characterized by weakness alone: the Duchenne and facioscapulohumeral dystrophies. The Duchenne type, which starts in the legs, affects boys only. The facioscapulohumeral type differs in genetic pattern (autosomal dominant), affects the two sexes equally, starts usually in adolescence, affects the shoulder, girdle, and face early, and may be much milder, compatible with an almost normal life span. Increasing evidence suggests that Duchenne dystrophy is due to a genetic fault of the muscle surface membrane.

A myotonic muscular dystrophy causes weakness, but has an additional and characteristic feature-myotonia. Myotonia is a delayed relaxation of the muscle after vigorous voluntary contraction, percussion, or electrical stimulation. The delayed relaxation is caused by repetitive firing of the muscle action potentials and is independent of nerve supply because it persists after nerve block or curarization.

The weakness seen in any myopathy is conventionally ascribed to degeneration of muscle fibers. At first, the missing fibers are replaced by regeneration, but ultimately renewal cannot keep pace, and fibers are lost progressively. As we have seen in electromyography, this leads to compound motor unit potentials of brief duration and reduced amplitude. The decreased number of functioning muscle fibers would then account for the diminished strength. The muscle damage does not invariably lead to weakness. Conversely, it is also possible that muscle weakness in some myopathies will be due to a biochemical or physiological abnormality instead of, or in addition to, loss of the muscle fibers.

Myotonia, being an impaired relaxation after a forceful contraction, is a manifestation of several inherited disorders. Weakness as well as myotonia characterizes myotonic muscular dystrophy.

3.1.9 Muscle Atrophy

Since the pioneering work of Tower [1937] it has been accepted that muscles that are paralyzed as a result of spinal cord injuries undergo atrophy and develop less force. The focus of this presentation is on three issues: 1) magnitude of muscle atrophy after spinal cord injuries and the distinction between denervation and disuse atrophies; 2) increased susceptibility of paralyzed muscles to fatigue; and 3) capacity of surviving motor nerves to sprout and reinnervate denervated muscle fibers in partially denervated muscles.

Muscle atrophy, a reduction in the size and/or number of muscle fibers, may be present as denervation atrophy or disuse atrophy [McComas, 1977; Greensmith and Vrbova, 1997]. Denervation atrophy results from injury to motoneurons in the ventral roots through which they exit [Kralj and Bajd, 1989; Solandt and Magladery, 1942]. Disuse atrophy occurs as a result of loss of muscle activation due to disruption of the central and segmental synaptic drive onto the surviving spinal motoneurons [Peckham *et al.*, 1976; Gordon and Patullo, 1993; Roy *et al.*, 1991].

Denervation atrophy. With spinal cord injuries, many neurons including the motoneurons in the ventral horn may be fatally damaged, and the ventral and dorsal roots may be traumatized even when the cell bodies are not directly affected. Thus the segmental trauma may lead to substantial denervation of muscles supplied by motoneurons in the spinal cord segment and by motor nerves that exit the spinal cord through the ventral roots at the level damaged.

The muscles that lose all of their innervation undergo drastic and rapid wasting [McComas, 1977; Greensmith and Vrbova, 1997; Roy *et al.*, 1991]. Generally, the proportion of muscles that suffer complete denervation after spinal cord injuries is small [Peckham *et al.*, 1976]. Many muscle fibers that receive their innervation from the affected spinal cord segments will suffer partial denervation because of the irreversible damage to their motoneurons. For example, in subjects with complete lesions at the C5 to C6 levels, the paralyzed thenar muscles lose as much as 50 percent to 90 percent of their normal complement of motor innervation [Yang *et al.*, 1990]. Prevention or reversal of denervation atrophy in these cases will depend on the capacity of the nerves of surviving motoneurons to sprout and reinnervate as many denervated muscle fibers as possible. The greater the sprouting, the better the reinnervation of denervated muscle fibers. Consequently, muscle fibers may survive and contract in response to artfully elicited activation (e.g., FES). The remaining motor nerves may not always succeed in reinnervating all the denervated muscle fibers; denervation atrophy may still contribute to the weakness of paralyzed muscles that receive their innervation from spinal segments at or near the lesion site.

Some reports have suggested that there may be a loss of motoneurons several segments below a spinal cord lesion in humans; the loss has been attributed to transsynaptic degeneration of motoneurons [Leeds *et al.*, 1990; Eidelberg *et al.*, 1989]. Because the remaining nerves sprout and reinnervate the denervated muscle fibers, denervation atrophy is unlikely to contribute to wasting of muscles that receive their innervation from spinal segments below the lesion site.

Disuse Atrophy

Muscle wasting after spinal cord injury is generally attributed to the muscle inactivity that ensues after loss of the synaptic inputs from higher centers and from spinal cord segments to spinal motoneurons [Pette and Vrbova, 1992]. Studies to date, however, suggest that much of the disuse atrophy of the paralyzed muscles should be attributed to concurrent changes in muscle length or loading conditions, rather than decline in neuromuscular activity [Gordon and Patullo, 1993; Roy et al., 1991]. The magnitude of disuse atrophy varies widely from study to study in both human and animals after spinal cord lesions but does not necessarily correlate with the decline in neuromuscular activity [Alaimo et al., 1984; Lieber et al., 1986a and b; Lovely et al., 1986; Martin et al., 1992; Roy and Acosta, 1986; West et al., 1986]. Neural activity that results in neuromuscular activity is generally reduced after spinal cord lesions but varies considerably depending on the type of lesion and the level of spasticity [Alaimo et al., 1984; Gordon and Patullo, 1993; Lovely et al., 1986; Roy et al., 1991; Stein et al., 1992].

Disuse atrophy is more pronounced in paralyzed muscle that normally bears weight especially those that cross single joints [Alaimo et al., 1984; Gordon and Patullo, 1993; Lovely et al., 1986; Roy et al., 1991; Stein et al., 1992]. These muscles often contain a large proportion of slow fatigue-resistant muscle fibers, which are largely responsible for maintaining posture and bearing weight [McComas, 1977; Greensmith and Vrbova, 1997]. For example, the soleus muscle, a postural muscle that extends the ankle, undergoes significant atrophy. In contrast, the atrophy may be negligible in other muscles in the lower limb that do not bear weight or that cross more than one joint. For example, the tibialis anterior (TA) muscle, which flexes the ankle and does not normally contract against resistance, does not atrophy as much as the Soleus muscle in a number of species, including humans [Gordon and Patullo, 1993; Roy et al., 1991]. The Medial Gastrocnemius (MG) muscle, which crosses both the knee and ankle joints, also undergoes less atrophy than the Soleus muscle although it is a synergist to the soleus muscle.

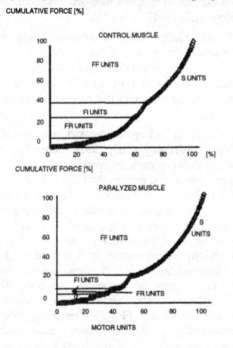

Fig. 3.6: Cumulative tetanic force of sampled motor units in normal and paralyzed Gastrocnemius muscle in a cat. FR - fatigue resistant, S - slow, FF and FI - fatiguing units. The recordings are after eight months of deafferentation of one leg, from a total of 350 motor units. Adapted from Gordon and Mao, 1994, with permission.

The principles carefully examined in animal experiments hold in humans [Gordon and Mao, 1994]. Non-weight-bearing muscles demonstrate little atrophy when paralyzed [Martin et al., 1992]. For example, subjects with complete C5 to C6 lesions;

the paralyzed thenar [Yang et al., 1990] and TA [Stein et al., 1992] muscles developed isometric forces very similar to those in able-bodied individuals. In contrast, the quadriceps femoris muscle, which normally lifts the lower limb by extending the knee, shows significant atrophy after spinal cord injuries [Kralj and Bajd, 1989].

A similar pattern of atrophy of limb muscles is seen after space flight, hind-limb suspension, limb immobilization, and other conditions in which muscles undergo shortening contractions that are not resisted by normal load [Gordon and Patullo, 1993; Roy et al., 1991; Baker, 1983]. These finding also suggest that changes in loading or length of paralyzed muscles after spinal cord lesions are responsible at least in part, for the atrophy that occurs.

The most severe disuse atrophy occurs in unloaded muscles that are immobilized at a shortened length or tenotomized [Baker, 1983]. Muscle fiber degeneration is particularly widespread in tenotomized muscles that undergo unopposed shortening contractions [Gordon et al., 1993b].

3.1.10 Fatigue in Paralyzed Muscles

The ability of muscles to sustain force over time depends on their fiber type composition, their metabolic profiles and the general nutritional and cardiovascular state of the organism. Slow-twitch muscles contain mainly slow oxidative fibers, which do not fatigue readily. Fast-twitch muscles contain a small proportion of the slow fibers and mostly fast fibers, which vary in their oxidative and glycolytic enzyme profiles, and the: corresponding susceptibility to fatigue [Burke, 1981; Enoka, 1988; Sargeant and Kernell, 1993].

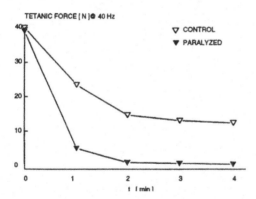

Fig. 3.7: Decline in tetanic force of medial gastrocnemius muscle as a function of time during a fatigue test before (open triangles) and 92 days after (closed triangles) paralysis unilateral deafferentation. The muscle was stimulated with 13 pulses at 40 Hz repeated every second for 4 minutes. Adapted from Gordon and Mao, 1994, with permission.

In paralyzed humans or animal models of spinal cord injuries (Figure 3.7), the capacity of paralyzed muscles to sustain contractions is dramatically reduced [Kralj and Bajd, 1989; Stein et al., 1992]. This effect of spinal cord injury on muscle endurance [Lieber et al., 1986a and b] is illustrated in an animal model of spinal cord injury. Within four minutes of repetitive activity, the tetanic force of paralyzed muscles declines to 3 percent of initial values as compared with 33 percent in the contralateral control muscles. The increased susceptibility to fatigue is accounted for by a reduced number of fatigue-resistant motor units in the paralyzed muscles, which, in turn, reflects a reduction in oxidative capacity of the muscle fibers (Figure 3.6).

Sprouting in Partially Denervated Muscles

Reversal of denervation atrophy in a partially denervated muscle depends on how many motoneurons survive the spinal cord injury and their ability to increase the number of muscle fibers that they supply by sprouting. Sprouting occurs from the terminal regions of the intramuscular nerve branches and serves to reinnervate denervated muscle fibers that lie nearby [Brown et al., 1981; Wernig and Herrarra, 1986]. Normally, motoneurons innervate hundreds or even thousands of muscle fibers. The motorneuron and its muscle fibers form a motor unit. Because of sprouting, each motorneuron supplies an increased number of muscle fibers, and activation of the motor unit generates more force than normal. In animal experiments in which the number of muscle fibers per motorneuron or the motor unit force, or both, were measured, the results showed that motoneurons can supply up to five times as many muscle fibers as they normally do [Gordon and Mao, 1994].

Evidence suggests that the limit in the number of muscle fibers per motorneuron is not set by the motorneuron itself but rather by physical constraints within the partially denervated muscle that limit the distance over which the sprouts can grow to reach denervated muscle fibers [Peckham, 1987]. Normally, the muscle fibers of a single-motor unit are distributed in a discrete area, and fibers belonging to different motor units are interspersed. In partially denervated muscles, the size of the unit territories do not increase significantly, but an increasing number of muscle fibers are incorporated in each territory. These observations indicate that motor nerve sprouts tend to reinnervate muscle fibers in close proximity. Under conditions of extensive denervation, nerve sprouts are therefore unlikely to grow far enough to reinnervate the many denervated, fibers that are outside their territory. This limitation may also account for the inability of nerve sprouts from one muscle to reinnervate adjacent denervated muscles.

3.1.11 Spasticity

The definition of spasticity is a subject of diverse opinions. A frequently used definition is that of Landau [1980] which includes: 1) decreased dexterity, 2) loss of strength, 3) increased tendon jerks, 4) increased resistance to slower passive muscle stretch, and 5) hyperactive flexion reflexes (flexor spasms). On the other hand, Knutsson [1985] described almost unlimited inter individual variation in subjects with spastic paresis. This is the basis for the opinion that spasticity has to be substituted by a detailed description of each particular subject's motor dysfunction. Studies applying refined biomechanical and electrophysiological measures have revealed a significant change in the passive properties of the spastic subjects [Herman, 1968; Lowenthal and Tobis, 1957; Thilmann et al., 1991; Sinkjær et al., 1993; Sinkjær and Magnussen, 1994]. Based on such observations, the idea that changes in the intrinsic muscle properties are largely responsible for spastic hypertonia has been accepted by some researchers [Dietz et al., 1981; Dietz, 1997; Hufschmidt and Mauritz, 1985]. Other investigators conclude, however, that the major cause of spastic muscle hypertonus is the widely accepted pathological increase in the stretch reflex activity [Ashby et al., 1987, Thilmann et al., 1991]. Here, a description obtained by analyzing different peripheral factors responsible for the "muscle tone" to passive stretch in subjects with their muscles relaxed or active is given to document changes in the organization of movement after central nervous system injury.

The resistance can be divided into: 1) an increase in the passive stiffness of tendons, joints, or muscles [Lowenthal and Tobis, 1957; Herman, 1970], 2) an increase in the intrinsic stiffness of the contracting muscle fibers [Dietz et al., 1981], and 3) an increase in the stiffness mediated by the stretch reflex [Ashby et al., 1987; Thilmann et al., 1991].

Phasic Response to External Perturbation - Spasms

In addition to the increased stiffness instant, very strong, firing of the muscles has been observed. This activity is triggered by a peripheral input (e.g., touching the skin at the leg, moving the leg passively, moving the foot passively, transferring). The tetanic contraction of muscles leading typically to simultaneous bilateral extension has been documented [Kralj and Bajd, 1989]. In most paraplegic and tetraplegic subjects both legs (hips, knees, and plantar flexion) will extend generating a painful and fatiguing pattern. The movement can be so strong that it "catapults" the body from the chair. This spasm is obviously centrally mediated and peripherally triggered. Experiments with standing of paraplegic subjects showed that these bilateral spasms are enhanced in low thoracic lesion (T11-T12), yet not so common in higher thoracic and incomplete cervical lesion subjects.

In children with cerebral paralysis, it was found that during a period of minutes or longer they developed strong tonus of extensor muscles (e.g., hip extensors, and knee extensors). The extension can be so strong that it sometimes prevents a child from sitting in the chair or prevents his/her walking with assistive systems. Some of the children are treated by a dorsal root rizotomy; that is the dorsal roots innervating the extensors in the legs are cut. This leads to unrepairable denervation of leg extensors, which is not necessarily positive. Pharmaceutical treatments can decrease to some extent the spasm, yet they interfere with some other behavior and are not always effective. The prolonged extension suggests that a higher central input that inhibits the extension is missing. Many connections are changed or missing after spinal cord injury developing very individual behavior; thus it is very difficult to generalize the motor changes, but spasms occur because the input of the higher CNS centers is missing to the part of the spinal cord below the lesion.

3.1.12 The Amputation

Accidents, disease, and congenital disorders cause amputations. Approximately 74 percent of all amputations are due to peripheral vascular disease (poor circulation of the blood) and cancer, 23 percent are due to accidents, and about 3 percent are due to a problem found at birth. The accidents most likely to result in amputation are traffic accidents, followed by farm and industrial accidents. Amputations in the case of disease are performed as a lifesaving measure. A congenital disorder or defect of a limb present at birth is not an amputation, but rather a lack of development of part or all of a limb. A person born with a limb deficiency, usually can be helped by use of an artificial limb.

Sometimes amputation of part of a deformed limb or other surgery may be desirable before the application of an artificial limb. There are about 0.15 percent of the total population ion the developed part of the world, and therefore almost one million amputees at the present time.

3.2 Assessment Methods of Sensory-Motor Disorders

To facilitate communication among professionals, who treat humans with disability, and improve the effects, several classification systems have been established. In many cases, the assessment methods lack numerical scoring, and consequently it is difficult to assess the efficacy of the treatment [e.g., Collins, 1962]. With few exemptions [Bard and Hirschberg, 1965; Bromstroom, 1966; Thoroughman and Shadhmer, 1999], researchers who have investigated the functional capacity of humans with disability have abstained from describing the neuromuscular capacity *per se* and apply specially designed activities of daily living (ADL) performance testing [Adler and Tal, 1965, Caldwell *et al.*, 1969; Dinken, 1967; Grill and Peckham, 1998; Moskowitz *et al.*, 1972]. Numerical scoring has been introduced for assessing ADL [Boureslom, 1967; Dinnerstern *et al.*, 1965; Shoenning *et al.*, 1965]. The common denominator of the mentioned methods of assessment is not standardization for the motor performances of humans with disability. Results from kinematic and dynamic studies [Winter, 1990] are a measure of motor performances, yet they are not standardized for assessing the functioning; hence, they cannot be used for predicting the course and outcome of the rehabilitation treatment. It should be noticed that although no standards for many behaviors exist, many recent studies quantify the level of disability and impact from the therapy [e.g., Cob and Claremont, 1995; Feng and Mak, 1997; Frigo *et al.*, 1998; Lum *et al.*, 1999].

3.2.1 Standards for Classifying the Sensory-Motor Disability

This classification is of specific interest for classifying paraplegic and tetraplegic subjects. As described in Section 3.1.3 spinal cord injury (SCI) deprives or eliminate traffic of neural signals from periphery to brain and *vice versa*. Examination of the dermatomes and myotomes provides information, which of the cord segments is affected by SCI, in other words which part of the spinal cord in damaged. From such an examination neurological level, sensory level and motor level (independently for right and left sides), sensory scores (pin prick and light touch), motor score and zone of partial preservation can be documented. The most recently adapted ASIA scale is replacing the modified Frankel classification since it provides a more detailed measure of the impairment [Maynard *et al.*, 1997]. It is noteworthy to consider the difference between the terms impairment and disability. The disability relates to functional deficit possibly very different between subjects diagnosed with the same impairment by using scales as ASIA [Ditunno *et al.*, 1994], Frankel [Frankel *et al.*, 1969], Fugl-Meyer [Fugl-Meyer *et al.*, 1975], etc. Therefore, it is instrumental to use functional measures that allow assessing the quality of life and ability to perform typical daily activities. The functional independence measure (FIM) is a possible method to measure the disability of a subject with SCI (Uniform Data System for Medical Rehabilitation, State University of New York, NY, USA). The quadriplegia index of function (QIF) is another valuable classification that could help in selecting the appropriate therapy or assistive system, but also in assessing the progress during the rehabilitation process and prediction on the long-term outcome. The FIM and QIF data describe disability and complement the more traditional neurological and impairment measures.

Sensory examination requires testing of key points in each of the 28 dermatomes on the right and on the left sides of the body. At each of these key points, two aspects of sensation are examined: sensitivity to pin prick and to light touch. Appreciation of pinprick and of light touch at each of the key points is separately scored on a three-point scale: 0 - absent; 1 - impaired (partial or altered appreciation, including hyperaesthesia); 2 - normal; and NT - not testable. The testing for pin sensation is usually performed with a disposable safety pin; light touch is tested with cotton. In testing for pin appreciation, the inability to distinguish between dull and sharp sensation is graded as 0.

The list of key points shown (Figure. 3.8) can be divided in four regions of the spinal cord: *C levels*: C2 - occipital protuberance; C3 - supraclavicular fossa; C4-top of the acromnoclavicular joint; C5 - lateral side of the antecubital fossa; C6 - thumb; C7 - middle finger; C8 - little finger; *T levels*: T1 - medial (ulnar) side of the antecubital fossa; T2 - apex of the axilia; T3 - third intercostal space (IS); T4 - fourth IS (nipple line); T5 - fifth IS (midway between T4 and T6); T6 - sixth IS (level of xiphistemum); T7 - seventh IS (midway between T6 and T8); T8 - eighth IS (midway between T6 and T10); T9 - ninth IS (midway between T8 and T10); T10 - tenth IS (umbilicus); T11 - eleventh IS (Midway between T10 and T12); T12 - inguinal ligament at mid-point; *L levels*: L1 - half the distance between T12 and L2; L2 - mid-anterior thigh; L3 - medial femoral condyle; L4 - medial malleolus; L5 - dorsum of the foot at the third metatarsal phalangeal joint.; and *S levels*: S1 - lateral heel; S2 - popliteal fossa in the mid-line; S3 - ischial tuberosity; S4-5 - perianal area (taken as one level). In addition to bilateral testing of these key points, the external anal sphincter should be tested; perceived sensation should be graded as being present or absent, *i.e.*, yes being incomplete lesion and no being complete injury. Position sense and awareness of deep pressure/deep pain (absent, impaired, normal) can be assessed, but this examination should be limited to only two joints (one at the hand and one at the leg).

Motor examination is performed through the testing of a key muscle in the ten paired myotomes. Each key muscle should be examined in a rostral-caudal sequence. The strength of each muscle is graded on a six-point scale [Brunnstrom and Dennen, 1931; Daniels and Wortingham, 1972]: 0-total paralysis; 1-palpable or visible contraction; 2-active movement, full range of motion (ROM) with gravity eliminated; 3-active movement, full ROM against gravity; 4-active movement, full ROM against moderate resistance; 5-normal active movement, full ROM against full resistance; and NT-not testable.

The following muscles are to be examined (bilaterally): C5 - elbow flexors (biceps, brachialis), C6 - wrist extensors (extensor carpi radialis longus and brevis), C7 - elbow extensors (triceps), C8 - finger flexors (flexor digitorum profundus) to the middle finger, T1 - small finger abductors (abductor digiti minimi), L2 - hip flexors (iliopsoas), L3 - knee extensors (quadriceps), L4 - ankle dorsiflexors (tibialis anterior), L5 - long toe extensors (extensor hallucis longus), S1 - ankle plantarflexors (gastrocnemius, soleus). For those myotomes that are not clinically testable by a manual muscle examination (*i.e.*, C1 to C4, T2 to L1 and S2 to S5), the motor level is presumed to be the same as the sensory level. In addition to bilateral testing of these muscles, the external anal sphincter should be tested based on contractions as being present or absent. This latter information is used solely for determining the completeness of injury. Other muscles could be examined, but their grades do not contribute to the ASIA motor score.

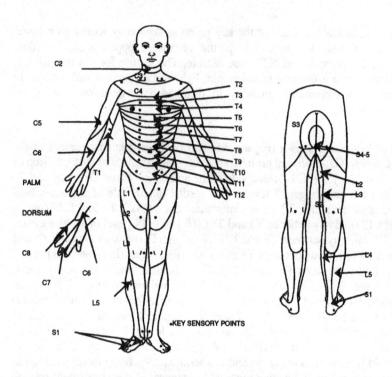

Fig. 3.8: Testing points to determine sensory loss due to spinal cord injury. The examination includes both left and right sides of the body.

Sensory scores and sensory level are obtained by using four sensory modalities per dermatome: R-pin prick, R-light touch, L-pin prick, and L-light touch. These scores should be summed across dermatomes and sides of body to generate two summary sensory scores: pinprick and light touch score. The sensory scores provide a means of numerically documenting changes in sensory function. *Motor scores and motor level* have two motor grades per paired myotome: right and left. The scores are summed across myotomes and sides of body to generate a single summary motor score. The motor score provides a means of numerically documenting changes in motor function. As shown in Section 1.1 each segmental nerve (root) innervates more than one muscle, usually two segments innervate most muscles. By convention, if a muscle has at least a grade of 3, it is considered to have intact innervation by the more rostral of the innervating segments. In determining the motor level, the next most rostral key muscle must test as 5, since it is assumed that the muscle will have both of its two innervating segments intact. For example, if no activity is found in the C7 key muscle and the C6 muscle is graded as 3, then the motor level for the tested side of the body is C6, providing the C5 muscle is graded 5.

ASIA impairment scale (modified from Frankel) [Tator *et al.*, 1982] uses the following grading of the degree of impairment: A - complete. No sensory or motor function is preserved in the sacral segments S4-S5; B - incomplete. Sensory but not motor function is preserved below the neurological level and includes the sacral segments S4-S5; C - incomplete. Motor function is preserved below the neurological level, and more than half of key muscles below the neurological level have a muscle grade less than 3; D - incomplete. Motor function is preserved below the neurological level, and at least half of key muscles below the neurological level have a muscle grade greater than or equal to 3; E - normal. Sensory and motor function is normal.

3.2.2 The Functional Independence Measure (FIM)

The FIM [Keith et al., 1987] focuses on six areas of functioning: self-care, sphincter control, mobility, locomotion, communication and social cognition. Within each area, two or more specific activities/items are evaluated, with a total of 18 items. For example, six activity items (eating, grooming, bathing, dressing-upper body, dressing lower body, and using toilet) comprise the self-care area. Each of the 18 items is evaluated in terms of independence of functioning, using a seven-point scale: 7 - Complete independence: The activity is typically performed safely, without modification, assistive devices or aids, and within reasonable time; 6 - modified independence: The activity requires an assistive device and/or more than reasonable time and/or is not performed safely. Dependent (human supervision or physical assistance is required); 5 - supervision or setup: No physical assistance is needed, but cueing, coaxing or setup is required; 4 - minimal contact assistance: Subject requires no more than touching and expends 75 percent or more of the effort required in the activity; 3 - moderate assistance: Subject requires more than touching and expends 50-75 percent of the effort required in the activity; 2 - maximal assistance: Subject expends 25-50 percent of the effort required in the activity; and 1 - total assistance. Subject expends 0-25 percent of the effort required in the activity.

Thus, the FIM total score (summed across all items; the maximum score is 126) estimates the cost of disability in terms of safety issues and of dependence on others and on technological devices. The profile of area scores and item scores pinpoints the specific aspects of daily living that have been most affected by SCI. In using the FIM with individuals who have experienced SCI, it should be kept in mind that the FIM was developed for the disabled population in general. It samples those areas of activity that have been found to be affected by impairment among diverse disability groups. Although basic issues of reliability and validity of the FIM have been explored by the developers, its validity as an instrument for precisely gauging changed functioning with all SCI subpopulations has yet to be demonstrated empirically. For example, it is not yet clear that the self-care items sensitively gauge changes in self-care functioning experienced by tetraplegic subjects during the course of rehabilitation. Further, the reliability estimates for the communication and social cognition areas have been found to be lower than for other areas assessed. The use of the FIM is relatively simple; it reflects functional issues of importance to SCI [Ditunno, 1992]. Specific instructions for use of the FIM can be obtained directly from the developers of the FIM (Uniform Data System for Medical Rehabilitation, State University of New York, NY, USA).

3.2.3 The Quadriplegia Index of Function (QIF)

The QIF is a functional assessment instrument designed specifically for use with quadriplegic persons by the Spinal Cord Injury Unit, Erie County Medical Center, Buffalo, NY, U.S.A. The QIF consist of two parts. One is composed of specific activities to be assessed by the evaluator. There are nine categories of functions to be assessed. Each activity under these nine categories is scored on a five scale (0 to 4) based on performance in order of increasing independence. The scores are: 4 - subject completely independent, needs no assistive device; 3 - subject independent with assistive device with no supervision; 2 - same as 3, yet supervision is required; 1 -

subject requires physical contact and human assistant to perform the task; and 0 - subject completely dependent, he/she is not able to do activity et all. The assessment is considering the ability of a subject to perform, not his daily behavior. Some activities are not assessed since they are sex related. The second part of the QIF is a questionnaire aiming to provide answers of the level of understanding of personal care variables; thus, cognitive independence is included in the scoring.

Nine categories are: 1) transfers (maximum 16 points). This includes transfers from bed to chair, from chair to toilet, from chair to vehicle, from chair to shower/tub; 2) grooming (maximum 12 points). Grooming comprises brushing teeth/managing dentures, brushing /combing hair, shaving, managing tampon; 3) bathing (maximum 8 points). Washing and drying upper body, lower body, feet and hair are included in four groups; 4) feeding (maximum 24 points). Drinking from cup or glass, using spoon and fork, cutting meat, pouring liquid, opening carton or jar, applying spreads to bread, preparing simple meals and applying assistive equipment are all parts of feeding; 5) dressing (maximum 20 points). Dressing is divided in upper clothes, indoor clothes, socks, shows and fasteners; 6) wheelchair mobility (maximum 28 points). Wheelchair mobility includes turning corners, reversing direction. locking the brakes, propelling on rough and uneven surface, maintaining sitting balance and moving and positioning in chair; 7) bed activities (maximum 20 points). Bed activities comprise changing and maintaining position (supine, prone, side), as well as long sitting8) bladder care (maximum 28 points). The bladder care relates to assessing voluntary voiding (toilet or commode), intermittent catheterization, indwelling catheter, ileac diversion, crede; and 9) bower care (maximum 24 points). Bowel program relates to assessing the ability for complete control (toilet and commode), suppository control, digital disimpaction, digital or mechanical stimulation.

The questionnaire, part of the QIF, relates to skin care, diet and nutrition, medication, equipment used for daily activities. It also includes physical and other plausible conditions such as autonomic dysreflexia, respiratory and other infections, deep vein thrombosis and other complication that follow tetraplegia. The final part of the questionnaire deals with human services that are available to a subject, some of them addressing the social and economical aspects of the life with SCI.

3.2.4 Muscle Assessment

The measurement of muscle strength appears to be an easy task, yet many difficult problems exist. Muscle forces are measured in isometric (length is constant), isokinetic (velocity of muscle contraction is constant) isotonic (tonus is constant) conditions. In current clinical practice, a physician or physical therapist subjectively makes most muscle strength measurements. The measurements are made by having the subject apply force against the manual constraint applied to the limb by the physician or therapist, or in some clinical end research facilities using computerized systems.

Manual Muscle Testing. The amount of restraining force needed to prevent movement of the subjects or the ability of the subject to move the limb against gravity can be manually assessed. The most popular rating system [Daniels *et al.*, 1956] uses a scale from 0 to 5 (Table 3.2). Except for grade 3, or fair, which requires a single motion through the full range of joint motion, the other tests have a large degree of subjectivity.

Isometric Testing. The quantitative testing of isometric muscle strength generally requires simpler instrumentation compared with dynamic testing. A force-measuring device needs to be positioned on the limb or portion of the body that is to be tested with a numerical readout of the measured force. The instrument may be a simple hand-held device or a more complete clinical or laboratory testing system that can measure forces associated with all the significant muscle groups from the neck down to the ankle. Hand-held devices have been reported in the literature and are commercially available either as a mechanical instrument with a mechanical readout or as an electronic instrument with a digital readout. These devices are satisfactory for the weaker upper extremity muscle groups and for most muscle groups in subjects with muscle weakness. For the stronger lower extremity muscle groups in normal or near-normal strength subjects, the testers cannot adequately resist the subject and provide satisfactory stabilization, thereby invalidating the test results [Smidt, 1984].

Table 3.1: The scale for manual muscle testing.

Number	LETTER	DESCRIPTION
5	N - NORMAL	COMPLETE RANGE OF MOTION AGAINST GRAVITY WITH FULL RESISTANCE
4	G - GOOD	COMPLETE RANGE OF MOTION AGAINST GRAVITY WITH SOME RESISTANCE
3	F - FAIR	COMPLETE RANGE OF MOTION AGAINST GRAVITY WITH NO RESISTANCE
2	P - POOR	COMPLETE RANGE OF MOTION WITH GRAVITY ELIMINATED
1	T - TRACE	EVIDENCE OF SLIGHT CONTRACTILITY; NO JOINT MOVEMENT
0	Z - ZERO	NO EVIDENCE OF CONTRACTILITY

Dynamic Testing. Dynamic measurement of the muscle performance is dominated by isokinetic testing. Hislop and Perrine [1967] first presented the measurement technique. CYBEX was an early commercial instrument produced to make the measurement. Several new instruments with similar characteristics have recently appeared commercially. Recording the force a subject exerts against a bar moving at a constant angular velocity makes an isokinetic measurement. The CYBEX II has a movable arm that can be adjusted to an angular velocity ranging from O to 300 degrees/s. The arm remains free until a force is applied which will move the arm up to the set angular velocity. When the bar reaches the set angular velocity any additional force will be resisted because the machine will not let the velocity increase. Because the bar must produce a reaction torque of a magnitude that prevents an increase in velocity, it is frequently referred to as having an accommodating resistance. The CYBEX also has a potentiometer attached to the shaft, which gives an electrical signal indicating angular position. The Ariel Tek systems represents one of the most advanced computer-controlled devices. Besides operating in the traditional isokinetic mode, it can be programmed to have a variable velocity, which can change as a function of the arm position. It can also operate in a variable resistance mode, which can change as a function of the arm angle. The OMNITRON system presents another type of dynamic muscle strength measurement device. KIM-COM and BIODEX are commercially available isokinetic instruments designed to measure eccentric as well as isometric and concentric muscle strength. These machines generate a positive output torque that can stretch an actively contracting muscle and can also move the joint through the range of motion for therapy [Farrell and Richards, 1986]. KIM-COM and Ariel Tek have a "force mode" which attempts to limit or control the maximum force.

3.3 Movement Analysis

Methods for acquiring data that describe human movement are called movement analysis. The data is needed to allow analyses of different behaviors and correlates those with physiological findings, but it is also required for synthesis of any control algorithm that can be used for systems aiming to restore movement as it will be shown in Chapter 5. The systems used for movement analysis aim to measure: 1) movement and forces acting to the body; 2) muscle activity during the movement; and metabolic functions such as blood pressure, heart rhythm, oxygen consumption and other metabolite status. The movement analysis also comprises calculation of derived mechanical characteristics such as joint torque and forces, power consumption of the system as a whole, distribution and transfer of power from one to the next segment in the system, and the mechanical work, and over all correlation between the mechanical and metabolic parameters.

3.3.1 Instrumentation for Data Capturing - Geometry

Interrupted Light Photography

Interrupted light photography was one of the first-introduced techniques [Murray *et al.*, 1964], which provides relatively accurate and inexpensive means of measuring movement. It utilizes a walkway that is non-reflective and preferably black. The studies are done in semidarkness. An open-shuttered camera records the data. Characteristic lines at the body are marked with silver Scotch-Lite tape or reflective fabric as the targets of interest (e.g., lateral aspect of the femur, lateral aspect of the calf). While the subject walks across the darkened walkway, each source of interrupted light produces discrete images at the rate determined by the number of flashes per second. Overhead mirrors permit simultaneous recording of mediolateral motion. The data analysis is time consuming and is done manually, which makes it very unpractical and time consuming.

TV and Infrared Camera (IC) Based Systems

These techniques follow the interrupted light photography. The systems use video camera connected to a computer; they vary from relatively unsophisticated video- or motion-camera systems that simply record the movement on film [Sutherland and Hagy, 1972], videotape or in digital form for later visual inspection, possibly in slow motion or more frequently frame to frame analysis. Sophisticated systems allow three-dimensional measurements of movement, and they, automatically process data to a form being of interest [Holzreiter *et al.*, 1993]. A system that uses video camera for recordings is for example PEAK Performance, CA, U.S.A. One (2D analysis) or more cameras (3D movement) are used for recordings; the software running in standard DOS, Windows or Unix based environment allows semi-automatic or automatic capturing of data and synchronize it with other recordings (e.g., EMG of force). The kinematic data has to be synchronized with other recordings, such as EMG, or ground reaction forces in the case of posture or walking analysis. All image-based system are in principle discrete, this is to say they record "steady" pictures at given times. The speed of recordings determines the sampling rate (e.g., 50 pictures for the PAL TV systems, or up to 120 pictures for 3D virtual reality goggle-type video display). The sampling rate has to be selected following the Shannon sampling theorem that says that

3 Pathology of Sensory-Motor Systems and Assessment of Disability

the sampling rate for analysis continuous signals has to be at least double of the highest frequency component in the signal [Anthonsson and Mann, 1985].

Higher sampling rate then required will not increase the quality of recordings; it will deteriorate it by introducing the noise (artifacts). Kinematics of movement of extremities comprises mostly low frequency data. The detailed frequency analysis of walking data [e.g., Winter, 1990] shows that approximation of the original signals with Fourier series having only components from 0 to 6 Hz captures up to 99.7 percent of the original. The frequency range is larger for analyzing sport and other powerful and fast movement, but is still low. Different camera based systems select a specific frequency as default (e.g., ProReflex Motion Capture Unit, Qualisys, Sweden uses 240 samples per second as the default value).

The Peak Motus® 2000 (Peak Performance Technologies Inc., CA, U.S.A) offers features and capabilities including user-customizable calculations, more graphics tools and improved automatic point identification. In addition, KineCalc™, a formula construction module that allows the user to set up algebraic, trigonometric or logical formulas for Peak Motus® to compute. KineCalc™ has a user-friendly point and click interface for entering mathematical formulas, which allows users to set up and modify complex equations without the need of specialized programming skills or detailed understanding of mathematics. Peak Motus® continues to be the only motion measurement system available today that provides the flexibility of both videotape-based and optical marker-based coordinate acquisition to measure and assess human and animal movement.

The SELSPOT system was one of the first systems introduced for movement analysis. It consists of infrared light-emitting diodes that are placed on the subject for skeleton markers. The diodes are pulsed at different times (time division multiplexed, only one at a time) by a control unit either worn by or connected to the subject. Opto-electronic cameras are placed along the walkway so that both cameras can see each diode. Due to each marker pulsing at its own time, the light detector in the camera samples the diode as a point in space at 315 Hz and can calculate the xy coordinates without further operator intervention. The data are then transmitted to a computer for three-dimensional calculations.

VICON (Oxford Metrics Ltd., Oxford, England) system uses retroflective markers that are placed on the subject and detected by the system via infrared strobes that are placed around the camera lenses. Up to 12 cameras record markers that are attached to selected points at the body. This data is used to calculate the position of each of the markers with respect to the external reference frame with reasonable precision ($\approx$ 1 mm). Once the markers are identified in two camera views, the three-dimensional calculations can be made. VICON offers two types of cameras: one with a sampling rate of 50 frames/s and one with sampling rates up to 200 frames/s utilizing a rotating shutter to freeze the movement. With Vicon's powerful and automated

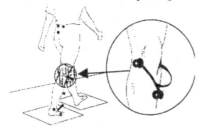

Fig. 3.9: Markers used for camera-based systems movement analysis. Adapted from Frigo *et al.*, 1998, with permission.

software, the use of 12 cameras and 50 markers is now no more complex than 6 cameras and 15 markers was a few years ago.

Northern Digital Optotrack, Waterloo, Ontario produces a variety of products. The OPTOTRAK (e.g., OPTOTRAK® 3020, 3D Motion Measurement) is a non-contact motion measurement system that tracks small infrared (IRED) markers, which are attached to a subject or object. The OPTOTRAK employs active marker positioned at the body. The OPTOTRAK Position Sensor is the main component of the system. Only one position marker is required to determine the 3D position of each marker, however, several position markers can be linked together to provide a larger, more flexible measurement volume. Several markers are used to compensate for periods when any of the markers go out of view. The OPTOTRAK position marker is able to distinguish the infrared light emitted from markers while ignoring interference from reflections and ambient lighting. The POLARIS family from Northern Digital Optotrack is another option for capturing movement. It is a set of highly versatile, low cost, real-time optical tracking systems. The POLARIS determines the real-time 6 degrees of freedom (DoF) transformations (positions and orientations) of tools based on measuring the 3D positions of markers.

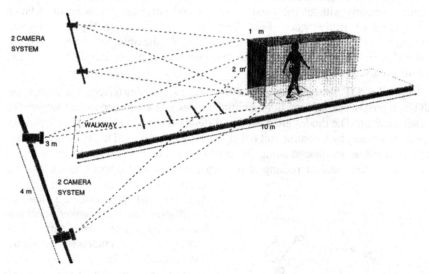

Fig. 3.10: The sketch of the gait analysis system. Adapted from Frigo *et al.*, 1998, with permission.

BTS, Bioengineering Technology and Systems, Milan, Italy is manufacturing ELITEplus (Figures 3.9 and 3.10), the new generation of fully automatic Motion Analyzers. Real time TV image processing and simultaneous collection of analog and digital signals makes ELITEplus a very quick system for multifactorial investigation of motion. Based on shape recognition of passive markers ELITEplus performs high accurate analysis of macro and micro movements. The whole system is controlled by a personal computer and is supplied with a wide range of user-friendly software packages designed for different fields of application. Thanks to computer vision techniques and to sophisticated algorithms, ELITEplus adopts the smallest markers and is environment insensitive; this leads to the highest dynamic accuracy. A modular system based on a master unit that can support up to seven slave units, ELITEplus can use up to eight TV cameras at 120 Hz. Marker detection is based on the pattern recognition technique and provides the system with great flexibility allowing its use even in the presence of disturbances brighter than markers in indoor as well as in outdoor applications (infrared flashes). ELITEplus software packages are modularly organized and provide solutions in accordance with the hardware system configuration and the customer's needs. The use of passive markers gives to the subject the greatest freedom of movements and allows the system the greatest flexibility of use with very small markers (less than 1 mm for small movements) or with large ones (up to 1 cm or more for large movements) simply by acting on zoom lenses.

Polhemus Incorporated, Colchester, VT, U.S.A. is manufacturing the Polhemus system, which employs magnetic tracking of the markers instead of visual tracking; thus the problem of "covered" markers is eliminated [Biryukova et al., 1998].

Goniometry

A goniometer measures joint angles. Electrogoniometers used in movement analysis are generally precision potentiometers that are firmly connected to a rigid mechanism, which is appropriately attached to the body; thus, when segments move, goniometers measure the rotation [Lamoreaux, 1981]. The mechanism carrying the joint angle transducer must follow the biological joint and should not constrain movement. This implies that both the transducer and the mechanism must be very light and that the leads connecting to the recording device long and flexible. The biggest problem is that the goniometer angle must be identical to the biological joint angle; this being difficult having in mind that biological joints are not simple hinge joints alike most transducers used as goniometers. Parallelogram type linkages are suitable as mechanisms to resolve the centering problem. A parallelogram mechanism allows that the axis of rotation of the transducer follows complex paths. The difficulties in using rigid structure goniometers, and needs to measure three-dimensional movement, forced the development of flexible goniometers (e.g., Penny & Giles Blackwood Ltd., UK). They use strain gauges as transducer and an intriguing design that allows the measurements to take place between two moving small plastic blocks. Flexible goniometers measure the angle between segments, thus the problem of centering of the goniometer axis to the biological one is eliminated. Similar principle for the design of a goniometer has been demonstrated by Japanese researchers several years ago; they used optical fibers to measure the deflection of the beam, being equal to joint angle. Attaching flexible goniometers is rather simple, however, not very reproducible. The accuracy of these devices is also rather low (e.g., Penny and Giles provide resolution of about 1 degree). Goniometers often use linear or taper potentiometers with continuously changing resistance that guaranty many cycles (e.g., 10000 times). Many other transducers such as relative or absolute encoders, Hall effect transducers, and gyroscopes are now incorporated in goniometers [Veltink et al., 1999].

Use of goniometers, especially with portable data acquisition systems [e.g., Popović M and Tepavac, 1992] allows prolonged measurements during normal activities. Goniometers can also use wireless communication, thus for example allow freely walking. Camera based systems provide precise results, yet they limit analysis of movement to the laboratory setting, which on the side of other problems introduces psychological constrains.

3.3.2 Gait Events Data Capturing Systems

Footswitches

Footswitches offer a fairly simple, rapid, and inexpensive approach to collecting data determining some phases of the gait cycle. Using binary information from switches mounted to determine force higher than a threshold allow calculations of walking speed, cadence, stride length, and limb support. The footswitches used in the VA-Rancho stride analyzer [Perry, 1981, 1992] are a good representative of these devices. Compression-closing switches are incorporated into flexible insole pads. The pads are divided at the forefoot-hindfoot junction to allow for differences in foot size. The insole pads can be taped to the subject's bare feet or inserted into shoes. There are four switches in each insole pad. Each one is located under the heel, the head of the fifth metatarsal, the head of the first metatarsal, and the great toe. In response to the compressive load of weight bearing, the switches close. Closure of an individual switch leads to a characteristic voltage change, which can be recorded. The four switches in the VA-Rancho system allow some determination of the foot contact pattern as well as identification of stance and swing phases.

In most footswitch systems, a pair of light beams is positioned along the line of walking progression. The light beams are arranged at a known distance from one another. As the walking subject passes each beam, a signal is received in the recording device. Thus, data about distance traveled and time are acquired in parallel with timing of switches.

Footswitches have disadvantages. Although minimal, attachment of devices to the subject is required and any attachment of instrumentation represents a modification of normal conditions. The biggest problem is the sensitivity.

Instrumented Walkway

The instrumented walkway offers a technique for determining the stride characteristics without attaching any devices to the subject at all. Sensors are all on the floor, not the subject. A representative device is the system developed at the University of Iowa [Brand et al., 1981]. A series of switches are mounted transversely along a walkway and covered by a protective mat. The switches are connected to a computer allowing time analysis of gait. The main problem with this system is that the walking is restricted to bipedal (no hand supports), and if both legs contact the same switch, this event can not be distinguished.

3.3.3 Instrumentation for Recording Contact Forces

Matrix insoles for pressure distribution and force measurement

The matrix insole method to capture distribution of forces and calculate the total force follows the footswitch application. The foot switch application provided the timing, but it was not capable of providing the amount of force information. The most frequently used system relies on thin imprints with number made of piezoresistive material. The force resisting sensors (FSR) have been used in various combinations, and provided reasonable, however, far from accurate recordings. The FSR (Interlink, CA, U.S.A.) has hysteresis, its output depends on the eventual bending of the sensor even if force is not applied, the resistance is dependent on the temperature and humidity and highly nonlinear, however, most problem can be compensated with intelligent processing of data.

The F-Scan system (Teckscan Inc., Boston, MS, U.S.A.) uses conductive and resistive inks on a flexible mylar substrate to form a matrix of 960 sensors on a disposable, 0.1 mm thick insole. Depositing a layer of conductive ink between two orthogonal conductors forms each 5 mm^2 sensing element. The matrix is scanned at 165 Hz per sensor with a resolution of 8 bits, yielding a sensitivity of ±4 kPa. Data are transmitted over a lightweight cable to a host computer.

Pedotti with coworkers [Dario *et al.*, 1983, 1984] used an insole from a film of the piezoelectric polymer, polyvinilylidene fluoride (PVDF). Circular aluminum disks of 6 mm diameters were deposited onto the film to form transducer at 16 sites. The recordings have been reproducible; ±3 percent differences were documented between different sensors and recording sessions.

Force plates

Advanced Mechanical Technology Inc. (AMTI), Newton, MS, U.S.A. supplies many research and clinical laboratories with systems to measure forces. An example is the OR6 Series force platforms. Specific uses include gait analysis, stability analysis, neurological analysis, prosthetics fitting, *etc.* The OR6 Series force platforms incorporate strain gages mounted on four precision strain elements to measure forces and moments. As with all conventional strain gauge transducers, bridge excitation and signal amplification are required. AMTI's amplifiers are high gain devices, which provide excitation and amplification for multiple channels. Automated data collection and reduction requires a computer and software are part of the system; thus the measured data allow precise automatic calculation of forces (three orthogonal force components along the X, Y, and Z axes), and the moments about the three axes, producing a total of six outputs. The high sensitivity, low crosstalk, excellent repeatability and long term stability of these platforms make them ideal for research and clinical studies.

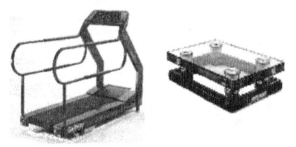

Fig. 3.11: The force platform instrumented treadmill (left) and the glass top force platform (right). Kistler Instrumente AG Winterthur, Switzerland.

Kistler (Kistler Instrumente AG Winterthur, Switzerland) is the pioneer in manufacturing force plates. The force transducers in Kistler platforms are piezoelectric devices. A portable multicomponent force plate measuring ground reaction forces and moments acting in any direction (9286 Slimline Force Plate) is frequently used in research and clinical facilities. The plates unique low-profile (35mm), light weight, wide measuring range, high center-of-pressure accuracy and low installed cost make it ideal for use in basic gait research and balance assessment. The following parameters can be measured and/or calculated using the software BioWare: force and moment measurements in all three axes, coordinates of the center of pressure, coefficient of friction, vertical (frictional) torque about center of pressure, power and energy, movement of center of mass in all three axes. The force plate is compatible with most movement analysis systems. The multicomponent force measuring plate (Figure 3.11, right) is also manufactures with a glass plate (9285 Multicomponent Glass-Top Force Plate) is designed for applications where video contact with the force platform while measuring ground reaction forces is needed. The outputs of the four 3-component force sensors are internally combined into 8 channels to allow force and torque measurements in all three axes.

Kistler is also supplying the Gaitway®, a piezoelectric ground reaction force measurement system housed in a commercially manufactured treadmill (Figure 3.11, left). What makes this treadmill unique is the ability to measure vertical ground reaction force and center of pressure for complete, consecutive, multiple foot strikes during walking and running. The instrumented treadmill system has been designed using a patented tandem force plate design (one plate in front of the other) and includes a patented algorithm which distinguishes left and right strikes. The Gaitway® allows collecting the data from the force sensors located in the bed of the treadmill, separates the left and right foot strikes, plots the results, and enables the user to selectively print and export data to other programs. The vertical force measurements allow for calculation of force, center of pressure, and temporal (time-based) gait parameters.

3.3.4 Energetics of Walking

The standard unit used in gait analysis for measurement of energy consumption is the amount of oxygen consumed by the body. The basis for this convention is the physiological production of metabolic energy from the combination of oxygen and carbon to form carbon dioxide. The oxygen consumption is determined by measuring the oxygen in expired air during steady state walking. Conversion to more convenient energy units is accomplished by the use of the equation $E = 4.92\ V(20.93 - O_e)/100$, where V is the volume of expired air in L/min, E is the energy in kilocalories/minute, and O_e is the percentage of oxygen in the expired air. The quiet-standing oxygen consumption rate for normal adults is 22.1 ± 1.68 cal/(min kg) for males and 19.9 ± 2.60 cal/(min kg) for females [Skinner et al., 1994]. This oxygen consumption rate is approximately 25 percent higher than the quiet-lying rate. Oxygen consumption increases during walking with the square of the velocity [Inman et al., 1981]. The quadratic relationship between velocity and oxygen consumption depends on the oxygen consumption being calculated per unit body weight.

Oxygen consumption can be expressed in the basic units noted above, or, alternatively, in two other useful units. The first of these is net cost in which the oxygen consumption is determined per meter traveled. This is useful as a means of measuring the gait efficiency. The other method is useful in estimates of endurance, particularly for subjects who are quite inefficient. For this method, oxygen consumption is expressed as a percentage of the maximal aerobic capacity. Since the anaerobic threshold (the maximum limit of continuous aerobic metabolism) is about 50 percent of the predicted maximal aerobic capacity, rates of oxygen consumption near this range indicate early fatigue and poor endurance.

Energy consumption measurements can be difficult to accomplish [Cavagna, 1975]. Oxygen consumption can be measured as an averaged quantity or in an on-line manner. The oldest and most reliable method is the Douglas bag technique. This method determines average oxygen consumption by collecting expired air over a period. The air is collected in a lightweight plastic bag as the subject inspires through a one-way valve and expires through another one-way valve connected by a tube to a mouthpiece. The nose is sealed with a clip. A thermistor can be used to measure respiratory rate. For safety, the electrocardiogram (ECG) is monitored by telemetry to obtain heart rate. Further, a heel switch is used to determine cadence, while velocity is an average over a prescribed distance and a measured time. It is important to obtain steady-state values, and monitoring heart rate and respiratory rate can assist in this. A large respiratory "dead space" must be avoided to prevent re-breathing carbon dioxide which would cause hyperventilation. The oxygen in the bag is measured by determining the total volume and percentage O_2. A standard laboratory blood gas meter can be used. On-line systems can be utilized instead of the Douglas bag. Beckman has a cart on wheels to measure the same parameters. This can be wheeled along next to a subject or alternatively used next to a treadmill. Similarly, Waters Instrument Corp. (Rochester, MN) has a portable metabolic unit utilizing an electrolysis technique to measure O_2 content.

The blood pressure and heart rate can be used as measures of the cardiovascular stress. Heart rate is easily obtained by ECG, and is readily amenable to telemetry. Burdett *et al.* [1983] suggested the use of a physiological cost index (PCI). The relation is PCI = $(H_w - H_r)/S$, where H_w is heart rate (beats/min) while walking, H_r is heart rate when resting, and S is average speed (m/min).

3.3.5 Capturing Muscle Activity - EMG

Recordings of muscle action during movement are useful for analyzing which muscles and at what times they are active. EMG recordings can be obtained with either surface-mounted electrodes or indwelling fine-wire electrodes. Surface electrodes are commercially available in various sizes and are used to gather muscle group activity or information from larger superficial muscles. When information about a specific muscle, a small superficial muscle, or a deep muscle is desired, indwelling fine-wire electrodes must be used.

Fine-wire electrodes are usually 50 μm in diameter; thus, they can be inserted easily through a single 25- or 27-gage disposable needle. The electrode makes the contact over the stripped insulation at the tip of the wire (<5 mm) [Basmajian, 1978]. When the correct placement is obtained, the needle is withdrawn and the wire ends protruding from the skin are connected to appropriate terminals.

Testing of electrode placement is accomplished by use of audioamplifiers, oscilloscopes, and, for the indwelling electrodes, muscle stimulators. Using muscle testing techniques [Beasley, 1961], the subject is asked to contract or use the muscle of interest, and the examiner evaluates the signal for appropriate interference patterns during the activity. When testing is satisfactory, then the EMG signals can be recorded during movement.

Beckman produces a popular type of surface electrodes. The Beckman electrodes come in two sizes (small- and large-diameter). Two electrodes can be fixed to a bar for ease of use, and so the electrode distance would always be the same. The EMG signals are vary small, and the interference noise large. Motion artifacts are specifically problematic because the wires are moving in the variable electromagnetic field. In order to minimize motion artifacts preamplifiers, being very small, to amplify the signal for about two to three orders of magnitude should be used as close as possible to recording electrodes. The Motion Control Incorporated, Salt Lake City, UT, U.S.A. is supplying surface electrodes built together with the preamplifiers having a gain of typically 350. This system is convenient because it can be easily applied and it guaranties excellent noise rejection. The amplifier built into the MCI electrodes requires external power.

The frequency content of EMG signals is up to about 1500 Hz; however, the maximum power is at much lower frequencies ($\approx$200 Hz). This information is relevant for selection of the sampling rate when collecting EMG. Typical cut-off frequency for EMG is at 1 kHz, but the actual decision is based on the analysis required.

EMG signals can be transmitted from electrodes to a computer for storing and analysis by using wires or radio-frequency wireless communication. Electrodes and preamplifiers can be directly connected to amplifiers and recording devices by cable. Cabled systems provide reliable data and clean signals. Mechanically, cabled systems are simple. It is important to use shielded cables to reduce movement artifacts. Cabled EMG amplifiers should have optical or transformer isolation as a safety precaution, to ensure those subjects cannot be injured from the EMG testing device.

During movement, cables used for signal transmission must be carefully fixed to allow free movement, and get out of the way. When walking this is a bigger problem since the wires must be long enough. There are several portable, multichannel systems that can capture EMG and other movement data using a microcomputer based system similar to Holter monitor [e.g., Tepavac and Nikolić, 1992]. Wireless communication allows the subject freedom of movement. Modern wireless transmitters are lightweight and easily attached to the subject. Routine dynamic electromyography using surface or wire electrodes can demonstrate the timing of muscle action during function.

3.3.6 Measurable Characteristics of Walking

Bipedal walking is an extremely complex motor control task. It requires the integration of the central nervous system with many peripheral sensory systems to control many muscles acting on a skeletal system with many degrees of freedom. The human mechanical system operates in a gravitational environment having a rather small base of support, a center of mass located at a considerable distance from the ground, making it difficult to ensure stable vertical posture. While walking, it is important to control the swinging leg to safely move without touching the ground and to provide gentle landing at the ground at the end of the swing. The regulation of such a system requires a neural control that has well defined total limb synergies, but is also flexible enough to respond to a wide variety of dangerous perturbations, and adaptable enough to anticipate changes sufficiently well in advance [Winter, 1991].

There are scores of variables that can be quantified allowing the insight to the control of walking. For the purposes of analysis, one can distinguish measurable and model based estimated variables. Measurable variables are: cadence, stride length, step length, joint angles, ground reaction forces, electrical activity of muscles (EMG), and

Table 3.2: Parameters of normal walking for male, female and 5 years of age child.

	FEMALE	MALE	CHILD (5 years)
VELOCITY [m/s]	1.4± 0.15	1.5± 0.2	1.05±0.05
DURATION T - GAIT CYCLE [s]	1.03± 0.08	1.06± 0.09	0.77± 0.06
CADENCE [step/s]	117± 9	113± 8	153± 11
STRIDE LENGHT [m]	1.37± 0.1	1.60± 0.18	0.86± 0.08
DURATION SSP [%T]	38± 4	40± 5	51± 10
DURATION SWING [s]	0.39± 0.03	0.41± 0.04	not measured
DURATTION STANCE [s]	0.64± 0.06	0.65± 0.07	not measured
LAT. MOTION OF HEAD [m]	0.04± 0.01	0.06 ± 0.01	not measured
VERT. MOTION OF HEAD [m]	0.04± 0.01	0.05± 0.01	not measured

metabolic energy cost and rate. Model based variables are: joint forces and torque, mechanical work and power, and mechanical energy. All of the listed variables are outcome measures, and because of the tremendous convergence and redundancy of the motor system, they do not lead to one ultimate answer about the organization of the natural control. It is possible, however, to build evidence that will eventually provide complete explanation of the organization of the natural control.

Walking over the flat, even terrain without obstacles results from cyclic movement of many parts of the body. The *gait cycle* is the elementary sequence of walking

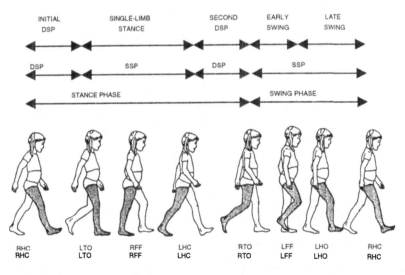

Fig. 3.12: Phases of the gait cycle. DSP – Double Support Phase, SSP – Single Support Phase, RHC – Right Heel Contact, LTO – Left Toe-Off, RFF – Right foot-Flat, LHC – Left Heel Contact, RTO – Right Toe-Off, LFF – Left Foot-Flat, LHO – Left Heel-Off.

(Figure 3.12). It starts when the heel of the ipsilateral leg touches the ground and ends just before the same heel touches the ground again. The heel contact is termed the initial contact; thus, the gait cycle is a period between two initial contacts. The duration of the gait cycle is often normalized to allow that specific events during the cycle can be expressed in percent. This allows inter-comparison between different individuals while walking under same conditions. There is no standard defining "normal" walking, because there are differences between male and female, different age groups, different races, and even within the same group of humans. There are common features, however, that are characteristic for all able-bodied subjects when walking. The gait cycle can be divided into two distinct phases: the stance phase, when the foot is at the ground, and the swing phase, when the foot is off the ground. The stance phase for normal, self-paced, level walking lasts for 60 to 65 percent of the gait cycle, while the swing phase lasts for the remaining 35 to 40 percent (Figure 3.12).

The patterns of walking are different for various environmental conditions (e.g., level, slope, stairs), directions of walking (forward, backwards, sideways, walking in circle), and different speeds of walking (slow, average, and fast).

The gait cycle can also be partitioned based on the number of legs contacting the ground (Figure 3.12). The period during which both legs have ground contact is called *double support phase (DSP)*, and the period during which only one leg is contacting the ground is called *single support phase (SSP)*. The gait cycle is composed of two DSPs and two SSPs. The first DSP starts simultaneously with the stance phase of the ipsilateral leg and lasts up to the moment when the contralateral leg starts the swing being between 16 and 20 percent of the gait cycle. The SSP is equivalent with the swing phase, and it lasts for 30 to 34 percent. The duration of the swing phase changes very little, in absolute terms, when the speed of walking changes; hence, the variation of the stance phase determines the duration of the gait cycle.

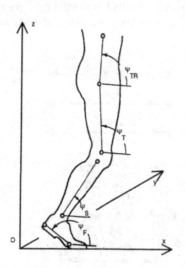

Fig. 3.13: Angles between the segments and the horizontal axis used to determine the joint angles.

The stance phase is sequenced to several sub-phases: *heel-contact, foot-flat, heel off,* and *toe-off*. Some use a terminology that distinguishes the stance phase to only three sub-phases: *early-, mid-,* and *late-stance phase*. The swing phase is sequenced to: *initial- and terminal swing, and initial-* and *terminal extension*, or using a different terminology to *earl-, mid-,* and *late swing*. The sub-phases of the gait cycle are fairly consistent for normal adults and children, yet altered in subjects with disabilities resulting from pain, spasticity, joint instability, or subjects walking with assistive devices (e.g., prosthesis).

The path along which the center of mass of the body moves during one gait cycle is termed the *gait stride*, and it is measured as the distance between the point contacted by the same heel in the two consecutive gait cycles. The *step length* is the distance between the heel contacts of the ipsilateral and the contralateral foot within the same gait cycle. The *cadence* is the number of steps per unit time (the number of times that both feet contact the ground). The reason for distinguishing the step from the stride is the walking symmetry. If the steps with the left and right leg are identical and time shifted for 50 percent of the gait cycle, the walking is symmetrical. A summary of normal values for stride characteristics of adults and children is found in Table 3.1.

Kinematics of Walking

In order to quantify the kinematics of walking, one has to select the system of reference. Movement of the segments can be defined in the external reference frame (e.g., the Descartes orthogonal coordinate system), in the internal coordinates (e.g., joint angles), or in the phase plane formed by arbitrarily selected state variables (e.g., joint angular velocities). If the walking pattern is known in one reference system, then it is possible, although not necessarily simple, to transform the change to the different reference frame by using transform matrices.

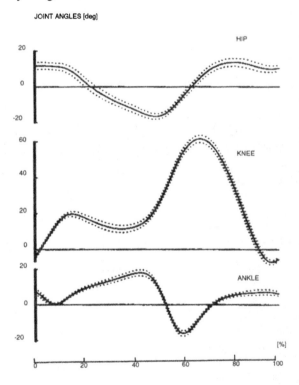

Fig. 3.14: Joint angle trajectories for normal walking of an able bodied subject. Dashed lines show standard deviation for 18 successive strides. Adapted from Winter, 1990, with permission.

The external coordinate system is typically positioned so that the Oxz plane (Figure 3.13) is parallel to the sagittal plane, and the direction of forward walking is along the Ox axis, Oz axis is vertical and anti-parallel to the gravity (Figure 3.13). The Oy axis is perpendicular to the plane Oxz. The Oy and Oz axes determine the frontal plane, while, the axes Ox and Oy determine the horizontal plane. The analysis of walking frequently considers a reduced, planar movement of the body. This reduction of the three-dimensional to two-dimensional movement assumes that all points of the body are moving in planes parallel to the sagittal plane, ultimately rotations of the segment are about the axes perpendicular to the sagittal plane.

Body movement can be described relatively to the neighboring segments, and in this case internal coordinates, the joint angles define walking. The body is composed of many bones, which form simple and complex joints. The walking involves most of the body segments, however, some are being dominant compared with others when analyzing movement. As one would expect, the leg segments are the most important for walking, which in no way should diminish the importance of the upper body and arms for the process. The joint angles are defined in reference to the position on neighboring segments (Figure 3.13). The segments of the body during the walking are assumed as rigid bodies; thus, the joint angles define the position of an arbitrary point of the body during walking.

The joint angles typically used for describing walking are (Figure 3.13):

$\varphi_A = \varphi_F - \varphi_S - \pi/2,$

$\varphi_K = \varphi_S - \varphi_T, \varphi_H = \varphi_T - \varphi_{TR}$

A typical record of trajectories of the hip, knee, and ankle is presented in Figure 3.14. This record relates to the reduced planar model of walking.

The phase space reference frame is used to characterize the inter-relationship, if any, between some internal or external coordinates during the walking. Figure 3.15 shows the state space representation of pelvis movement. Two different walking sessions of the same subject are presented. In the first one, the subject was walking slowly, at an average speed of v = 1.25 m/s, while in the second series he walked at average speed v = 1.9 m/s. The phase space diagram does not include the time explicitly. The state space trajectory shows implicitly how a specific point is moving in time. The full circles show right heel contact, empty square the left toe-off,

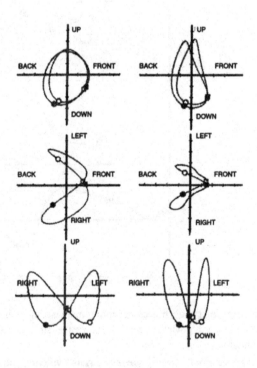

Fig. 3.15: Phase space diagram showing the hip movement for two speeds. See text for details. Adapted from Cappozzo, 1991, with permission.

empty circle the left heel contact, and the full square the right toe-off. The diagrams show the repetitive nature of movement.

Ground Reaction Force

There are two major external forces acting during walking: gravity and the ground reaction force. The media resistance and viscous drag will not be discussed since they play a significant role only under special conditions (e.g., walking with the legs under water, walking when exposed to a very strong wind). Some authors include inertial forces, but one should remember that those are fictive forces, *i.e.*, just the terms used within the methodology introduced by D'Alembert. Inertial forces and torque are fictive dynamic variables that are defined based on the inertial properties of the body and accelerations in general sense. Inertial forces and torque are terms making it possible to transform dynamic equations of movement into the form of equilibrium equations [e.g., Goldstein, 1957].

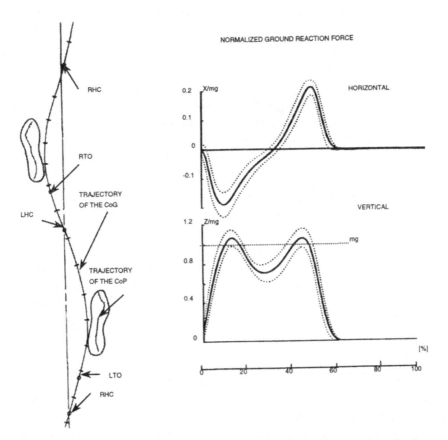

Fig. 3.16: The trajectory of the Center of Gravity (CoG) (left), and the ground reaction forces normalized to the bodyweight of the subject during normal walking. Adapted from Winter, 1990, with permission.

The force of interest for analyzing the walking is the ground reaction force. The ground reaction force is a passive force except in the case that the support is moving with some acceleration relative to the body. The ground reaction force is a reaction of the ground to a walking human. The normal component of the ground reaction exists as the consequence of gravity, while the transversal component is a result of friction. The friction force is always smaller or equal to the product of the normal ground reaction force and the coefficient of friction. The friction force, being passive, is the only external force that acts at the body in the direction of progression (level walking). A typical record of ground reaction forces in vertical and the direction of walking is presented in Figure 3.16 (right panel). The force is equal to zero during the swing phase of the gait cycle.

Walking is a dynamic process, where the small bases supports the whole body during the SSP, and then the body weight is transmitted to the other leg/foot during the DSP. The ground reaction force is distributed over the surface touching the ground. Using techniques of vector operations developed for mechanics, one can replace all the component forces acting at one foot with only one force and one moment-of-force (torque). The point through the force crossing the sole is called the *center of pressure (CoP)*. The center of pressure is constantly moving over the sole, while walking or standing. Gravity acts to all masses composing the body, and for the purposes of analysis, they can all be replaced with a single resultant force acting at the point called the *center of mass (CoM)*.

The center of mass is projecting to the ground, and it is called *center of gravity (CoG)*. During quite standing the CoG must belong to the surface determined with feet, so-called support base (see Chapter 2). In contrast, during walking the CoG rarely belongs to the zone where the sole contacts the ground. During the DSP the CoG is within the area determined with feet (Figure 3.16, left panel). During the SSP, the CoG is out of the zone determined with the sole of the supporting foot. This all supports the concept that walking is a cyclic process during which a human intentionally leans to an unstable (falling) position, and then by activating muscles puts the leg in a position that prevents a fall. During this "falling" phase, the center of mass accelerates; the body is gaining kinetic energy because of the gravity. Once the "new support leg" prevents the fall, the center of mass starts going up against the gravity; the kinetic energy is now transformed to the potential energy. This process is repeated at every step (twice during one gait cycle). Some kinetic energy will be lost at impact of the foot with the ground (heel contact), and this is the reason why the foot must gently touch the ground. Part of the impact energy will be stored in the elastic elements of the foot and shank, and recuperated during the push-off phase. One can easily see the effects of impact and recuperated energy by walking on the hard and soft supports (e.g., unpacked sand).

Energetics

Metabolic energy is required for muscle contractions. Muscular contractions result with forces that act on body segments and generate movement. The amount of energy consumption is directly related to the amount of oxygen used by the body. The energy consumption rate can be estimated by measuring the volume of oxygen consumed per unit time. The amount of oxygen is expressed as its volume (m^3); hence the rate is expressed in m^3/s, while the energy rate is expressed in Joules (J) per second (s). In order to have measures that are easy to memorize and use by clinicians, the energy rate is usually expressed in Kcal/min, and instruments for measuring flow of gasses show the amount of oxygen in liters per minute. The rate of 0.2 liters of oxygen per minute corresponds to an energy rate of 1 kilocalory/minute. In addition, the energy consumption is expressed per distance that was covered, and this is termed energy cost per distance.

Energy cost and rate can be expressed in a number of different ways when walking is considered. The energy costs of walking per unit distance, per unit body mass, or per step are all used in clinical practice. When energy consumption per unit body weight is expressed as a function of velocity, there is a minimum in the energy consumption at approximately 1.4 meters per second. For able-bodied adults the average velocity of normal level walking is included in the Table 3.1. Walking slower or faster leads to the increased metabolic cost. Similarly, greater mass increases the energy consumption, and it should be noticed that this energy increase is more pronounced if the mass increase is on the lower extremities rather than attached to the trunk. This follows the earlier description of the locomotion where it was concluded that the trunk behaves as a quasi-conservative system. The energy exchange (coming from muscles) is very small between the legs and the trunk (Figure 3.17). Most of the energy is used to provide posture (static work). The metabolic energy cost is higher for slower walking because muscles have to slow down ballistic and inertial movements, and it is higher for faster walking because then the muscle must generate large forces to produce adequate acceleration of segment. Furthermore, the transfer of energy rises between the legs and the trunk.

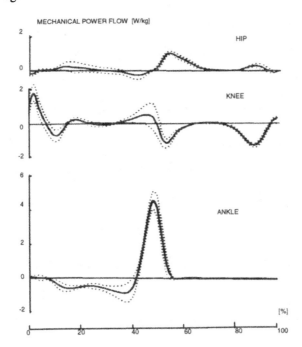

Fig. 3.17: The mechanical power at the ankle, knee and hip joints. See text for details. Adapted from Winter, 1990, with permission.

The energy cost and energy rate should not be confused with mechanical work and power. Mechanical energy that is contributing to walking is changing from kinetic to potential because of the action of muscles, gravity, and ground reaction force.

Muscle Function

The act of walking is a carefully orchestrated process in which the muscles, acting across each joint, are carefully tuned to provide efficient motion. Other muscles at both joints to provide proper action at the desired joint at the appropriate time must balance muscles that cross two joints. The action of muscles creates torque around the joints of the lower limb, which with other external imposed torque results in a net torque that

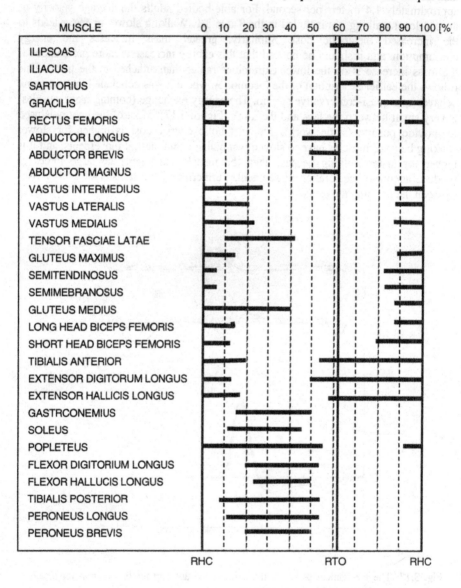

Fig. 3.18: The timing of the muscles of the leg during one gait cycle for normal walking at speed of v = 1.5 m/s [Popović, 1981].

results in movement of the skeletal structure. As it would be the case in an orchestra, the conductor has to give the rhythm and get each and every instrument that is at his disposition to play at right times with the appropriate dynamics. The conductor has to adapt to the availability and skills of players, and based on the task select a preferred tune. The perfection can be achieved only if sufficient training is allowed, and sufficient flexibility is built to ensure correction if some unpredicted event occurs. In an organism, muscles have limited strength and range of speed that they can generate, after being used for some time they can be fatigued, and certainly an injury or disease may cause that they dramatically change their performance.

It is impossible to measure individual muscle forces and other characteristics in vivo with the techniques available now. It is, however, possible to assess when they are active and estimate the level of activity by measuring the electrical activity, so-called electromyogram (EMG) (Figure 3.18).

Dynamic electromyography has permitted evaluation of the time relations of muscle function during gait. Application of electrodes to the skin surface overlying muscles can provide a measure of activity of all muscles that are contributed to the electrical signal measured at the skin. It is very difficult to record EMG from deeper muscles or distinguish between muscles that are very close from surface recorded EMG. Alternatively, fine-wire electrodes inserted into the muscles permit the recording of the electrical activity produced by any individual muscle during the walking. The electrical activity corresponds to the time of muscle contraction as well as its level of activity [Winter, 1992]. Recording of EMG has permitted a determination of the muscle function at each joint during each portion of the gait cycle.

EMG, however, is not helpful in determining whether a muscle is shortening or lengthening during its activity. In general, the motions of the lower-extremity segments place the muscles in a situation so that their length is elongated to provide the most effective function. The muscles of the lower extremity and their timing during gait are given in Figure 3.18. Most muscle activity is present at the beginning and termination of the stance and swing phases of gait because acceleration and deceleration of the segments are occurring as body weight is transferred from one foot to the other. Conversely, during mid-stance and mid-swing, little electrical activity is occurring in the muscles. The schematic shows only the timing in order to avoid ambiguity.

Joint Forces and Torque

Joint forces and torque are internal, dynamic variables that exist because of the external forces and muscle contractions (Figure 3.19). Joint forces and torque always come in pairs of anti-parallel equal vectors, acting at neighboring segments. The sum of all internal forces and torque for any given system of rigid bodies is equal to zero. Joint force and torque are the net outcome of all muscle forces and their moments in addition to the forces and torque contributed by the external forces acting at a joint being considered. Figure 3.19 shows a typical sequence of joint torque for normal walking. Joint force and torque can be estimated from measurements, yet very difficult. The muscle acts to the segment via tendons. If a cocontraction is taking place as a given joint, the analysis yields only the net effect of both agonist and antagonistic muscles.

A friction exists at any joint, but it cannot be measured *in vivo*, neither separated from the net value. Increased friction reduces the effective torque generated by muscles. The stability of a joint is secured with ligaments. Ligaments play an important role when the movement reaches the end of the physiological range; the ligaments oppose and prevent further motion. At low speeds and within the mid-range of movement, ligaments do not contribute much to the joint torque and force. The torque caused by the ligament can be measured only when the muscles are silent. The joint torque is of interest for analyzing movement, while the joint force plays a role when designing replacement parts such as artificial extremities or endoskeletal prosthesis (e.g., hip prosthesis). The methods for calculating joint forces and torque are described in Chapter 5.

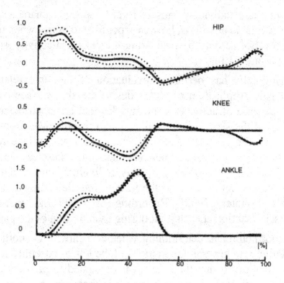

Fig. 3.19: Normalized joint torque for the normal walking pattern of a male able-bodied subject at speed v = 1.5 m/s. Adapted from Winter, 1990, with permission.

The joint torque projected to an axis is an oriented scalar variable; it is determined with its intensity and direction (Figure 3.19). The simplest way to deal with this scalar is to add the sign to the intensity; positive sign means that the projection of the torque is congruent with the axis, and if negative, then the directions are opposite. The direction of rotation of the segment can be the same as the torque, and these directions can be opposite. The same holds for angular velocities. For planar movement, the integrated product of the joint torque and the angle of rotation for a selected interval are equal to the mechanical work at the joint, and the product of the joint torque and the absolute angular velocity is the mechanical power at the joint. The products, ultimately the integrals, can be positive or negative which could lead to the conclusion that since the work is negative, energy is "produced". In both cases, the work is the result of activity of muscles; hence, metabolic energy is the source. A negative work or power means that the segment observed "receives energy" from the neighboring segments via the joint analyzed.

All data shown are all for able-bodied subjects, and it is termed normal walking, and used for comparison with data recorded in subjects with sensory-motor disorders.

4. Restoring Movement: State of the Art

> "Everything may die, nothing may be regenerated. It is for the science of the future to change, if possible, this harsh decree."
> Santiago Ramon y Cajal [1890]

The state of the art of rehabilitation technology for restoring movement is described in this chapter. The first two sections, Neuroregeneration and Neurorehabilitation, review methods to repair and/or restore natural control by surgical and therapeutic procedures. These techniques fully rely on comprehensive understanding of the organization of the organs and tissues, which are preserved, deprived, or missing after an injury or disease and utilization of the biotechnology to regain lost function. The third section, Neuroprostheses presents the functional electrical stimulation (FES) principles and tools for restoring movement. This is followed by a description of FES systems and a combination of FES with external skeleton orthoses used in humans with motor disability. The section Neuroprostheses also summarizes problems (e.g., muscle fatigue, spasticity, and low energy efficiency when standing and walking) still not resolved, which are preventing wider clinical and home usage at this time. The final section of this Chapter 4 discusses the state of the art of artificial legs, arms, and hands.

4.1 Neuroregeneration

Neuroregeneration is a technique aiming to restore neural tissues, which is lost because of the trauma or disease. There are two major issues regenerating the neural substrate and providing that once it is anatomically restored to become functional. For long time, surgery of peripheral nerves (e.g., radial and ulnar nerve repairs) allows humans to regain part of their functions after a period of time and adequate therapy and training. Many neurons after the nerve repair are not connecting to the original pathways, yet the plasticity of the nervous system allows later limited functioning [Mc Pherson, 1991]. The neuroregeneration of the central nervous system is still controversial, but the development of neural and genetic engineering will very likely make it feasible and very attractive in the future.

"Unlike peripheral nerves, axons (nerve fibers) in the brain and spinal cord do not regenerate naturally" is a typical sentence in most articles dealing with neuroregeneration of the central nervous system. The good news is that each of these articles goes on to describe some new strategy to overcome this natural self-restraint, and to report success in achieving regrowth in a laboratory test situation.

The advances in neuroscience during the last years have been astonishing. Today's breakthroughs depend on access to molecules that were first imagined nearly a century ago. Hundreds of factors (e.g., biologically active molecules) are now known, and they prove to be instrumental to promoting spinal cord regeneration. In 1906, the Nobel Prize in Physiology/Medicine was granted to two men, Camillo Golgi and Santiago Ramon y Cajal, on opposing sides of the debate about the "neuron theory." Their battlefields were the developing, degenerating and regenerating brain, spinal cord and optic nerve, in one word the central nervous system (CNS). Even these early researchers were preoccupied by the contrast between lush regrowth in peripheral nerves and failure of regeneration in the CNS.

Ramon y Cajal [1890] deducted that nerve fibers (axons) grew via a structure at their tip that he called the growth cone, writing, "*From the functional point of view, one might say that the growth cone is like a club or battering ram endowed with exquisite chemical sensitivity...*". His brilliant deductions from anatomical still-pictures were confirmed later by studies of living tissues. He concluded that the "frustrated and aborted" regeneration was due to lack of guidance factors. These seemed to be supplied in peripheral nerves by Schwann cells being absent from the CNS. In Cajal's laboratory pieces of nerve have been grafted into the CNS, proving that the nerves could regenerate when Schwann cells provide a nourishing environment [Tello, 1911].

The trophic factors needed for regeneration were unknown for many years, and new data contradicting early theories moved to investigating of dense scarring, lack of blood flow, and the overall failure of regeneration in the CNS. In parallel, spinal cord injury rehabilitation was born in England during the World War II, and many casualties were taught how to live with the disability, despite the lack of hope for recovery [Guttman, 1973]. The CNS regeneration was simply seen as unachievable. Scientists concentrated, instead, on how embryonic nerves find their targets. They analyzed growing of cells toward signals radiating from distant sources. It appeared that a well marked path is "written" at the cellular level in developing systems, where distances were small, and a few sign-post cells could guide a growing axon from point A to point B. The implications for regeneration of nerves remained bleak. If guidance depended on short distances or timed cues, then there might be little hope for rewiring the adult CNS, which is thousands of times bigger, and where carefully timed meetings between the growing fibers seems out of the question. Although the theory of long-range chemical attraction seemed more plausible, not a single attractant had been discovered.

Cajal [1928] predicted the discovery of the first growth factor. The breakthrough was the discovery of the substance that could rightfully be called the Nerve Growth Factor (NGF). Purified NGF has been analyzed and its protein structure defined. Though suspected to exist, other factors proved hard to find because they occur in such small quantities that makes experimental analysis difficult. During the seventies a new factor [Barde, 1988], acting on a different population of nerve cells than NGF, was discovered, and it is called the "brain derived neurotrophic factor" (BDNF).

In the next few years, the new factors were discovered so quickly that they were simply numbered: neurotrophins [Heumann, 1994]. The pace of scientific discovery had gone from almost forty years for NGF to little more than a decade for BDNF, to only a few years for new members of the neurotrophin family and several other such families. Human nervous systems work via accurately mapped nerve connections. Effective regeneration will depend on understanding the cues growth cones used to locate their targets during development. Signals lie in the cellular terrain. The growth cones detect and grow along other cells or on proteins that surround them (extracellular matrix, seeking out surfaces that promote growth. Several promoters on cells, called cell adhesion molecules, have been identified. When the cells touch, the cell adhesion molecules on their surfaces stick, as happens when axons grow in bundles through the CNS.

The attention was focused for most of the century on long and short-range attractive (tropic) or nutritive (trophic) molecules. Failure of regeneration in the CNS was attributed to the lack of these or to mechanical barriers. In the mid-eighties Schwab [Schwab and Caroni, 1988] showed that CNS myelin actually repels growth cones. Much excitement has surrounded the findings suggesting that blocking these blockers to hide them from growing nerve fibers can improve regeneration.

Other inhibitors were soon found in myelin, on other cell surfaces. For example, proteoglycans, form chemical barriers around injuries, preventing even growing axons from crossing the region. Very recent work shows that some growing axons that escape these barrier zones can grow long distances, even when other inhibitors are present.

Studies of Schwann cells led Bunge [Bunge *et al.,* 1993] to propose that these growth-promoting cells, derived from a patient's nerves, could be used to bridge CNS injuries clinically (Figure 4.1).

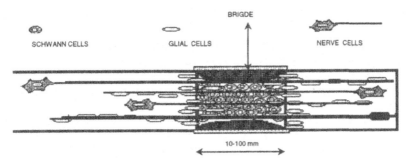

Fig. 4.1: Schwann cell bridge for grafting peripheral nerves into the spinal cord. Schwann cell bridge and ensheathing glia cells have been placed and after about six weeks some nerve cells "grow" through the bridge. Modified from The Miami Project to Cure Paralysis Newsletters: The Project, XI(2), 1998.

Aguayo and his colleagues [Aguayo, 1985] revisited the work in Cajal's Laboratory [1928] of grafting peripheral nerves into the spinal cord. They showed that grafted nerve segments allow damaged spinal nerve fibers to grow through the graft to the CNS border. Using new techniques to trace nerve fibers, they proved conclusively that CNS regeneration is possible in adult mammals.

Two grafting strategies emerged as promising for spinal cord injury (SCI): fetal spinal cord and peripheral nerves Schwann cells. Both were based on the idea of substituting the barren CNS environment with one that naturally supports nerve growth. Fetal tissues offered the possibility of replacing nerve cells as well as providing support cells (glia), as demonstrated by Reier and coworkers [Reier and Houle, 1988, Goldman, 2000]. The use of fetal human tissue would be difficult for both technical and ethical reasons, yet initial trials are taking place in SCI persons with expanding cysts to determine the safety of the procedure and survival of the grafts. Schwann cell and peripheral nerve grafts do not replace nerve cells, but do show a unique capacity to bridge gaps in spinal tissue. Recently, emphasis has been on why nerve fibers grow long distances within these bridges, but stop at the CNS/peripheral nerve junction (Figure 4.2).

Adding growth factors enhances both strategies. Bregman [Bregman et al., 1993, 1994] and Kuhlengel [Kuhlengel et al., 1990] reported that fetal grafts regenerate best into spinal Schwann cell or peripheral nerve grafts when growth factors are added. Cheng and Olson [Cheng et al., 1996, 1998; Olson et al., 1998] reported that a complex combination of peripheral nerve Schwann cells, a growth factor, a blood product, and surgical stabilization promote regeneration from cells in the rat brain through and beyond a complete injury, improving locomotion. This result, however, has not been reproduced in other laboratories testing the technique, but researchers agree that some combination of strategies will probably be needed for substantial regeneration and restoration of function to be accomplished.

It has been demonstrated that the adult human spinal cord is rewiring somewhat after SCI. Stepping motions, coordinated by spinal nerve circuits, can be enhanced with training (see the following section). It is clear that a person with SCI will not need to regrow all the damaged spinal cord connections to regain some function. Rather, fibers carrying some information from above the site of injury to nerve cells below it could improve the functional status significantly by influencing the spinal nerve circuits. Growth within the cord tissue beyond the injury will be needed, and this may require overcoming CNS inhibition.

Researchers show understandable caution in transferring the techniques from basic laboratory to human trials. Clinical researchers agree that a first step in human trials is assessing the safety of new treatments. A new treatment then will be accepted if it is proven to significantly improve the function in randomly selected patients. Proving effectiveness requires rigorous and objective follow-up; anecdotal or vague claims of improvement rarely pan out. The strongest tools are systematic studies that separate chance occurrences from real effects of a treatment. Misinterpreting cases of natural recovery from SCI as being the effect of an experimental treatment can lead to costly and possibly debilitating procedures that do not offer real hope for recovery, and may diminish the chance to pursue better proven therapies later.

Fulfilling the promise of regeneration research by moving to clinical treatments is a long process, because there are still many unknowns. The studies described here overturned the dogma that CNS regeneration cannot occur, but further work is needed before applying these strategies clinically. Human injuries are each unique, so clinical scientists take great care in transferring experimental results to use in patients.

"The cure" is likely to be a combination of strategies that restore function – no single therapy will qualify. Treatments involving protecting the CNS at the time of trauma, complex transplantation strategies, and subsequent rehabilitative retraining that includes assistive systems will probably yield the most successful results in restoring function after SCI.

4.1.1 Techniques to Regenerate CNS Structures

Among the array of strategies being tested, the problem of bridging a gap in the spinal cord by grafting peripheral nerve helper cells (Schwann cells) into the site of injury seems to be a promising method [Xu et al., 1995]. They are well known to stimulate axon regeneration by making proteins that promote the nerve growth either on contact, or at a distance (by secreting "growth factors"). By bringing the cells that create the growth-promoting environment in nerves supporting the regeneration into the spinal cord, Bunge and her colleagues [Guénard et al., 1992] provided a scaffold for regrowing nerves and restoring communication between the brain and paralyzed regions of the body. A cable of Schwann cells grafted into the spinal cord inside a "guidance channel" stimulates thousands of nerve fibers to regenerate across the length of the bridge.

Early tests proved that Schwann cells are much more effective in eliciting the growth of distant nerve cells (located in the brain) if other growth-promoting proteins are added to the bridges. Specific growth factors (scientists have identified dozens of proteins that could be effective), used in combination with Schwann cell bridges or peripheral nerve grafts, augment regeneration and attract growth from nerve cells that modulate movements, affect autonomic functions, and carry sensory messages.

Despite the success of the bridging strategies, a barrier awaits the regrowing axons at the point where the bridges end. In order to make functional connections with the nerve circuits beyond the bridge, the growing nerve fibers must leave the supportive bridge and grow into the "hostile" spinal cord environment. The spinal cord environment contains proteins that stop regenerating axons. Schwab and colleagues [Rubin et al., 1994] attempt to overcome this inhibition using antibodies that prevent the axons from seeing these stop signals. Using the basic guidance channel model, a second type of helper cell just outside the bridges can be transplanted. These helper cells, called olfactory ensheathing glia, are found only in nerves that carry odor sensations to the brain. Ensheathing glia share some characteristics with Schwann cells, including some of their growth-promoting properties, but they may also express traits that resemble astrocytes, a helper cell in the CNS that can inhibit axon growth. Unlike either cell type, ensheathing glia also migrate extensively within the CNS. Throughout life, ensheathing glia usher growing axons across the barrier between the peripheral nerve environment and the brain.

Raisman [1997] also indicates that ensheathing glia are an important new strategy for improving regeneration. His group used ensheathing glia to stimulate the growth of nerve fibers from the brain (specifically, the cerebral cortex) past a very small area of damage in their spinal cord pathway. Although the exact connections made by the regrowing axons are not yet known, these investigators also reported that the ensheathing glia accompany the growing fibers. Importantly, the ability of the rats to use their forepaw in a reaching task significantly improved, indicating that some functional connections must have been made.

In summary, the transplantation of suspensions of Schwann cells has been employed quite successfully for repair of some fiber pathways within the brain structures [Kromer and Cornbrooks, 1985; Montero-Menei et al., 1992; Stichel et al., 1995]. When implanted after SCI, Schwan cell suspensions have been associated with improved peripheral nerve graft/host spinal cord union [Wrathall et al., 1982] and decreased cavitation and reactive gliosis [Martin et al., 1993], but not with definitive repair of interrupted spinal cord pathways. When tissue gaps exist within the spinal cord, there is a need for presentation of regeneration substrates in a form that provides stable physical contacts between the regions of the injured parenchyma.

Another important finding is that providing artificial guiding channels is effective [Guest et al., 1997]. The PAN/PVC, a patented name of a specially treated polyvinyl chloride, guidance channel, seeded with a defined cell population, provides one type of controlled regeneration environment. The channel is highly biocompatible, offers substantial tensile strength due to its trabecular outer wall, reduces invasion of mesenchymal cells into the enclosed transplant, and limits the molecular exchange between the graft and the external wound environment due to its permselective smooth inner membrane [Aebischer et al., 1988, 1989 and 1990]. Following transaction at the thoracic level in the nude rat, human Schwann cells grafted inside distally capped

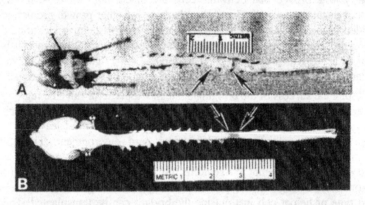

Fig. 4.2: Experimental work in animals to regenerate nerve tissue *in situ*. Perfused neural axes with performed grafts placed with or without channels. A) 4 mm long graft is used to bridge the 6 mm gap with the channel at the T8-T10 spinal cord level (arrows); B) 3 to 4 mm (arrows) graft without a channel at the T8 spinal cord level. Adapted from Guest et al., 1997, with permission.

channels survived and supported the regeneration of substantial numbers of neuronal processes, including propriospinal, sensory, motor, and brainstem neurons important for locomotion [Guest and Bunge, 1995]. Previous investigators using other rodent strains have not demonstrated such ingrowth of brainstem neurons unless an erogenous source of neurotrophin was supplied [Xu et al., 1995], methylprednisolone was administered following injury [Chen et al., 1996], or the graft was placed at the cervical level [Richardson et al., 1984]. Most regeneration studies have emphasized the need for functional reconnection of long descending pathways to effector neurons. The potential for regenerating propriospinal neurons to contribute to functional recovery has not been extensively explored for transplantation strategies in the mammal.

There are possible adverse effects of channels; thus, employing the PAN/PVC channel is only to form and organize the spinal cord cable, knowing that it could then be removed and implanted without the channel. This strategy would enable formation of the initial graft but not control of the ongoing regeneration environment. Transplantation could be performed with much less trauma to the cord stumps and less bone removal, thereby diminishing instability.

4.1.2 Surgery to Provide Muscle Innervation - Grafting Peripheral Nerves

More than any other form of trauma, nerve injuries complicate successful rehabilitation, because mature neurons do not undergo cell division [Fields *et al.*, 1989]. Under the right conditions, however, axon extensions can regenerate over gaps caused by injury, reconnecting with the distal stump, and eventually reestablishing functional contacts. Peripheral nerve injuries that result in long gaps require surgical implantation of a bridge or guidance channel between the proximal nerve end and the distal stump in order to restore function and organ reinnervation.

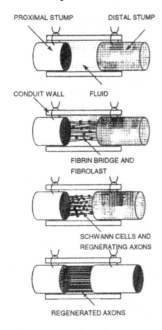

Fig. 4.3: Silicon chamber model showing the progression of events during peripheral nerve regeneration. See text for details. Adapted from Heath and Rutkowski, 1998, with permission.

When the nerve is cut or crushed, and nerve function is lost, the portion of the nerve distal to the injury dies and degenerates; the proximal segment may be able to regenerate and reestablish nerve function. A crush often leaves a continuous tubular structure through which the axon can regrow, but a cut creates a gap across which the growth cone of the regenerating axon must navigate. To improve recovery, severed nerves can be surgically sutured end-to-end over small gaps; large gaps, however, must be repaired with a graft inserted between the proximal and distal nerve stumps as a guide for the regenerating axon. When they reach the distal stump, the growth cones enter endoneurial tubes, that is columns of Schwann cells surrounded by basal lamina. In contact with the Schwann cells and the basal lamina, the growth cone proceeds towards its target. The effectiveness of the regeneration process depends on whether the axons enter the appropriate endoneurial tubes and reconnect with the correct target.

The typical graft of choice is the autograft, which is a segment of nerve removed from another part of the same body. This procedure allows only a small proportion of axons to make functional and physiological connections (10 percent). Disadvantages of the nerve autograft also include a second surgical procedure, limited availability, and permanent denervation at the donor site. Allografts, that is grafts from other living species, have also been used, but then immuno-suppression was required, and very poor success rates have been recorded [Mackinnon and Dellon, 1990]. Autologous and autogenous blood vessels [Chiu *et al.*, 1988] and muscle fibers [Glasby *et al.*, 1986] have also been used as conduits for nerve regeneration with varying levels of success, but these still suffer from some of the same disadvantages as auto and allografts [Doolabh *et al.*, 1996]. Conduits have also been formed from other biological materials, with collagen showing the greatest potential for success [Archibald *et al.*, 1995].

Avoiding the problems of availability and immune rejection, a promising alternative for extending the length over which nerves can successfully regenerate is the artificial nerve graft, frequently called a nerve guidance channel. The artificial graft is a synthetic conduit that bridges the gap between the nerve stumps, directs, and supports the nerve regeneration. The conduit may be implanted empty, or it may be filled with growth factors, cells or fibers. An artificial graft can meet many of the needs of regenerating nerves by concentrating neurotrophic factors, reducing cellular invasion and scarring of the nerve, and providing directional guidance to prevent neuroma formation or excessive branching.

Nonresorbable Artificial Nerve Grafts. Because of its inert and elastic properties, silicone tubing was one of the first and most frequently used synthetic materials for nerve grafts. Clinical intubulation of regenerating nerves, however, often leads to long-term complications including fibrosis and chronic nerve compression, requiring surgical removal of the conduit. Despite diminishing clinical use, the silicone chamber and other nonresorbable materials such as polyethylene have been useful for studying nerve regeneration in vitro. This allowed spatial and temporal examination of the regeneration process. For example, early experiments using the silicone-chamber model indicated a maximum gap length between the proximal and distal ends of 10 mm (for rat neurons) across which regeneration could occur [Lundborg *et al.*, 1982]. Only by filling the graft with one or more neurotrophic substances, longer distances could be bridged [da Silva *et al.*, 1985].

The chronological sequence of nerve regeneration was also elucidated from silicone-chamber experiments (Figure 4.3). In the case of rat sciatic nerve, fluid from the nerve stumps, which contains compounds exhibiting neurotrophic or neurite-supporting activity, fills the chamber within the first day. Within a week, a fibrin bridge forms between the proximal and distal nerve stumps, and fibroblasts begin infiltrating the bridge from both ends. At the same time, changes are taking place in the distal stump. The process by which the damaged axonal materials are removed and recycled by Schwann and other cells, preparing the environment for axon regeneration, is known as Valerian degeneration. By the second week, Schwann cells and axons begin migrating along the bridge. Because of their many functions, Schwann-cell migration into the chamber matrix is critical to successful regeneration across the gap. In contact with the Schwann cells, the axons grow into the distal stump and proceed towards their targets. Finally, over a period of two to eight weeks, Schwann cells myelinate the axons [Fields *et al.*, 1989].

In order to enhance regeneration further, the artificial nerve graft may be filled with one or more substances. Although some gels may impede axon extension, filling the chamber with phosphate-buffered saline or dialyzed plasma enhances regeneration. Supplementing the fluid in the silicone chamber with growth factors and erogenous matrix precursors, many of which are produced by Schwann cells, has also been shown to promote regeneration across larger gaps (15-20 mm) than would be repaired by empty tubes. Some of the compounds that have been shown to enhance nerve regeneration in conduits are laminin, collagen, nerve-growth factor (NGF), acidic and basic fibroblast growth factors, and fibronectin [Jenq and Coggeshall, 1987].

Semipermeable tubes possess advantages over impermeable silicone tubes if they still prevent infiltration of cells. Increased exchange of nutrients between the lumen and the outer environment is believed to be responsible for the improved regeneration observed with selectively permeable tubes [Aebisher *et al.*, 1988].

Resorbable Artificial Nerve Grafts. Although artificial nerve grafts constructed from nonresorbable materials have shown good motor and sensory recovery over the short term, long-term complications often mean that a second surgical procedure is necessary to remove the conduit. Shortly after the axons penetrate the distal stump, the nerve guide may actually become detrimental because of its toxicity or its tendency to constrict the nerve. A graft made of bioresorbable materials is a promising alternative for promoting successful long-term recovery, as has been seen both experimentally and clinically, because after serving as an appropriate scaffold for regeneration, the conduit eventually degrades. Many resorbable materials have been examined for nerve and other tissue-engineering applications such as Polyester, Polyglacictin, Polyactic acid, and others [Rosen *et al.*, 1990; Heath and Rutkowski, 1998]. The most important concern in designing a resorbable graft, apart from biocompatibility, is choosing a material and processing conditions that will result in a graft that degrades slowly enough to maintain a stable support structure for the entire regeneration process, yet it will disintegrate later without polluting the organism. The time required for regeneration will be a function of the nerve location, the species and age of the patient, and the gap length. For example, based on information gained from the silicone-chamber model, a biodegradable graft for a 10 mm gap in the rat sciatic nerve should maintain its strength for eight weeks or longer in order to ensure that axons have entered the distal stump and been myelinated. In addition, the graft should be flexible and its wall should have a thickness sufficient to hold a suture connecting the nerve epineurium and the graft. To avoid nerve compression, the inner diameter of the graft should be large enough to accommodate polymer swelling during degradation, which is seen with some polymers [den Dunnen, 1993]. When using porous materials, the nominal pore size will determine which molecules will pass through the graft between the surrounding tissue and the regenerating nerve.

Grafts may also be constructed of two layers, of the same or different materials, to achieve the desired support and retention properties [den Dunnen, 1993]. A thin, nonporous skin on the inner surface of the tube is the primary permeability barrier and serves to retain neurotrophic factors. A thicker, porous external layer provides structural support. This model is analogous to the structure of anisotropic ultrafiltration membranes used for separating proteins from cells and/or smaller molecules.

Bioresorbable grafts also have the significant advantage because as they degrade, a growth or trophic factors are trapped in or adsorbed to the polymer. With controlled release, compounds with short *in vivo* half-life can be supplied slowly to the regenerating axons over the life of the graft. The extended release of basic fibroblast growth factor has been shown to enhance the growth of myelinated and unmyelinated axons across a 15-mm gap in the rat sciatic nerve compared with conventional tubes.

Bioartificial Nerve Grafts. Although controlled release is one way of supplying factors to enhance nerve regeneration in a synthetic conduit, providing the necessary quantities and types of compounds at the rates most conducive to regenerate on will surely be a challenge. Many of the neurotrophic factors that have been or will be considered for controlled release are made by Schwann cells, which serve several important roles in nerve regeneration: Schwann cells secrete neurotrophic factors and express cell-adhesion molecules that enhance nerve regeneration; they form an endoneurial sheath, which serves as a guide for axonal growth; they aid in clearing debris and create a suitable environment for nerve growth; they myelinate axons [Bunge, 1994]. Experiments have shown that Schwann cells stimulate axons to elongate faster and over longer distances than it is possible on acellular matrix. In essence, the presence of Schwann cells may be the single most critical factor in promoting axon regeneration in the milieu of the regenerating peripheral nerve. New procedures aimed specifically at the isolation of Schwann cells from adult rat [Morrissey et al., 1991], and human [Rutkowski et al., 1992] cultures have also been developed, making the addition of syngeneric cells to grafts possible.

4.1.3 Surgery to Provide Muscle for Movement - Tendon Transfer

Early trials of surgery to improve paralytic hand function in tetraplegia began after the Second World War. These surgeries were often based on experience with subjects having peripheral nerve injuries. Individuals with tetraplegia have different and usually more profound motor and sensory deficits compared with humans with peripheral nerve injuries. The tendon transfer is more effective in tetraplegics compared with humans with peripheral lesions; there are many more intact muscles available and appropriate for tendon transfer in tetraplegics.

Reliable techniques for surgical improvement of hand function have been developed and accepted in the two decades since Moberg [1975] demonstrated that a simple surgical reconstruction could restore lateral pinch. The development of the "key grip" procedure has generated interest in hand surgery programs for tetraplegia [Moberg, 1990]. He estimated that 60 percent of subjects who have tetraplegia benefit from operative procedures on the upper extremities. It remains essential, however, that the surgeon is experienced in hand reconstruction for individuals with tetraplegia and that a team experienced in hand rehabilitation is available postoperatively.

Generally, the motion in a distal joint can be surgically restored by transferring the tendon of a muscle having active function in such a way that it restores motion in a joint having no function. Or it can be restored by tenodesis of the tendon of a paralytic muscle spanning two joints in such a manner that voluntary motion at the proximal joint (over which the subject has active control) causes the distal joint to move purposefully. Surgical reconstruction may involve not only restoration of pinch and grasp, but also thumb and finger openings. It is not possible to simultaneously restore active opening and closing in one surgical procedure because in the healing phase the joints must be held in a position of flexion or extension to avoid tension on the tendon anastomosis until adequate tendon healing has occurred. Consequently, procedures to provide both finger/thumb openings and pinch and grasp require two separately staged procedures.

Surgical Procedure

Many clinicians consider three categories of hand functions as the most important: sensing, gripping, and human contact. The reconstructive procedure must aim to restore these functions as much as possible, but not hinder the abilities preserved. The importance of sensing and gripping is well recognized, yet the human contact function of the hand is of paramount importance (e.g., shaking hands, eliminating claw-like hands, and providing soft contact). Soft pliable hands are an asset even with no active grip, and can under no circumstance be given up [Moberg, 1975]. Another basic principle that must guide the planning of treatment is the requirement that any procedure performed must be reversible.

After thorough examination and evaluation, the surgeon must explain to the subject in detail what is and is not possible (Table 4.1).

Table 4.1: Clinical classification of the tetraplegic hand. Observation on 97 patients. BB - Biceps Brachialis m; ECRL and ECRB - Extensor Carpi Radialis Longus and Brevis m; EDC - Extensor Digitorum Communis m; EDQ - Extensor Digiti Quinti m; ECU - Extensor Carpi Ulnaris m; FDP - Flexor Digitorum Profundus m; EIP - Extensor Indicis Proprius m; EPL - Extensor Pollicis Longus m; FCU - Flexor Carpi Ulnaris m. The percent shows the fraction of the population from the total of 97 subjects [Zancolli, 1975].

Clinical Group	Lowest Functioning Cord Segment	Basic Functioning Muscles	SUBGROUPS				Function Achieved by Surgery
Flexor of the elbow 13%	5	BB	A	Without Brachioradialis			
			B	With Brachioradialis			Weak Lateral Pinch
Extensor of the Wrist 74%	6	ECRL, ECRB	A	Weak Wrist Extension			Weak Lateral Pinch and Grip
			B	Strong Wrist Extension 82%	1	without PT and FCR (76%)	Effective Lateral Pinch and Strong Grip (best in 3)
					2	without FCR with PT (16%)	
					3	with PT, FCR and TR (8%)	
Extrinsic Extension of the Fingers 6.8%	7	EDC, EDQ, ECU	A	Complete Extension of Ulnar Fingers and Paralysis of Radial Fingers and Thumb			Lateral and Pulp Pinch, Strong Grip (better in B)
			B	Complete Extension of All Fingers and Weak Thumb Extension			
Extrinsic Flexor of the Fingers and Thumb Extension 6.2%	8	FDP, EIP, EPL, ECU	A	Complete Flexion of Ulnar Fingers and Paralysis of Flexion of Radial Fingers and Thumb. Complete Thumb Extension			Excellent Pinching and Grasping (better in B)
			B	Complete Flexion of All Fingers and Weak Thumb Flexion. Weak Thenar Muscles. Paralysis of the Intrinsic Muscles of the Fingers without or with Flexor Superficialis			

Timing and Selection Criteria. Surgery should be performed after the subject has completed a program of rehabilitation of the upper extremity, including proper posturing by means of splints and active and passive range of motion, and before adequate time has been allowed for psychological adjustment to the injury [Zancolli, 1975]. Delay of surgery for one year generally allows adequate time not only for neurological stabilization, but also provides sufficient time for psychological recovery and social stabilization. Candidates must be highly motivated and cooperative to comply with the postoperative recovery and rehabilitation processes.

The subjects also need to be aware of the commitment to the postoperative rehabilitation process that is necessary for an optimal outcome. The subjects may benefit from additional rehabilitation to learn new activities of daily living skills. The subjects regain significant motor function after surgery. Consequently, they have the potential to perform tasks not gained in the initial rehabilitation program. Special attention needs to be given to individuals who anticipate returning to work as caretakers or full-time employees, since more extensive planning may be necessary to accommodate the relatively long postoperative recovery and rehabilitation time.

Examples of Tendon Transfer Surgical Procedures

The minimum requirements to restore key grip are sensory information (afferent input), one mobile joint in the thumb, and one muscle [Moberg, 1978]. The wrist joint and proximal joints in the arm are necessary; these joints are part of the reaching-grasping function. The minimum information (afferent input) is provided either by vision or by cutaneous sensibility in the thumb or index finger if the two-point discrimination is at ten to twelve millimeters or better. The minimum motor prerequisite is a Grade 4 brachioradialis muscle. If the wrist extensors (Extensors Carpi Radialis Longus and Brevis m.) are good enough, the brachioradialis muscle can be used in another way, for example to provide a thumb abductor. If the wrist extensors are present but too weak, they must be reinforced by the brachioradialis.

An example of effective surgery for elbow extension is posterior deltoid (DE) to triceps tendon transfer in C5 tetraplegia (Figure 4.4). If the posterior DE strength is 4 or 5, then its transfer to triceps will be effective. At surgery, the border between the posterior and middle DE is identified by the oblique orientation of the fibers of the posterior deltoid in contrast to the vertical fibers of the middle DE. The distal end of the DE is attached to a free tendon graft from the leg (anterior tibialis tendon or flexor hallucis longus) and attached to the triceps

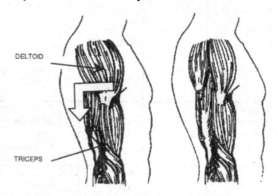

Fig 4.4: Transfer of the Posterior Deltoid m. to the Triceps m: before surgery (left) and after the surgery (right). Adapted from Waters *et al.*, 1996, with permission.

tendon. This procedure allows for active elbow extension, enabling subjects to stabilize themselves for sitting and while transferring. It has been reported [Raczka *et al.*, 1984] that in 14 out of 22 subjects who received this treatment, the functional improvement and level of independence raised. The subjects reported functional improvements in the areas of grooming and personal hygiene, pressure relief, writing speed and clarity, and self-feeding.

Brachioradialis m. to Extensor Carpi Radialis m. transfer demonstrated that active wrist extension could be provided in subjects with wrist extensors lacking strength for tenodesis grasp (Figure 4.4). It is difficult to determine the strength of the Brachioradialis (BR) muscle by manual muscle testing because it is not possible to isolate its contribution to elbow flexion from the Biceps and Brachialis m. Moberg recommended performing surgery under local anesthesia, detaching the tendinous insertion of the BR and connecting it to a tensiometer. The strength of the BR is measured at surgery to determine if it is suitable for transfer. The literature reports that subjects having 1 or 2 out of maximum grade 5 wrist extension strength preoperatively have adequate strength of BR for the transfer [Waters et al., 1996a].

After surgery, it is easier for subjects to utilize hand orthoses since precision of hand placement is enhanced by the restoration of active motion at the wrist [Waters et al., 1985a]. Although wrist extensor strength following BR to extensor carpi radialis brevis (ECRB) transfer is sufficient to provide some wrist control, it may not provide sufficient strength to achieve 4 or 5 grade (active movement against gravity with moderate resistance).

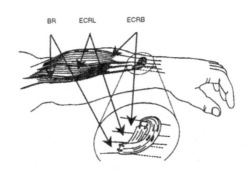

Fig 4.5: Transfer of the Brachioradialis m. to the Extensor Carpi Radialis Brevis (ECRB) m: BR - Brachioradialis m; ECRL - Extensor Carpi Radialis Longus m. Adapted from Waters, 1996, with permission.

Moberg [1978] suggested the key grip procedure to augment and/or provide passive Flexor Pollicis Longus (FPL) tenodesis. He observed that lateral or "key" pinch between the thumb and side of the finger was often present in subjects who had developed a "natural" tenodesis of the FPL due to spasticity or contracture. His procedure replicates what he observed as often occurring "naturally." Bunnel originally recommended flexor tenodesis of the thumb and finger flexors [Bunnel, 1949]. He demonstrated that functional pinch could be easily achieved between the thumb and side of the index finger since this often occurred naturally in C6 tetraplegia if spasticity or contracture in the FPL was present (Figure 4.6).

Moberg's key-pinch procedure (Figure 4.6) is the simplest type of hand reconstruction in a C6 tetraplegic. To restore the lateral or key grip in subjects without a natural tenodesis, Moberg surgically created FPL tenodesis by securing the proximal end of the tendon to the distal radius. To prevent thumb Interphalangeal (IP) joint flexion, an intermedullary screw was percutaneously inserted via the distal tip of the thumb and placed across the IP joint. The Extensor Pollicis Longus and Brevis tendons are secured proximal to the metacato-phalangeal joint to prevent excess flexion.

Reiser and Waters [1986] reported on the long-term follow-up of the Moberg procedure. Seven of the nine subjects who had undergone the Moberg procedure for an average of 7.4 years, earlier continued to report enhancement of function. The functional activities most commonly improved were grooming, eating, writing, and desktop skills. The function in the early postoperative period was not compared with functional status at the follow-up time of the study.

Most surgeons now agree that, when possible, transfer of an active motor to the FPL to provide lateral pinch and to the finger flexors to provide grasp allows better function and is preferable to FPL tenodesis [e.g., Waters et al., 1985a]. With passive tenodesis, control of distal function by proximal joint movement eliminates a degree of freedom of hand placement and precision of movement, since wrist motion must simultaneously accompany pinch. Because pinch can be obtained independently of wrist position after active tendon transfer, the precision, versatility, and usefulness of pinch are enhanced in comparison with FPL tenodesis.

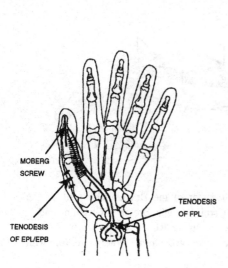
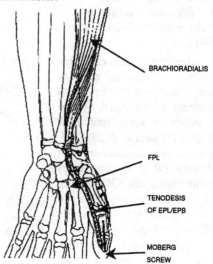

Fig 4.6: Moberg's key grip procedure: FPL - Flexor Pollicis Longus m; EPL and EPB - Extensor Pollicis Longus and Brevis m. Adapted from Waters *et al.*, 1996, with permission.

Fig 4.7: Transfer of the Brachioradialis m. to the Flexor Pollicis Longus (FPL) m. for active lateral grasp: EPL - Extensor Pollicis Longus m; EPB - Extensor Pollicis Brevis m. Adapted from Waters *et al.*, 1996, with permission

To provide the lateral pinch, the tendon transfer of the BR to the FPL (Figure 4.7) became almost a standard procedure [Waters *et al.*, 1985a]. To provide finger flexion, tendon transfer to the Flexor Digitorum Profundus (FDP) has been the procedure of choice, as it provides grasp and a firm surface for lateral or palmar thumb pinch (Figure 4.7). The Flexor Carpi Radialis, Pronator Teres, and the Extensor Carpi Radialis Longus have all been used as motors for lateral pinch and for finger flexion [Freehafer *et al.*, 1987].

Waters and associates [1996a] reported a functional improvement in 15 of 17 hands following transfer of the BR to the FPL. Twelve subjects reported at least four functional activities (hygiene, grooming, mobility, and writing) that they were able to perform more efficiently after surgery. Nine subjects were able to pick up a pen and write, and the five subjects who required a wristband orthosis preoperatively were able to grasp objects without it after surgery.

Mechanisms for the Integration of Command after Tendon Transfer

The mechanism of integration of motor commands after tendon transfer remains obscure despite some experimental studies in animal or man. The recent demonstration of cortical and spinal neural plasticity and recent advances in motor control theories may serve as a basis for considering this question.

Tendon or nervous transfers were used soon after the injury as an experimental mean to test the plasticity of motor command in animals [Jeannerod and Hecaen, 1979]. Sperry [1947] studied locomotion of rats and observed that the muscular patterns were not modified after nervous or tendinous crossover. He concluded that the command of locomotion did not adapt to a modification of the effectors, and reported an adaptation of upper limb voluntary movements in the monkey and concluded that goal-directed movement is adaptable. Forssberg and Svartengren [1983] studied the transfer of ankle extensor muscles on flexor muscles in cats and observed that the muscular activation pattern was little modified but that locomotion could adapt correctly to the transfer. They conclude that the spinal flexion-extension pattern is robust, yet there may exist a more complex adaptation at cortical level characterized by the necessity of a learning.

All analyses of the plasticity after tendon transfers in humans rely on EMG analysis. Close and Todd [1959] suggested that the old pattern of the transferred muscle seldom disappears; hence, a transfer of a synergistic muscle is more likely to be efficient. Leffert and Meister [1976] studied 19 patients who had tendon transfers after an upper-limb peripheral nerve paralysis. They concluded that the transferred muscle was active soon in its new function and demonstrated that a part of a muscle could be transferred and that it could become functionally isolated from the remaining part. The transferred muscle keeps most part of its previous behavior, but it is also able to produce a different pattern. Similar findings have been confirmed in an independent study of Illert with coworkers [1986].

It is likely that the clinical improvement after the tendon transfer and rehabilitation is due to the cortical plasticity of the central command. Plasticity has been demonstrated in somatosensory as well as in motor cortex [Nudo et al., 1997, Xerri, 1998]. Both sensory [Merzenich et al., 1983] and motor [Sanes et al., 1990] cortical maps show plasticity. The reorganization of somatosensory and motor maps was evidenced in man by functional imaging methods [Elbert et al., 1995] and by cortical magnetic stimulation cartography [Hallet et al., 1993]. In tetraplegic or amputee subjects, the cortical areas activating shoulder muscles are enlarged suggesting that the motor areas corresponding to the distal, paralyzed or absent muscles became appropriate for the remaining shoulder muscles [Levy et al., 1990; Ojemann and Silbergeld, 1995]. Neural plasticity has also been suggested at the level of subcortical and in particular spinal structures [Mendell, 1988, Wolpaw and Carp, 1990]. The most important element allowing neural plasticity to take place is the intensive exercise, which is task oriented and with the augmented feedback [Barbeau and Rossignol, 1987].

4.2 Neurorehabilitation

The neurorehabilitation comprises methods and technology for maximizing the efficiency of preserved neuro-muscular structures in a human with motor disability. Maximizing function relates to developing new movement strategies that benefit from the preserved, but without the treatment unused sensory and motor systems. The most important step for effective neurorehabilitation is to timely assess the regional, selective, and nonselective functions of the nervous system, and based on the findings develop a protocol and apply restorative procedures to upgrade the functions [Dimitrijević, 1988].

The term *neurorehabilitation* was introduced following the outcome of the rehabilitation of subjects with head injuries. Many subjects have a temporary motor activity deficits due to focal damage to the hemispheres of the brain [Jennett and

Taesdale, 1984]. In subjects with a severe brain injury, motor deficit remains even after many years (e.g., examination of 300 subjects, who had experienced unconsciousness or posttraumatic amnesia for a week or more, found that 40 percent exhibited a slight hemiparesis, 20 percent brainstem syndromes, 5 percent brainstem pseudobulbar symptoms, and 35 percent had no neurologic deficits), as reported by Roberts [1976].

Central nervous system provides the basis for structuring neurorehabilitation activities to promote and enhance recovery of function following the injury or disease. Spontaneous recovery occurs through the process of compensation, substitution, diaschisis, and dynamic reorganization through training. The organization of learning within the cerebral cortex results from the repeated activity on the part of the individual and becomes organized into a functional system of behavior. The repeated activities could also change the neuronal connections and their function at lower levels of the central nervous system. These processes lead to new types of integrated multiple sensory modalities, which directly affect the abilities for voluntary motor control.

The primary objective of the neurorehabilitation is to promote and develop processes underlying sensory and motor systems and change the dynamics of "learning" by providing the substrate that in normal circumstances would not be available. The effectiveness of neurorehabilitation activities is dependent upon and relates to the degree of disability, but even more to the specificity of losses of neural connections of each individual subject. The experience gained in applying the neurorehabilitation in both subjects with brain damages and spinal cord injuries suggests that consistent and direct feedback to the subjects about their performance is an essential element in achieving effects.

The key issue in neurorehabilitation is to identify which parts of the neuronal circuits are still preserved, yet partially disconnected so that they cannot generate motor and sensory functions [Geschwind, 1985]. The actions in the actual application of the neurorehabilitation to the subjects with central nervous system lesions include the following: training on a one-to-one basis, providing of constant and systematic augmented feedback, insisting on a prolonged and intensive training directed to tasks that require integration of potentially functional structures, progressive increase of the difficulties of the training task, and ensuring of successful endeavors.

Neurorehabilitation has been originally developed for stroke subjects, yet the procedures have been applied to other types of motor disabilities. Studies of human recovery after spinal cord injury are limited in most cases to clinical neurological assessments and recordings of somatosensory evoked potentials. Most subjects after spinal cord injury are not aware of all the intrinsic resources that may still be available to them if they are appropriately developed and used in a functional manner. It has been shown that extensive training is capable of speeding up the process of recovery, if any is to follow.

The recovery in functioning of the muscle after clinically diagnosed complete mid-thoracic spinal cord lesion (Figure 4.8) is following the program of intensive training [Dimitrijević, 1988]. The training has been introduced after careful and comprehensive tests such as polyelectromyography of phasic and tonic stretch reflexes, effects of reinforcement maneuvers on the motor unit activity of paralyzed muscles and volitional activity [Dimitrijević *et al.*, 1984], recordings of somatosensory evoked potentials [Dimitrijević *et al.*, 1983], and mapping of sensory cutaneous functions [Lindblom, 1981].

The restorative neurology program at the Baylor College, Houston, Texas, USA, studied residual function in spinal cord injured subjects aiming to assess and treat disability. The simultaneous electromyographic recordings from several muscles documented phasic and tonic stretch reflexes, withdrawal reflexes, somatosensory evoked potentials, and other responses to pain, cold, *etc.* One of many interesting results is shown in Figure 4.8; a subject with an injury at C4 level caused by a motor vehicle accident was followed for several years. Ten weeks after the injury there was neither volitional movement at the ankle joint, nor EMG activity in muscles shown. In the second 10 weeks, the beginning of the well-organized dorsi- and plantar flexion was observed. This activity became organized with increased amplitude, better reciprocity, and a more sudden onset and cessation of muscle activity. The patterns remained throughout five years of the follow-up.

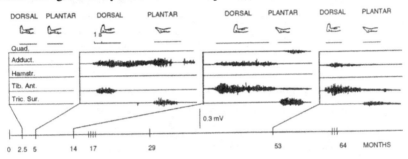

Fig. 4.8: EMG activity recorded from the right Quadriceps, Adductors, Hamstrings, Tibial Anterior and Triceps Surae m. at four times (2.5, 5, 14 and 53 months after the injury). The task was to voluntary dorsi and plantar flex the ankle joint. The first recordings have been done 2.5 months after the injury, and no activity could be recorded. The recordings after 64 months (not shown) remained stable. Adapted from Dimitrijević, 1988, with permission.

The intriguing question, posted many years ago, deals with the potential use of centers in the spinal cord that are intact, and may serve as central pattern generator (CPG) circuitry, thereby, allowing locomotor behavior. The results are rather controversial, because it is very difficult to eliminate sensory input when trying to generate locomotor behavior by stimulating the spinal cord directly (phasic input).

As described in Chapter 2, human walking depends upon neuronal mechanisms within the spinal cord that can act even in the absence of any afferent input (CPG). Until recently, it was thought that stepping movements could not occur in humans with spinal cord injury [Barbeau *et al.*, 1999]. However, involuntary stepping movements have been documented in a human after spinal cord injury, indicating that a spinal motor program generator exists also in humans [Calancie *et al.*, 1994]. The finding came after the subject with spinal cord injury at cervical level "complained" after many years of various therapies that he noticed cyclic movement of the legs while lying on the back. This behavior could be replicated in the laboratory condition with the frequency of 0.3 Hz while he was standing. A sensory input triggered the alternative flexion and extension, and it was possible to affect the frequency of alteration. The sensory input was coming from the hip extension. The cyclic, locomotor-like activity measured in the self-triggered locomotion activity (supine position) is shown in Figure 4.9.

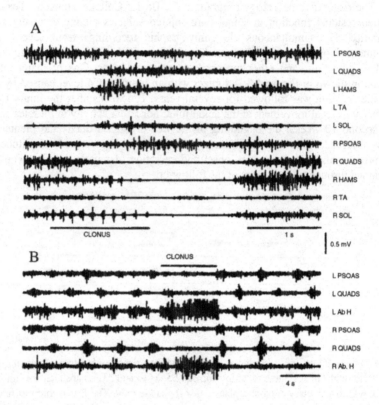

Fig. 4.9: Two records of involuntary stepping with the incomplete C4 subject supine, undisturbed by external sensory input or voluntary contraction. Clonus, lasting for about 1.5 seconds, has been observed in distal muscles of the right leg (A), and it spread from left side to the right side (B) lasting for about 4 seconds. The abbreviations are L - left, R - right, PSOAS - Iliopsoas m; QUADS - Quadriceps m; HAMS - Hamstrings m; TA - Tibialis Anterior m; SOL - Soleus m; Ab - Abductor m; H - hip. Adapted from Calancie et al., 1994, with permission.

Calancie and coworkers [1994] also showed that the EMG recordings (Figure 4.10) from the same subject in whom the involuntary locomotor-like movement occurred, while in supine position, can ambulate in parallel bars. This walking occurred after the subject was standing for some time in the parallel bars, and considerable extensor spasticity and clonus ceased. Only slow and moderate EMG activity has been recorded during voluntary walking. The involuntary stepping was completely shut down when the subject loaded his legs by supporting his body weight through his legs and maintaining the balance with his arms.

In humans without voluntary movement in their lower limbs resulting from a spinal cord injury the threshold to elicit the flexion reflex is often markedly reduced. This reflex consists of a "stepping" movement involving flexion of all the limb joints, and its presence implies that the coordinating neuronal circuits have persisted in the isolated spinal cord. Moreover, in able-bodied humans and in spinalized animals, depending on the precise phase of the gait cycle, stimulation of non-nociceptive afferents facilitates the activity of ipsilateral flexors or extensors. Furthermore, it has an effect on the contralateral limb as well and an indication of the gaiting mechanisms at spinal level driven by signaling load of afferents and hip joint angles.

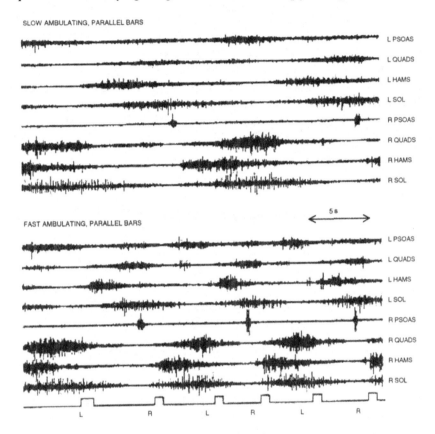

Fig. 4.10: The EMG recordings from eight muscles simultaneously while the incomplete C4 tetraplegic subject ambulated in parallel bars at slow (top) and his most rapid rates (bottom). The bottom trace shows the onset of the stance phase for each leg during fast walking. The abbreviations are L - left, R - right, PSOAS - iliopsoas m; QUADS - quadriceps m; HAMS - hamstrings m; SOL - soleus m. Adapted from Calancie *et al.*, 1994, with permission.

4.2.1 Neurorehabilitation of Walking

It is a common clinical finding that neurologically impaired subjects have difficulties with weight bearing through their affected legs during standing and walking [Visintin and Barbeau, 1989]. One of the limitations of conventional walking retraining is that it is done under full weight bearing conditions, most of the time using parallel bars and walking aids to alleviate the load on the legs. A dynamic and task specific approach consisting of progressive increase of weight bearing during treadmill walking could be an effective strategy to retrain the walking. The clinical implications and advantages of such a strategy are numerous. The three components of gait: weight bearing, balance, and stepping could be retrained simultaneously under dynamic conditions. Walking retraining could be initiated early in the rehabilitation period, providing as much body relief as needed to provide vertical posture and allow for assisted or unassisted stepping of legs. Other means of enhancing movement could be integrated such as electrical stimulation that is timed to drive the appropriate muscles. In short, this neurorehabilitation technique provides an environment that is well suited for relearning movement because it eliminates the needs for non-existing strong contraction of postural muscles; thus, increases the safety attitude; therefore allows other networks to reconnect if any of this is to happen.

Stepping on the motor driven treadmill has previously been described in a variety of other mammals after complete (primates) and incomplete low spinal transaction (animals) [Grillner, 1981; Gossard and Hultborn, 1991; Eidelberg et al., 1981; Eidelberg and Yu, 1981]. It has been demonstrated that prolonged training [Gossard and Hultborn, 1991] can enhance the amount and quality of spinal stepping, while the animal is supporting its body weight.

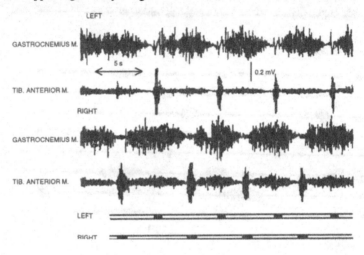

Fig. 4.11: Simultaneous EMG recordings from main flexor and extensor muscles in the legs of a paraplegic walking on a static surface between parallel bars. Bottom traces show stance (open) and swing (black fields) in right and left leg. Phasic activities in both legs are well pronounced in four consecutive. The recordings have been made after prolonged intensive treadmill walking. Paraplegic subject has right leg functionally paralyzed, and left leg functional. Adapted from Wernig and Müller, 1992, with permission.

Wernig and Müller [1990] started inducing the walking in humans with paraplegia and tetraplegia on the treadmill. Wernig and Müller studied [1992] nine subjects with spastic paresis resulting from spinal cord injuries. They showed that prolonged treadmill walking training was effective in permitting or enhancing locomotion movement of legs, in absence of voluntary movements. This study also showed that locomotion, which is learned on the treadmill under conditions of reduced body weight, could subsequently be executed on a static surface with full body weight beard by the paralyzed limb. Five of them had complete functional paralysis in one leg, *i.e.*, they were unable to actively move their limbs from a resting position, while the other four subjects had a less severe paralysis. In all subjects skin sensibility and proprioception were present to different degrees in both limbs. One of the five severely paralyzed subjects trained independently by ambulating in parallel bars over a period of ten years; other subjects have been trained on a commercial motor driven treadmill with a variable speed control. A parachute harness suspended from the ceiling by a set of pulleys, which allowed free movement of legs and arms, and provided a variable degree of body weight support, supported the subjects. Speed was set each time to be the most comfortable for each subject. The usual training time was 30 minutes daily in a single session, five days a week. The training was enhanced by therapists moving the legs to provide swing of the leg and to control the leg not to be in the hyperextension once it was in the stance. To quantify progress in endurance, each daily training session included two testing rounds. A testing round was defined as the maximum continuous period during which a subject could perform unaided bipedal stepping. The results from this study indicate that this walking is feasible. Phasic activity of prime flexor and extensor muscles of both legs has been documented (Figure 4.11). The main result is that all non-ambulating subjects, being able to stand for a prolonged time without bracing with only arm support over parallel bars or even crutches when starting the program, achieved walking at the end.

Paraplegics improve the walking capacity mainly by augmenting the hip flexion, knee extension, and balance. In addition, treadmill locomotion improves muscle strength and enhances cardio-respiratory fitness. Therefore, the treadmill locomotion is of benefit to spastic paraplegic persons with different degrees of paralysis [Dietz et al. 1995, Wernig and Müller, 1992].

Barbeau and Rosignol [1994] studied the walking of subjects who have been supported with a harness, thereby, their body-width has been reduced. To elicit the flexor-like stepping movement in the paralyzed limb, the subjects were instructed to load the fully extended limb during stance and to unload and shift the body weight onto the contralateral limb shortly before swing. Therefore, care was also taken that the arm support provided by a lateral frame was used merely to maintain balance; not to provide body weight support [Barbeau and Rossignol, 1994]. Endurance of the stepping movements to some degree correlated with the spastic muscle tone present, which varied during the study. Barefoot walking and pinching of the limb facilitated stepping and were occasionally applied during the first weeks of training.

The body weight support was initially set at 40 percent, later reduced to 20 percent, and finally eliminated (zero percent) when a plateau in endurance became visible. After several weeks of treadmill training in some subjects walking on a static surface was attempted once a week; thus, replacing the treadmill session. Initially, when necessary, a subject was supported by two therapists, one on each side, yet after a period of training two canes or a walker were sufficient. Apart from treadmill training and over the ground walking, patients participated in the regular rehabilitation program provided in the clinic.

Four subjects with functionally complete paralysis in one limb learned to walk on a static surface after prolonged periods of training although active limb movement in the resting position remained absent. None of these subjects could sufficiently activate the hip flexion or knee extension in the paralyzed limb to allow movement against gravity. Locomotor movement of the paralyzed limbs was initiated and maintained by spinal reflexes or motor programs. Typically, to start locomotive movements the paralyzed limb extended in the hip joint to more than 180 degrees has first to be fully loaded and then, by shifting body weight onto the contralateral limb, unloaded.

In three subjects stepping on the treadmill was achieved only after several training sessions in which the therapist moved the paralyzed limb in a stepping pattern

[Barbeau and Rossignol, 1994]. Similarly, even with automatic stepping, knee extension had to be performed passively for some time (several days to weeks) before it occurred unaided.

The results indicate that despite the nearly complete loss of time locked voluntary movements in one (or both) limb(s) due to spinal cord injury, humans can learn to perform bipedal stepping with joint stabilization and body weight bearing. Possibly, even unilaterally remaining descending connections coordinate the extension and flexion pattern in each limb and manage interlimb coordination.

It was shown that this is the optimal time to start the walking training. In a screening program involving chronic paretic subjects it was found that in three out of six comparable candidates the flexion pattern was evokable within minutes of treadmill walking, and the body weight support indicated that successful training might be started years after the initial spinal cord lesion.

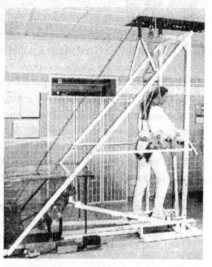

The modern concept of motor learning favors task specific, repetitive training. The repetitive walking training on the powered treadmill, with the additional requirements of reducing the body weight, moving the legs by therapists, and providing lateral stability, led to the development of an advanced mechanized gait trainer.

The device (Figure 4.12) includes several features that allow hemiparetic subjects to have normal like kinematics: harness that provides necessary body weight reduction and vertical excursions of the center of mass, lateral movement of the pelvis to facilitate the frontal plane postural balance, and the most important powered foot plates that move the foot alike in an able-bodied human while walking.

A single electrical motor, with the appropriate mechanism, moves the feet supports allowing variable speed of walking

Fig. 4.12: Hemiparetic subject practicing on the advanced gait trainer. Adapted from Hesse et al., 1999 with permission.

and guarantying normal distribution between the stance and swing phase of the gait cycle. The neurorehabilitation comprises methods and technology for maximizing the efficiency of preserved neuro-muscular structures in a human with motor disability.

The data shown (Figures 4.13 and 4.14) are from a hemiparetic subject (male, 55 years of age). The hemiparesis was caused by an ischemia in the territory of the left middle artery weeks before assessment. The subject could walk independently, yet still needed firm physical assistance for balancing and supporting his weight on the paretic limb. On the treadmill he required a support of 15 percent of his body weight through the harness, and two therapists facilitated a more normal walking by moving his leg and helping him with the postural balance during the paretic limb stance. Both the weight relief and basic cycle parameters remained identical to those when walking on the treadmill. A single therapist controlled that the paretic knee did not hyperextends during stance.

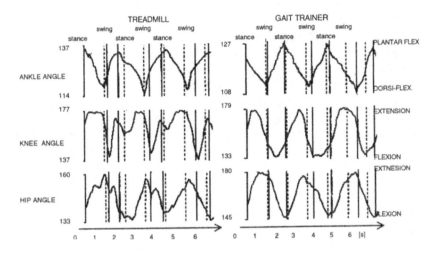

Fig. 4.13: Averaged and normalized sagittal kinematics of the right ankle, knee and hip joints of a right hemiparetic subject while walking on the powered treadmill (left) and on the advanced gait trainer (right). Adapted from Hesse *et al.*, 1999 with permission.

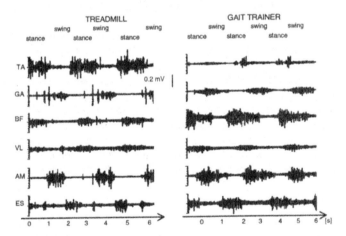

Fig. 4.14: Raw EMG signals of the right Tibialis Anterior (TA) m, Gastrocnemius (GA) m, Biceps Femoris (BF) m, Vastus Lateralis (VL), Adductor Magnus (AM), and Errector Spinae (ES) m. of a right hemiparetic subject while walking on the powered treadmill (left) and on the advanced gait trainer (right). Adapted from Hesse *et al.*, 1999 with permission.

The advance gait trainer presented here did not have control of the ankle joint; thus, there was no plantar flexion during the loading of the heel after the heel contact and no dorsiflexion during the initial and mid swing phases of both legs. The advanced gear mechanism can be enhanced to include the ankle movement.

By analyzing the EMG data a pronounced Gastrocnemius muscle activity due to spasticity related clonus was noticed. On the gait trainer, the activity of Gastrocnemius m. and the Tibialis Anterior m. was decreased with respect to the activity recorded during the treadmill walking. The activation pattern of the thigh muscles (Biceps

Femoris m, Vastus Lateralis m, and Adductor Magnus m.) was comparable between treadmill and gait trainer.

Hesse and coworkers [1995, 1997, 1999] also compared the energy rate of walking: the amount of oxygen used per unit mass and unit distance was 0.47 ml/(kg m) and 0.30 ml/(kgm) for the treadmill and gait trainer respectively. The energy cost of walking is therefore reduced with about 40 percent.

The gait trainer and eventual similar training systems allow a non-ambulant subject to practice walking repetitively without overstraining therapists, but the biggest advantage is the provision of able-bodied like walking pattern (e.g., lateral and vertical movement of the pelvic region being symmetric, symmetric leg movement during both stance and swing phases, variable relief of the body weight through the harness system). Further and detailed clinical studies are still to come to show the applicability and effectiveness of this neurorehabilitation method. The maximizing function relates to developing new strategies that can benefit from the preserved, yet unused systems.

Hemiparetic subjects typically have excessive extensor synergy with a strong adductor muscle component; thus frequently exhibit a narrow base of support while walking, leading ultimately to instability and increases the risk for falling. Although the central nervous system obtains error signal information regarding inappropriate body movement through sensory feedback loop, such input may be enhanced by extrinsic visual or auditory information [e.g., Colbourne *et al.*, 1993; Hanke, 1999]. A special walkway to measure all the temporal and distance parameters of gait and a walker have been designed to provide feedback in improving pathological walking [Hirokawa and Matsumura, 1989]. Simple systems are favorable for clinical use; thus Aruin [Aruin *et al.*, 1999] designed an auditory feedback based on a portable device measuring the distance between the knees of a walking subject. When the distance becomes too narrow (variable threshold), an auditory signal warns the hemiparetic subject; thus he/she can adjust the posture to increase the distance between the knees and maintain the safe support base [Aruin *et al.*, 1999]. The improvement in walking has been statistically significant and both immediate and carry over effects noticed. The learning of this safer walking was three times faster compared with verbally instructed subjects, indicating that the provision of biofeedback is effective.

4.2.2 Neurorehabilitation of Standing

As described in Chapter 1 postural control (standing) is a complex motor activity. Standing is a prerequisite for walking, yet it is also *per se* important providing many medical benefits to humans with disability [e.g., Klose *et al.*, 1997]. In humans with leg paralysis, proprioceptive and cutaneous input coming from legs is deprived and modified, therefore, the vestibular and visual information is not "mixed" with the necessary flavor of what the legs are doing; thus, maintaining vertical posture is very challenging. A clear distinction must be made between paretic and paralyzed subjects. In principle, paretic subjects have potentials in their neuro-muscular system to be retrained; thus they are potential candidates for independent, arm-free standing. The leg muscles in paralyzed humans are diminished; thus standing requires some kind of fixation of the leg joints in the erect position (e.g., FES of joint extensors, knee-ankle-foot orthosis, and standing frame), but they can still benefit from neurorehabilitation because they could "relearn" the functions of the non-paralyzed body segments that fit the functioning of the external assistive system.

Hemiparetic subjects, in most cases caused by stroke, show reliable correlation between isometric muscle strength of the leg and ratings of postural balance [Bohannon, 1989]. Since the balance depends on bilaterally symmetric responses to the disturbances [Horak and Nashner, 1986] and the fact that hemiparetic subjects have asymmetric weakness, their balance disturbance could primarily be a matter of scaling down the muscle strength on the paretic side making them asymmetric [Hamrin et al., 1982].

The difference in muscle strength causes the posture to be asymmetric: 60 percent of the body weight is carried by a non-paretic limb [Bohannon and Larkin, 1985], the paretic knee is slightly flexed, and the foot of the paretic limb is placed in front of the body line (increasing the support base and moving the center of pressure to the forefoot zone of the non-paretic leg).

Striking changes occur in the neuronal networks within the central nervous system after stroke. Hemiparetic subjects have difficulties to cope with posture disturbances. Anteroposterior stability is deprived, and subjects cannot tolerate typical perturbations. It is interesting that the muscle synergies remain reasonably symmetric in both paretic and non-affected legs. Wing and coworkers [Wing et al., 1993] analyzed the stability in the frontal plane, by generating lateral perturbations. A significant loss of balance was reported when comparing to the matching age control subjects, specifically expressed in asymmetric responses. Stroke subjects have also problems in dealing with the forces that are created by their own actions. If during quite standing stroke subjects are asked to shift the center of mass and maintain it for short time in this new position, (e.g., 10 seconds) returning back to the "equilibrium", then they could do the task only for few centimeters, about 20 percent of the magnitude of shift recorded in the control subjects [Dettmann et al., 1987].

In summary, stroke often results in weak, slow, uncoordinated, asymmetric muscle action, possibly compounded by sensory deficits so that many aspects of balance may be impaired.

Helping the hemiparetic subject to change the performance by facilitating practice and giving structured feedback about performance, followed by the assessment of the contribution that this augmented training has made, is currently accepted concepts for restoring posture. The feedback can be provided about the position of the center of pressure, joint angles, acceleration of some part of the body, *etc.* One of the important elements in providing the learning environment for restoring posture is the safety. In this context safety comprises two elements: 1) sensations provided to the hemiparetic subjects, allowing them to relearn standing without fearing to fall; and 2) safety that the training does not lead to any deterioration of preserved functions or further injuries. The rehabilitation can perhaps be speeded up if the training device is powered to allow randomized perturbations that are typical for daily activities, but also if the relearning is competitive requiring maximal involvement of the subject while practicing.

A Multi-purpose Standing Frame. A standing biofeedback training device, which includes a height adjustable work table, weight bearing sensors, and a real-time visual and auditory feedback, has been developed for postural training [Lee et al., 1996]. The application of the device in many stroke subjects showed faster relearning of postural control. Novel compliant standing frame (Figure 4.15) has been developed for neurorehabilitation; it supports standing subjects with disability from falling in multiple directions (antero/posterior and medial/lateral). The rectangular frame holds the subjects' hips allowing two degrees of freedom (rotation around the vertical axes is constrained). The frame is the top of two rigid bars connected with two degrees of freedom joints to the support base [Mihelj et al., 1999]. The knee fixation is required for humans with paralyzed legs since the machine does not hold the subject in the vertical direction. The major feature of this device is that the movement of the hip frame is externally controlled with hydraulic actuators. The actuators control movements and stiffness of the joints that hold the vertical bars of the frame [Matjačić and Bajd, 1998a and b]. The external (machine) ankle mechanisms operate in parallel with the human ankle joints; thus, the machine controls the stiffness of the ankle joints of the standing human.

In a limited number of paraplegic subjects the system has been applied for several daily sessions [Matjačić and Sinkjær, 1999]. Subjects having difficulties in maintaining the balance when standing have been requested to learn the "new sensation" of increased stiffness in the ankle joints and move their upper body to bring their body (the frame) into the neutral, vertical position. After only about a week, subjects learned how to move the upper body, allowing the therapists to reduce the stiffness of the ankle joints. The initial values were in the range of 18 Nm/degree, decreasing to about 3 Nm/degree. This low value of stiffness can be relatively easily provided to subjects without the machine (e.g., stiff ankle shoes); thereby the subjects would be able to stand arm-free for extended periods of time because of the newly developed system for controlling the posture.

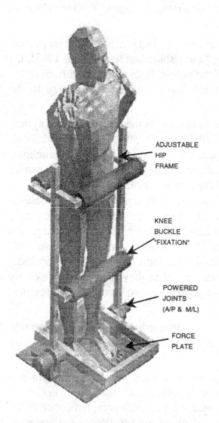

Fig. 4.15: The sketch of the multi-purpose standing frame for neurorehabilitation of postural control. A/P – antero/posterior, M/L – medio/lateral movement. Adapted from Mihelj et al., 1999, with permission.

The experiments indicate that paraplegic subjects, when provided with safety, can learn how to use their preserved neuro-muscular mechanisms and ultimately improve their functioning.

In addition, humans with paralysis can be supplied with information about the state of their feet legs. As mentioned earlier, the stability of bipedal standing is labile, requiring that the projection of the center of mass to the support base is as close as possible to the center of pressure, and that both of these points are more or less in the center of the support base. If the information about the position of the center of pressure is provided to the patient, he/she may be able to move his/her upper part of the body (voluntarily) and "balance" back to the safer posture by moving the center of mass.

Several available feedback channels can be used to "inform" the subject. A SwayWeigh (Ramar Ltd, Oxon, U.K.) provides a quantitative indication of weight distribution using visual feedback [Shumway-Cook et al.; 1988].

The subjects learn how to position their body in order to have a symmetrical distribution of the ground reaction forces between the legs. The visual display (needle pointing the approximate direction of the center of pressure to the center of mass) provided indication as to which leg is more loaded; thus when shifting the body to ensure even loading the needle on the meter comes into the vertical position. This is a low cost, portable device, which leads to immediate improvement, but also shows carry-over effects [de Weerdt et al., 1989].

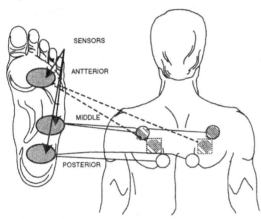

Fig. 4.16: Cognitive feedback system for enhancing balance control in a standing paraplegic. Three pairs of electrodes provide electro-cutaneous feedback about the position of the center of pressure. The position is calculated in real-time based on pressure distribution measured with piezoresistive based insoles. Courtesy of Dr. Zlatko Matjačić, Aalborg University.

Only a few simple sensory systems have been tested to improve the cognition of standing. Petrofsky and Phillips [1983a] used a vibrotactile feedback to the chest of a paralyzed subject to "let him know" the distribution of ground reaction forces. Matjačić and Bajd [1998a and b] used a single channel auditory feedback in arm-free paraplegic standing. Andrews et al. [1988] suggested electro-cutaneous signaling to the subject whenever inclination in the sagittal plane exceeded a predetermined threshold angle. The common conclusion from all studies is that the provision of information leads to a better postural control and reduces the body swaying. Recently, Matjačić (personal communication) tested an apparatus consisting of the following elements: a sensory system to assess the pressure distribution under the feet and perform feature extraction, an encoding algorithm, an electro-cutaneous interface to the unimpaired part of body, and the visual display. The visual display was used to develop cognition of the subject on the electro-cutaneous information.

Electro-cutaneous interface is realized with three pairs of skin stimulation sites, symmetrically placed with respect to both sides of the upper body. The information brought to the cognition included: Anterior, Middle, and Posterior regions at the sole (the two sites for the anterior and middle zones are at the back, one for the anterior zone at the chests), and Left, Balance, and Right (Figure 4.16). The results when providing paraplegic subjects with electro-cutaneous feedback indicate that the encoding scheme could be interpreted reliably after an appropriate training. It was also shown that the residual sensory system of the upper non-paralyzed part of the body could not track different postures consistently if the feedback was not provided.

4.2.3 Upper Extremity Augmented Feedback

At present, little technology is used in the rehabilitation of upper extremities. Reinkensmeyer *et al.* [1999] described a robotic "smart exercise partner". This is a self-ranging robot requiring the subject to be capable of moving independently or using the contralateral limb to move or guide the impaired arm. Lum *et al.* [1999] described the design of a robot "rehabiltator" focused on bi-manual tasks to promote motor recovery. The basis of the work is PUMA robot augmented by better sensors and Motor Image Movement Enabler, which is cloning movement of one to the other arm.

Hogan with his colleagues [Krebs *et al.*, 1998] introduced MIT-MANUS back-drivable robot for augmented training. The system has undergone extensive clinical trials [Aisen *et al.*, 1997]. The system is effective for both diagnosing and delivering meaningful therapy via engaging "video games". MIT-MANUS is a robot designed for safe, stable, and compliant operation in close physical contact with humans. This is achieved using impedance control, a key feature of the robot control system [Hogan, 1985].

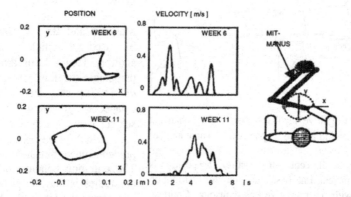

Fig. 4.17: A hemiplegic subject drawing clockwise circles after six and eleven weeks of practicing with his affected arm. The hand-holder connects the arm to the MIT-MANUS robotic assistance (shown right). Adapted from Krebs *et al.*, 1998 © IEEE.

Its computer control system modulates the way the robot reacts to mechanical perturbation from a subject or clinician and ensures a gentle compliant behavior. MIT-MANUS can move, guide, or perturb the movement of a subject's arm and can record movement motions and mechanical quantities such as position, velocity, and forces applied. The device is portable and exceeds applicable safety standards for operation in a clinical environment [Krebs *et al.*, 1998]. The planar module has two degrees of freedom for elbow and forearm motion. It also permits a small range of passive vertical motion through a set of springs. A three-degrees of freedom module mounts on the end of the planar module and provides movement of the wrist.

One of the studies showing the efficacy of the MIT-MANUS included 20 stroke subjects, and the goal was to measure the recovery of functions when subjects played video games controlled by the robot arm. The games included drawing circles, stars, squares, diamonds, and navigating Windows. Some games required predominantly shoulder motion, while others required predominantly elbow movement. Additional games required the coordination of both shoulder and elbow joints. The games have been selected to maximize correlated sensory feedback, including visual, audio, and proprioceptive stimuli.

The procedure lasted for about seven weeks, and consisted of daily exercise with the normal arm and three packets of 20 repetitions with the robot guided affected arm. If the subject was not able to complete the task with the impaired arm, he assisted it with the normal arm.

The individual improvement in functioning is presented with an example (Figure 4.17). The task was to draw a smooth circle. The analysis of the velocity profile (middle panels, Figure 4.17) indicate that after six weeks the subject made discrete movement; and the drawing is a polygon with curved sides (Figure 4.17, left panels), yet after 11 weeks the movement became much smoother. The velocity profile still shows that the movement is segmental.

The summary data for all subjects using MIT-MANUS show that there is an universal improvement in functioning (FIM reduced to upper extremities, described in Chapter 3) for 14.1±9.7 out of 66, compared with 9.9±11.2 in the control group. This result fits into the results that have reported positive outcomes with different therapies (repetitive passive exercises [Bütefisch *et al.*, 1995], forced use of paretic limb by restraining the contralateral limb [Taub *et al.*, 1993; Wolf *et al.*, 1989], biofeedback [Wolf and Binder-Macleod, 1983], and functional electrical stimulation [Smith, 1990]). The efficacy of these different therapies is controversial. Studies examining the differences of the outcomes between the techniques showed little variation [Dickstein *et al.*, 1986].

Wittenstein Aktiv Technologies has developed other systems with similar goals. The devices developed use measurements of the operator's forces for synthesising the commands to a servo system. The force displacement characteristics and dynamic behavior can be accurately controlled. The systems have originally been developed for aircraft and simulator control sticks. The systems have been adapted to provide different interfaces to the human body. One of devices used for rehabilitation is for the control of elbow movement and has three degrees of freedom, each controlled by an integrated motor/gearbox servo system.

The linkage, which controls the arm movement is maximizing the movement range of the arm whilst maintaining appropriate force levels to control movement. To give the best dynamic response the system has high natural frequencies.

4.2.4 Electrical Therapy

FES of paralyzed muscles holds promise as a strategy to assist humans in executing functional movement after central nervous system injuries. Muscle atrophy is one of the problems that must be addressed for this method to be successful. Electrical stimulation can be effective for preventing atrophy or building the muscle from its atrophied stage.

Facilitation of Voluntary Movement

The facilitation of a voluntary movement implies learning of the diminished movement by means of electrical stimulation allowing eventual regaining of voluntary control of some muscles. Candidates for this type of therapeutic electrical stimulation are subjects who have reduced voluntary control of muscles due to a prolonged fixation of the joint. The facilitation is very productive in hemiplegic and incomplete paraplegic subjects. It has been suggested that therapeutic electrical stimulation helps also in "learning" a new movement after the transposition of tendons. Although electrical stimulation itself exerts an influence upon the afferent nervous system, better effects are achieved if a subject takes an active part in the therapy. In the simplest case the subject watches a movement and triggers it himself. Therapeutic electrical stimulation restores voluntary movements even more successfully, if combined with other conventional rehabilitation therapies (e.g., physical, hydro).

Strengthening of Atrophied Muscles

Training methods with electrical stimulation vary for different muscles, particularly with respect to the duration of stimulation, the loading of contracting muscles, and the muscle type. A short stimulation duration and muscle loading regimen is exemplified in a situation in which the subject rides an exercise bicycle that provides loading to the quadriceps femoris muscle while receiving 30 minutes of electrical stimulation daily [Petrofsky and Phillips, 1983a]. In other regimens, electrical stimulation is applied for longer duration (e.g., one or two hours per day) to the same muscles, but with less loading [Kralj and Bajd, 1989]. The duration of stimulation may be as long as eight hours on a daily basis for muscles in the upper extremities [Peckham et al., 1976a and b], whereas two-hour sessions are effective in increasing the endurance of lower-limb muscles without external loading [Stein et al., 1992]. Outcome measures are difficult to compare from study to study because the variables for stimulation are different for each subject.

Low-frequency stimulation paradigms that increase muscle endurance have had different effects on muscle strength, depending on conditions of stimulation. The results of many animal studies, in which muscles were stimulated at low frequencies (10-20 Hz) for two or more hours per day, show that an increase in muscle endurance and oxidative capacity is often accompanied by an undesirable decrease in muscle fiber size and muscle force [Gordon et al., 1993a]. For example, endurance of the medial gastrocnemius muscle of the cat was dramatically increased by 20 Hz stimulation for 12 hours per day, but the peak tetanic force of the muscle was significantly reduced. These results are consistent with the normal reciprocal relationship between endurance and strength in normal motor units [Gordon and Patullo, 1993]. In human subjects, daily sessions or at least three sessions per week of low-frequency stimulation increased the muscle endurance and strength when the stimulated muscles contracted against set resistances [Bajd et al., 1989]. The muscle strength did not increase significantly under conditions in which the stimulated muscles did not contract against a load, for the muscles tested [Stein et al., 1992].

Several factors may influence the muscle strength and should be considered in designing training regimens. These factors include: muscle length, activity, loading, muscle type, and function, and the interaction of these factors [Roy et al., 1991].

Muscle Length. Goldspink [1977] showed that both innervated and denervated muscles pinned at long length underwent substantially less atrophy initially than muscles fixed at short length. Others have confirmed and extended these original findings. Generally, there is an inverse relationship between the initial degree of atrophy and the amount of stretch imposed on an immobilized muscle [Roy et al., 1991].

Muscle Activity. Salmons and Vrbova [1969] first demonstrated that increased activity could convert fast-twitch muscles to slow twitch muscles. Using the cat model in which the spinal cord has been hemisected and the ipsilateral hind limb deafferented, Kernell et al. [1987a and b] were able to greatly reduce the spontaneous nerve act and study in detail the effects of stimulation on muscle properties. Increased amount of stimulation to cat peroneus longus muscle induced an increase in fatigue resistance, decrease in muscle strength [Kernell and Eerbek, 1989]. Superimposing a brief period of high frequency stimulation (100 Hz for 0.5 percent of the day) on continuous stimulation (10 Hz for of the 24 hours) prevented most of the loss of strength. Attempts to reproduce these findings in human subjects, however, have not been successful (Popović D, unpublished observations). The conclusion of Kernel agrees with the experimental work of applying doublets and N-lets [Karu et al., 1995; Burke et al., 1973]. The short bursts of high frequency activation, or so-called intermittent stimulation, is able to produce a much larger force for short periods of time, but it does not decrease the fatigue resistance, and does not fatigue the muscle. The basic of this behavior is described in Chapter 1.

Muscle loading. It is generally accepted that to build strength a muscle must get close to the maximal forces for short periods of time, whereas to improve endurance a muscle must maintain small forces for long periods of time [e.g., Salmons and Henriksson, 1981]. Thus, isometric or even eccentric forceful contractions are necessary for building strength, whereas concentric contractions against light loads may increase the endurance.

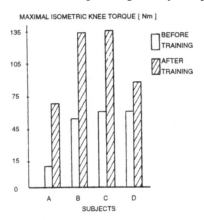

Fig. 4.18: Maximal isometric knee net joint torque before and after six weeks of 30 minutes daily FES of quadriceps muscle with surface electrodes at 25 pulses per second.

Muscle Type and Function. As previously described, a general finding in both subjects with spinal cord injuries and animal models is the more severe atrophy of extensor muscles, especially slow-twitch muscles that cross a single joint [Gordon and Patullo, 1993]. These muscles are largely responsible for maintaining posture and bearing weight. In subjects with paralysis of legs, the quadriceps femoris muscle undergoes more significant atrophy than the tibialis anterior muscle. The strength of the quadriceps femoris muscle does improve after retraining [Kralj and Bajd, 1989], and the strength of the tibialis muscle changes very little [Stein et al., 1992].

Interactions. Although some of the factors discussed earlier have been individually studied, little is known about the interaction among them. For example, a muscle contracting at a long length would produce a greater load because of the passive length-tension properties of muscle. Unloaded muscles lose weight and are less forceful even if they are exercised or stimulated for 20 minutes per day [Gardiner and

Lapointe, 1988]; the muscles are only able to maintain weight and force if changing joint angle [Goldspink and Goldspink, 1975] passively stretches them. Also, physiological extensors that maintain body posture against gravity are activated more

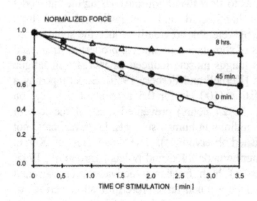

Fig. 4.19: The mean values of force decay of the ankle dorsiflexor for five paraplegic subjects, who received intermittent stimulation for six weeks 0, 45 minutes and 8 hours) daily. Adapted from Stein et al., 1992, with permission.

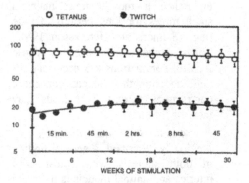

Fig. 4.20: The tetanic and twitch forces measured during the isometric ankle dorsiflexion. The stimulation parameters have been selected by assuring that the M-wave response is constant. Adapted from Stein et al., 1992, with permission.

Candidates for the strengthening of atrophied muscles are not necessarily subjects with spinal cord injury, but also subjects with orthopedic problems (artificial joints) and arthritic subjects whose muscles are atrophied either as a result of the immobilization of a joint by a plaster cast or due to pain in a joint. In all subjects the muscles have weakened since they are not used as a result of a lesion in the central nervous system or other reason. In hemiplegic subjects the therapy will be applied to muscles and muscle groups, which are antagonistic to the muscles that are typically spastic (e.g., knee extensors will be stimulated with subjects with a predominant flexion synergistic pattern in the standing position). The strengthening of muscles in humans with paralysis by electrical stimulation is highly advisable due to the fact that a continuous muscle contraction promotes better blood circulation and prevents pressure sores [Kralj and Bajd, 1989].

The strengthening of the knee extensor muscles for four subjects (Figure 4.18) shows effects after 6 weeks of 30 minutes daily exercise. An increase of the net joint torque at the knee joint is variable, yet bigger than 25 percent in all. The exercise has been performed against the load at the ankle. The data for quadriceps stimulation are from the clinical evaluation of the electronic stimulator manufactured by the company "Medicina TS", Belgrade, in the Rehabilitation Institute, Belgrade, Yugoslavia [Popović et al., 1997].

It is desirable, but not required that subjects cooperate in the strengthening program. During the training of atrophied muscles subjects can do other things, since the exercise is boring. It is of interest to say that the pain threshold changes with time, and that the levels that subject are ready to tolerate if they have sensation change dramatically over the application of electrical stimulation

The strengthening of atrophied muscles can be even more effective when electrical stimulation is combined with various classical rehabilitation aids such as exercises with weights, pulleys, and other mechanical systems offering resistance to an electrically induced torque. In general, isotonic strengthening is more effective than the isometric one. Isometric strengthening must be applied with arthritic subjects where a joint movement inflicts an unbearable pain.

One of the most comprehensive studies on selecting the preferred stimulation regimen was done by Stein et al. [1992]. Without going into details the results of this study will be discussed. Figure 4.19 shows the normalized force vs. time of stimulation for the Tibialis Anterior m. averaged over five subjects after six weeks of daily stimulation for different periods of time.

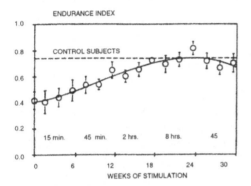

Fig. 4.21: Endurance index is a fraction of force still being generated after 3.5 minutes of intermittent stimulation. The endurance increased progressively. Open circles are means measured every two weeks. Adapted from Stein et al., 1992, with permission.

The other result relates to the maximum twitch and tetanus force. The ankle net joint torque does not change after the stimulation compared to the measurements before the training (Figure 4.20), being different from the chronic stimulation of the quadriceps muscle (Figure 4.18). The difference in the maximum net joint torque between subjects is noticeable; however, the increase in the force is congruous over the population studied.

The effects of stimulation are mostly pronounced when analyzing the endurance, that is the fatigue resistance cause by the changes in the muscle structure. At the beginning of the stimulation program the muscles fatigue very fast. However, after chronic stimulation muscles can generate large forces even after prolonged periods of time, that are comparable with the muscles of able-bodied subjects.

Stein et al. [1992] studied in details the endurance of the dorsiflexor muscles (Figure 4.21). The chronic stimulation has been applied for more than 39 weeks, and the protocol remained the same, yet the duration of daily stimulation changed from 15 minutes all the way to eight hours. The conclusion of the study was that the endurance does not differ very much between the two-hours and eight-hours daily stimulation. However, there is a noticeable drop of the endurance when the stimulation time was decreased to 45 minutes. Measuring the strength and endurance in subjects six weeks after they stopped the daily chronic simulation showed both measured quantities will return to the almost base line (before the strengthening started).

The endurance test has been performed by recording force using the known geometry of the ankle joint and measured torque. The test has been performed by intermittent stimulation, two second on, followed by two seconds of no stimulation for a period of 3.5 minutes. The stimulation parameters have been adjusted to ensure that the M-wave is constant, to eliminate the variability imposed by different positioning of electrodes, impedance, etc. Figure 4.22 shows the force profile measured at the beginning and at the end of the test in a paraplegic subject.

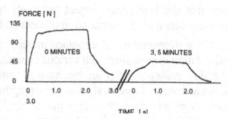

Fig. 4.22: Tension was produced by a train of stimuli to common peroneal nerve at 40 Hz for two seconds, followed by two seconds of no stimulation. The recordings have been performed for 3.5 minutes. Adapted from Stein et al., 1992, with permission.

Increasing the Range of Movement

Contractures are typically seen in most immobilized subjects (e.g., hip contractures because of the prolonged sitting in wheelchair, elbow contracture because of immobilization due to the fracture splint). The contractures limit the range of joint movement. This anomaly results from both an affected joint and from a shortening, thickness, and fibrosis of muscle fibers. Contractures also appear because of a permanent unbalance between the antagonistic and the agonistic muscle. In case of the contracture the muscle group (antagonist) should be stimulated to correct the position.

Electrical stimulation provides movement, and this exercise is beneficial because it improves the metabolic use of calcium, which when unbalanced is the major reason behind contractures. By stimulating muscles active movements are induced, and calcium pumps will be activated (described in Chapter 1). Contraction of muscles will result with the rotations of body segment around joints. The stimulation program should last more than one-hour daily (e.g., two or three session of 20 to 30 minutes) [Stefanovska et al., 1989]. Muscle contraction provoked by electrical stimulation has to be strong enough to move a joint throughout the entire range of motion. It should be taken care, however, that too strong stimulation might cause an excessive movement and consequently pain. Spasticity may greatly interfere with this exercise routine, yet there is indication that this program actually can decrease the spasticity.

Electrical stimulation can be applied even in the case that a splint immobilizes the joint. It is clear that in this case the stimulation results in isometric contractions. With paralyzed subjects therapeutic electrical stimulation may be applied even before the contractures have set in. Approximately 30 minutes of daily exercise by means of cyclic stimulation suffices to preserve joint mobility. A subject can perform such a program alone without the help of the physiotherapist or his family members [Kralj and Bajd, 1989].

Moderation of Spasticity

Various reports on the application of electrical stimulation with hemiplegic subjects and subjects with a spinal cord injury have proven that spasticity is moderated as a result of electrical stimulation. Some reports state, however, that muscle tonus increased after the subject had undergone a program of therapeutic electrical stimulation. These are primarily subjective reports of subjects and their therapists. Quantitative measurements of spasticity performed on subjects with spinal cord injury show that in about 50 percent cases electrical stimulation considerably moderates spasticity and that the influence of electrical stimulation remains for quite some time after stimulation. In other subjects an increased spasticity was noticed immediately after applying stimulation (e.g., low thoracic spinal cord lesions) being counter productive and affecting the quality of life. In some subjects after stroke, a long term carry-on effect has been indicated, allowing them to walk much easier at faster pace [Stefanovska et al., 1989].

Spasticity is discussed in more details in the last section of Chapter 4.

Electrical Stimulation in Case of Peripheral Nerve Lesions

The purpose of therapeutic electrical stimulation is to slow down the progress of muscular atrophy, which would develop before an eventual regeneration of the peripheral nerve, which lasts some months. In determining the indications for the application of electrical stimulation in case of peripheral nerve lesions we should be extremely careful, as medical opinions are not unanimous in this point. It seems that the stimulation of a completely denervated muscle prevents the development of collateral re-innervation, which means that it can be noxious. In many cases only a partial impairment of peripheral nerves occurred, and then the electrotherapy is undoubtedly useful. Stimulating a denervated muscle is much more complex. The amount of electrical charge to activate the muscle is several order of magnitude larger compared with the same innervated muscle (see the following section about neuroprostheses). By applying stimulation voltage of about 100 V, at pulse duration of 50 to 80 ms and stimulus frequency of 7 to 10 Hz, fused contraction may be obtained in some denervated muscles, but sometime the pulse duration must be as long as 300 to 500 ms, and the frequency at about 1 or 3 Hz. A considerable amount of energy is transferred via electrodes to the muscle tissue; thus biphasic pulses, where a negative one follows a positive stimulus, and large skin electrodes should be considered [Kralj and Bajd, 1989].

Use of Biofeedback in Therapy with Electrical Stimulation

The combination of a biofeedback and therapeutic electrical stimulation improves the voluntary control, which is evident from the augmented isometric torque and range of motion. Biofeedback training of subjects who have had a stroke is often rather difficult because they could have cognitive and concentration problems, however, imposing it is extremely effective for improving the functioning.

4.3 Neuroprostheses

A neuroprosthesis is a system for replacing or augmenting a function that is lost or diminished because of the injury or disease of the nervous system. The basic principle for operation of a neuroprosthesis is the stimulation of neuro-muscular tissues, *i.e.*, activation of sensory or motor systems. FES is at this time the essence of neuroprostheses. FES elicits controlled neural activation by delivering low level electrical currents. It is also possible to use a time varying magnetic field, and thereby induce pulsatile currents directly; this technique is not yet developed efficiently enough for functional usage.

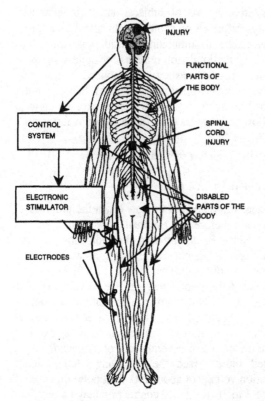

Figure 4.23 shows the principle of FES based neuroprosthesis. After an injury or disease of the central nervous system (e.g., stroke, paraplegia, tetraplegia) as described in Chapter 3, parts of the body will be functioning normally, but parts of the body will be paralyzed. The paralysis leaves some muscles without connection to the central nervous system (CNS); these muscles will be denervated and without surgical procedure they cannot be used for NP. In contrast, many muscles will be connected to the CNS below the level of injury; thus, they are innervated, but not controllable volitionally. These muscles can be used for the movement restoration. In parallel, many sensory pathways are connected to the CNS, yet their function is lost or modified because they do not reach the corresponding center within CNS. The NP can be considered as a bypass of the damaged sensory-motor structure. The FES system comprises an interface to the sensory and motor systems of he body and controllable stimulator.

Fig. 4.23: Principle of operation of the motor neuroprostheses (NP). Components of the NP are: control system, stimulator, sensory feedback (not shown) and electrodes.

4.3.1 Functional Electrical Stimulation (FES) Principles

The literature dealing with NP frequently uses other terms than FES, such as neuromuscular electrical stimulation (NMES) and functional neuro-muscular stimulation (FNS), aiming to precisely describe the application of electrical stimulation; the term FES is used throughout this book.

FES systems aim to achieve sensory-motor integration; thereby a better function of humans with paralysis. FES activates motoneurons or reflex pathways by stimulating sensory nerve fibers. The electrical stimulation can also be applied to sensory nerve fibers eliciting a perceived response in the skin, which may be used to provide sensory cues [Peckham *et al.*, 1988]. Many other applications are considered within the so-called neuromodulation (e.g., epidural stimulation for pain).

Chapter 2 describes mechanisms of contraction and discusses how muscle contraction can be graded and controlled: size principle, recruitment order, frequency of activation, *etc*. All these elements must be followed precisely in order to achieve a natural-like sensory-motor function. Although a variety of electrodes and stimulus waveforms may be utilized to excite the tissue, basic physiological properties favor one over the other.

FES can be delivered using so-called monopolar or bipolar configuration (Figure 4.24); this is relevant only when multi-channel stimulation is applied. In the bipolar configuration two electrodes are positioned in the vicinity of the neuro-muscular system that is to be stimulated, and the electrical circuit is closed between these two electrodes (e.g., channels A and B, Figure 4.24). In the monopolar configuration active electrodes (e.g., channels 1 to 4, Figure 4.24) are positioned in the vicinity of the structures to be stimulated, while a single *common* electrode is positioned relatively distant to the stimulated structures, yet somewhere along the neural pathway to the CNS.

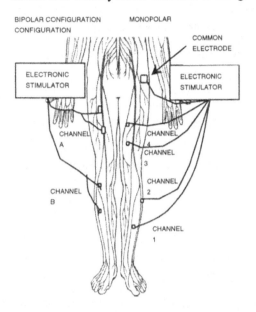

Fig. 4.24: Schema of the monopolar (right) and bipolar (left) configuration used in NP.

FES delivers trains of the electrical charge pulses, mimicking to an extent the natural flow of excitation signals generated by the CNS in non-impaired structures. FES operation can be modeled with a relatively simple electric circuit: generator, electrodes, and tissue. The tissue is an ionic conductor with an impedance of about 10 to 100 Ω, and electrodes are capacitive conductors whose electrical properties depend on many variables, but their impedance is from 500 Ω to 5 kΩ, and they induce a phase shift of about 10 to 30 degrees. The generator can work as a current- or voltage-regulated device.

The amplitude and duration of stimulus pulses, output impedance of the generator, and impedance of electrodes determine the electrical charge that will be delivered to neuro-muscular structure. Generators (stimulators) are usually referred to as constant-current or constant-voltage devices. High-output impedance devices will deliver the desired current to the tissue, regardless of the changes in electrode properties up to the voltage capacity available. These constant-current stimulators are correctly termed current-regulated stimulators.

The electrical charge delivered to the stimulated structure depends on the impedance of electrodes to tissue interface when the stimulators that have a low-output impedance, or so-called constant-voltage or voltage regulated devices, are applied. This is the reason to use the current regulated electronic stimulator so that the consequences of typical impedance changes can be ignored. Figure 4.25 shows the patterns of the voltage and current for the current regulated (A) and voltage regulated (B) stimulators. Since the electrode-skin interface has electro-capacitive properties, the voltage regulated the stimulation results with uncontrolled electrical current (Figure 4.25B); thus, although the voltage may be substantial, the actual charge delivered to the tissue may be very small. This may result in pain, yet no or very week muscle contraction. In contrast, current regulated stimulators precisely control the charge delivered to the tissue (Figure 4.25A). The issue that has to be considered is that the current regulated stimulator may cause tissue damage if the surface of the electrode is too small.

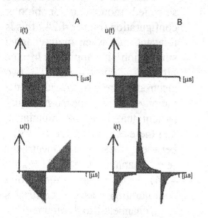

Fig. 4.25: Current regulated stimulation (A), and voltage regulated stimulation (B). The top panels are the output of the stimulator, the bottom the the current and voltage applied to the tissue.

The stimulus waveform selected for the excitation process must take into consideration the desired physiological effect (action potential generation), potential damage to the tissue, and potential degradation of the electrode. The process is discussed in detail by Mortimer and collaborators [Mortimer, 1981; Scheiner et al., 1990; McCreery et al., 1995]. The waveform selected is generally rectangular. A nonrectangular pulse could be utilized, but the rise time must be sufficiently fast so that the nerve membrane does not accommodate and fails to open its channels. The stimulus waveform may be unidirectional (monophasic) or bidirectional (biphasic) as shown in Figure 4.26. Biphasic stimulus is recommended for several reasons. Surface stimulation is more comfortable with biphasic than monophasic stimulation. For implanted electrodes, the potential for damage to the tissue will be lessened with the biphasic stimulus. Tissue damage is significantly related to the pH change at the electrode tissue interface. At the cathode, the pH may increase due to the production of OH^-, while at the anode the environment will become more acidic [Scheiner et al., 1990]. While some buffering capacity for pH changes exists in the tissue, the changes with monophasic stimulation are greater than those with biphasic stimulation. Although reactions at the electrodes are not completely reversed with the biphasic stimulation, this stimulus allows significantly greater charge injection before tissue damage is encountered [Mortimer, 1981].

The shape of the secondary pulse is also important. Conceptually, one would like the electrode reactions to be totally reversible, suggesting a rapid current reversal in the secondary phase. With the metallic conductors presently used, the electrode reactions are not completely reversed. The biphasic pulse limits the extent of irreversibility of the reactions. Balanced charge stimuli are generally used in which equal charge is delivered in each half-cycle. Some degree of imbalance may be allowed, but this issue is still being studied.

Both electrodes receive a pulse of each polarity (Figure 4.26). By convention, the electrode that receives the negative stimulus pulse first is called the cathode. During

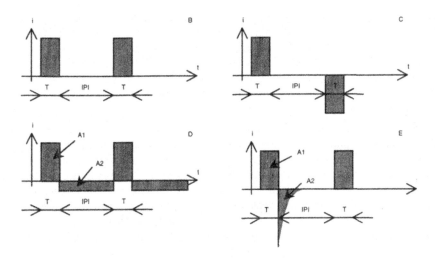

Fig. 4.26: B) Monophasic constant current; C) biphasic constant current; D) biphasic balanced constant current; and E) biphasic compensated constant current patterns of stimulation. Surface A2 (electrical charge) has to be at least 80 percent of the surface A1 for safe subcutaneous stimulation. T is the pulse duration, IPI is the inter-pulse interval, and the height of the shaded squares is the amplitude of the pulses I.

the cathodic phase (assuming a monopolar configuration) the charge is delivered first to the active (working) electrode, which is near the depolarization site. This is important in order to minimize the risk of possible tissue damage. The anodic pulse is then applied after a short interphase delay following the cathodic pulse.

This second pulse will allow the action potential to fully develop on the nerve since immediate current reversal may stop the firing of a nerve fiber, which is just at its threshold. This prevents the electrode potential developed on the working electrode from corroding due to the application of excessive anodic potentials. The cathodic pulse does not contribute to the corrosion of the electrode. For example, using non-noble intramuscular electrodes, the cathodic amplitude may be 20-40 times greater than the anodic phase.

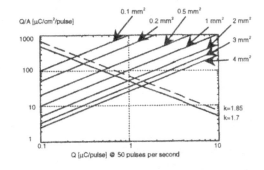

Fig. 4.27: Safe electrical charge vs. the area of electrode in contact with the tissue. The stimulus parameters being lower of the k=1.7 are safe.

The surface area of the electrode is important in defining the safety of the stimulation (Figure 4.27). The geometric surface area may be many times less than the real surface area, depending upon the surface structure of the stimulating electrodes.

Large surface areas will diffuse the current and may not effect the excitation desired. A small surface area may result in a high charge density and current density. When selecting an electrode one must know these values to assess the safety of the stimulation. Although absolute safe levels of stimulation have not been established for all electrode types and all stimulus waveforms, the values presented by Grill and Mortimer [2000] provide the investigator with estimated safe levels for neural stimulation. With intramuscular electrodes, safe stimulation is demonstrated at a charge density of 2.0 $\mu C/mm^2$ in the cathodic phase using balanced biphasic monopolar stimulation with a current-regulated stimulus with a capacitively coupled recharge phase (panel E in Figure 4.26).

Figure 4.27 summarizes the results of many studies [e.g., Grill and Mortimer, 2000]. The lines pointed with arrows and numbers correspond to the surface of the active electrode. The safe zone is left (Figure 4.27) from the line denoted with k=1.7. The diagram shows the safe parameters of stimulation when using monopolar stimulation with implanted electrodes, once the size of electrode is known, or *vice versa* the minimum size of the electrode if the parameters are known. The electrical charge over the surface of the electrode and pulse is at the vertical axis, and the charge per pulse at the horizontal axis of Figure 4.27. Note that the diagram is for the 50 Hz stimulation, yet the diagram for other frequencies typical for FES is similar.

Either amplitude modulation (AM) or pulse width (duration) modulation (PWM) may govern the level of recruitment. A comparison of the method of recruitment modulation to be selected should include consideration of recruitment linearity, charge injected (for safety reasons), and ease of implementation and control of the circuitry that generates the stimulus pulses. This comparison has been made for intramuscular electrodes. The results were that, in consideration of recruitment, the differences between AM and PWM were small. PWM utilized a slightly lower charge density than AM to evoke a response of equal magnitude, a result that has been theoretically confirmed. Since timing circuits (*i.e.*, regulating pulse width) can be easily constructed and controlled with a resolution of 1 μs or less, many designers of stimulator use this technique.

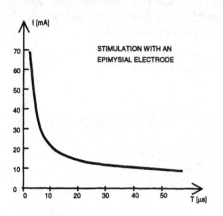

Fig. 4.28: Amplitude-duration (I-T) diagram for the gastrocnemius m. Adapted from Popović *et al.*, 1991a, with permission.

As shown in the amplitude-duration (I-T) curve (Figure 4.28) relatively short stimulus rectangular pulses result in the muscle nerve being excited. Much larger charge is required to stimulate the muscle directly. Therefore, FES utilizes short pulses, generally less than 200 μs, resulting in the activation of the nerve.

The threshold for excitation of the fibers of a peripheral nerve is proportional to the diameter of the fiber as described in Chapter 1. Since the nerve is composed of a mixture of afferent and efferent fibers with a spectrum of fiber diameters, short pulses of constant amplitude will excite large afferent and efferent fibers. Longer pulses may also excite smaller fibers, including afferents normally carrying information of noxious stimuli, and therefore may be painful to the subject. For this reason and in order to minimize the electrical charge injection, short pulse duration is preferred.

The regulation of the strength of a motor response is done through the number of active motor nerve fibers and the rate at which they trigger action potentials (see Chapter 1). In voluntary control, these two mechanisms are called recruitment and temporal summation, respectively. The same terms are utilized to describe electrically elicited events, despite the fact that the origins of the events are different than in a voluntary contraction. When the stimulus is sufficiently large, an action potential will be elicited in the nerve. The action potential will propagate in both directions (up and down) from the site of stimulation. The minimum stimulus level to achieve the action potential response is known as threshold. A single muscle action potential generates a twitch response in all of the muscle fibers innervated by the same nerve. The magnitude and time course of the twitch contraction depends upon the number and type of muscle fibers in the motor unit and recent stimulation history (e.g., potentiation, muscle fatigue). The duration of the mechanical response of a twitch contraction lasts for less than 40 ms in motor units composed of fast, glycolytic muscle fibers longer than 100 ms in slow, oxidative motor units.

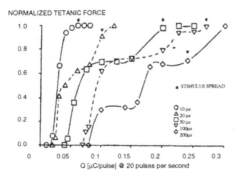

Fig. 4.29: Force developed in medial gastrocnemius muscle in a cat vs. electrical charge per pulse. Shorter pulses required less charge to elicit force, but the recruitment range is very small and higher amplitudes are required. Longer pulses are less effective, and produce nonlinear recruitment. Adapted from Popović et al., 1991a, with permission.

Most, if not all, FES systems activate a number of motor units. The number of motor units that are active (*i.e.*, the level of recruitment) is regulated by the electrical charge injected. The electrical charge is the integral of the current over the duration of the stimulus. In case of using rectangular pattern of stimulation, the electrical charge per pulse can be calculated by multiplying the stimulus pulse amplitude, I, and the pulse duration, T.

In a physiological contraction, the recruitment order is fixed; slow, fatigue-resistant motor units are active at a lower voluntary effort than larger, fast, fatigable units. In an electrically induced recruitment, the recruitment order is not known *a priori*, but depends upon the variables of position and geometry as well as fiber size. An inverse order of electrically induced recruitment is typical when applying FES; the largest fibers are being easily excited, compared with small fibers. This implies that the recruitment has to be considered at all times in order to provide controlled and graded externally induced activation. The recruitment of nerve fibers with increasing stimulus pulse amplitude or duration is nonlinear as shown in Figure 4.29. For this reason, a linear increase of muscle output force cannot be achieved by a linear change in the input. The selection of the most effective parameter for regulation of recruitment has been studied by many [e.g., Bajzek and Jaeger, 1987; Baratta *et al.*, 1989; Baratta and Solomonov, 1990; Crago *et al.*, 1974, 1980; Gruner and Mason, 1989; Popović *et al.*, 1991a].

The second mechanism effecting the overall force developed by the muscle is temporal summation (see Chapter 1). Stimulus pulses applied in rapid succession to the nerve will produce a mechanically additive effect of the twitch response. At low frequencies the response is unfused, and variations of the muscle force are noticeable. As the mechanical responses sum with increasing frequency, the force variability ceases, and the force increases (Figure 4.30).

The frequency at which the mechanical responses produced are sufficiently smooth is known as fusion frequency.

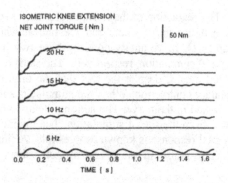

Fig. 4.30: The isometric knee extension net joint torque in a paraplegic subject (T8) elicited by stimulating quadriceps muscle (surface electrodes, pulse duration T = 300 μs, current intensity I = 100 mA).

At this frequency sufficient smoothness of muscle force is expected. The point at which fusion is achieved depends upon the speed of contraction of the activated muscle fibers, and therefore ultimately upon the level of recruitment. In most human upper extremity muscles, the fusion occurs at less then 20 Hz. Increasing the stimulus frequency above the fusion frequency to the level of tetanus results in a further increase in force. Up to 40 or 50 percent of the maximum muscle force may be regulated by temporal summation from fusion to tetanus. Temporal summation leads to temporal modulation being inversely proportional with the frequency (f) of stimulation. In order to grade the force the muscle temporal modulation of the interpulse interval (IPI = 1/f), or a combination of recruitment and temporal modulation can be selected.

4.3.2 Instrumentation for FES

A functional diagram of the FES system (Figure 4.31) shows the main components required for restoring motor function after an injury of the central nervous system (e.g., brain infarction, spinal cord injury). The stimulator receives command signals, generates trains of pulses of electrical charge, and delivers those to the excitable tissues via electrodes.

Each of the components has to be selected or built based on the eventual application (e.g., lower extremities, upper extremities, single-channel, multi-channel, transcutaneous, percutaneous, and fully implanted systems).

Electrodes

Surface electrodes [e.g., Bowman and Baker, 1985] are placed on the skin surface over the area where the stimulus is to be delivered. McNeal and Baker [1988], McNeal and Reswick [1976], Sagi-Dolev et al. [1995] described the criteria for surface electrodes: low impedance and even distribution of current, flexibility to maintain good skin contact, ease of application and removal, and suitable mounting for days without irritation of the skin. A surface electrode has three elements: the conductor, the interfacial layer, and the adhesive. The earliest electrodes used metal plates for the conductor, gel- or saline-saturated fabric for the interfacial layer, and tape or circumferential bands for maintaining position. Substantial improvements of these electrodes have been directed toward resolving some of the problems, such as drying of the conductor, difficulties in application and maintaining position and good electrical contact of the entire electrode surface, especially on the skin surfaces with a large radius of curvature (back and abdomen). Usage of conductive polymer (silicone rubber filled with carbon) and conductive adhesives proved to be effective for clinical and home usage.

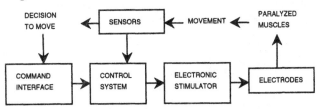

Fig. 4.31: Instrumentation for FES system: Command interface, control system, electronic stimulator, electrodes and sensors. Decision to move is at the voluntary level of the user. The arrow from sensors to the decision to move is indicating possible augmented feedback discussed in Section 4.2.

Surface electrodes for most applications have a rather large surface area of 5 cm^2 or more. They could be applied in either a monopolar configuration or a bipolar configuration. In the monopolar configuration, the working electrode (cathode) is placed over the muscle or nerve to be excited and the indifferent electrode (anode), which can be larger in the surface area, is placed remotely. In the bipolar configuration, the most common for surface stimulation, both electrodes typically are the same size and are placed over the site to be excited. In larger muscle groups, three or more electrodes can be applied for the same muscle [Petrofsky and Phillips, 1983b]; the central electrode is the anode, while the proximal and distal electrodes are cathodes. This method, if sequential stimulation of different cathodes is applied, allows a decrease of the frequency of stimulation of 50 percent since different motor units will be recruited asynchronously.

The stimulus parameters required for activation by using surface electrodes depend on the stimulus waveform, the surface area, electrode materials, placement, skin impedance, and other factors. Typically, for the rectangular pulsatile waveform frequently used, threshold values are 30 mA or greater for a pulse width of 100-300 μs. Stimulus pulses shorter than the 50 μs cause stronger unpleasant sensation (pain); thus, they are not used. The impedance of surface electrodes is between 1 and 5 kΩ.

The primary limitation encountered with surface electrodes is that small muscles generally cannot be selectively activated, and deep muscle cannot be activated without first exciting muscles that are more superficial. Furthermore, fine gradation of force can be difficult because relative movement between the electrode and muscle will alter the stimulation-force relationship. Physical movement of the electrode can cause such movement, from length changes in the muscle induced by the contraction process, or from internal change in the nerve-electrode geometry during isometric contraction. The pain is definitely a limiting factor in applying surface electrodes in subjects with preserved sensory and diminished motor functions.

Subcutaneous electrodes can be divided into those in which the electrode is secured to the muscle exciting the motorneurons, and those, which are contacting the nerve that contains the motoneurons. The advantages of subcutaneous electrodes vs. surface electrodes are better selectivity, repeatable excitation, and permanent positioning. The sensation to the users is much more comfortable since the electrodes are placed away from the pain receptors, and the current amplitude is much lower. The potential disadvantage of implanted electrode is the damage that can result from improper design and implantation (e.g., irreversible deleterious effects to the neural tissue, physical failure of an electrode requiring an invasive revision procedure).

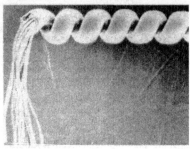

Fig. 4.32: A coiled intramuscular electrode made of multistrand stainless steel with Teflon insulation. The insulation is stripped down at the tip of the electrode (left). Adapted from Triolo *et al.*, 1996, with permission.

The mechanisms of failure of subcutaneous electrodes may be separated into three categories: physiological, biological, or physical [Mortimer, 1981; Scheiner *et al.*, 1990]. The physiological criteria include insufficient strength, poor recruitment properties (such as nonlinearities), stimulus thresholds that are excessively high or low, poor repeatability, insufficient selectivity of activation of the desired muscle or muscle group, and adverse sensation [Crago *et al.*, 1974; Gruner and Mason, 1989; Popović *et al.*, 1991d; Grandjean and Mortimer, 1986]. The biological failures include those mechanically induced at surgical installation, excess encapsulation, infection or rejection, and those induced with stimulation [Mortimer, 1981]. The physical failures are those of the conductor, such as electrochemical degradation or mechanical failures (breakage), and of the insulator. Categorization of electrode failure requires, if possible, identification of the failure mechanisms to at least this level [Scheiner *et al.*, 1990; Smith *et al.*, 1994].

Subcutaneous electrodes which are secured to the muscle, include two types: the intramuscular electrode [Bowman and Erickson, 1985; Handa *et al.*, 1989a; Prochazka and Davis, 1992; Smith *et al.*, 1994], which can be injected using a hypodermic needle either nonsurgically through the closed skin or through an open incision, and the epimysial electrode [Grandjean and Mortimer, 1986], which is fixed to the muscle surface and must be placed surgically. The intramuscular electrode is a helical coil fabricated from a multiple-strand wire (Figure 4.32). Such a configuration provides a structure, which is able to sustain multiple flexion without fracture. Generally non-noble alloys are employed (e.g., type 316L stainless steel) and wire insulation is Teflon. The electrode is a thin wire that fits in the lumen of a 19-gage hypodermic needle. A hook formed at the end of the coil keeps the electrode from being pressed out of the needle during insertion and assists in securing the electrode when the needle is withdrawn.

The intramuscular electrode is used as the cathode electrode in a monopolar configuration with a surface electrode as the indifferent (anode) electrode. Bipolar configurations have not been used because the anodic potentials are sufficient to induce corrosion on the anode intramuscular electrode. Although it would be possible theoretically to change the material to one, which is less subject to anodic degradation (e.g., platinum), the candidate materials have not demonstrated sufficient strength to withstand the forces induced during cycling. The intramuscular electrode is implanted, using the hypodermic needle as the carrier, into a site near a motor point of the target muscle. Stimulation applied through the needle shaft assists in identifying the position of the needle tip. Positioning of the electrode within an individual muscle can be achieved in 80 percent of the injections by an experienced investigator, although the absolute position will vary somewhat from one injection to the next in the same muscle.

Placement of multiple intramuscular electrodes within a single muscle enables one to employ sequential stimulation techniques on rather small muscles, since the extent of recruitment can be quite focused and restricted.

Electrodes are either inserted directly through the skin with the needle (the target muscle is near the skin interface), or implanted and tunneled subcutaneously (the target muscles extended distances of 15 cm from the skin interface. Intramuscular electrodes generally elicit a maximal muscular contraction with a 20 mA, 200 µs stimulus. This is on the order of 10 percent of the stimulus charge required by surface electrodes. The impedance of the intramuscular electrode is typically 300 Ω, but the entire load impedance of tissue and surface anode may be as high as 1.5 kΩ. The probability of functional operation of intramuscular electrodes in the upper extremity is 80 percent after one year. Of the failures one-third are physical failures. In the case of a fracture, the broken segment will remain in place and the external segment will be withdrawn. Two-thirds of failures are due to an altered physiological response, believed to be caused by a physical displacement of the electrode, and present modifications on electrode design are under way to correct both problems.

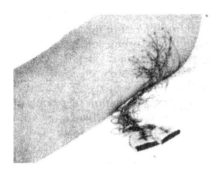

Fig. 4.33: Several percutaneous stainless steel electrodes with Teflon insulation exiting the upper arm of a tetraplegic subject. Adapted from Triolo *et al.*, 1996, with permission.

The primary disadvantage of percutaneous electrodes is the maintenance of the skin interface (Figure 4.33), yet reports show that only few infections occurred in implantation of over 2000 electrodes, some implanted for more than five years [Peckham, 1988]. Granulomas at the skin interface are infrequent, but they are treated with local cauterization. The advantage of percutaneous (intramuscular) electrodes over surface electrodes is that they provide a means of eliciting focused, repeatable responses over time with a nonsurgical technique.

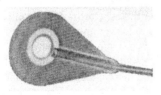

Fig. 4.34: An epimysial electrodes used as part of the Freehand system. Courtesy of NeuroControl Corp., Cleveland, Ohio, U.S.A.

The epimysial electrode [e.g., Grandjean and Mortimer, 1986] is a disk-shaped metal with a reinforced polymer for shielding the surface away from the muscle and for suturing to the muscle (Figure 4.34). The electrode is surgically placed on the muscle near the motor point. The conductive surface of the disk is 3 mm in diameter. In contrast to the intramuscular electrode because the placement is surgical and small size is not so essential, the lead may have a more mechanical redundancy than the intramuscular lead.

This electrode can be replaced quite easily in a surgical procedure in case of failure, into either the original site or an adjacent position. The stimulation levels required and impedance are similar to those of the intramuscular electrode. The physiologic characteristics of stimulation over this electrode are also similar to the intramuscular electrode. That is, the recruitment is nonlinear with either pulse-amplitude or pulse-width modulation and may be approximated by piece-wise linear segments. The recruitment may also be length-dependent, meaning that the force output changes with muscle length due to changes in the electrode to nerve coupling. This is in addition to the length-tension properties of the muscle.

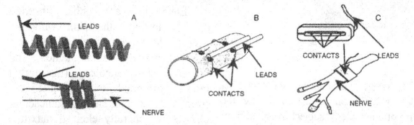

Fig. 4.35: A) Huntington type helix nerve electrode; B) circular cuff electrode with a longitudinal slit; C) flat cuff electrode for selective stimulation.

Another types of surgically placed electrodes are nerve electrodes (Figure 4.35). Nerve electrodes have the potential for producing the most desired physiological response [Sweeney and Mortimer, 1986; Naples *et al.*, 1988; Rutten *et al.*, 1991; Sweeney *et al.*, 1990; Loeb and Peck, 1996]. The electrode must be designed with an appreciation for the sensitivity of the nerve to mechanical trauma, manifest by swelling, its longitudinal mobility during muscle movement, and the necessity of maintaining a constant orientation between the nerve fibers and the electrode.

The nerve electrodes are characterized by their placement relative to the nerve: adjacent, encircling, or intraneural. *Adjacent electrodes* are placed next to the nerve, usually by suturing to the epineurium (Figure 4.44). This electrode can be installed through a relatively simple surgery, yet suffer from poor repeatability.

Cuff electrodes encircle the nerve; they have either tube (Figure 4.35, B and C) or spiral configuration (Figure 4.35, A). The latter is a loose, open helix, which is wrapped around the nerve in a monopolar configuration. Cuff electrodes come in a variety of configurations; they all have a longitudinal opening to allow installation on the nerve without damaging it. The cuff is formed of a polymer (usually silicone rubber or recently polyamide), sometime reinforced with Dacron. The electrodes within the cuff are made out of metal, usually being circumferential around the inner surface of the cuff. A self-wrapping cuff [Naples *et al.*, 1988] uses the same materials, yet it is self-sized; thus eliminates the problem of selecting the appropriate size. Both cuff and spiral electrode configurations may be used in various monopolar, bipolar, or tripolar configurations [Sweeney and Mortimer, 1986; Naples *et al.*, 1988].

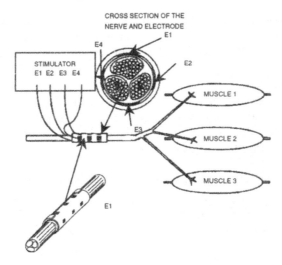

Fig 4.36: Idealized 12 contact circular cuff electrode (with a longitudinal slit) for selective stimulation with a four-channel stimulator. Adapted from Sweeney *et al.*, 1995, with permission.

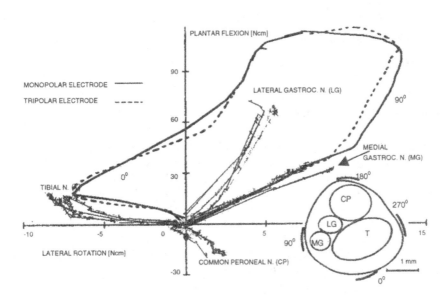

Fig. 4.37: Selective activation of four fascicles with a four polar cuff electrode positioned around the sciatic nerve of a cat. Appropriate voltages applied to four polls result with desired activation; thus, the activity of several muscles can be controlled by a single cuff and four-channel stimulator. Adapted from Sweeney *et al.*, 1995, with permission.

With the choice of the proper geometric relationship between the nerve and electrode and the configuration, it is possible to restrict the direction of current flow and generate action potentials that propagate unidirectionally along the nerve. Encircling cuff electrodes typically requires one-tenth the charge required with muscle (intramuscular or epimysial) electrodes, with maximal responses elicited with stimulus amplitudes on the order of 2 mA and pulse widths of 300 μs. The recruitment gain is often higher compared with the intramuscular electrodes, and similar nonlinearities are encountered.

For some time the development of cuff electrodes is oriented towards stimulation of some regions within the large nerves (e.g., sciatic nerve, tibial nerve). The main idea is to use multipolar cuff electrodes and vary the potentials between these points [Sweeney et al., 1995, Veraart et al., 1993]. Figure 4.36 shows the multipolar cuff electrode for selective stimulation of nerves.

Experiments have been done with a tripolar electrode (12 contacts), and monopolar (4 contacts) cuff electrodes and a four-channel stimulator (Figure 4.37). It has been shown that by using "intelligent" control it is possible to stimulate several muscles by activating corresponding fascicles within a sciatic nerve of a cat [Qi et al., 1999] and peripheral nerve of humans [Haugland and Sinkjær, 2000].

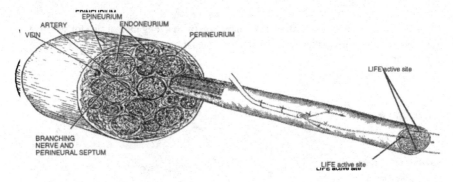

Fig. 4.38: Longitudinal Intra-Fascicular Electrode (LIFE). See text for details. Courtesy of Dr Yoshida K, Aalborg University, 2000.

The impedance is in the range from 300 Ω to 3 kΩ. Surgical installation of a cuff electrode requires careful dissection to identify the nerve and place the electrode around the nerve. It has been recommended (although disputed) that the inside diameter of the electrode should be 20 to 50 percent larger than the nerve diameter to minimize nerve compression and necrosis due to postsurgical swelling and fibrous tissue ingrowth. The structure of the nerve may not allow selective excitation of individual muscles, depending upon the location where branching of the nerve occurs. Longitudinal surgical dissection to partition the nerve into separate components is typically not desirable because of the trauma induced.

It is noteworthy to acknowledge the 15 years of clinical success by using cuff electrodes, however only in limited number of humans. These electrodes, which are regarded as stiff by most investigators today, were placed on the relatively mobile peroneal nerve to correct foot-drop in hemiplegia [Waters et al., 1985b].

Intraneural electrodes utilize a conductor that invades the epineurium. Many studies have been done with intraneural electrodes. There is sufficient evidence that maximal contraction is elicited at stimulation levels an order of magnitude lower than with nerve cuff electrodes (200 μA, pulse duration 300 μs). The variations of such a design would be a valuable clinical tool, yet the connectors, fixation, and neural damage are still not resolved to allow clinical usage.

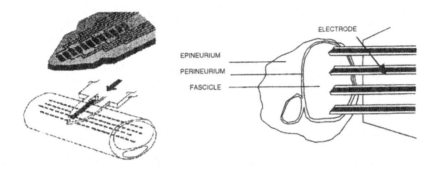

Fig. 4.39: Intraneural multipolar "sword" type electrode made out of solid silicon with golden contacts (left) and (right) intrafascicular metal electrode. Adapted from Rutten et al., 1991, with permission.

For some time the longitudinal intrafascicular electrodes have been investigated. Nannini and Horch [1991] showed that a single electrode implanted within a nerve fascicle could produce axonal recruitment with almost no excitation of muscles that are not targeted (neutral size specificity). The electrodes are positioned inside of the perineurium (Figure 4.38); thus, the current and charge requirements for stimulation are very low compared with externally placed electrodes [Nannini and Horch, 1991]. It was also shown that the intrafascicular electrodes are safe for long term usage; the tissue damage is minimal and the longevity of electrodes is substantial. The recent version of intrafascicular electrode is called longitudinal intrafascicular electrode - LIFE [Yoshida and Horch, 1993].

Rutten with coworkers [1991] and Meier et al. [1995, 1998] demonstrated that the *sword type electrodes* (Figure 4.39) are selective, therefore, they could minimize the needs for using many electrodes for the activation of different muscles that are innervated from a single nerve. The intraneural electrode can thus reduce the surgery procedure and risks associated with them, reduce the hardware that has to be implanted and minimize the charge that has to be developed.

Intraspinal stimulation. In order to maximize the usage of the preserved neural networks after the injury of CNS it would be beneficial to stimulate higher CNS structures, rather than to directly activate the last-order motoneurons. There is evidence in humans that the neural circuitry of the spinal cord is capable of generating complex behaviors with coordinated muscle activity [Pinter and Dimitrijević, 1999, Dimitrijević et al., 1998]. This method is currently receiving more attention [Tai et al., 2000; Mushahwar and Horch, 1997, 2000]. Clinical applications in the motor system include stimulation of the sacral anterior roots for bladder function [Brindley et al., 1986; Davis et al., 1997; Rushton et al., 1990]. The behaviors that can be mediated by the isolated spinal cord include reaching-like limb movements [e.g., Tresch and Bizzi, 1999; Lemay and Grill, 1999], standing [de Leon et al., 1998], walking [Barbeau et al., 1999]. Spinal circuits can be activated by epidural and intraspinal electrical stimulation [Grill et al., 1999]. Two methods are equally appealing: intraspinal microstimulation enables direct activation of spinal neurons, and afferent input makes synaptic contacts on spinal neurons; thus, they also could be used for stimulation of CNS.

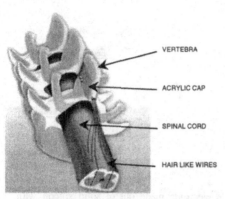

Fig. 4.40: The schema of using very fine metal wires to directly micro stimulate the spinal cord, thereby activate movement. Courtesy of Dr. Arthur Prochazka, University of Alberta, Edmonton, Canada.

A promising new interface to stimulate spinal cord neurons has been developed: microwires finer than a human hair [Mushahwar and Horch, 1997] have been tested in animal experiments (Prochazka, personal communication). The microwires were implanted in the spinal cord of animals for up to six months (Figure 4.40). The implants caused no pain or discomfort, and the motor activity remained normal, indicating that the wires had not damaged the spinal cord. When trains of electrical micro-pulses were delivered through the microwires, the stimuli were not perceived, yet strong coordinated limb movements were produced, sufficient to support body weight. This indicates that spinal cord microstimulation could generate useful movement in people with paraplegia or tetraplegia.

Subliminal microstimulation, insufficient to cause muscle contraction on its own, was found to boost weak voluntary contractions. This could be important, since 80% of spinal cord-injured people has a weak voluntary control over some muscles. Subliminal microstimulation may allow these people to activate more muscles and thereby regain more control over their own movements. For the same reason, subliminal microstimulation may eventually be useful in augmenting the benefits of spinal cord regeneration, when techniques for this succeed in humans. The results show that microwires implanted in the spinal cord are stable in place, and microstimulation through these electrodes produces strong, controllable movements, but it could also evoke spasticity.

Intraspinal microstimulation can activate groups of spinal neurons and may enable activation of these spinal circuits and generation of subsequent motor behaviors. Giszter et al. [1993] demonstrated that microstimulation of the gray matter in spinal frogs generated organized patterns of endpoint forces (force fields) which were similar in structure to endpoint force patterns generated during natural motor behaviors. The force fields generated at the endpoint by microstimulation of the spinal cord were organized into a few limited types, some of which produced convergence to a single point in space where the net endpoint force was zero, and the limb was inherently stable. Further, co-stimulation of independent sites generated superposition of the individual force fields and new points of convergence [Mussa-Ivaldi et al., 1994; Lemay et al., 1997]. Similar experiments in spinal rats revealed that organized motor responses may also be evoked by intraspinal microstimulation in mammals [Tresch and Bizzi, 1999].

Lemay and Grill [1999] analyzed the endpoint forces elicited by intraspinal microstimulation. The characteristics of the force fields differed between ventral *versus* dorsal and intermediate locations. Endpoint forces at dorsal or intermediate locations varied both in direction and magnitude with changes in endpoint position.

For some stimulation sites, the endpoint forces varied as to the production of a force field which converged to a point in the workspace where the net active endpoint force was zero. Electromyographic records indicated that the convergent fields were produced by co-activation of multiple muscles. In contrast, while the magnitude of endpoint forces evoked by ventral microstimulation varied with limb position, their directions were largely invariant, and the resulting force fields were parallel or divergent. Similar parallel or divergent patterns were evoked by intramuscular stimulation of individual muscles.

Endpoint force measurements revealed that intraspinal microstimulation can generate organized, multiple-joint, multiple-muscle motor responses, which were not obtained by direct stimulation of muscles or by intraspinal stimulation of motoneurons. Organized motor behaviors evoked by microstimulation support the hypothesis that intraspinal microstimulation and activation of spinal interneuronal circuitry may simplify neural prosthetic control of complex motor behaviors [Barbeau et al., 1999].

Electronic Stimulators

Many stimulators have been designed for FES application; almost every research center developed its own unit to allow flexibility when developing different applications [e.g., Arabi and Sawan, 1999; Belikan et al., 1986; Bijak et al., 1999; Brindley et al., 1978; Borges et al., 1989; Buckett et al., 1988; Donaldson, 1986; Ilić et al., 1994; James et al., 1991; Maležič et al., 1978; Minzly et al., 1993; Smith et al., 1987; Thrope et al., 1985]. The differences are in selecting the components that will be used, the number of channels, and over all the control structure. Many stimulators are directly PC-computer based, yet they have a self-standing modality allowing its application by eventual user at home. Parastep I, manufactured by the Sigmedics, Chicago, IL, was the first surface stimulator to be FDA approved in 1994, followed by the Handmaster (NESS, Ra'anana, Israel), and Freehand System (NeuroControl, Cleveland, OH). The first two stimulators are approved for therapeutic use, yet they are frequently used as assistive systems. The Freehand system received the approval for restoring grasping in C5-C6 tetraplegic subjects.

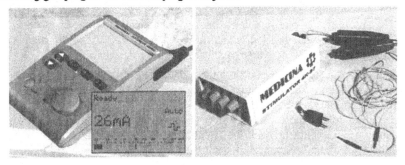

Fig. 4.41: Two commercially available stimulators for use with surface electrodes. The stimulator Danmeter, Denmark (left) is used for therapy, and the stimulator 4K-TS (right), Medicina TS, Belgrade, Yugoslavia for standing and walking.

There are several companies that distribute one- and two-channel stimulators for correcting foot-drop (e.g., MicroFes, Ljubljana, Slovenia; Odstock stimulator, Salisbury, UK; COTAS, Denmark). Few multichannel systems that are applicable for paraplegic subjects can also be used in clinical studies (Figure 4.41) and controlled home usage (e.g., Parastep, Sigmedics, IL, U.S.A; Parastim, Ljubljana, Slovenia; Quadstim, Biomech Design, Edmonton, Alberta; Medicina 4TS, Belgrade, Yugoslavia).

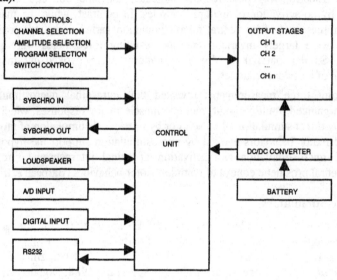

Fig. 4.42: Block diagram of the electronic stimulator. "Synchro in" and "synchro out" are the interface with other stimulators or devices used in the same subject. RS232 input/output is a serial communication to host PC-based computer. See text for details

An electronic stimulator for FES application has to be a self-contained device with a low power consumption, small, light, and must have the simplest possible user interface [Bogataj et al., 1989]. The stimulator should be programmable, and the programming can be done by wireless communication with the host computer, although using wires is acceptable. The stimulator needs a set-up mode; mode of programming when communicating with the host computer. Once the programming is finished, the stimulator should be turned to the autonomous mode.

The description of one stimulator for surface applications [Ilić et al., 1994] illustrates the principles that apply for other devices. The main parts of the stimulator are (Figure 4.42) the DC/DC converter, output stage, and controller.

The output stage generates constant current pulses of both polarities, controls the amplitudes and duration of positive and negative pulses, controls the delay between positive and negative pulse, and regulates the frequency of stimulation ($f=1/IPI$). All these features follow the earlier described "biological" activation of muscles (except for the orderly recruitment) with the intention to ensure minimal tissue damage and minimize unpleasant sensations during and after the use.

The power source is used to convert the low battery voltage to the high voltage needed for stimulation. The battery operated power supply unit generates galvanically isolated high voltages, two per output stage. The DC/DC converter was designed for high efficiency, small size, and small weight.

The current programmed flyback configuration is adopted as the suitable solution; simplicity, simple realization and low cost are advantages of the flyback topology. The programming via current feedback with constant space and variable operating frequency provides a simple converter control circuit, stable control loop, and reliable overload protection [Ridley, 1990]. The efficiency of the stimulator can best be described by the duration of possibly fully loaded operation. The described stimulator can run on a 1 Ah, 6 V rechargeable battery for 6 hours. During these 6 hours all 4 channels are simultaneously firing at 50 Hz, 500 µs pulse duration, with the current of 140 mA at a capacitive load with the impedance of 1.2 kΩ.

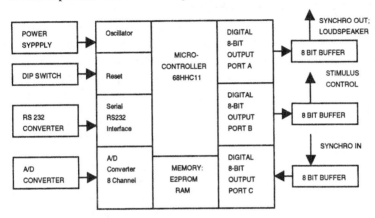

Fig. 4.43: Schematic organization of the control unit based on 68HC11 microcontroller. Adapted from Ilić *et al.*, 1994 © IEEE.

The control unit is shown in Figure 4.43. The 68HC11 Motorola microcontroller is the core of the device. The microcontroller operation is supported by the reset and supply voltage monitoring circuits and by the RS232 converter that provides standard voltage levels for asynchronous serial communication. The switch is used to change the operation mode of the 68HC11 microcontroller. The bootstrap mode is used to download programs in the E2PROM memory of the microcontroller from the host computer by using the serial RS232 interface.

The programming on the PC-based host computer uses Windows type interface with menu and graphical support. The single chip mode microcontroller operation is used when the stimulator operates in the autonomous mode. The A/D converter input of micro-controller can accept up to eight analog voltages within the range of 0 to 5 Volts, with the maximum sampling rate of 100 Hz. The digital input has been used to accommodate digital sensors such as AD202 accelerometer. Digital output ports through buffers drive the output stages, the loudspeaker and the synchronization output. The synchronization input and push buttons are buffered and connected to the digital input port of the microcontroller.

The pulse duration and interpulse interval are controlled by software loops. Therefore, pulses at different types of output cannot be generated simultaneously as they appear in sequence. There are three programs that are originally designed: 1) periodic pulse generation at the desired frequency is possible using a timer with four output compare registers, one for each output channel; 2) the input synchronization pulse disables the periodic output pulse generation and generates output pulses; and 3) sensory driven applications being part of the rule-based program.

An effective interface between stimulator and user is achieved through push buttons (command signals), and a loudspeaker (feedback). The host computer interface is realized by serial RS232 interface. Synchronizing input and output are used to connect several stimulators. In such a case the stimulator delivering synchronization pulses works as a master unit, while the others operate in the slave mode. The A/D input serves as an interface to be used for closed-loop control. The stimulator at this stage can accommodate up to eight analog and eight digital types of input.

Electronic Stimulators for Implanted Systems

Implantable stimulators for FES may be separated into single- or multichannel devices. Single-channel implants, which have been fabricated, are all radio-frequency powered and controlled devices (Figure 4.44). They use relatively few discrete components and have a receiving antenna, which is integrated into the circuitry. The packaging materials are epoxy or glass-ceramic. The most common single-channel configuration is one in which lead wires are used to place the electrode away from the site of the receiver unit. Avery and Medtronics have employed this design for neuromuscular applications in commercially available devices many years ago.

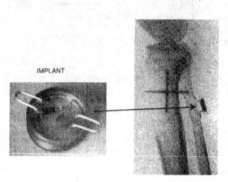

Fig. 4.44: The early version of the single-channel foot-drop implant designed in Ljubljana. Modified from "Functional Electrical Stimulation manual" Jožef Štefan Institute, Ljubljana, Slovenia, 1983.

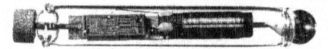

Fig. 4.45: BION - the microstimulator with anodized Tantalum (left) and Iridium surface activated ball (right) electrodes. The electronic circuitry is hermetically sealed with glass beads in the glass capillary tube (length 13 mm, diameter 2 mm). Courtesy of Loeb GE, 1996.

Alternatively, the electrodes may be an integral part of the packaging of the circuitry, allowing the entire device to be placed adjacent to the nerve such as it is in the Ljubljana designed implantable foot-drop system [Strojnik et al., 1987].

Two alternative schemes have been considered for multi-muscle excitation. It is possible, in principle, to use several one-channel units that are controlled from one controller [Cameron et al., 1997, 1998a and b; Strojnik et al., 1987], or to use a single implantable stimulator that will connect with multiple electrodes [Holle et al., 1984; Thoma et al., 1978; Rushton, 1990; Strojnik et al., 1990; Smith et al., 1996; Davis et al., 1997].

The single channel devices have been developed originally for foot-drop correction and implanted in many subjects with positive experience, yet the development was continued in a different direction, i.e., towards multi-channel stimulators [Strojnik et al., 1990, 1993]. The wireless single channel stimulator has been developed for extensive use in restoring motor functions, and up to now animal experiments show great promises [Cameron et al., 1997]. The BION, single channel wireless stimulator is sealed with glass beads and uses an anodized Tantalum and surface activated Iridium electrodes to minimize tissue damage (Figure 4.45).

The diameter of the glass tube is 2 mm, and the length of the whole device is 13 mm. The BION is powered by inductive coupling from an external coil at 2 MHz. A total of 256 units can be driven from a single control based on the Motorola 68HC11 microcomputer. The pulse width control is from 3 to 258 µs with the increment of only 1 µs, the pulse amplitude control from 0.2 to 30 mA in two ranges of 15 linear steps. The stimulator delivers charge balanced monophasic pulses, allowing for selection of a square of exponential discharge tail.

The problem with all implantable devices without batteries, which require lot of power to drive sensory and motor systems, is low efficiency of radio-frequency transmission. In order to transmit energy the emitting and receiving antenna must be close and aligned; this being very difficult if a stimulator is injected into a deep muscle.

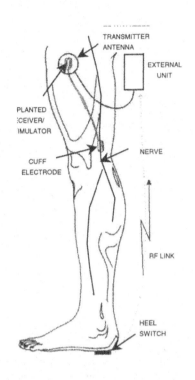

Fig. 4.46: The use of the miniature implantable two-channel stimulator for selective stimulation of the nerve fascicles via multipolar cuff electrode. Two-channel stimulator is packaged with the receiving antenna to receive signals via radio frequency from the external unit (power and control signals). Adapted from Haugland et al., 2000, with permission.

The alternative solution, accepted by most other research teams developing electronic stimulators is a miniature, implantable, multi-channel device that will excite as many muscles as needed. The difficulty is that such a stimulator will be remote from the stimulation points, therefore, connectors and leads have to be used between the stimulator and stimulation points.

The use of long leads should be eliminated after the technique of selective nerve stimulation, including potential stimulation of the spinal cord directly, or spinal roots is perfected. The experiments conducted at Aalborg University with the two channel fully implanted RF driven stimulators [Haugland, 1997; Gudnason et al., 1999], integrated in the cuff electrode (Figure 4.46) suggest that this is a viable technique. Selective activation of different muscle groups has been achieved in a sitting and walking subject.

Almost ten years ago Rushton [1990] demonstrated the feasibility of multi-joint movement and posture control by stimulating spinal roots. This development has been continued, and a better understanding of the motor control will help in bringing this technology to effective usage.

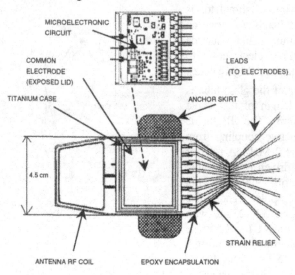

Fig. 4.47: Sketch of the multichannel implantable system with wireless communication. Adapted from Smith *et al.*, 1998, © IEEE.

A Stimulator-Telemetry Multi-Channel Device. The stimulation-telemetry system presented recently [Smith *et al.*, 1998] is an excellent example of the state of the art of technology in implantable systems (Figure 4.47). The device can be configured with the following functions: 1) up to 32 independent channels of stimulation for activation of muscles (or sensory feedback), with independent control of stimulus pulse interval, pulse duration, pulse amplitude, interphase delay (for biphasic stimulus waveform), and recharge phase duration (for biphasic stimulus waveform); 2) up to eight independent telemetry channels for sensors, with independent control of sampling rate and pulse powering parameters of the sensor (power amplitude and duration); 3) up to eight independent telemetry channels for processed (rectified and integrated) myoelectric signals (MES), with independent control of the sampling rate and provisions for stimulus artifact blanking and processing control; 4) up to eight independent telemetry channels for unprocessed MES channels, with independent control of sampling rate; and 5) up to eight independent telemetry channels for system functions, providing control or sampling of internal system parameters, such as internal voltage levels.

Due to overall timing constraints, implant circuit size, implant capsule size, number of lead wires, circuit and sensor power consumption, and external control and processing requirements, it is not practical to realize a single device having the maximal capabilities outlined above. However, the intent of the stimulator-telemeter system is to provide the means of realizing an optimal implantable device having all the necessary circuitry and packaging to meet the anticipated clinical applications, without requiring design or engineering effort beyond that of fabricating the device itself. For example, a basic upper extremity application would require, minimally, eight channels of stimulation for providing palmar and lateral grasp and sensory feedback, along with one joint angle transducer as a command control source.

The stimulation-telemetry implant device comprises an electronic circuit that is hermetically sealed in a Titanium capsule with feedthroughs. A single internal radio frequency (RF) coil provides transcutaneous reception of power and bidirectional communication. The lead wires connected to the feed-through holes extend to the stimulating electrodes, to the implanted sensors, or to the recording electrodes. The later two connections are used as control input The circuit capsule, coil, and lead wire exits are conformably coated in epoxy and silicone elastomer to provide physical support for the feedthroughs and RF coil, and stress relief to the leads making it suitable for long-term implantation.

The functional elements required to realize the system include the following: 1) an RF receiver for recovering power and functional commands transmitted from an external control unit; 2) control logic circuitry to interpret the recovered signals, execute the command function, and to supervise functional circuit blocks; 3) multichannel stimulation circuitry for generating the stimulus pulses that are sent to the stimulating electrodes; 4) multichannel signal conditioning circuitry which provides amplification, filtering, and processing for the signals to be acquired (MES and sensor signals); 5) data acquisition circuitry for sampling and digitizing these signals; 6) modulation circuitry for telemetering the acquired data through the RF link; 7) power regulation and switching circuitry for selectively powering the included functional blocks of the circuitry, as needed, to minimize power consumption of the device; 8) system control circuitry to allow interrogation or configuration of the operation of the device.

Sensors for FES Systems

Sensors for FES applications should provide to both the system and the user information regarding the conditions of the neural prosthesis. In some cases, it is not obvious that the user does need instant information (e.g., if automatic execution follows the desired trajectory), yet if anything unexpected is happening, the sensory warning may prevent catastrophic consequences. Sensors are needed in FES systems for the command interface (e.g., activating the neuroprosthesis, changing the mode of operation).

Some neuroprostheses rely on control systems that are sensory driven, using a so-called rule-based control [Willemsen *et al.*, 1990a and b). The rules are *If-Then* relations, where *If* relates to the sensory information; hence, in order to apply this control, the sensory signal is instrumental. Closed-loop control is based on minimizing the error at the output, therefore a sensor is essential to provide the signal to be used for comparison with the desired sensory value. The sensory system to be used should provide information of various kinds, such as the contact force or pressure over the area of contact (grasping, standing, and walking), the position of the joints (prehension, reaching, standing, and walking), and perhaps the activity of the muscle. The dynamic range, resolution, and frequency response of sensors must be determined upon the application. For example, force sensors for walking and standing must withstand several times body weight under dynamic loading and joint position sensors must allow unrestrained movement over the entire range of motion of the joint.

The constraints imposed on the sensors for FES systems are significant; they must be cosmetically acceptable and easy to mount, they should be self-contained, have low power consumption, and must provide adequate information. In most available FES systems sensors are placed externally. The sensor positioned at the surface of the body is not a suitable solution for many situations (e.g., an external-force sensor on the digits of the hand requires donning and needs a cable to communicate with the control box, and it should work in variable temperature conditions and hazardous environment). The alternative is to use implanted sensors. They have to meet the same performance specifications while functioning in a more hostile environment. These sensors should communicate with the remote control box, and the device must be powered via radio-frequency (RF) link. The ultimate solution is to use available sensor in the organism; to record from nerves and muscles and process the information in a real-time useful signal. This solution requires the ability to interface without the nerves and interpret the signals they are supplying to the central nervous system.

Artificial Sensors for Neuroprostheses

The technology is making huge steps in life sciences by providing better and more effective use of solid state silicon based devices. Micromachining and microelectronics allow the transfer of what is a dream today, into a commercial product tomorrow. Manufacturing of devices that include millions of transistors or similar arrays is relatively simple, and reasonably inexpensive. The automotive and space research contributed a great deal to the market of sensors and actuators. The precision, reproducibility, longevity, and other characteristics of silicon based devices are excellent. This is to say that sensors of many kinds are available (Figure 4.48), but in order to benefit from them, intelligent control and integration into the biological control are necessary.

Selecting sensors for the application has to start from the considerations of the dynamic characteristics of the plant and the process; range of operation, frequency content of the signal to be recorded, accuracy requirements. In Sections 1.3 to 1.5 somatosensory systems available to the central nervous system have been described. These systems are highly redundant, information is combined from many noisy signals in not completely known ways, and decisions on what and how to control are made at different levels using the richness of the hierarchical and parallel organization of the systems. This cannot be replicated with sensors available today, and most probably it should not be cloned.

In order to control the position of the extremity, it is of interest to know the joint angles and joint angular velocities, and if in contact with the environment, the contact forces. The most commonly used sensors for measuring joint angles are potentiometers. However, joint angle can be effectively measured with optocouplers, optical fibers, strain gages, Hall effect transducers, magneto-transistors as well as many other transducers.

The field effect transistor (FET) is a micro-miniature electronic device in which the current amplification depends on the applied voltages. In principle the FET transistor has three zones, source, gate, and drain. The actual width of the gate determines the gain of the transistor. The width of the gate in these applications is controlled by an electric signal. The arrays of FET devices mounted on specially designed support rely on the change of the gate width provoked by mechanical factors, *i.e.*, the force. One of the advantages of such a device is the ability to measure micro strains and displacements in addition to the recording of finite displacements. A single FET could record small displacements; multiple devices built in a single semiconductor support are convenient for measuring bigger displacements.

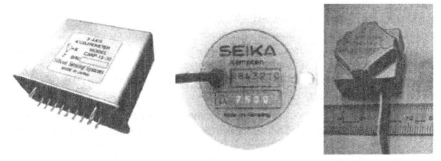

Fig. 4.48: Commercially available solid state based sensors: 3-axis accelerometer from the Silicone Sensing Systems, U.S.A (left), tilt sensor from the Seika, Germany (middle) and the ratemeter from the Silicon Sensing Systems (right).

Maalej *et al.* [1987] have investigated the Interlink manufactured Force Sensing Resistors (FSR) (Figure 4.49, left), based on elastomer material. With the instrumentation capable of dealing with the hysteresis and nonlinearity, the sensor was suggested as a valuable asset for neuroprosthetics. The FSR sensor certainly does not qualify if using the data presented in Table 4.2.

Table 4.2: Estimated requirements of physical transducers for neuroprostheses. Dynamic response specifications are 3 dB points. E/F -extension/flexion, Lat - lateral movement. [Popović *et al.*, 1990].

Application	Measured Variable	Range	Resolution	Dynamic Response
		degrees		*Hz*
Standing	Knee Angle	-5 to 20	1	10
	Ankle Angle	-10 to 15	3	10
Level Walking	Knee Angle	-5 to 70	1	20
	Ankle Angle	-10 to 20	3	50
Stairs Climbing	Knee Angle	-5 to 100	1	100
	Ankle Angle	-10 to 50	3	100
Standing/ Walking	Hip Angle - E/F	-15 to 80	3	25
	Hip Angle (Lat)	-40 to 20	5	25
Hand funct.	Joint Angles	-20 to 120	.3	100
		N		*Hz*
Walking/ Standing	Foot Contact	5 to 1500	5	1000
	Force of Arms	5 to 400	0.1	100
Hand Function	Contact Force	0.1 to 80	0.1	100
		cm		*Hz*
	Linear movement	25	0.1	100

The piezoresistive sensors are very frequently used in recording of displacements, *i.e.*, forces and pressures (Figure 4.50, right). The most frequently used sensors are strain gauges, yet they are often unsuitable for neuroprosthetics because of the size, power consumption, and temperature variability (Figure 4.49, right). The use of polymer elastomer is effective for recordings of the forces and pressures. The elastomers can be stretched or compressed appreciably, but they return to their original shapes after the stress is removed. The elastomers are made conductive by impregnating them with metal powders or carbon black. The electrical conductivity of elastomers using metal fillers is good, but elastomers exhibit nonuniformly large hysteresis, and poor tensile and compression properties. Moreover, it was found that the hardness of the rubber cannot be made independent of the metallic loading for a given conductivity [Webster, 1988].

This is the reason why most of the sensors implemented so far have used carbon-loaded conductive elastomers. The resistance of a conductive silicone-rubber sensor depends on the contact resistance between the conductive rubber and the metal plate (or between two pieces of conductive rubber) (Figure 4.49, left). In the unstressed state the resistance is at maximum; however, when compressed, the resistance decreases because of an increase in the contact area. These sensors can be implemented as discrete or array sensors. A commercially available insole based on the piezoresistive sensors is shown in Figure 4.50, and known under the name Tecscan F-scan insole in parallel with the discrete FSR sensor manufactured by Interlink, CA, U.S.A.

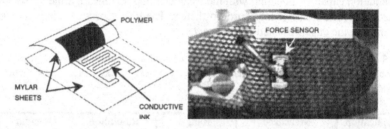

Fig. 4.49: Scheme of the force-sensing resistor (left) and force sensor (full bridge, 4 strain gauges) installed in the sole of the foot of the Belgrade Transfemoral Prosthesis (right).

It is also possible to use piezoelectric sensors. The high level of piezoelectricity was obtained by poling vinylidene-fluoride-based polymers. Polyvinylidene fluoride (PVF2) became a popular sensor [Dario et al., 1983]. PVF2 films mechanically appear the same as a thin sheet of plastic. These films are flexible and durable. Their flexibility allows them to be manufactured in large thin sheets or complex shapes, depending on the application. The material is also very light and thin. PVF2 can be manufactured in thickness ranging from 6 to 2000 μm. Because Young modulus for this material is low (2 GPa), PVF2 very closely follows the distribution of the forces applied to it. The film is relatively unbreakable. It can be stretched up to 14% before yielding [Hausler et al., 1980]. The PVF2 is highly temperature sensitive because of its pyroelectric properties.

Optical fibers can be used for measurements of displacements. The compactness, sensing ability, relative durability, and light-ray conducting properties make optical fibers good candidates for the use as miniature, wearable tactile sensors. Optical fibers can withstand tensions of up to 690 kPa. They are noise and corrosion resistant and very compact. A typical optic fiber sensor bundle is 1.3-3.2 mm in diameter and composed of individual fiber elements, each with an approximate diameter of 75 μm [Coulombe, 1984].

Optocouplers may be used in many different devices for measurements of force, pressure, and displacement. A load cell described by Maalej and Webster [1988] is designed for forces between 0 and 50 N. The light emitting diode is bonded to the

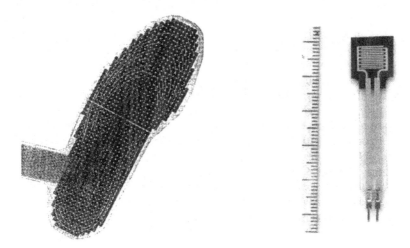

Fig. 4.50: Tecscan F-scan (left) insole with 960 piezoresistive fields (sensors) that can be scanned at 165 Hz per sensor (Cobb and Claremont, 1995, with permission), and discrete 1 x 1 cm force sensing resistor (FSR) (Interlink, California, U.S.A).

support in such a way that it is only partly visible from the phototransistor mounted at the same U shaped frame. Once the frame is loaded, then it bends; the amount of light falling to the photo-transistor changes, and the output voltage at the phototransistor is highly correlated to the force loading the U shape frame. The nonlinearity of such a device can be compensated with the adequate electronic circuitry, and the measurements are reproducible. The device has small hysteresis, the random error is small, and the thermal drift is only minimal; the drawback is low spatial resolution.

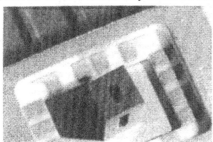 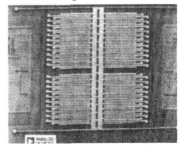

Fig. 4.51: A three-axial accelerometer mounted in a 5x5x5 mm^3 tungsten housing [Bergveld, 1999, with permission] and the ADXL05 single axis accelerometer structure (Analog Device, U.S.A).

The capacitive changes can be used for measurements of pressures and forces. The series of multielement capacitive sensors was fabricated using specially designed capacitor films that had contacts at each end [Seow et al., 1988; Crago et al., 1986b]. The sensor is an array of 8 x 8 fields. Each of the fields has the capacity of only 5 pF. The small capacity imposes series problems coming from parasite capacitance. The sensor was designed for force feedback control in grasping of tetraplegic subjects with an implanted system.

The implantation of artificial sensors introduces a series of constraints [Ko, 1986]. The following elements have to be considered: 1) size and weight have to be small; 2) the transducer must work in hazardous environment; 3) the noise rejection must be very high; 4) devices must be reliable, yet rugged; 5) sensors must withstand sterilization; and 6) the material in contact with the body has to be nontoxic and biocompatible. With solid-state electronic technology, transducers can be designed satisfying the uniformity of the device performance, high reliability, low cost, and integration with the electronic circuits that interface with other signal processing or computing circuits. Two examples of this technology used for accelerometers are shown in Figure 4.51. The specific role of micromachining technology, development of biocompatible polymers, and hermetic packaging has to be pointed out. Wet etching, using chemical and electrochemical techniques, has been developed. Dry etching techniques using plasma, ion beam, and spark erosion have been reported and can be used to machine three-dimensional structures from a substrate, either semiconductor or others. Silicon diaphragms, micro-cavities, beams, and bridges in micron scales have been fabricated in laboratories. The bonding of semiconductors and glass materials allows hermetically sealed unit design. Metal compounds have also been used as a brazing material to seal silicon to metal, ceramics, *etc.* [Ko, 1986]. In addition, the plasma etched holes, laser drilled holes, spark erosion holes, and other micromachining techniques improved very much the quality of sensors. Nevertheless, the number of implanted sensors is rather limited.

Hall effect transducers for general purposes are commercially available. Hall effect transducers are used for angular displacement, force and proximity sensing. The Hall effect is expressed when a semiconductor crystal with a current I is positioned in an external magnetic field. When the direction of the flow of the current differs from the direction of the applied external magnetic flow, each of the moving particles will be drifted from the direction of the current because it is exposed to a Lorentz force. The Hall voltage will be created in orthogonal to the plane of the current and the magnetic

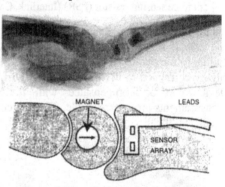

Fig. 4.52: The implantable Hall effect based transducer. The transducer is implanted at the wrist joint (upper panel) the schematic (bottom panel) shows the components. Adapted from Johnson *et al.*, 1999, © IEEE.

field. Hall voltage depends on so-called Hall coefficient R_H, external current I, magnetic field B, and physical dimensions of the sensor. Hall coefficient R_H depends on the concentration of the carriers. The temperature sensitivity and extreme nonlinearity of the Hall transducer are main disadvantages of the device.

The first application of the implanted sensor based on Hall effect was to measure the knee joint angle [Troyk *et al.*, 1986]. The transducer comprised the samarium-cobalt magnets (B_{max}=140 mT). The poles of the magnets were placed opposing so that when the knee rotated, the polarity of the magnetic field imposed upon the transducer changed from north to south. It was found that the spacing of approximately 1.5 cm produced a near linear response from 0 to 50 degrees of the knee angle. In

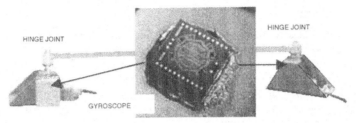

Fig. 4.53: Optical gyroscopes integrated in the goniometric system for the knee and ankle joints [Fuhr and Schmidt, 1999, with permission]. A commercially available gyroscope (middle) fabricated by MicroSensors Incorp, Costa Messa, CA, USA.

comparison, the same linearity with a single magnet is in the range from 0 to 30 degrees. Recently, the Cleveland research team introduced the implanted Hall effect transducer in the wrist joint (Figure 4.52) for volitional control of the Freehand system [Johnson et al., 1999].

The use of optical gyroscopes has been recently introduced for measuring joint angles and angular velocities (Figure 4.53)

Natural Sensors for Neuroprostheses

Natural sensors, such as those found in the skin, muscles, tendons, and joints present an attractive alternative to artificial sensors for FES systems (Figure 4.54). The natural sensors are distributed everywhere in the body and comprise information used for natural control, thereby they are ideal to be integrated in the artificial control. Most

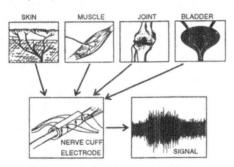

Fig. 4.54: Sensors in skin, muscle, joints, and bladder recorded by a whole nerve cuff electrode might be useful for control of neural prostheses. In many applications the electrodes are made with multistrand wires or thin platinum plates cast into the inside wall (not visible in the figure). The insulating nerve cuff is made of flexible silicone rubber (silastic). A silastic sheet flap adhered over the cuff opening ensures a tight seal. Sutures attached to the outside of the cuff are used to close the cuff after the nerve is placed inside. Adapted from Haugland and Sinkjær, 2000, with permission.

of the peripheral sensory apparatus are still viable after brain and spinal cord injuries, yet not connected to the appropriate higher centers of the central nervous system.

Cuff Electrode for Recording of ENG Activity

Stein and co-workers [Stein et al., 1975] were among the first to use the cuff electrode for chronic recording from peripheral nerves. Hereafter it has been used in a variety of applications. Cuff electrodes have been applied as a tool in studies analyzing peripheral nerve and spinal cord function in animals [Hanson et al., 1987; Hoffer et al., 1981; Hoffer et al., 1987; Hoffer, 1990, 1988; Hoffer and Loeb, 1980; Hoffer et al., 1995; Milner et al., 1991; Little, 1986; Loeb et al., 1987; Loeb and Peck, 1996; Palmer et al., 1985; Stein et al., 1977; Stein et al., 1981], the activity in axotomized or regenerating nerves [Davis et al., 1978; Gordon et al., 1980; Gordon et al., 1991; Hoffer et al., 1979; Krarup and Loeb, 1987; Krarup et al., 1988; Krarup et al., 1989], and the clinical use in FES applications in animals [Edell et al., 1982; Haugland, 1996; Haugland and Hoffer, 1994a and b; Haugland et al., 1995; Hoffer and Sinkjær, 1986; Nikolić et al., 1994; Popović et al., 1993] and humans [Popović and Raspopović, 1991; Sinkjær et al., 1994; Haugland and Sinkjær, 1995; Haugland et al., 1999; Sinkjær et al., 1999].

A nerve cuff electrode for recording is similar to the cuff based stimulating electrodes described earlier. It consists of an insulating cuff typically made of a flexible silastic tubing and circumferential metal electrodes, covering approximately 80 percent of the perimeter, placed at the inside wall of the cuff (Figure 4.55). The nerve is placed inside the cuff through a longitudinal slit; the slit allows opening of the cuff (pulling on sutures glued to the outside of the cuff) for easy implantation. After the cuff has been placed around the nerve, the sutures are tied in order to keep the cuff closed in the time after implantation, where connective tissue will grow into the cuff.

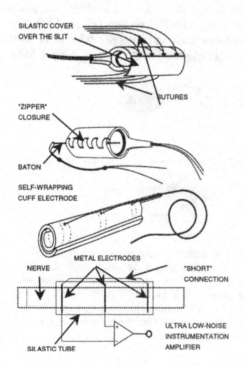

Fig. 4.55: Typical cuff electrodes with the longitudinal slit. See text for details.

The metal contact to nerve is made by locally stripping the insulation from the multistrand wires (stainless steel or Pt_{90}/Ir_{10} alloy) and sewing it to the inside wall of a prefabricated cuff. A new fabrication technique made it possible to use thin platinum plated casts into the inside wall of dip-coated cuffs [Haugland, 1996] and to use a "zipper" closure [Kallesøe et al., 1996]. The self-coiling cuff (Figure 4.55) is yet another design, which in part uses the fabrication techniques first described by Naples et al. [1988]. After installation, the silastic sheeting comprising the self-coiling cuff wraps with several overlapping turns around the nerve. The novel design of a self-wrapping cuff made of polyamide and silicon rubber (silastic), with gold contacts printed at the polyamide is shown in Figure 4.56. The prestretched silicon layer over the polyamide allows the self wrapping around the nerve, and self-fitting of the diameter of the electrode to the size of the nerve.

To avoid the pulling force transferred via the lead wires to the cuff, the wires are often routed into a loop where they leave the cuff.

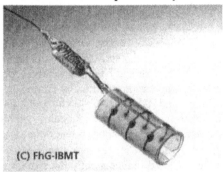

Fig. 4.56: The novel self-wrapping polyamide multipolar electrode for selective recording/stimulation of the whole nerve developed for the EU project GRIP. Courtesy of Stieglitz T, Fraunhofer Institute, St Ingbert, Germany, 2000.

The silastic tube provides electrical insulation that captures the weak neural currents to the tube. The longer the cuff, the less current will leak through the tissue surrounding the cuff; thus, the recorded signals have bigger amplitude with increases in the cuff length. The optimal cuff length for recording from large myelinated afferents is more than 4 cm [Stein et al., 1975; Marks and Loeb, 1976]. A 4 cm long cuff contains about 95 percent of the maximum signal strength that could be recorded with the longer cuff [Thomsen et al., 1996]. There are many nerves that cannot be separated from the surrounding tissues for 4 cm because of the anatomy; hence, shorter electrodes are imposed. Electrodes being 2 cm long yield useful signals in both animal and human applications [Sinkjær et al., 1994; Haugland et al., 1999]. Stein with coworkers [1977] concluded that the length of the electrode, i.e., the distance between the recording sites in the cuff, should be at least 25 percent of the wavelength of the compound action potential.

The signal-to-noise ratio is more favorable when recording from small-diameter nerves than from larger nerves; this is because narrower nerve cuffs around thin nerves produce a more restrictive internal path for the flow of the discharge currents. The power of the signal is inversely proportional to the cross sectional surface of the nerve [Stein et al., 1977].

Cuff electrodes record the current between the two contacts; this current results from the voltage generated by all sources in the surroundings. The currents generated by action potentials of larger fibers are higher than those from the smaller fibers; thus the recorded potential of larger fibers is dominating at the recording site. The typical configuration of contacts in cuff electrodes includes three metal contacts, which are positioned close to the ends and in the middle of the cuff (Figure 4.55, bottom panel). The outer electrodes are shortened to minimize the effects of external electrical field entering the cuff (e.g., EMG of the surrounding muscles). This layout allows differential recordings between the middle electrode and the end electrodes. New developments suggest that the use of two additional conductor rings at far ends of the cuff, being shortened and not used for recordings, increases the signal to noise ratio (Struijk, personal communication, 2000).

To obtain better recording access to the fascicles lying deeper in a trunk nerve, cuffs have been applied with electrodes mounted radially so that they tend to insinuate themselves into the nerve (*i.e.*, in between the fascicles), as reported by Tyler and Durand [1996] in their work to develop a cuff for selective stimulation of nerve fascicles. These designs and others seek to incorporate mechanical effects that try to remodel the morphology of the whole nerve to facilitate a spatial isolation of the component fascicles of the nerve.

Nerve damage in long-term implants

The issue of nerve damage is important, especially with regard to the applications of nerve-cuff electrodes in human subjects. Connective tissue covers the cuff electrodes, and the shape of the nerve changes so as to completely fill the cuff [e.g., Larsen *et al.*, 1998]. According to Hoffer [1990], the cuff should be at least 20 percent larger than the diameter of the nerve to prevent compression neuropathy caused by post-surgical edema [Davis *et al.*, 1978; Strain and Olson, 1975]. Compression neuropathy affects the larger fibers most severely [Gillespie and Stein, 1983; Sunderland, 1978]. The self-wrapping design overcomes this problem because the size of the electrode will follow the swelling [Naples *et al.*, 1988]; yet they could easily allow connective tissue to grow inside, open the cuff, and reduce greatly the signal to noise ratio.

Recently, a large histological study with a total of 40 rabbits including experimental, sham-operated, and control animals was performed [Larsen *et al.*, 1998]. Animals were assigned to a long-term implant group (16 months) and a short-term implant group (14 days).

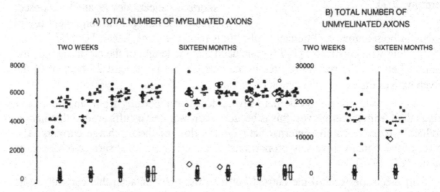

Fig. 4.57: Left and middle panels show total number of myelinated axons at two weeks and sixteen months. Circles show the numbers for the treated animals. The open diamonds indicate result from one animal. Triangles refer to sham-operated animals, and squares to control animals. The cross-section level is shown at the bottom with icons, and horizontal lines indicate the group mean. Right panels show the number of unmyelinated axons. Adapted from Larsen *et al.*, 1998, with permission.

The cuff electrodes were placed on the tibial nerve, just distal to the knee. The traction of the wires on the electrode was minimized by having the wires exit the electrode distally and routing them, via a loop just proximal to the knee, to a subcutaneous connector placed in the groin. At the conclusion of the studies, transverse nerve sections were made at levels proximal to the cuff, at the mid-cuff level, and distal to the cuff.

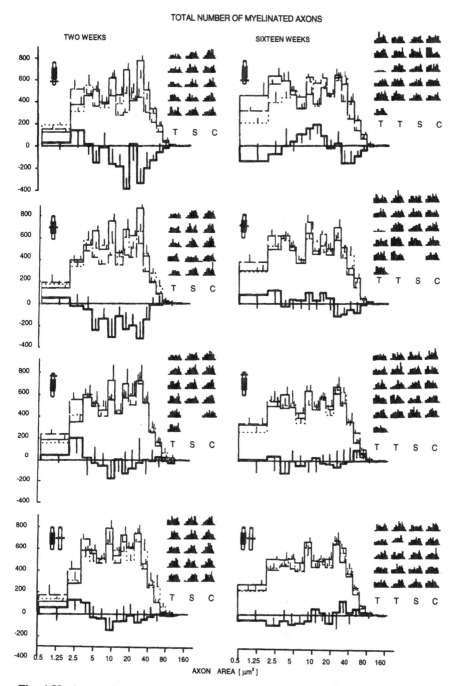

Fig. 4.58: Averaged absolute size distributions of myelinated axons at two weeks and sixteen months. Dashed lines show treated animals, dotted lines sham-operated animals, and solid lines control animals. Vertical bars show SEM. The thick solid lines show the difference between treated and control distributions, *i.e.*, the distribution of the loss of myelinated axons. The ordinate shows the absolute (total) number of axons in each class; abscissa is logarithmic. Adapted from Larsen *et al.*, 1998, with permission.

Sections from the nerve in the contralateral leg served as additional control material. Nerve fiber diameter histograms could thus be obtained at various places with respect to the nerve cuff.

The histological study [Larsen et al., 1998] showed that there was a statistically significant loss of myelinated fibers inside the cuff of 27 percent (p=0.002) and distal to the cuff of 24 percent (p=0.01) 14 days post-surgery, whereas the numbers of fibers proximal to the cuff and in the contralateral leg nerve were unchanged (all numbers compared with the 14-day control group). The sham-operated animals showed no significant loss of fibers. Sixteen months post-surgery there was no longer any significant decrease in the total number of myelinated fibers. No change was found in the number of unmyelinated fibers at either two weeks or sixteen months after implantation (Figures 4.57 and 4.58).

The initial loss (after 14 days) appeared to be non-specific for fiber size, except for sparing of the unmyelinated fibers. After 16 months, although the total number of fibers was the same as in the control group (Figure 4.57, left), there appeared to have been a shift from the largest fiber group (the largest 20% of fiber diameter) towards the smaller fibers, probably indicating that the fibers regenerated, but not to their original diameter. This effect was most pronounced distal to the cuff, but also visible inside the cuff. Proximally and contralaterally there was no change. The results demonstrate that implanted cuff electrodes may cause initial loss of myelinated fibers, which subsequently regenerate. This implies that long-term implantation is possible without a significant loss of nerve fibers.

Processing of Nerve Recordings

The electroneurogram has a relatively small amplitude; when recording the activity from skin receptors in human applications, it is typically below 5 µV [e.g., Haugland et al., 1999]. The amplitude of noise in the surrounding tissues is often several orders of magnitude higher.

The electroneurogram is to be used for two plausible functions (Figure 4.59): cognitive feedback to the subject and feedback within the sensory driven control. An ultra-low-noise differential preamplifier must be used with a high common-mode rejection ratio [Nikolić et al., 1994]. The biological noise that is partly picked-up by the cuff electrode comes from EMG of the surrounding muscles, therefore, filtering with a higher order filter above the frequency of EMG is required. The nerve cuff and the amplifier configuration reject a large fraction of the external noise. However, when nearby muscles are stimulated, the cuff will still record some of the artifacts.

Figure 4.60 shows data recorded from a digital nerve in a human subject while the Flexor Pollicis Longus (FPL) muscle was stimulated at a fixed rate of 20Hz. Stimulation artifacts appear as large spikes saturating in both positive and negative direction. Attempts to blank the artifacts by shorting or disconnecting the input to the amplifier as it is often done when recording EMG during stimulation [e.g., Knaflitz and Merletti, 1988] cannot be recommended. If this is done to an amplifier with this high gain, it can easily cause even larger artifacts due to switching noise and changes in source impedance.

If the stimulated muscles are very close to the cuff, evoked EMG responses may also be picked up. These responses can selectively be suppressed by highpass filtering as they contain frequencies mainly below 1kHz, and the nerve signal (depending on

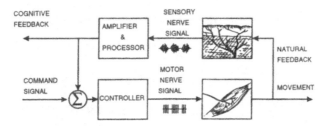

Fig. 4.59: Schema of the various steps in providing a reliable feedback signal from natural sensors for restoring sensory and motor systems in disabled humans.

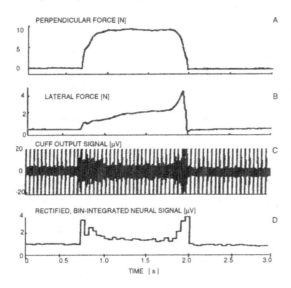

Fig. 4.60: Signal recorded from cutaneous nerve while stimulating nearby muscles electrically. Force is being applied to the skin within the innervation area of the nerve by a hand-held force probe. A) Force applied perpendicularly on the skin. B) Lateral force applied along the skin. In this case the lateral force was increased so that the probe slipped across the skin at the end of the trial. C) Signal recorded from the nerve. D) Signal after rectification and bin-integration of the artifact-free periods. Adapted from Haugland and Sinkjær, 2000 with permission.

the exact dimensions of the cuff and the type of nerve fibers in the nerve) usually contains frequencies above 1kHz.

The cuff electrode can be connected directly to an implanted amplifier. The gain of the amplifier should be approximately 120 dB. The amplified signal can be transmitted using radio frequency communication to the external unit. The bandwidth of the transmission channel should be at least 10 kHz. The same transmission link must provide energy for the amplifier to operate, since the implanted device should not have batteries. It uses a technique known as morphogonostic coils. This technique is based on shaping the coils so that the summed magnetic flux from one inductive link going through the coils of the other is zero. This is done by making the coils (implanted and external) for the power transmission in a rectangular form and the coils of the signal link in the shape of a figure eight. Each of the links runs at separate frequency.

The amplifier and the antenna must be small enough to fit into the region close to the electrode in order to minimize the noise picked up by the leads. The device designed for a totally implanted foot-drop neuroprosthesis [Haugland and Sinkjær, 2000] has been implanted in one subject so far (Figure 4.61).

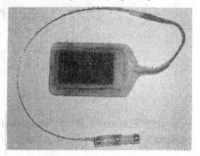

Extracting Sensory Signals from Cuff Electrode Recordings

Fig. 4.61: The implantable amplifier and the cuff for recordings of the neural signals. Adapted from Haugland *et al.*, 2000, with permission.

The information contained in the cuff recorded nerve signal appears to be stored in the variance of the amplitude of the signal [Jezernik and Sinkjær, 1999] rather than in the frequency content. A simple way to assess the amplitude is to filter, rectify, and integrate the signal in bins containing all the data between two stimulation artifacts. Haugland and Hoffer [1994b] have described the method of high-pass filtering and bin-integration of nerve cuff signals.

There are potential benefits for real-time control yielded through the application of sophisticated signal analysis such as a Singular Value Decomposition (SVD) to perform an orthogonal decomposition of "noise" and wanted signal [Upshaw and Sinkjær, 1998] an d Adaptive Logic Network [Popović *et al.*, 1993; Kostov *et al.*, 1999] to extract reliable event markers from whole nerve cuff afferent recordings. The results lead to an improved Signal to Noise Ratio (SNR), improved detection rate, and estimators needed for real-time control.

Algorithms Based on a Singular Value Decomposition (SVD)

The method is intimately related to the method for extraction of the envelope of the signal, and is in essence based on Rectification followed by Bin-Integration (RBI) of the signal during noise-free periods.

In addition, an estimate of the standard, Toeplitz, autocorrelation matrix has to be computed. The orthogonal decomposition of this matrix is performed using a SVD, resulting in singular (eigen) values, which provides an ordered measure of the relative importance (in a least-squared energy sense) of the principal signal components in the eigen-spectrum domain [Haykin, 1991]. The eigenvalue-spread (the difference between the largest and smallest eigenvalues) can be used as a measure of the separation of the signal and noise subspaces. A small spread means that there is little statistical difference between the orthogonal signal components, indicating a purely stochastic (*i.e.*, noise-only) signal. Conversely, a large spread points to the presence of a signal component (*i.e.*, the signal and noise case)

Unfortunately, this separation of noise and signal and noise subspaces is complicated when the noise is "colored" (non-white). Although methods for modifying the standard 2nd order decomposition methods have been described (pre-whitening, for example), another solution is the use of a higher-order (greater than 2nd) statistic of the signal as a basis for a subspace decomposition. The 3rd order cumulate (which is equivalent to the 3rd moment for zero-mean signals) is shown to be immune to the contribution of all symmetrically distributed signals (e.g., Gaussian), [Nikias and Petropulu, 1993]. Thus, 3rd order cumulates provide a measure of the "skewness" (difference from a symmetric distribution) of a signal. If the distribution of the noise subspace is symmetric, as it is the case with the nerve signals (where the noise follows a Gaussian distribution), then it is suppressed in the 3rd order cumulate domain. It is important to note that this noise suppression also holds for colored noise sources, such as the 1/f noise of the typical amplifier.

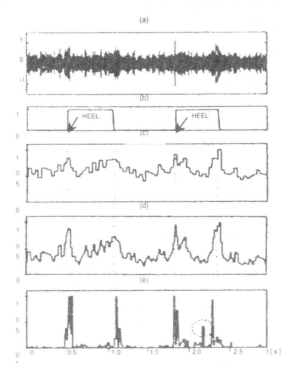

Fig. 4.62: (a) The filtered (1.6-1.9 kHz) nerve signal recorded during FES assisted walking. (b) The output from the heel switch: 1 – heel contact, 0 – heel off. (c) The output of the RBI algorithm processed in real time on the DSP system. (d) and (e) The output of the 2nd and 3rd order algorithms (respectively), processed off-line. Note, 3rd order algorithm provides recognition of events such as heel contact and heel-off, yet false detection could occur (dashed line circle in the bottom panel). Adapted from Upshaw and Sinkjær, 1998, © IEEE.

As with the 2nd order subspace decomposition method, it is possible to use an estimate of the true 3rd order cumulate value, obtained by selecting an appropriate subset of the 2-D cumulate matrix [Rangoussi and Carayannis, 1995].

Figure 4.62 compares the performance of the SVD algorithms when applied on human sensory nerve signals recorded during FES assisted gait. The traces show from the top: a) the original nerve recordings from the sural nerve in a walking human; b) the output of a switch-sensor placed in the subject's shoe where a "high" level indicates stance phase; c) the rectified bin integrated (RBI) signal from panel (a); d) 2nd order detector, and e) the 3rd order detector obtained by SVD, respectively. Note that the raw signal contains short "bursts" of activity, corresponding to the change (derivative) of the applied mechanical stimuli. This is evident in the output from all three processing algorithms as a marked increase in level within a short window around the onset/offset of heel contact (the "edges" on the top trace, indicated with dashed lines).

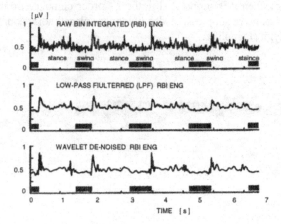

Fig. 4.63: Processed recordings from a cuff electrodes at the sural nerve of a walking human. Four consecutive steps are presented: RBI ENG (top), low-passed filtered RBI ENG (middle), and wavelet do-noised RBI ENG (bottom). Black bars are heel-switch data. Adapted from Kostov *et al.*, 1999, with permission.

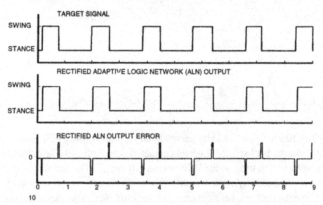

Fig. 4.64: Target signal (top panel) and ALN estimated signal (middle panel) after applying blanking and restriction rules (see text for details). The bottom panel shows timing errors, that is delays between the original and predicted intervals. See text for details. Adapted from Kostov *et al.*, 1999, with permission.

A method for processing RBI ENG and extracting features was investigated by Hansen *et al.* [1998] for the detection of heel contact and heel off from a walking human with a cuff implanted on the sural nerve. Adaptive Logic Network (ALN) training was done using one data set and tested (evaluated) on another [Kostov *et al.*, 1995]. A target was a heel switch signal (black bars in Figure 4.63) recorded along with the ENG. The target was used both for the training and as reference for evaluation. All parameters were optimized with regard to the detection performance, which was calculated as the percentage of correctly detected samples compared with the target signal.

Low pass filtering (Figure 4.63, middle panel) and wavelet de-noising (Figure 4.63, bottom panel) have been investigated as two pre-processing methods for separation of signal and noise. Low pass filtering has the advantage of simple calculation, which would offer better applicability in a real-time implementation; however, wavelet de-noising has the advantage of filtering signals by removing signal components smaller than a certain size, regardless of their frequency. Batch processing using different filtering in the cut-off frequency range 2-15 Hz and filter order range 1 to 40 revealed that a 1st order Butterworth filter with a 6.5 Hz cut-off frequency offers the best ALN performance.

In order to perform pattern recognition on time-varying data, it is necessary to have the temporal dimension represented in the input domain (Figure 4.64). An experiment was performed processing batches with and without the first derivative as additional input signals [Kostov et al., 1992]. Varying a configuration of previous samples, which are added to the input domain, revealed information of optimal temporal information configuration. The experiment included zero to five previous samples equally spaced in the range of one to ten samples, which is equal to time information ranging to 500 ms. Figure 4.64 (bottom panel) shows the timing errors, the values −1, 0, and 1 show that the ALN predicted signal is preceding, matches the timing, or it is delayed compared with the original signal respectively.

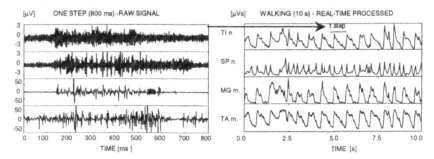

Fig. 4.65: Raw (one step) and real-time processed recordings (10 seconds) from the Tibial (TI) n, Superficial Peroneal (SP) n, Medial Gastrocnemius (MG) m, and Tibialis Anterior (TA) m. in a cat walking on a powered treadmill. The recordings were applied for rule-based control of FES supported walking. Both EMG and ENG signals (natural sensors) have been used for control. The cuff and epimysial electrodes have been implanted in cats for more than 3 years; the recordings remained stable throughout the experiments. Adapted from Popović et al., 1993, © IEEE.

The use of cuff electrodes for recordings of neural activity in freely moving cats, in parallel with recordings of the EMG activity of leg muscles with epimysial electrodes in order to test the control based on finite state models of locomotion [Popović et al., 1993] provided further insight in the reliability and stability of implanted electrodes and using natural sensors. Several cats have been implanted for up to 3.5 years, and the recordings have been stable and reliable. The recordings have been processed with a portable, battery powered device [Nikolić *et al.*, 1994], which provided amplification, filtering, and BIN integration; thus real time use of natural sensors for control was facilitated. Figure 4.65 (right panel) shows 20 seconds of the processed recordings from nerves and muscles in a walking cat. The left panel shows the original recordings from only one stride (indicated with the arrow in the right panel). The recordings have been used for a rule-based controller. The information that could be reliably extracted was based on the threshold detection. Since two nerve recordings have been captured simultaneously, and a separate threshold level was adopted for each nerve, four pieces of information were available.

Extraction of Position Information from Nerve Cuff Muscle Afferents Recordings

Normal motor function relies heavily on signals from muscle afferents for information about the static and dynamic forces acting about the joints. It might be useful for future FES systems if control signals could be derived from recordings of this afferent activity, and initial successes in this area by Yoshida and Horch [1996] lend support for this effort. Using the rabbit ankle as a model for the human ankle, Riso *et al.* [2000] characterized the responses evoked in a pair of complementary mixed nerves (the tibial and peroneal components of the sciatic nerve) that carry muscle afferents from the main ankle extensor and ankle flexor muscles. Simultaneous recordings were obtained using tripolar cuffs installed around the two nerves. For the initial study, a servo apparatus was used to rotate the ankle with ramp and hold movements that alternated from flexion to extension. Figure 4.66 shows the basic responses to this passive motion. Dorsiflexion (see '2') movement stretches the extensor muscles, and after a position threshold '3' is exceeded, evokes vigorous activity in the tibial nerve. At the start of the plateau (hold) phase ('4'), there is a reduction in the tibial activity because the dynamic response from the spindle primary

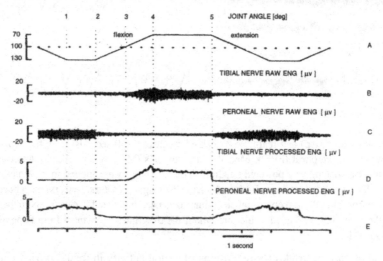

Fig. 4.66: Joint angle and nerve activity recorded from the tibial and peroneal nerves in a rabbit during passive ankle movement over a range of 60 degrees. The nerve activities before processing are in B and C, while D and E are the rectified and integrated signals using a moving window average. Adapted from Riso *et al.*, 2000© IEEE.

afferents is curtailed, leaving only the spindle secondary (static) afferents discharging and possibly some contribution from the Golgi tendon organ afferents. At '5' the motion reverses direction toward extension with two consequences: the activity halts abruptly in the tibial recording (since the spindles are being shortened), and in a complementary manner, an increase is seen in the afferent activity recorded from the peroneal nerve.

The most rudimentary analysis of the dual nerve recordings reveals the direction of the movement of the joint. Moreover, if the rate of the motion is increased, then the dynamic response is also increased. Calibration of the dynamic response, however, has been difficult to achieve because it depends strongly on the initial stretch (*i.e.*, related to the starting position) of the responding muscles [Jensen *et al.*, 1998; Riso, 1998; Riso *et al.*, 2000]. A final consideration with regard to the intended application for FES concerns the effect of contractions within the muscles whose afferents are being recorded, since it is well known that contractions unload the spindle receptors and interrupt their activity. At the same time, however, the Golgi tendon receptors will be activated by the contraction. The activity recorded by the cuff will represent a summation of these opposing effects, and studies have shown that only at very high muscles stimuli does the contraction of the muscle fibers change the sensitivity of the recorded whole nerve afferent signals [Jensen *et al.*, 1998]. In such situations one way of circumventing the complications of muscle contractions would be to not apply FES to some muscles around each joint so as to receive passive movement signals from them. In situations where FES is given only to the muscle(s) on one side of a joint at any given time (*i.e.*, co-contraction of antagonistic pairs is avoided), the muscles opposite to the FES muscle will be passively stretched.

Micera *et al.* [1999] attempted to extract position information from the whole nerve muscle afferent signal using a Neural Fuzzy Model (NFM). This hybrid structure is able to integrate the positive features of neural networks and fuzzy systems.

The position of the joint was extracted using a dynamic neuro-fuzzy predictor trained using the gradient descent algorithm. The fuzzy system used a non-singleton fuzzification method to transform the real input values into a set of fuzzy input values, which were then processed by the network. This method is very useful when noise is present in the available data. Moreover, the history-sensitive behavior of the Fuzzy System (FS) due to its recurrent structure makes it suitable to model complex and dynamic processes better than the standard feed-forward systems. The results indicate that the selected FS is able to predict the ankle position from the recorded nerve signals; the low prediction error suggests that the neuro-fuzzy predictor might be useful in a closed-loop functional neuromuscular stimulation system to control joint position. Because of the reduced number of implemented rules, the FS can run as a real-time controller. Future work will be in the direction of testing the robustness of the NFM using different passive and active trajectories [Micera *et al.*, 1999].

EMG Signals for Control of Movement

EMG signals have for quite some time been used for artificial hands in so-called myoelectric control as described in Section 4.4 and Chapter 5. Here, the methods are described as to how electrical activity of a muscle (EMG) can be used as a natural sensor. The EMG signal is related to the muscle force, yet this relation is not direct and reliable [Bigland and Lippold, 1954; Edwards and Lippold, 1956; Millner-Brown and Stein, 1975]. The amplitude of the EMG is nonlinear upon the length of the muscle,

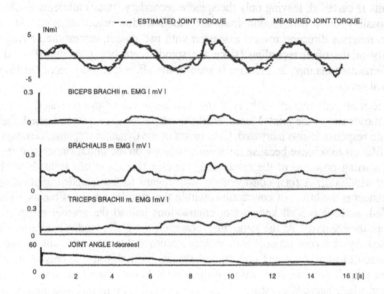

Fig. 4.67: Recorded and estimated net joint torque at the elbow joint from the real-time processed surface recorded EMG activity of Biceps Brachii m, Brachialis m, and Triceps Brachii m. Adapted from Meek *et al.*, 1990, with permission.

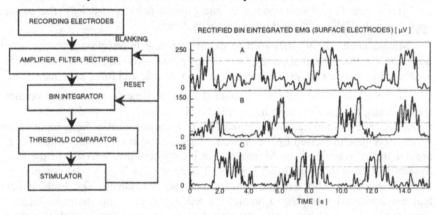

Fig. 4.68: The EMG processing (left) and recordings (right) from the wrist extensor in three tetraplegics (A, B, and C) during their contraction of the wrist extensors (the finger flexors are stimulated at 20 Hz). Adapted from Saxena *et al.*, 1995, with permission.

velocity of the shortening of the muscle, and the fatigue level [Philipson *et al.*, 1981]. The frequency content of the EMG also changes with the fatigue, and it is not related to the force in a meaningful manner. It is, however, possible to use modeling and simulation and thereby estimate the relation between the EGM signals and the joint torque [Meek *et al.*, 1990]. In order to develop a control, which allows transhumeral amputees to use powered elbow and hand prosthesis and over all controls the arm at the subconscious level, it was essential to develop the estimation procedure of the elbow joint based on the EMG recordings from the elbow flexor and extensor muscles (e.g., Biceps Brachii, Brachialis, and Triceps Brachii muscles).

Figure 4.67 shows the measured and estimated net joint torque at the elbow joint, based on the recordings from the elbow flexor and extensor muscles. The estimate is based on the modeling and experiments with able-bodied humans, who moved their forearm against the measure load, while the EMG was recorded with intramuscular electrodes.

EMG signals could also be used for the control of a neuroprosthesis; several systems have been designed and tested in clinical environments [Keller *et al.*, 1998; Rakoš *et al.*, 1998; Sennels *et al.*, 1997; Tepavac and Medri, 1998]. For example, an EMG controlled grasping system has been developed and evaluated [Saxena *et al.*, 1995]. The sensory system (Figure 4.68, left panel) includes an ultra low-noise, high impedance; high common mode rejection ratio preamplifier. The preamplifier is realized with a pair of JFET transistors at the input, followed by the instrumentation amplifier (CMRR > 100 dB, A = 100, f ∈ 100-10000 Hz). The signal was further fed to a cascade of a RC high-pass filter with gain (f > 100 Hz, A = 100), full-wave precision rectifier, and a blanking device. The blanking device switches the output of the amplifier to the ground when the stimulation pulses are delivered to the appropriate motor nerves. During the blanking period the input to the integrator is zero.

The signal was then BIN integrated, with 10 ms intervals, and fed to the input of a comparator. The second input of the comparator can be set to a predetermined level. If the integrated EMG crosses the preset threshold level (Figure 4.68, right panels, dashed horizontal lines), then the comparator output goes "high". This control signal changes the state of a flip-flop that turns on the NP. Typical recordings in presence of strong stimulation of the surrounding muscles are shown in Figure 4.68 (right panel).

Recording from the Cortex - Brain Interface

Recently the possible use of recordings from higher cortical structures is attracting attention from many researchers. One possible method is to use the focal recordings using the EEG instrumentation [McFarland *et al.*, 1998; Wolpaw *et al.*, 1998; Vaughan *et al.*, 1998]. The other, rather invasive technique is much more attractive because it will provide direct access to the structures that are directly delegated for sensory-motor functions. A multi-electrode system with 100 needles made out of silicon has been tested for both recording and stimulating brain and peripheral neural structures (Figure 4.69).

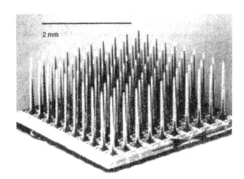

Fig. 4.69: The intracortical electrode array (100 electrodes) made of solid silicon. This array is for stimulating motor and recording from sensory systems. Courtesy of Dr. Richard A Norman, University of Utah, Salt Lake City, UT.

Norman with colleagues tested the system in animal experiments aiming to provide a possible tool for visual prostheses [Norman *et al.*, 1999; Rouche and Norman, 1999]. The electrode is only 2.5 x 2.5 x 2 mm^3 and provides 100 independent

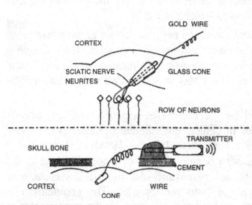

Fig. 4.70: The cone electrode. Drawing is not to scale. Bottom panel shows the final configuration of the implanted cone electrode. See text for details. Adapted from Kennedy, 1989, with permission.

stimulation or recording points. The system can be implanted in the cortex by using a special tool, which allows the device to penetrate into the brain or peripheral nerve (Norman, personal communication, 1999) and, if properly installed, to remain there without any special attachment. The longer-term experiments indicate that the neural tissue is slowly pushing the implant out; thus, it is likely that after some time, the electrode will not operate.

The design of a recording electrode from the brain, which has been tested in many animal experiments [Kennedy, 1989; Kennedy et al., 1992], relies on golden electrodes mounted in the small glass cone (Figure 4.70). The recordings from the cone electrodes will stabilize over the time (Figure 4.71), and there is no guarantee and method to select the exact neurons, whose activity will be recorded.

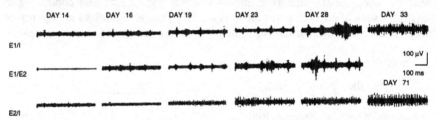

Fig. 4.71: Recordings from the monkey cortex using a cone electrode. The firing rate is increasing over time, and then remains stable. See text for details. Adapted from Kennedy, 1989, with permission.

The electrode is biocompatible, and it is installed into the brain by generating (intentionally) a small injury and putting the cone into the injured structure. The neurons will promote through the cone. The actual electrodes are glued inside the cone; thus, a single neuron activity will be recorded with one cone electrode. The firing rate of cells is the information of interest.

In Chapter 2 it was shown that the direction of the firing rate of cells within the motor cortex correlates with the direction of hand movement; the preferred direction of increased firing rate is the direction of the distal segment of the hand [Georgopoulos et al., 1982]. Schwartz with coworkers [Schwartz and Adams, 1995; Lin et al., 1997] showed that there is very high correlation between the three-dimensional movement and the firing rate using fine wire electrodes. Fine wires are not convenient as a chronic interface because they migrate. Although the recordings from many electrodes implanted in the brain suggest that the percentage of electrodes operating is unchanged over time, the fact is that the recordings are often from different cells on different days, which makes the technique difficult to apply directly.

Command Interface for Neuroprostheses

Effective application of a neuroprosthesis requires that the user "has" a decisive command of the activities that he/she is planning, as well as of the manner in which he/she is anticipating to execute those. In upper-extremity systems the user has to select the mode of grasping (e.g., lateral, palmar, and pinch), the level of the grasp force based on the object to be grasped (e.g., weight, friction coefficient between the hand and the object), and to control the prehension (size of the object). The upper extremity systems, if used to assist reaching comprises many more variables to be controlled (e.g., the wrist movement with two degrees of freedom, elbow movement having one degree of freedom, and the shoulder joint with three degrees of freedom). Both, the hand and the arm controls require variable level of cocontraction of agonist and antagonist muscles to ensure sufficient stiffness and eliminate jerky movement. It is obvious that it would not make much sense to provide command interface for all of these activities, yet some of those are essential. The immediate answer is that a combination of continuous and discrete control input would work the best. The terminology of automatics classifies such control systems into so-called hybrid systems [Lima and Saridis, 1999].

Several devices have been tested for the command interface; none being ideal so far [Hart et al., 1998]. The discrete control has to be provided with a switch. The difficulty of using a switch is its positioning and providing its operation at the subconscious level. Humans learn fast; thus, the second issue is much less of a problem, but a cosmetic, reliable, and reproducible mounting is not simple. In many applications a single switch was insufficient; hence, a multi-button interface is required (e.g., control of elbow NP as described by Popović and Popović [1998a]). The voice control could be used, as shown many years ago [Nathan, 1989]. The Japanese group used the respiratory control for their multichannel intramuscular electrode system [Hoshimiya et al., 1989; Handa et al., 1989b]. The Freehand system [Hart et al., 1998] uses a switch mounted at the chest to turn on and off the system and select between grasps, as it will be described in the next section. The NESS Handmaster [Nathan, 1997] and the Belgrade Grasping System [Popović and Popović, 1998b] use two switches; one is mounted at the hand, while the parallel switch is mounted at the control box (device). This redundancy allows the user to select which switch works better for him/her while performing different activities. The alternative solution is to use natural signals from muscles, and set a single threshold or multiple thresholds that operate as a switch as shown earlier [e.g., Saxena et al., 1995].

The other command interface has to provide a continuous signal (e.g., grading force, opening the hand during the prehension). Meek et al. [1990] developed a system where EMG sensors operate in a continuous mode. They control the elbow action of a powered transhumeral prosthesis. There is yet no efficient system based on EMG, which can use the continuous mode for NP although many systems are described in the literature [e.g., Graupe and Kline, 1996].

Different types of joysticks mounted at the contralateral shoulder, ipsilateral wrist, or in some cases being mounted at the wheelchair frame have been tested and used with variable successes. The selection of the most appropriate position of the joystick is individual and depends entirely on the user's ability to control it, because in parallel he/she must monitor what the neuroprosthesis is doing. It is not likely that a tetraplegic subject is capable of using visual input for both grasping and controlling the joystick; thus, the control input must come from the part of the body that has somatosensory feedback channels still operating.

The NP for walking requires at least a command input for selecting the mode of activity: standing up, sitting down, start walking, change of the modality of walking (e.g., stairs, slope, change of the velocity). So far switches of different kinds have been used for triggering a specific phase of the gait cycle (e.g., the swing phase of each leg [Kralj and Bajd, 1989], or the whole gait cycle [Kobetič and Marsolais, 1994]. The switches have been controlled by hands, or positioned in the shoes, or realized using the threshold detection of the EMG from the non-paralyzed muscles [Graupe and Kohn, 1988]. Since the walking is considered as a cyclic activity, there was very little attention to a possible interface that would allow continuous input to the leg movement. It is likely that such interface will become necessary once the walking NP start providing more function than they do today.

4.3.3 Neuroprostheses for Restoring Grasping and Reaching

NPs for upper-limbs are being developed to establish and augment the independence to the user. The target population for many years is tetraplegics with diminished, yet preserved shoulder and elbow functions, lacking the wrist control and grasping ability [Triolo et al., 1996]. Controlling the movement of the whole arm has lately received more attention [Crago et al., 1998; Grill and Peckham, 1998; Lemay and Crago, 1997; Popović and Popović, 1998a, b, 2000a and b; Smith et al., 1996]. The feasibility of restoring upper extremity function to individuals with high cervical spinal cord injury (C4 or higher) using FES and/or reconstructive surgery has been evaluated. Externally controlling movement to these individuals is challenging and not very successful for two primary reasons: 1) the number of retained voluntary functions is so low that there is a minimal opportunity to substitute for lost functions or even to use these motions to control external devices; and 2) individuals with C3 or C4 level spinal cord injuries exhibit extensive denervation of the shoulder and elbow muscles, which limits the possibility of using FES to restore movement.

Available NP can be divided upon the source of control signals to trigger or regulate the stimulation pattern into the following groups: contralateral shoulder movement [Hart et al., 1998], voice command [Nathan, 1989; Nathan and Ohry, 1990], respiratory activity [Handa et al., 1989b], contralateral hand controlled joystick [Rudel et al., 1984], wrist movement [Prochazka et al., 1997; Hart et al., 1998], EMG activity of agonistic muscles [Saxena et al., 1995; Thorsen et al., 1998], and switches mounted at various places at the body [Popović et al., 1998b; Nathan, 1997]. The division can also be made upon the method that the patterned electrical stimulation is delivered to: one to three channel surface electrode systems, multichannel surface stimulation system, multichannel percutaneous systems with intramuscular electrodes, and fully implanted systems with epimysial electrodes [e.g., Triolo et al., 1996].

The first grasping system used to provide prehension and release [Long and Masciarelli, 1963] had a splint with a spring for closure and electrical stimulation of the thumb extensor for release. This attempt was unsuccessful mostly because of the technology used, but also because of muscle fatigue and erratic contractile response. Rudel et al. [1984] following the work of Vodovnik [Reberšek and Vodovnik, 1973] suggested the use of a simple two channel stimulation system and a position transducer (sliding potentiometer). The shift of the potentiometer forward from its neutral position caused opening by stimulating the dorsal side of the forearm. The backward movement of the sliding potentiometer caused closing of the hand by stimulating the volar side of the forearm.

The follow-up of initial FES system use was systematically continued in Japan [Hoshimiya et al., 1989; Handa et al., 1989b]. This effort resulted in the only FES clinic in the world, located in Sendai, Japan. Many subjects have been implanted with up to thirty percutaneous intramuscular electrodes per extremity. These electrodes are connected to a thirty-channel device that delivers a pre-programmed sequence of stimulation pulses. The preprogrammed sequence is prepared based on the activity of muscles recorded in able-bodied subjects. The intramuscular EMG determined the pattern of muscle activity in able-bodied subjects. The stimulation in the Sendai Hospital is applied in most cases as a therapy, not to assist grasping and reaching. The thirty-electrode system is used to control muscles required for both grasping and reaching. So far, it has been applied to several hundred individuals in Japan, and the target population includes mostly subjects with complete, high cervical spinal cord lesion (C4).

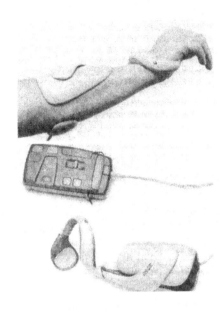

Fig. 4.72: The Handmaster NMS1 grasping device. Courtesy of Dr. Roger Nathan, Ra'anana, Israel.

An early version of the system has been demonstrated for functional reaching and grasping [Hoshimiya et al., 1989]. The command interface of subjects with such high lesions is very restricted; thus, a voice or suck/puff control and preprogrammed EMG based stimulation patterns have been selected.

A different method has been used at Ben Gurion University, Israel [Nathan, 1989]. They applied a voice controlled multichannel surface electrode system. As many as 12 bipolar stimulation channels and a splint have been used to control elbow, wrist, and hand functions. There is very little practical experience with the system, because of the complexity of tuning it for the needs of every single user. Surface stimulation does not allow control of the small hand and forearm muscles necessary to provide dexterity while grasping. Daily mounting and fitting of the system has been problematic.

Based on accumulated experience with developing reaching and grasping systems and the above outlined principles, the Handmaster NMS1 system was designed by Nathan [Nathan, 1997], and recently approved for the therapy of humans. The approval for marketing and home use follows the claims that it improves grasping functionality of humans after stroke by long term, carry-on therapeutic effects. The Handmaster is a three-channel stimulation system (Figure 4.72).

The surface electrodes are housed in a nicely designed, rigid plastic orthosis that supports the wrist in a limited volar flexion. The thumb is free to move. One channel stimulates the Extensor Digitorum Communis at the volar side of the forearm, and the second channel is applied over the Flexor Digitorum Profundus and Superficialis. The third electrode activates the thumb opposition. A switch on the stimulator box turns on, with adjustable delay, the grasping function. The grasping function consists of opening of the fingers, period of no stimulation, followed by the stimulation of both the thumb and finger flexors. The next switch operation triggers the release function. This switching starts the stimulation of the finger extensors for a short period (adjustable), followed by turning off the stimulation. A duplicate, parallel switch is mounted at the plastic wrist orthosis to allow the user to operate the system single-handed. By "hitting" the switch to the desk, or some other solid object, the desired operation starts.

Although the Handmaster NMS1 neuroprosthesis has been approved for humans with hemiplegia as a therapeutic device, it is used both as therapy and as orthosis. The clinical evaluation of the electrical stimulation effects concluded that both long-term and orthotic effects are noticeable, and a comprehensive analysis of the effects of the FES systems used for arm and hand after stroke [Hines et al., 1995] indicated modest, but positive carry over therapeutic effects.

Wrist motion is essential for augmenting the fine motor control of the fingers and hand [Tubiana, 1984]. Positioning of the wrist in the direction opposite that of the fingers alters the functional length of the digital tendons so that maximal finger movements can be attained, and this is called tenodesis. Conversely, some flexion of the wrist puts tension on the long extensors, causing fingers to open automatically and aiding full finger extension. The wrist extension is caused by two groups of muscles: 1) Extensor Carpi Radialis Longus and Brevis (extension of wrist, radial deviation); and 2) Extensor Carpi Ulnaris Brevis (extension of wrist, ulnar deviation). The range of wrist movement required for normal functioning is [Brumfield and Champoux, 1984]: 10-degree flexion and 35-degree extension. This range was determined for the following seven functional activities: lift glass to mouth, pour from pitcher, cut with knife, lift fork to mouth, use telephone receiver and push dialing button, read newspaper, rise from chair; and seven personal care activities (touch of head occiput and vertex, shirt neck, chest, waist, sacrum, and shoe). When the wrist was immobilized [Volz et al., 1980], the best performance was achieved having the wrist in a 15-degree extension.

Some tetraplegics retain wrist movements, and they can grasp by using a tenodesis. However, the grasp generated with a tenodesis is rather weak, and the handling of heavier objects (e.g., opening the door, picking up a camcorder battery or VCR tape, holding a book, *etc.*) is frequently not feasible. In addition, to hold an object by using tenodesis, it is necessary to maintain the wrist extension during manipulation, and this is difficult or even impossible. Subjects who are able to use tenodesis for limited grasping have typically innervated finger flexors, but they are not controllable volitionally. Some devices rely on this rather simple principle, and they can improve the grasping function, by augmenting the flexion of the fingers, including the control of a thumb position. The differences between the systems are command signals to trigger tenodesis, or stop it once it has been activated artificially.

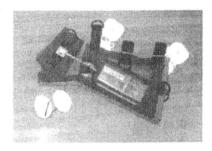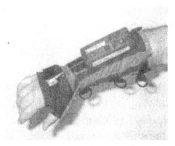

Fig. 4.73: The Bionic Glove; the surface stimulation grasping device (palmar grasp) comprising three stimulation channels and n controlled by the dorsal/volar wrist flexion.

Prochazka et al., [1997] suggested the use of wrist position to control the stimulation of muscles to enhance the tenodesis grasping, and designed a device, the so-called Bionic glove (Figure 4.73), later modified and called Tetron. A sensor is used to detect wrist movement, and trigger opening and closing of the hand. A microcomputer is built into the battery operated stimulation unit, which detects movements and controls three channels to stimulate thumb extensors and flexors, and finger flexors. The user volitionally triggers the opening of the hand by flexing the wrist for an angle that is bigger than a pre-selected threshold value (the Extensor Digitorum Communis muscles are stimulated). The closing is initiated by extending the wrist to an angle that is bigger than a pre-selected threshold. A dead-zone (hysteresis) allows movement of the wrist once the "open" or "close" stimulation pattern is activated. An easy-to-use push 3-button interface allows setting of the parameters, and the optional audio feedback facilitates the learning process. In the clinical evaluation [Popović et al., 1999a] it was indicated that the stimulation is beneficial to tetraplegic subjects (therapy effects and orthotic assistance), but that the overall acceptance rate for long time use is at about 30 percent of potential users. One of the conclusions was that the control, donning and doffing should be improved, as well as its cosmesis. The Tetron, novel version of the Bionic Glove, incorporates several motor programs for grasping, which the user can select, and the hardware has been improved and minimized.

Myoelectric control is effective for artificial arms and hands, and the technology is available. Using EMG signals above the lesion to control FES systems has received much attention. Most systems use the EMG signal only as a trigger. In this way, the EMG is only replacing a mechanical switch. The reason for replacing a simple switch with a complex EMG recording unit and additional hardware is that it can be controlled automatically at the subconscious level. The use of myoelectric signals from the above lesion sites (forearm wrist extensors) to trigger the stimulation of thumb and finger flexors has been presented [Saxena et al., 1995]. A threshold discrimination of the EMG is done, which activates the proper stimulus pattern to be applied to the surface electrodes (Figure 4.74).

The EMG recordings depend upon the placement of the electrodes, skin, and electrode impedance. The analysis of the processed recordings from the same subject in day-to-day sessions, when mounting electrodes into more or less identical positions (the electrode positions were marked at the skin), showed a reproducible pattern of EMG [Saxena et al., 1995]. An EMG signal changes both amplitude and frequency content. The amplified, rectified, and BIN integrated EMG recordings show a peak when the subject elicits and maintains a voluntary muscle contraction compared with the recordings when resting. The variability of recordings, although being wide, can be eliminated by a threshold method to be set by the user on a daily basis. The effect of muscle fatigue has to be taken into account. During sessions lasting 60 minutes, the peak of the integrated rectified EMG signals dropped to about 60 percent compared with its maximal value at the beginning of the test [Lenman et al., 1989].

A different version of controller that uses a multi-threshold principle was tested [Saxena et al., 1995] to allow users to vary the strength of the grasp. The clinical result favors the simple, single-threshold system because of the difficulties in tuning of the internal components, variability of EMG recordings, and even more because of the lack of feedback about the strength of the grip.

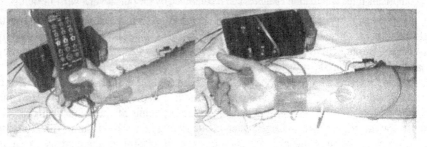

Fig. 4.74: The EMG controlled grasping device developed at the Miami Project to Cure Paralysis. Adapted from Saxena et al., 1995, with permission.

A new laboratory version of the myoelectric control of a grasping system has been developed and tested by the ParaCare group at the University of Zurich, Switzerland [Popović MR et al., 2000]. The system controls grasping based on: 1) analog EMG control that uses recordings from the deltoid muscle from the ipsilateral arm; 2) discrete (digitally processed EMG based on the coded series of integrated, rectified, and compared with threshold signals; 3) push button interface; and 4) sliding potentiometer (proportional control).

The group at the Institute for Biokibernetik, Karlsruhe, Germany, suggested the use of EMG recordings from the muscle, which is stimulated [Vossius et al., 1987]. The aim of this device was to enhance the grasping using weak muscles. Hence, in principle, it could be possible to use retained recordings from the volar side of the forearm to trigger on and off the stimulation of the same muscles. In this case it is essential to eliminate the stimulation artifact, and the evoked potential caused by the stimulus, in order to eliminate positive feedback effects, which will generate a tetanic contraction that cannot be turned off using the method presented. Thorsen and colleagues [1999] have further developed this approach.

The Belgrade Grasping/reaching System (BGS) is a four-channel system [Ilić et al., 1994] allowing two modalities of grasping: side and palm grasps by generating opposition and control of elbow movement. A preprogrammed sequence is triggered using a switch interface, similar to the Handmaster system. The grasping is separated into three phases: 1) prehension (forming the correct aperture); 2) relaxing (allowing the hand to get good contact with the object; and 3) closing the hand by opposing the palm and the thumb or the side of the index finger and the thumb (Figure 4.75). The releasing function includes two stages: opening of the hand and resting. It is possible to select the duration of each of the phases of the grasp/release upon the individual characteristics of the subject, as well as his/her preferences. The BGS comprises a reaching controller. The initial version of the system used so-called scaling law, the new version uses synergistic control based on mapping of the angular velocities at the shoulder and elbow joints, as it is described in Chapter 5.

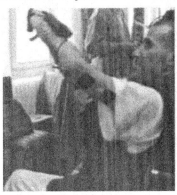 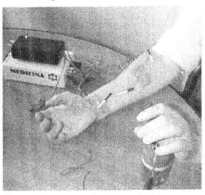

Fig. 4.75: The Belgrade Grasping System (BGS) used by an incomplete tetraplegic (C5) for reaching and grasping (left). The position of electrodes for grasping function (right).

The most advanced, and by all standards most promising grasping NP follows from more than twenty years of dedicated work by Peckham and many coworkers from the Case Western Reserve University (CWRU), Cleveland, Ohio [Peckham et al., 1980a and b]. A fully implantable stimulation device (Figure 4.76) is approved for human use under the name Freehand system, distributed by the NeuroControl Corp. of Cleveland, Ohio. The system has an external unit (control box, power source) and an implantable part (remotely powered and controlled stimulator, leads with epimysial electrodes, and a sensory system) [Smith et al., 1987].

The system has been initially developed and used for a long time with percutaneous, intramuscular electrodes. The Freehand system is implanted when the neuro-muscular structure needed to support its capacity is available. In many cases, a surgery, which includes tendon transfers, pining some joints, or other procedures developed to augment functioning of humans with upper-limb disability, precedes the use of the system.

The objective of this system is to provide grasp and release for individuals with C5 and C6 level spinal cord injuries. Coordinated electrical stimulation of paralyzed forearm and hand muscles is used to provide lateral (key pinch) and palmar grasp patterns. The subjects obtain proportional control of grasp opening and closing by voluntary movement of either the shoulder or wrist. An external transducer is mounted on the chest to measure the shoulder motion; or on the dorsum of the wrist to measure the wrist flexion/extension. The novel version of the wrist sensor can be implanted [Kilgore et al., 1997; Hart et al., 1998]. The control signal is sent to an external control unit, which converts the signal into the appropriate stimulation signals for each electrode. These signals are sent across an inductive link to an implanted stimulator receiver, which generates the stimulus to the appropriate electrode. Seven epimysial electrodes, sewn onto the muscle surface through surgical exposure, are used for muscle excitation. Sensory feedback regarding the control state is provided through an eighth implanted electrode placed in an area of normal sensation.

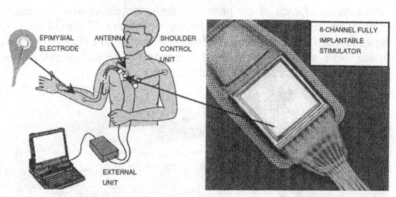

Fig. 4.76: The Freehand system. Multichannel stimulator is implanted (inset) and connected with epimysial electrodes as described earlier. Adapted from Smith *et al.*, 1998, © IEEE.

The electrode leads are tunneled subcutaneously to the implanted stimulator located in the pectoral region. The surgical procedures to enhance both voluntary and stimulated hand functions are often performed in conjunction with the stimulator implantation. More than 200 tetraplegics have received the Freehand NP at more than a dozen sites around the world. The subjects have demonstrated the ability to grasp and release objects and to perform activities of daily living more independently when using the neuroprosthesis. The subjects utilize the device at home on a regular basis. NeuroControl Corp. of Cleveland, Ohio, USA, coordinates the clinical trials.

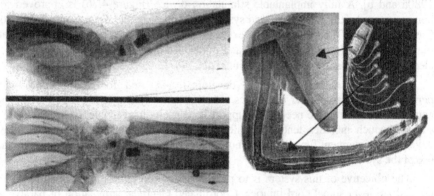

Fig. 4.77: Xerogram of the implanted wrist joint transduced based on the Hall effect (left) and the whole system (right). Adapted from Hart *et al.*, 1998, © IEEE.

A next-generation of implantable NP is developed at the CWRU. The implantable stimulator/telemeter extends the capabilities of the existing Freehand stimulator by increasing the number of stimulus channels available. Telemetring information about the implanted signal from transducers, muscle activation, and operational status to an external computer is now possible. The increased number of stimulus channels allows: increased flexibility to control muscles, active extension of the elbow joint, and improved sensory feedback strategies. The system also includes a new implantable transducer for sensing movement of joints such as the wrist or shoulder. Implanted transducers replace external ones, sensing command control movements from the wrist for persons with C6 level injuries, or the shoulder in C5 level injuries. In C5 injuries, an implanted wrist transducer would provide feedback signals to control wrist muscle stimulation, freeing these individuals of forearm orthoses.

The initial implementation of the advanced stimulator/telemeter provides ten channels of stimulation and one implanted joint angle transducer (Figure 4.77). The stimulator/telemeter unit has been implanted in several individuals. Clinical tests of the implanted joint angle transducer began in 1997. The transducer has been implanted in the wrist, allowing the individual to control grasp opening and closing through voluntary movement of the wrist.

A prototype of sixteen channels of stimulation, one implanted joint angle transducer, and two channels of myoelectric signal transduction is developed. This system will be applicable to individuals with C5 level injuries, with placement of the joint angle transducer in the shoulder joint. The myoelectric signal obtained from arm or neck muscles will be used to control various features of the grasp and/or arm movements.

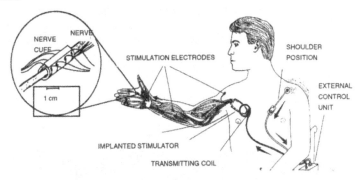

Fig. 4.78: Drawing of instrumented arm in a 28-year old tetraplegic male. Nerve cuff electrodes used to record activity from cutaneous mechanoreceptors at the radial aspect of the index finger are shown in the inset. Lead wires from the cuff are routed subcutaneously to a site on the volar forearm where they exit via a small connector. The cuff is located on a branch of the palmar digital nerve. Signals recorded from the cuff are processed and fed to the control unit. A radio-frequency link is used to provide power for the implanted circuitry.

The Freehand system utilizes the individually tuned cocontraction map to provide palmar and lateral grasp. The user voluntarily selects between these two grasps, and controls the prehension proportionally [Peckham and Keith, 1992]. The additional feature of the system is the ability to "lock" the stimulation pattern at any of the preprogrammed combinations. Visual feedback and experience gained through the usage help the subject to perform daily activities [Wijman et al., 1990]. The joystick mounted on the contralateral shoulder or some other position at the body controls the preprogrammed sequence of stimulation. The palmar grasp starts from the extended fingers and thumb (one end position of the joystick), followed by the movement of the thumb to opposition and flexing of the fingers (other terminal position of the joystick). The lateral grasp starts from the full extension of the fingers and the thumb, followed by the flexion of the fingers and adduction of the thumb. The system is applicable if the following muscles can be stimulated: Extensor Pollicis Longus m, Flexor Pollicis

Longus m, Adductor Pollicis m, Opponens m, Flexor Digitorum Profundus m. and Superficialis m, and Extensor Digitorum Communis m. An important feature of the grasping system is related to daily fitting of the joystick (zeroing the neutral position), and going to hold mode from the movement mode. The hold mode is the regime where the muscle nerves are stimulated at the level at which the same force is maintained, and the user selects the level.

The initial CWRU system suggested the use of myoelectric signals obtained from a site with some regaining voluntary activity. Scott and colleagues [1996] evaluated the myoelectric control to drive the CWRU system, and these results are integrated in the development of the next generation of the Freehand system. Using muscles that are not affected and easily controllable, a bilateral control of the CWRU system might be possible.

Closed Loop Control for the Freehand Grasping System with Natural Sensors

In able bodied humans tactile mechanoreceptors in the hand relay detailed information about respond to mechanical events on the glabrous skin such as changes in contact force, skin stretch, and slips [Srinivasan *et al.*, 1990]. During precision tasks, an able-bodied person produces grip forces just sufficiently larger than the minimum force required holding an object. If the grip force is insufficient and the object starts to slip, low-threshold mechanoreceptive units exhibit sharp activity bursts

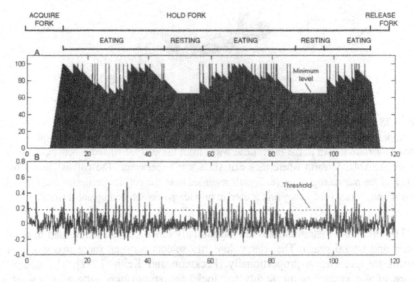

Fig. 4.79: Use of nerve signals from cutaneous mechanoreceptors to control a hand grasp neuroprostheses in an eating task.. A) Command signal. "100" is maximal stimulation of the involved muscles in the lateral grasp. "0" is a minimal preset stimulation level. B) Processed nerve signal originating from the cutaenous mechanoreceptors in the index finger. At the time the processed nerve signal exceeded threshold the command signal was increased to 100 which caused a maximal stimulation intensity at twice the instantaneous stimulation frequency to the involved finger muscles. After this initial reaction the command signal was set to a higher level than before the event, linearly depending on the amplitude of the processed nerve signal. In periods when no neural events exceeded the threshold the command signal was automatically decreased using a slow linear ramp.

[Westling and Johansson, 1984; Vallbo and Johansson, 1984]. A short-latency reflex of cutaneous origin is usually elicited by a slip so that within 80 ms of the start of a slip, the grip force increases and the object is held securely again [Johansson and Westling, 1987]. These rapid corrective responses are automatic, and do not involve conscious participation by the subjects.

In tetraplegics the activity patterns of tactile mechanoreceptors in the hand are usually not affected [Thomas and Westling, 1995], but the person cannot perceive sensation due to the lack of connective networks. In laboratory experiments, it has recently been shown that neural activity from low-threshold mechanoreceptive units in the skin of the index finger can be recorded with long-term implanted nerve cuff electrodes. The nerve signal contains information that allows detection of the occurrence of slips, thereby the signal to stimulate the thumb flexor/adductor muscles and stop the slip is available. The control operates without any prior knowledge about the strength of the muscles and the weight and surface texture of the object [Haugland et al., 1999].

Such signals, when implemented within an artificial reflex, give reliable and useful feedback signals to a hand grasp neuroprostheses. The application of this control is for daily activity tasks (e.g., self-feeding) that a tetraplegic cannot do, if not provided with a neural prostheses. A nerve cuff electrode and the stimulation system (NeuroControl Corp., Cleveland, USA) were implanted in two subjects as shown in Figure 4.78.

A "standardized" eating task, where the tetraplegic subject used a normal fork, was used to evaluate the system. The timing of the task and the number of objects were chosen based on a video analysis of several meals while the subject was eating in a social environment with the system in closed-loop control mode.

Figure 4.79 shows in parallel the recordings from the cuff electrode and automatically adjusted level of stimulation. This level of stimulation corresponds to the position of the proportional controller (joystick) between 0 (open hand) and 100 percent (closed hand). An adequate grasp force was maintained at all time without any need the subject to interact with the system once he intentionally opened the hand and closed it around the fork.

The increase in the command signal depended on the recorded activity from the cutaneous mechanoreceptors. When an event was detected; i.e., the nerve signal exceeds a preset threshold (shown in Figure 4.79B), then a command signal automatically increases in order to maintain a safe grasp. During the resting phases (Figure 4.79A), the controller automatically decreases the command signal to a predefined minimum level, at which the fork was kept in the grasp with a minimally needed muscle stimulation.

With the system in closed-loop mode, the mean lateral pinch force was about 40 percent lower compared with the operation in the open-loop control. Using less force should allow the subject to delay the onset of muscle fatigue.

4.3.4 Neuroprostheses for Restoring Standing and Walking

NP started to be used for walking assistance in Ljubljana, Slovenia [e.g., Vodovnik et al., 1967, 1981; Kralj and Grobelnik, 1973; Kralj and Bajd, 1989; Bajd et al., 1982, 1983, 1985, 1986, 1989; Kralj et al., 1980, 1983, 1987; Gračanin et al., 1967, 1969]. The available surface NP systems use various numbers of stimulation channels.

The simplest NP to assist walking, from a technical point, is a single channel system. This system is only suitable for stroke subjects and a limited group of incomplete spinal cord injured subjects. These individuals can perform limited ambulating with the assistance of the upper extremities without a FES system, although this ambulating may be both modified and/or impaired. The FES in these humans is used to activate a single muscle group. The first demonstrated application of this technique was in stroke subjects [Gračanin et al., 1969], even though the original patent came from Liberson et al. [1961]. The stimulation is applied to ankle dorsiflexors so the "foot-drop" can be eliminated.

The Odstock Foot-drop Stimulator (ODFS, the Department of Medical Physics and Biomedical Engineering, Salisbury District Hospital, Salisbury, Wiltshire, UK), the single channel foot-drop stimulator manufactured by COTAS, Denmark, and MicroFES and FEPA10 peroneal stimulators, Ljubljana, Slovenia, are among the few FES systems in clinical use. At the time of writing in excess of 450 people had used the ODFS, more than 3000 COTAS stimulators are sold, and more than 1000 Ljubljana systems have been distributed over more than 20 years.

The ODFS is a new technology that follows the work of Lieberson et al. [1961]. It is a single channel stimulator providing electrical stimulation to the tibialis anterior muscle or the common peroneal nerve [Granat et al., 1991, 1996; Maležič et al., 1984, 1992; Stein et al., 1993; Sweeney and Lyons, 1999; Wieler et al., 1999]. The stimulation, timed to the gait cycle by using a switch placed in the shoe, causes ankle dorsiflexion with some eversion and/or could elicit a flexor withdrawal reflex [Burridge et al., 1997a and b]. The reflex comprises ankle dorsiflexion, hip and knee flexion, with external rotation of the hip. The components of the movement may be varied by adjusting the electrode position and stimulation amplitude. The ODFS stimulator gives an asymmetrical biphasic output of maximum amplitude 80 mA, with a 300µs duration of the pulse and the interpulse interval of 40 ms. Stimulation is applied by means of skin-surface electrodes placed, typically, over the common peroneal nerve as it passes over the head of the fibula bone and over the motor point of tibialis anterior. The output of the stimulator is normally triggered after heel rises from the ground on the affected side and continues until heel strike occurs. Stimulation can also be triggered by heel strike from the contralateral leg, which is a useful function if heel contact is unreliable on the affected side. It may also be possible to stimulate for a fixed time, again useful if heel contact was inconsistent. The rise and fall of the stimulation envelope can be adjusted, an essential feature as a sudden contraction of the tibialis anterior could cause a stretch reflex in the calf muscles. Additionally, adding an extended ramp at the end of the stimulation can prevent "foot flap" due to the premature ending of dorsiflexion.

A randomized, controlled trial has been performed in subjects with hemiparesis of different origin (e.g., stroke, spinal cord injury, ad multiple sclerosis) when using ODFS. After reaching neurological stability, the subjects were divided into two groups: subjects who used the device and received 10 sessions of physiotherapy, and a control group who only received the 10 sessions of physiotherapy [Taylor, 1997].

The key for the success of a rehabilitation device is the adequate application, i.e., the selection of subjects who could benefit from the NP. The subjects have been judged suitable for treatment if their dropped foot was due to an upper motor neuron lesion and was corrected by electrical stimulation. The subjects for the ODFS study could move from sitting to standing unaided and could walk at least 10 meters with appropriate aids. The subjects understood the basics of the operation of the ODFS. Tolerance of the sensation of the stimulation was required. Stroke subjects showed a mean increase in walking speed of 27 percent and reduction in Physiological Cost Index (PCI) of 31 percent with stimulation and changes of 14 percent and 19 percent respectively whilst not using the stimulator. The measured differences in walking with and without stimulation were statistically significant in the stroke subjects.

The age (mean ± standard deviation) of the subjects was 55.4±18.2 years, and the time since stroke was 5.4±10.7 years. Among 111 subjects 58 had a left, and 53 had a right hemiplegia. The study also included eight subjects with incomplete SCI (42.1±13.2 years). The effect of the foot-drop stimulation for this group of subjects was an increase in walking speed of 19 percent (6 m/min) and a drop in PCI of 20 percent (0.22 beat/m).

Some users of the ODFS showed a reduction in quadriceps spasticity, measured by the Wartenberg Pendulum Drop Test [Burridge et al., 1997a and b]. The treatment group also showed a reduction in depression score on the Hospital Anxiety and Depression scale suggesting an improvement in quality of life.

Two stimulation channels; restricting the muscle groups to the anterior tibialis and either the hamstrings or posterior tibial, (calf) muscle groups have been used to correct the foot-drop problem [Taylor, 1997]. The stimulation is initiated and terminated using footswitches. A novel programming design allows fine control of timing and parameters of each stimulation channel, yet simple to use by a trained physiotherapist. This follows the application of the Compustim-10B, two channel, microcontroller based, neuromuscular stimulator. It was found that stimulating the hamstring and calf muscles (in addition to the anterior tibialis muscle) is most effective.

The study was designed to use the subjects as their own controls. Three phases, each lasting for twelve weeks comprised: the use of only one channel of the Compustim-10B applied via the common peroneal nerve (weeks 0-12 and 24-36), and phase "B" (weeks 12-24), with two channels active. During weeks 8 to 12 the second muscle group and optimum control algorithm were selected based on clinical observation during experiments performed in the laboratory. During this period subjects continued to use the Compustim-10B in a single channel mode at home. Between weeks 12 and 24 subjects used two-channel stimulation at home, and progress was reviewed at four-weekly intervals.

At each session, data was collected with no stimulation, one channel, and when applicable, with two channels. A clinical improvement in gait was observed in all 12 subjects. In 11 subjects, it was considered by the clinician that the identified gait abnormality had been improved by application of a second channel of stimulation. Six subjects used hamstring stimulation, but only one subject showed the anticipated improvement. In five subjects, no change has been noticed. There was no significant change in walking speed or PCI, during the 8 weeks prior to using the Compustim-10B. Stimulating the second muscle group with the Compustim-10B was shown to have a significant therapeutic and orthotic effect on walking speed. The comparison between walking speed with two-channel stimulation at week 24 and with walking with no stimulation, before the second channel was introduced, showed a mean increase of over 20 percent. There were, however, no significant changes in the PCI over time and the different systems.

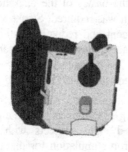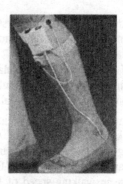

Fig 4.80: Sketch of the Walk-Aid (left), a single-channel, self-contained stimulator to correct foot-drop problem (Adapted from Da Silva *et al.,*1997). The mounting shell is easy to model to the leg shape and it comprises sensors, electrodes, stimulator and the battery. The KDC 2000A, Cotas, DK (right) peroneal stimulator to correct foot-drop problems.

Stein and colleagues [Dai *et al*, 1996] have designed an appealing self-contained system. The system integrates a single channel stimulator and a tilt sensor; thus, eliminates a foot switch, which was not fully reliable, because it easily generated false triggering and malfunctioning (Figure 4.80). The stimulator has been commercialized, yet the distribution failed to make it a market success.

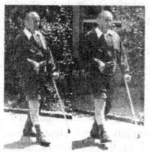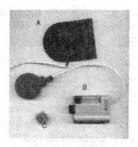

Fig. 4.81: Hemiplegic subject walking with the stimulator turned off (left) and on (middle). The stimulator (right) is fully implantable (Ljubljana, Slovenia) and comprises: a heel switch (A), an external stimulator with a single AA battery, an emitting RF-antenna (B); and the implant receiver-electrodes (C) that is attached to the common peroneal nerve.

The systems used most frequently in clinical practice follow the principles that are initially integrated in the peroneal stimulator Fepa 10, Soča, Ljubljana, Slovenia. The fully implantable stimulator IPPO (Figure 4.81) has been tested in more than 20 subjects after they had already used the surface stimulation system. The walking pattern did not change with the implanted stimulator compared with the surface electrode based device, however, the ease of application, reproducibility, and cosmesis improved greatly. The implantation is relatively simple, and it is performed in daily surgery.

Medtronic Corp., Minneapolis, MI, developed an implantable version of the stimulator with nerve electrodes to deal with foot-drop almost 30 years ago. Waters with colleagues implanted a series of these devices and reported effective and safe operation of the nerve electrodes (no failures), yet Medtronic Co. decided to stop this line of research [McNeal and Bowman, 1985; Watters *et al.*, 1985b]. Rozman and colleagues [Kelih *et al.*, 1988; Rozman *et al.*, 1994] developed a two-channel implantable stimulator for correcting foot-drop. A single channel stimulator receives power via a radio frequency (RF) link. The stimulator that incorporates electrodes is attached close to the common peroneal nerve just below the knee joint. The external unit is controlled with a switch mounted in the insole worn in the shoe of the plegic leg. Both the wired connection and a RF link with the switch in the shoe have been tested. The dual channel stimulator is used to correct eversion/inversion of the foot in addition to the dorsiflexion.

The rationale for implanting a cuff electrode on a cutaneous nerve innervating the foot is to remove the external heel switch used in existing systems for foot-drop correction.

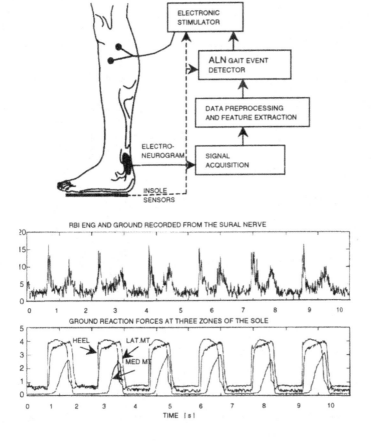

Fig. 4.82: Closed-loop control scheme applying sensory nerve signals from the sural nerve to detect foot contact and clearance (top); example of sural nerve activity (middle) and three foot sensors (bottom) during walking. Arbitrary units. The three external foot sensors are placed at medial (MED MT), lateral (LAT MT) metatarsal, and heel zones. An implantable telemeter recorded the nerve signal. Adapted from Kostov *et al.*, 1999, with permission.

Thereby, it is possible to use such systems without footwear and to prepare them to be totally implantable systems. After processing the nerve signal heel contacts can be detected using the afferent nerve signal information alone [Hansen et al., 1998; Kostov et al., 1999] for deciding when the muscle that prevents foot-drop must be stimulated during gait. Figure 4.82 shows an example where the nerve cuff electrode is placed around the sural nerve just proximal to the ankle joint. The signal is passed to an amplifier, and through an Adaptive Logical Network (ALN), and a trigger signal is extracted that decides when to stimulate the peroneal nerve during the swing phase of walking [Kostov et al., 1999]. The use of ALN for mapping sensory signals and motor action is described in Chapter 5. During a step, the nerve signal is modulated with a distinct peak at heel-contact. In the swing, when the foot was in the air, the neural activity decreased to the background noise level. Exactly when the foot touched the ground, the nerve responded with a sharp peak of activity as the skin innervated by the sural nerve was stretched. This peak was followed by a second burst in the late stance phase of the step that coincided with an increase on the forefoot at push off. Applied in combination with the implantable telemeter for nerve recordings [Zhou et al., 1998] and implantable nerve stimulators (e.g. [Kljajić et al., 1993]), a full implantable NP to prevent foot-drop might be clinically acceptable in the future.

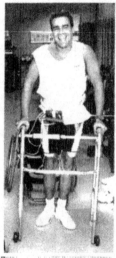
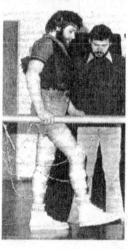

Fig. 4.83: A paraplegic subject participating in the Miami Project to Cure Paralysis study of walking with the Parastep I system, (Sigmedics, Chicago, IL).

Fig. 4.84: The use of a six-channel stimulator to restore standing and walking with support over a parallel bars, walker, and crutches [Kralj and Bajd, 1989]. Switches are used to trigger the swing phase of the walking.

A multichannel system with a minimum of four channels of FES is required for ambulating of a subject with a complete motor lesion of lower extremities and preserved balance and upper body motor control [Kralj and Bajd, 1989]. Appropriate bilateral stimulation of the quadriceps muscles locks the knees during standing [Bajd et al., 1982; Jaeger et al., 1989]. Stimulating the common peroneal nerve on the ipsilateral side, while switching-off the quadriceps stimulation on that side, produces a flexion of leg. This flexion combined with adequate movement of the upper body and use of the upper extremities for support allows ground clearance and is considered as the swing phase of the gait cycle. Hand or foot switches can provide the flexion-extension alternation needed for a slow forward or backward progression (Figure

4.83). Sufficient arm strength must be available to provide balance in parallel bars (clinical application), and with a rolling walker or crutches (daily use of FES). These systems evolved into a commercial product called Parastep-1R (Sigmedics, Chicago, IL), which has been approved for home usage in 1994 by the Food and Drugs Administration [Graupe and Kohn, 1997; Guest *et al.*, 1997; Jacobs *et al.*, 1997; Needham-Shorpshire *et al.*, 1997; Nash *et al.*, 1997; Klose *et al.*, 1997].

A dual-channel stimulator (The "Jožef Štefan" Institute, Ljubljana, Slovenia) was developed almost 20 years ago for standing and walking; one stimulator is required per leg (Figure 4.84). A stimulator comprises three leads for two channels (monopolar stimulation). Stimulating the quadriceps muscle the extension of the knee and plantar extension are generated; stimulating the peroneal nerve results in a flexion (withdrawal) reflex. A stimulator has a push-button, hand-control that switches between the extension (stance phase) and flexion (swing phase) at timings volitionally determined by the user. The system has a safety feature preventing the user to accidentally press flexion function simultaneously in both legs. The switches are mounted in the handles of a walker or crutches and both a wireless and the flexible lead connection of switches to the stimulator are available. The use of this assistance for standing and walking has been tested in Ljubljana, Slovenia, in more than 100 subjects over a long time [Kralj and Bajd, 1989], and based on the results many other rehabilitation research clinics around the world accepted the treatment and built their own similar stimulators.

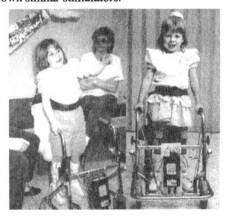

Fig. 4.85: A young girl after a motor vehicle caused paraplegia uses the Quadstim stimulator (Biomech Design, Edmonton, Alberta, Canada) in combination with an ankle-foot orthosis for standing and limited walking.

The research that relies on the four-channel stimulation system includes testing of automatic control of walking, use of different sensors, augmented feedback to provide information on the phase of locomotion, but these components have been used only in the laboratory settings, and in principle they do not differ from the point of view of the user.

Biomech Design Ltd. from Edmonton, Canada, manufactures the Quadstim, a four-channel stimulator, which has been used in several rehabilitation centers in Canada for restoring and studying the assisted standing and walking [James *et al.*, 1990].

The user controls the intensity by sliding potentiometers; the frequency and pulse duration of the current regulated pulses are adjusted by the therapist or engineer before the device is given to the user. The system comprises three push-button switches for selecting which channels are active (Figure 4.85), and allows a standby mode. The stimulator incorporates an interface for the communication with a microcontroller; thus, different control schemes can be implemented if necessary.

Multichannel percutaneous systems for gait restoration with many channels were suggested [Marsolais and Kobetič, 1983, 1987; Kobetič and Marsolais, 1994; Kobetič

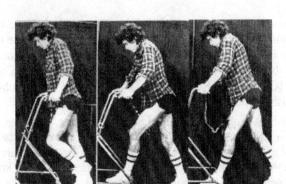

Fig. 4.86: Paraplegic subject walking with a 16-channel stimulator applied via percutaneous intramuscular electrodes [Marsolais and Kobetič, 1987].

et al., 1997]. The main advantage of these systems is the plausibility to activate many different muscle groups. A preprogrammed stimulation sequence is used for timing and intensity variation of up to 16 channels. The sequence is cloned from the EMG pattern recorded in able-bodies subjects. A 16-channel stimulator has been applied over as much as 64 percutaneous electrodes. Some electrodes are stimulating at very low intensity muscles that are still voluntarily controlled in the abdominal region to provide proprioceptive feedback to the user about the operation of the system. The experience of the Cleveland research team suggested that 48 channels are required for a human with a complete spinal cord injury at mid thoracic level to achieve a reasonable walking pattern. Initially, the method used excluded external bracing, and claimed that FES *per se* will be adequate, but this method has been changed towards combining the stimulation with some orthotics. Fine-wire intramuscular electrodes were positioned by using subdermal needles, and tunneled towards a point where an external connector from several electrodes is attached (externally). These intramuscular electrodes serve as the cathodes, positioned close to the motor point of selected muscles. Knee extensors (Rectus Femoris m, Vastus Medialis m, Vastus Lateralis m, and Vastus Intermedius m.), hip flexors (Sartorius m, Tensor Fasciae Latae m, Gracilis m, Iliopsoas m.), hip extensors (Semimembranosus m, Gluteus Maximus m.), hip abductors (Gluteus Medius m.), ankle dorsiflexors (Tibialis Anterior m, Peroneus Longus m.), ankle plantar flexors (Gastrocnemius Lateralis m, Gastrocnemius Medialis m, Plantaris M, and Soleus m.), and paraspinal muscles are selected for activation. A surface electrode has been used as a common anode. Interleaved pulses are delivered with a multichannel, battery-operated, portable stimulator. The hand controller allows the selection of the walking modality. The ethics committee of the CWRU and Veterans Administration Hospital in Cleveland, Ohio, approved these systems for clinical studies, and the protocol included the removal of the complete hardware after the study. The application was investigated in complete spinal cord lesions and in stroke subjects [Marsolais *et al.*, 1990]. The same strategy and selection criteria for implantation were used for both stroke and SCI subjects. This system allowed selected humans to walk up to 1.1 meter per second, and walk distances of almost one thousand meters (Figure 4.86). The preprogrammed stimulation sequence included the following walking modes: standing up, sitting down, quite standing, walking, walking stairs or curb, walking backwards.

Recent projects somewhat changed the initial emphasis of research with implanted systems at the CWRU/VA Center, Cleveland, OH, USA, [Kobetič *et al.*, 1999; Sharma *et al.*, 1998]. Providing a device to exercise, stand, and maneuver in the vicinity of the wheelchair to individuals with spinal cord injures (SCI) through the application of FES is now the primary goal; a system named Freestand (Figure 4.87), which follows the design of the Freehand, is approved for clinical studies (Figure 4.87). A comprehensive approach to the prescription and installation of surgically implanted FES systems for individuals with varying levels of preserved volitional movement is to be employed. A single 8-channel CWRU/VA implanted receiver-stimulator (IRS-8) will be used for exercise and standing in individuals with complete motor deficits, and to facilitate walking in selected individuals with partial paralysis. The protocols for applying and evaluating the FES standing system are developed for the distribution of the system to other sites to allow a multi-center clinical trial. A 16-channel stimulation system is under development, and it will be offered to qualified users of the standing system with complete injuries who are interested in a short distance stepping with FES. The target group is limited to T4 to T11 spinal cord injured persons. The plan is also to combine both 8- to 16-channel implanted muscle stimulator with a trunk-hip-knee-ankle-foot orthosis with programmable joint locks. The purpose is to provide more immediate mobility to paraplegic individuals and to study functional mobility requirements using the implantable devices currently available.

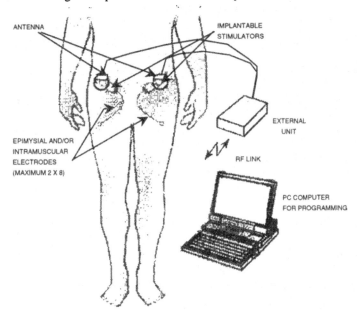

Fig. 4.87: The sketch of the fully implantable FreeStand system that uses intramuscular and/or epimysial electrodes. Adapted from Kobetič *et al.*, 1999, © IEEE.

A different approach to use multichannel totally implanted FES system [Thoma *et al.*, 1978, 1987] was proposed and tested in a few subjects. This system used a 16-channel implantable stimulator. The electrodes have been attached to the epineurium of the selected nerves. Femoral and gluteal nerves were stimulated for hip and knee extension. The so-called "round-about" stimulation was applied in which four electrodes were located around the nerve and stimulated intermittently. This stimulation method was selected to provide physiological-like firing rate to reduce muscle fatigue. The method is finding its extension with the new electrode design that allows selective stimulation of specific fascicles within a nerve.

In 1991 the first 22 channel FES system based on the Nucleus FES22, Cochlear Ltd., Australia, was implanted in a T10-paraplegic male. After a considerable time of training and fitting the program it was possible to achieve sensory feedback driven standing for about one hour [Davis et al., 1997]. The sensory signals were acquired from the electro-goniometers at the knee joints. Stance stability was assisted with the Andrews' Anterior Floor Reaction Orthosis. The closed-loop control minimizes the time of stimulation; only about 10 percent of the total standing time the muscles are externally activated.

In 1998, a second T10-paraplegic male was implanted with an updated 22-channel stimulator with telemetry (FES24-A, Neopraxis Pty Ltd, Lane Cove, N.S.W., Australia). 18 channels are connected to epineural electrodes on nerves for muscle activation and limb movements thereby allowing exercise and open-loop standing for 30 minutes. Over seven months, the thresholds for stimulation changed in only five of the total of 13 nerves for less than 10 percent.

Praxis FES24-A is a multi-functional stimulator. 10 electrodes are thin flexible platinum cuffs (Flexi-Cuff), sized at least twice the diameter of encircled nerve. Eight other electrodes are button-shaped, made of platinum, and placed on the epineurium. Each button has an attached Dacron mesh that is used to suture the electrode to the adjacent connective tissue. The stimulation originates from an external, battery operated, belt worn controller, called Navigator, which uses the Motorola 68332 micro-controller. The stimulation is delivered via an external RF linked antenna that is magnetically held to the skin by an underlying magnet in the implant. The stimulation parameters are 6.0-8.0 mA, 25-500 µs pulse width, and frequency of up to 60 Hz per electrode. The user can select different strategies via a menu driven protocol based on a simple LCD and keypad interface. A remote RF-linked button is being developed for finger control to compliment the keypad. The sensory system comprises two accelerometers and a rate gyroscope. The safety is achieved by using a trunk vest with shoulder straps connected to an overhead standing frame (Maine AntiGravity Systems, Portland, ME). The suspension system provides sufficient slack for a 40 degrees knee buckle with full weight support.

Two subjects who received multi-channel nerve stimulation systems can do some one-handed tasks including reaching for and holding a 2.2 kg object at arm's length. These tasks were achieved while in the "C"' posture with no activation to the lower extremity muscles and balance maintained by the other upper extremity.

This study indicates the plausibility that the implanted FES system operates safely and reliably for long period; the first implant works for more than 7.5 year.

4.3.5 Orthoses - External Skeleton Neuroprostheses

The rehabilitation devices that replace or assist diminished or lost bodily functions are termed the orthoses, also called braces or splints. The term orthosis comes from the Greek word *Orthos*, meaning straight or correct. The original meaning of the term relates to an appliance used to straighten, correct, protect, support, or prevent musculo-skeletal deformities. An orthosis is a functional substitute (augmentation) of the function, in contrast to prosthesis that is both a morphological and functional replacement of the body part and its function. This section deals with orthoses used for control of posture and movement of extremities.

Orthoses are made from many materials, in almost infinite number of designs and constructions. Orthoses are sometimes used as short term assistance (e.g., bone healing, stress relief), yet in other cases they are used for long-term, sometimes life-long application. Orthoses can be rather simple (e.g., fixation of a joint or several joints at a desired position), or highly complex (e.g., powered external skeleton for reaching/grasping and/or standing/walking). Some orthoses limit the range of movement, some provide physiological-like movement, and the most advanced ones are in fact the articulated robots able to drive the arm or the leg. Articulated robots for rehabilitation must have anatomical human-like segments because they have multiple contacts with the body in most applications.

The main difficulties when applying orthoses are: 1) the interface; 2) the weight; 3) the size of the device; and 4) the control that must be integrated into the preserved natural mechanisms of the non-paralyzed parts of the body.

An orthosis has to tightly fit to the form of the body. The interface must be soft in order to minimize potential high pressures that could cause an injury. The orthosis has to be secured in place close to the body; thus, the straps made out of soft material are usually a part of an orthosis.

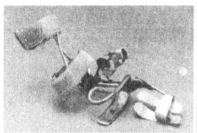 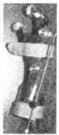 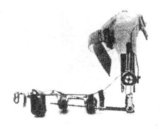

Fig. 4.88: The tenodesis orthosis (left and middle panels), the elbow/wrist body powered orthosis (right). The mechanical linkages flexes and extends the distal joints based on the active movement of the proximal joints (e.g., when the wrist is flexed, the hand opens, and

The joints of an orthosis should duplicate the movement of human joints. Biological joints are polycentric structures; hence, the external joints moving in parallel should replicate the natural counterpart. Tendons and ligaments, in addition to the joint capsule impose many constraints that are difficult to match by mechanisms. It is possible do design a perfect "copy" of the structure found in nature, as it is the case with artificial joints (e.g., the endoskeletal hip and knee joint prostheses), however, this does not apply for an orthosis. The orthotic and the correspondent body joint must rotate in parallel (around the same axis); hence, it is a condition *sine qua non* to provide polycentric features.

The orthosis must be robust, yet light and cosmetically attractive, because it is an essential part of the daily life. New polymer and composite materials that include graphite and Cevlar resolve the requirements to some extent. The orthotic joints are still made almost exclusively out of metal (e.g., stainless steel, titanium, and some other light alloys).

Non-powered, yet active orthoses can be used to control some degrees of freedom (e.g., the knee cage provides stability in the lateral direction and allows flexion and extension). Active orthoses can use body power of joints that are non-paralyzed to drive the paralyzed one (e.g., tenodesis brace, Figure 4.88). Bodily powered orthoses use the principles and methods described in Section 4.4.1 on bodily powered prosthetics. Externally powered orthoses use actuators to generate joint movement.

Arm and Hand Orthoses

Arm and hand orthoses are designed to provide the posture and control of movement in the shoulder, elbow, and wrist joint, and in addition for controlling the opening and closing of the hand. The mechanics of the arm is described in Chapter 2.

To allow a person with impairment preventing him/her to move objects against gravity (shoulder and elbow movement), an orthotic device for mechanical guidance of the arm counteracting effect of gravity has been designed. The complexity of the developed prototypes has ranged from simple, passive, counterweighted devices that support the arm against gravity [James and Orr, 1984] to complex, powered exoskeletons with many degrees of freedom [e.g., Vukobratović and Stokić, 1981]. Powered orthosis prototypes suffer from difficulties relating to cost, power consumption, weight, user acceptance, and the control interface.

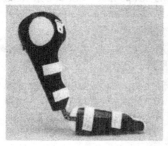
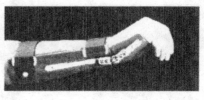

Fig. 4.89: Orthosis to provide control and support to arm joints. Many similar designs, most from prefabricated modules and thermoplastic material (formed to fit the body shape) with Velcro bands are used mostly as temporarily relief from stress and prevention of injury.

Two examples of commercially available orthosis with articulated, however, non-powered joints are shown in Figure 4.89. The two representative elbow and wrist orthoses, which can be locked in a position or where the joint angle can be limited to a certain range, follow the principle of modularity. Prefabricated elements are made in different sizes, and the custom made interface from thermoplastic or composite materials to fit the user. Both orthoses have a spring stainless steel lateral and medial joint constructions, which are attached to acrylic and silastic lamination.

The wrist fixation orthosis is frequently applied in tetraplegic subjects and combined with FES based neuroprosthesis [Peckham and Keith, 1992; Keith *et al.*, 1988].

Lower-Limb Orthoses

Varieties of mechanical orthoses have been used in the past, and they continue to be used. They vary from a Swivel Walker, which is almost like a standing frame with a limited facility to move from place to place, to Ankle-Foot Orthosis (AFO).

Ankle-Foot-Orthosis (AFO)

Only one orthotic system of this variety has been described for ambulatory use in paraplegics [Lyles and Munday, 1992]. The Vannini-Rizzoli Stabilizing Limb Orthosis (V-RLSO) comprises a pair of polypropylene orthoses shaped to fit the lower legs. An orthosis on each side partially encloses the lower leg from about 2 cm below the lower pole of patella to tips of the toes. A pair of specially designed leather boots fit over the orthoses.

The V-RLSO has a flat rigid sole externally, and the inside of the orthosis is 10 to 15 degrees plantar flexed in order to shift the ground reaction in front of the ankle and knee during standing. When using this system, the subject controls static equilibrium by maintaining hips and knees in extended position and head held high. During ambulating, the subject can shift the center of mass forward and then with the help of walking aids is able to move the unweighted foot forward in a pendulum fashion by shifting the upper torso slightly towards the side and forward.

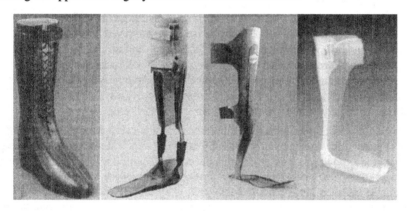

Fig. 4.90: Four types of Ankle Foot Orthosis (AFO). V-RLSO (left), two types of composite material based orthoses (middle two panels), and an AAFO with a spring mechanism for the ankle joint (left).

Most AFO systems are made out of light composite materials (Figure 4.90). Plastic AFO can support the shank allowing limited dorsiflexion, yet it can be made very stiff in order to immobilize the joint. Andrews et al. [1987, 1989] introduced an orthosis proven effective for standing, and it is named floor-reaction orthosis (FRO). The FRO forces the shank into a five degrees of flexion, bringing the hips forward; thus, the center of gravity is in front of the center of pressure. This leads to a so-called "C" posture, which is intrinsically stable and does not need the knee extensors for standing. The C posture may lead to a knee joint injury; the knee cage could protect the knee.

Knee-Ankle-Foot-Orthosis (KAFO)

Knee-Ankle-Foot-Orthoses, as the name suggests, provides stabilization of the knee along with stabilization of the ankle and foot. This is achieved by application of three forces. The first is applied in front of the knee preventing it from buckling under the body weight, and the other two forces are applied in an opposite direction to that of the first, *i.e.,* posteriorly, one at the upper posterior thigh and the other at shoe level.

In the past, KAFOs were extensions of below knee double iron orthoses. Traditionally they were attached at the lower end to a firm lace up shoe through a stirrup or a round caliper. The ankle joint provided medio-lateral stability; it was similar to traditional AFO, in that, it had a posterior stop to prevent plantar flexion but allowed dorsiflexion. A knee joint, with or without lock, was added at the level of the knee. Most KAFOs used for paraplegic locomotion have knees with locks so that they are locked during standing or walking, but could be unlocked during sitting. The simplest lock is a drop lock, which is unlocked after sitting down. A bale or Swiss lock provides easier locking and unlocking mechanism. The most essential bands on a KAFO are posterior calf and upper thigh bands. A large variety of other combinations of thigh and calf bands has been described. However, Lehmann and associates [1969, 1976] showed that most of these additional bands are often unnecessary. Some KAFOs are fitted with pelvic bands in order to help stabilize the pelvic girdle. Theoretically these orthoses are Hip-Knee-Ankle-Foot variety (HKAFO) and should not be classed as KAFOs (Figure 4.91).

Scott [1971] described several modifications of traditional KAFOs, making them lighter in weight and giving more stable base with improved balance to the user. Supporting bands were discarded except a thigh band and an anterior rigid patellar tendon strap. The knee was offset eccentrically, and the ball locks have been retained. The shoe plate was extended beyond the metatarsal heads to provide better support. A solid ankle was set at 5 to 10 degrees of dorsiflexion. This KAFO is one of the commonly prescribed orthosis for paraplegics.

Ambulating with knees locked in full extension in a swing-through or a swing-to fashion requires lifting the center of mass up at every step. This increases the energy cost of walking, however, it is an acceptable trade-off with the increased amount of safety due to locked and stable knees. Locked knees allow the subject to lean backwards to stabilize hips. Leaning backwards, with locked knees, places the center of mass of the trunk behind the hip joint resulting in tightening of the anterior hip capsule providing internal stabilization of the hip.

Swivel Walker was established as a means of ambulating for severely disabled children by Motlock and Elliott [1966] in early sixties. Rose and Henshaw [1973] have described an updated and somewhat improved version. The Swivel Walker allows humans with spinal cord injury at thoracic and cervical levels up to C6 to maintain the upright posture without the use of any other walking aid. The device consists of a rigid body structure that provides stability to hips, knees, and ankles via a frame with three points of fixation. The extrinsic stability is provided by a pair of swiveling footplates mounted beneath the body frame. These feet plates provide mobility. The center of mass of the system projects slightly forwards of the foot-plate bearing center; hence, when inclined to one side it causes progression of the center of mass due to the gravity and ground reaction force. Walking is achieved by alternately sideways rocking of the trunk so that one footplate is lifted off the ground, the frame then automatically swivels forward on the contralateral footplate. This process is repeated cyclically with the opposite leg. The orthosis is available in standard sizes and designed in modules that can be interchanged.

The Swivel Walker provides some independence in getting around, the walking is extremely slow, and the energy consumption very high. Humans can walk only on an even level surface. Transferring to upright posture needs to be carried by helpers.

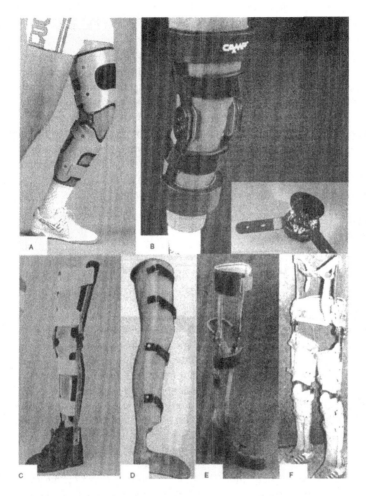

Fig. 4.91: Different types of the knee-ankle orthoses (A and B), Knee-Ankle Foot Orthoses (KAFO) (C, D, and E), and Hip-KAFO (HKAFO) orthoses (F).

Following a thorough analysis of requirements of reciprocal walking for humans with paralyzed legs, Rose [1979] evaluated a system comprising specially designed hip guidance articulations. The orthosis was initially called the *Hip Guidance Orthosis*, yet it is now known as the *ParaWalker*. The orthosis has a rigid body brace that is attached to two KAFOs via the specially designed hip joints (Figure 4.92, left). The KAFOs are in minimal abduction at the hips in relation to the trunk. The orthosis has three support points. A support point on the chest is provided by a leather chest strap. A support point on the buttocks is provided by a polypropylene band attached on either side directly to the joint housing. It has low friction hip joints with flexion/extension stops. A release mechanism for the stops is provided to allow the user to sit down. The KAFOs stabilize the knees and ankles. The knee of either side is held in extension by an anterior strap at the level of upper end of the Tibia reacted by the posterior thigh band and a vertical extension on the rear of the shoe plate. These two together provide the third support point for the main orthosis. The orthotic knee joints are normally locked during walking, but have release mechanisms to enable user to sit down. A shoe plate incorporating a rocker sole is fixed to the either KAFO with an appropriate amount of dorsiflexion.

The system allows reciprocal walking for subjects with thoracic level lesion using crutches. The rigid body brace of the ParaWalker can resist the adducting moments about the stance hip in the coronal plane. A push on the crutch to tilt towards the stance side allows the subject to clear the swing leg. As soon as the swing leg is clear off the ground, the gravity causes it to move forward through pendulum action causing flexion at the hip. This is possible because the center of mass of the leg lies behind the hip joint axis when it is in extension. The flexion is limited by stops on the hip joints. When the swinging leg contacts the ground, it is in flexion. Force is required to raise the trunk upwards and pull it forwards during stance. The force has to be generated by the user, through the same crutch, which tilts him sideways.

Reciprocating Gait Orthosis (RGO). The principle of linking hips together to allow reciprocal movement of both hips in HKAFO was first developed in the late 1960s. At the Ontario Crippled Children's Center in Toronto, Canada, Motlock and his colleagues described a mechanism based on the use of gears [Motlock, 1992]. In England, David Scrutton [1971] described the use of a pair of Bowden cables to control the motion of orthotic hip joints in a reciprocating brace with poly-planar hip hinges used for spina bifida children.

The reciprocating gait orthosis, which is a refinement of the original design described by Scrutton, was jointly developed by the Louisiana State University Medical Center and Durr-Fillauer Medical Inc. [Douglas *et al.*, 1983]. The orthosis includes trunk support, a pelvic assembly and bilateral KAFOs. The thoracic support consists of extensions of upper side members of hips up-to or just above the level of the xiphoid process of sternum with 5 centimeter wide adjustable anterior and posterior encircling straps (Figure 4.92, right). The extension prevents uncontrolled collapse of the trunk and yet allows the user to move upper extremities freely. The rigid pelvic assembly consists of a pelvic band covering the gluteal and sacral areas with special thrust bearing hip joints coupled together with a cable and conduit. The KAFOs have posterior offset of the knee joints with drop locks on the lateral sides. The AFOs and thigh sections are made of Polypropylene. The AFOs are each reinforced in the ankle area with an insert made of a composite material to assure resistance against dorsiflexion. The most important feature of the system is the cable coupling of the left and right leg movement. The coupling provides hip joint stability during standing by preventing simultaneous flexion of both hips; yet, it allows flexion of one hip and simultaneous extension of the other when a step is taken. The cables can be disengaged to sit down.

Solomonow and his associates [1989, 1997a and b] described several limitations of the original orthotic system which were encountered during its usage and suggested modifications to the system. In their experience most subjects were able to doff and don the orthosis independently, but were unable to stand up without assistance. Many paraplegics have some degree of Hamstrings contracture and hence their knees cannot reach full extension. Since the automatic knee locks operated only in full extension, these subjects were unable to remain upright. Another major concern was the inability to negotiate ramps or driveways with mild to moderate inclinations.

A ratchet knee joint was incorporated into the design. This knee joint extends freely, but locks in any position short of full extension. This prevents the knee from flexing during the process of standing up even if it is not fully extended and supports the subject's weight. Force applied to the knee at heel strike of the first step brings it into full extension. The ratchet knee joint has a ball type lock which can be operated to allow free flexion to enable the subject to sit down.

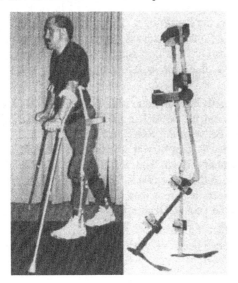
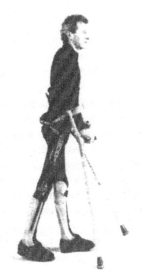

Fig. 4.92: Hip-Guidance Orthosis (HGO) – left, and Reciprocating Gait Orthosis with the Bowden cable connecting the hip joints (middle and right).

A different hip joint within RGO has two locking positions. One is the standard position at full hip extension to attain normal upright posture. The other position allows 20 degrees of flexion from the previous position. This allows the subject to move the center of mass of upper trunk forward so that while walking on the ramp it would remain in front of the support area preventing loss of balance posteriorly.

Whittle [1989] studied orthotic gait of subjects using the RGO and the ParaWalker as a part of comparative biomechanical assessment of these two orthoses. He found similar walking velocities for both orthoses. The total excursion of the leg in the sagittal plane (flexion/extension) was significantly greater with the RGO. However, the stride length was similar for both orthoses, because in the ParaWalker gait, the smaller leg excursion was compensated with greater pelvic rotation in the transverse plane. In addition, during the ParaWalker gait there was significantly greater abduction of hip on the swing side and smaller adduction of hip on the stance side, making it easier to use with the crutches. The subjects were unable to use crutches with the RGO. The force through the legs was a little higher with the ParaWalker. The force through the arms was probably higher with the RGO.

Advanced Reciprocating Gait Orthosis (ARGO). Although the crossed Bowden cables are a simple and effective way to produce reciprocal hip joint movement, they may not be the most efficient mechanical coupling. Since the cables are secured only at each end, some of the energy associated with the active hip extension is wasted in the unwanted cable friction. In addition, since a cable needs to be in tension to transmit large forces effectively, only half of the system is being used at a time. A modified version of RGO is called Advanced Reciprocating Gait Orthosis (ARGO). The hip joints are modified and are interconnected using a single Bowden cable encased in a tube in an attempt to reduce friction. Its major advantage over the RGO is that it allows the user to rise from sitting position and to sit down from standing position with relative ease. The user can stand up directly from normal sitting position with flexed knees without having to extend them manually before commencing to stand up as is necessary with the RGO as well as with the ParaWalker. This is achieved by mounting a compressed gas strut on the thigh side link on each side providing a knee extension moment to augment standing and control hip flexion during sitting down. The hip and knee joints on each side are connected via a knee lock actuating cable so that the hip mechanism releases the knee lock.

During the development of the ARGO, Jefferson and Whittle [1990] tested a subject using the ParaWalker, RGO, and the ARGO in parallel. They found similar motion in pattern and in magnitude between the RGO and ARGO. In the ARGO, however, the pelvis appeared to be shortly stationary at a particular instant during the gait cycle enhancing its jerky movement pattern. The walking with the ParaWalker showed marked differences from that of the other two. It showed greater smoothness before and after movements. The subject's legs remained more or less parallel to each other in the coronal plane allowing better ground clearance.

Motlock [1992] suggested another modification to the RGO known as the Isocentric RGO; the Bowden cables have been replaced with a centrally pivoting bar and tie rod arrangement.

Powered Orthoses

Attempts to design externally powered skeleton to be used to "carry" the subject and move his/her legs following the nature-like pattern characterize the early seventies,

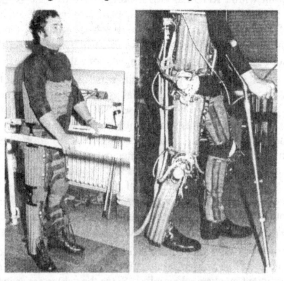

Fig. 4.93: The modular non-actuated (left) and powered (right) exoskeleton (AMOLL) used for training and exercise of the walking. Courtesy of Dr. Pierre Rabishong, France.

when bipedal robots became popular [e.g., Hristić et al., 1974, 1981; Vukobratović, 1974, 1975]. This development resulted with heavy, rigid, cosmetically unacceptable, and inappropriate assistive systems for paraplegics. The so-called *soft orthosis* has been introduced by the company Aerozur, Paris; long tubes that could be filled with compressed air created "high" trousers reaching mid-thoracic level. Once the tubes were blown up, the subject had erect posture. The pressure applied to skin, inability for skin to breath through the costume, need to depressurize the system every time a subject wanted to sit, and essential use of the compressor every time he/she wanted to stand up made the system obsolete.

The modular brace that inherited compressed air tubes, but only to form modules around the shank, thigh, and trunk (Figure 4.93), provided soft interface at points of contacts with the body, yet used metal joints [Rabishong et al., 1975]. This orthosis has been implemented for the gait training in the rehabilitation institution using a master-slave control; the therapist walked with one orthosis (master), while the other (slave) followed the kinematics and carried the paraplegic subject.

A modular orthosis, where the textile cuffs (trunk, thigh, shank) connected the mechanical joints, has been designed for muscular dystrophy subjects and tested in a small number of subjects [Hristić et al., 1981].

The powered Self-Fitting Modular Orthosis (SFMO) was introduced [Popović et al., 1979, Tomović et al., 1978; Popović, 1990a] to be a part of a hybrid assistive system [Schwirtlich and Popović, 1984, Popović and Schwirtlich, 1993].SFMO was designed based on the following principles: 1) modularity; 2) self-fitting to the body; 3) soft interface; 4) self-centering of orthosis joints to the leg joints during walking; and 4) partial powering (Figure 4.94). The modules have been designed to allow the integration into a lateral hip-knee-ankle orthosis, and integration of the left and right side. The integration has been accomplished by wearing modified types of jeans. The SFMO allowed a selection of the joints with a mechanical brake, electrically controllable brakes, and powered joints by so-called cybernetic actuator [Popović M and Popović, 1983]. The SFMO has been evaluated; the results show that the standing and walking, when using passive SFMO, are comparable with functioning with conventional orthoses, however, the use of the powered SFMO was assessed as too complicated and unacceptable for paraplegic subjects.

The advantages of the SFMO are the small weight, modularity, and over all self-fitting. The modularity proved to be a favorable feature; during the treatment modules could be added or removed depending on the needs.

4.3.6 Hybrid Assistive Systems

In order to minimize problems because of the muscle fatigue and to increase the safety, a combination of a mechanical orthosis and FES was suggested. The resulting orthosis is called Hybrid assistive system or Hybrid orthosis [Tomović et al., 1973]. The support, stability of the joints, and constraint to unwanted motion of the joints are provided by the mechanical component of the orthosis, while FES provides propulsion. Schwirtlich and Popović [1984] suggested a hybrid orthosis, which consisted of the SFMO and surface electrodes FES to provide the knee extension and swing of the leg during walking (Figure 4.94, left). A four-channel stimulator was used. The user initiates steps by triggering flexion, and this is followed by sensory driven knee extensor activity. The SFMO uses brakes activated by a micromotor. The shoe insole switches, inclinometers, and joint angle sensors provided necessary information for automatic, rule-based control described in Chapter 5.

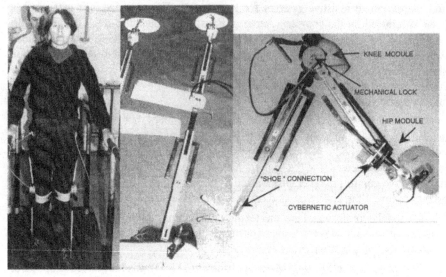

Fig. 4.94: An active, partially powered Self-Fitting Modular Orthosis (middle and right) designed for usage in Hybrid Assistive Systems (left). The cybernetic actuator shown at the hip is applicable for all joints if necessary (ankle, knee or hip) [Popović, 1981].

Andrews and Bajd [1984] suggested two variants of hybrid orthoses. One consisted of a combination of a pair of simple plastic splints used to maintain the knee extension and a two-channel stimulator per leg. One channel stimulated Gastro-soleus muscles, and the other provided flexor withdrawal response. Since the knee was held in extension only dorsiflexion of the foot and flexion of the hip were obtained. The other hybrid system comprised the KAFO and two-channel stimulation per leg. The quadriceps and common peroneal nerve were stimulated on each side. The quadriceps stimulation caused knee extension, and the peroneal nerve stimulation produced synergistic flexor response. The mechanical brace incorporated knee joint locks, which were remotely controlled by a solenoid actuator or a Bowden cable. Andrews [1986] also described a short leg orthosis in combination with FES. A Floor Reaction Orthosis (FRO) was fabricated using high-density polypropylene in a usual fashion, except that the ankle joint was set in approximately 5-degree plantar flexion. This has the advantage of being able to stabilize the knee joint when the ground reaction vector passes anterior to the knee joint axis. The FRO cannot stabilize the leg when the vector passes through or behind the knee joint axis. The FES control system was added to react appropriately, whenever a destabilizing situation arose, and to activate Quadriceps muscles. A sensor was incorporated in the calf strap of the FRO to feedback the status of the ground reaction vector. Andrews and associates [1988] suggested a different way of using the FRO in conjunction with FES. This consisted of a rigid ankle foot orthosis, a multichannel stimulator with surface electrodes, body-mounted sensors, a rule based' controller, and an electro-cutaneous display for supplementary feedback. The finite state controller reacted automatically to destabilize shifts of the ground reaction vector by stimulating appropriate anti-gravity musculature to brace the leg. The system also featured a control mode to initiate and terminate flexion of the leg during forward progression. A simple mode of supplementary sensory feedback was used during the laboratory standing tests to assist the subject in maintaining the posture.

In the cases of Reciprocating Gait Orthosis and Hip Guidance Orthosis used in combination with FES, other control methods were used. In the case of RGO the inbuilt mechanism to provide propulsive forces was not adequate. Solomonow and associates [1989] found that ambulating with the modified RGO at the Louisiana State University (LSU), so-called LSU RGO (Figure 4.95), was associated with high energy cost, and most subjects were unable to stand up without assistance. Considerable arm strength was required for the subject to attain an upright position by pressing down on the handlebars of their walker. Most subjects were unable to generate such a force. To reduce the stress over upper extremities and to reduce the energy requirements during walking an electrical stimulation system was designed. Surface stimulation of Rectus Femoris and Hamstrings muscles was used. The stimulation electrodes were incorporated in a plastic polymer cuff.

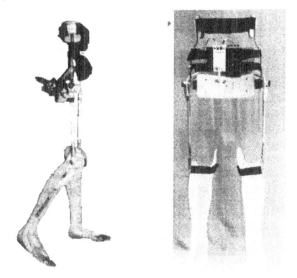

Fig. 4.95: The LSU RGO based hybrid system for restoring standing and walking. The system comprises an RGO, an electronic stimulator, and surface electrodes. FES is added to RGO to enhance movement generated with the upper part of the body, thereby decrease the energy requirements for walking.

The electrode cuffs were secured on the thighs with Velcro straps. A four-channel stimulator was worn on a belt. Finger switches were mounted on the handle bars of the walker. The subject controlled the stimulation himself. To stand up without assistance the subject stimulated both Quadriceps and both Hamstrings simultaneously. The Quadriceps extended the knees, and the Hamstrings extended the hips pushing the subject in an upright position. During walking the subject simultaneously stimulated the right Quadriceps to produce right swing and left Hamstrings to produce left forward push, then again simultaneously stimulated the left Quadriceps and right Hamstrings to produce left swing and right forward push, respectively. Phillips [1989] described a similar system; in addition to the stimulation of Hamstrings, the stimulation of ipsilateral Gluteal muscles was also suggested to improve hip extension of the stance leg. Four two-channel stimulators were used. The entire bulk of Quadriceps was stimulated using three-electrode configuration with two channels of one stimulator for each leg. The other two stimulators were used to stimulate Hamstrings and Gluteal muscles on each side.

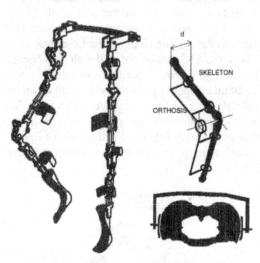

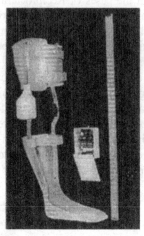

Fig. 4.96: The sketch of the Controlled-Brake Orthosis (CBO), an orthosis with brakes in the knee and hip joints (left), and model of parallel action of the orthosis and the skeleton (right). Adapted from Goldfarb and Durfee, 1996, © IEEE.

Fig. 4.97: The Dynamic Knee Brace System (DKBS) and the control circuitry. A wrap-spring clutch mechanism is controlling the knee joint state at any angular position. Adapted from Irby et al., 1999, © IEEE.

A research group in the Netherlands is currently working on the development of Modular Orthosis with multichannel Surface Electrical Stimulation (MOSES) system. It is proposed that the orthotic component of the system will be of HKAFO variety with a modular construction. The trunk support will be removable to facilitate wheelchair usage and transfers to and from wheelchairs to other places in a sitting position. In addition, the knee joint mechanism will provide automatic unlocking of the joint during the respective swing phase while remaining locked during the respective stance phase. Actuation of this mechanism will be provided from the hip on the same side. This is in an attempt to reduce the energy requirements of locomotion and at the same time improving kinematics of locomotion. Electrical stimulation of the stance side hip extensors will provide propulsion. The system is currently undergoing clinical evaluation [Hermens et al., 1994].

An important element in hybrid assistive systems is the possibility of controlling joints of the orthosis. Goldfarb and Durfee designed and evaluated a magnetic particle brake for FES-Aided walking [1996].

The design of the system considers the feature that has been neglected by most other researchers; the fact that the external skeleton operates in parallel with the body skeleton (Figure 4.96) and that the movement of the orthosis is not identical to the movement of the body. The orthosis will generate forces that will be transferred to the body through the visco-elastic connections, and the orthosis will move relatively to the body even during the quite standing, *i.e.*, swaying around the vertical posture [Popović, 1981].

Irby *et al.*, [1999a and b] suggest a wrap-spring clutch to be used within a KAFO system (Figure 4.97). The wrap-spring clutch is a principle that is proven in transmission of rotational movement. The effects of friction when a flexible body is surrounding a non-movable body are amplified in the exponential manner; thus, a small force at one end can hold a large force at the other end. This design allows minimization of the device, and over all small energy consumption when compared with other brake systems used in orthotics. There are two braking mechanisms used for the SFMO: a spring loaded pin brake that can be released by hand or micro motor, and the use of cybernetic actuator where the braking is applied using the telescopic mechanism (ball-screw).

4.3.7 Issues Impeding the Effective Use of Neuroprostheses

Restoring movement by activating the paralyzed neuro-musculo-skeletal structures is one of the promising methods, especially when combined with extensive neurorehabilitation, which is goal oriented intensive therapy. The usage of neuroprosthesis allows many humans with disabilities to improve their quality of life. NP is an external system that interfaces the preserved bodily functions, and provides necessary drive to the paralyzed structures. The technology available for NP is improving in parallel with the body of knowledge how and what to assist; thus, interface to natural mechanisms becomes more appropriate. There are some neuro-musculo-skeletal issues that has to be dealt with in the future in order to make NP suitable and applicable for many more users and their daily independent life. Available NP in many cases do not provide adequate function because of the inherent problems to the neuro-musculo-skeletal system when exposed to external activation after the injury: muscle fatigue, reduced net joint torque when generated by NP in comparison with the torque activated by CNS in able-bodied subjects, modified reflexes, spasticity, joint contractures, osteoporosis, and stress fractures [Commar *et al.*, 1962].

NP activate synchronously motor units at frequencies above the physiological values typical for natural control, thereby cause muscle fatigue [Bigland-Ritchie *et al*, 1979; Bigland-Ritchie and Woods, 1984; Kralj and Bajd, 1989; McNeal *et al.*, 1989; Solomonow *et al.*, 1983]. In principle, physiological sequence of stimulation of the muscles can be generated [Baratta *et al.*, 1989], yet it has not been integrated in the available NP. Control schemes are still not good enough to limit the duration of stimulation and thereby minimize the chance for muscle fatigue to occur. The modeling and methods that can overcome the issues related to muscle fatigue are discussed in Chapter 5.

Spasticity. Redundant muscle groups can not be externally controlled in the way identical to biological, that is central nervous system functions have not be successfully cloned so far. A central nervous system injury results in modified reflexes [e.g., Stein and Capaday, 1988], so numerous unexpected situations may occur, resulting in inappropriate antagonist contraction. In addition, the CNS changes are responsible for the reorganization in tonic and phasic properties of different muscle groups, *i.e.*, spasticity [Stefanovska, *et al.*, 1989; Dimitrijević and Nathan, 1971]. Some subjects with paralysis cannot benefit from NP because it is impossible, or extremely difficult to create functional movement because of the spasticity.

The definition of spasticity is a subject of diverse opinions. A frequently used definition is that of Landau [1980] which includes: 1) decreased dexterity, 2) loss of strength, 3) increased tendon jerks, 4) increased resistance to slower passive muscle stretch, and 5) hyperactive flexion reflexes (flexor spasms). Knutsson [1985] described almost unlimited inter individual variation in subjects with spastic paresis; therefore a detailed description of each particular subject's motor dysfunction is required. Studies applying refined biomechanical and electrophysiological measures have revealed a significant change in the passive properties of the spastic subjects [Herman, 1968; Thilmann et al., 1991; Sinkjær et al., 1993; Sinkjær and Magnussen, 1994]. Based on such observations, the idea that changes in the intrinsic muscle properties are largely responsible for spastic hypertonia has been accepted by some researchers [Dietz et al., 1981; 1995; Hufschmidt and Mauritz, 1985]. Other investigators conclude, however, that the major cause of spastic muscle hypertonus is the widely accepted pathological increase in the stretch reflex activity [e.g., Ashby et al., 1987]. Here, a description obtained by analyzing different peripheral factors responsible for the "muscle tone" to passive stretch in subjects with their muscles relaxed or active is given to document changes in the organization of movement after central nervous system injury.

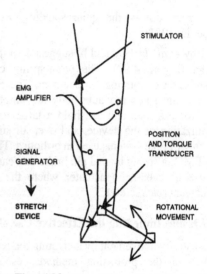

Fig. 4.98: A schema of the setup for studying spasticity during sitting, standing and waling in the plantar and dorsiflexors. For details see Sinkjær, 1997.

The resistance can be divided into: 1) an increase in the passive stiffness of tendons, joints, or muscles [Lowenthal and Tobis, 1957; Herman, 1968], 2) an increase in the intrinsic stiffness of the contracting muscle fibers [Dietz et al., 1981], and 3) an increase in the stiffness mediated by the stretch reflex [Ashby et al., 1987; Thilmann et al., 1991].

To study the importance of the different components, a brief passive stretch can be applied to the isometric muscle of interest during different voluntary activities in able-bodied and spastic hemiplegics. These studies should be performed by imposing well-defined angular displacements (Figure 4.98) around a joint. The measured forces and/or changes in electrical activity of the muscle [Gottlieb and Agarval, 1970; Hunter and Kearney, 1982; Allum and Mauritz, 1984; Sinkjær et al., 1988] can then provide information to understand the pathology, and resolve the problems that it causes.

The increase in ankle joint torque in the spastic and contralateral plantar flexors of a hemiplegic subject after imposing passive dorsiflexion was measured. The total torque increment is the sum of the reflex-mediated torque and the non-reflex mediated torque. The non-reflex torque increment was measured during a continuous electrical stimulation of the tibial nerve innervating the ankle plantar flexors. The electrical stimulation abolishes the stretch reflex [Sinkjær et al., 1988; Toft et al., 1991]. The net

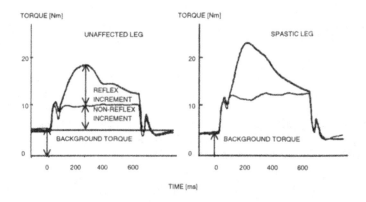

Fig. 4.99: Total and non-reflex torque responses to a stretch of the plantar flexors in a hemiplegic subject: A) unaffected, contralateral leg; B) affected, ipsilateral leg. The non-reflex torque was measures when stimulating the tibial nerve at 10 Hz. This stimulation generated plantar flexion (contraction) and the stretch reflex suppression. Adapted from Sinkjær, 1999, with permission.

reflex torque obtained when the non-reflex torque has been deducted from the total torque exceeded the non-reflex torque with nearly two times in the contralateral (unaffected) and spastic leg (Figure 4.99). The reflex net torque and the non-reflex net torque in the spastic leg both exceeded the ones in the contralateral leg. The non-reflex muscle component part of the torque opposing the stretch stems from the properties of the collagen tissue (passive properties) and the contractile apparatus in the stretched muscles (intrinsic properties). The sum of the passive and intrinsic properties is termed the non-reflex properties. The passive stiffness at a joint is reported to be several times bigger in spastic subject than those in able bodied subjects depending on the joint, joint position, subject group, and applied method [Thilman *et al.*, 1991; Sinkjær and Magnussen, 1994; Malouin *et al.*, 1997; Mirbaghei *et al.*, 1998]. Sinkjær and Magnussen [1994] found an increase in passive stiffness of up to 40 times in the spastic ankle during fast passive dorsiflexion, and an increase of about 100 percent in the passive stiffness of the contralateral leg.

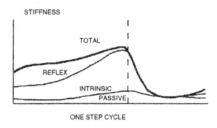

Fig. 4.100: A sketch of the passive, intrinsic and reflex mediated stiffness during walking. See text for details. Adapted from Sinkjær, 1999, with permission.

When the passive stiffness was measured in a more acute stage [Malouin *et al.*, 1997], an increase in passive stiffness of about 39 percent has been found in the affected leg three months after stroke. These increases are all with respect to ankle passive stiffness in age-matched able-bodies subjects. Malouin *et al.*, [1997] found a low correlation between the increased passive stiffness and factors such as the range of movement, the Ashwort score, and the Fugl-Meyer lower extremity motor score. This indicates that the early changes in the mechanical response to stretch in plantar flexors occur without regard to the level of disability. The changes in passive stiffness may be due to changes in collagen tissue, tendons, joint capsules, and the muscles possibly leading to clinically observable contractures [Lowenthal and Tobis, 1957; Herman, 1968; Hufsehrnidt and Mauritz, 1985].

Given the different Young's module of muscle and tendon, the large proportional length (six to eight times), and the small cross-sectional area (about 140 times) of the tendon, the changes in the Achilles tendon have most likely led to the observed increase in stiffness [Thilmann et al., 1991]. This does not exclude that changes in other collagen tissues [Toft et al., 1989a and b], or muscle fibers themselves [Dietz et al., 1986] add to the increased passive stiffness.

Changes in the muscle fibers should be reflected in the intrinsic stiffness (Figure 4.100). Sinkjær et al. [1993] found a significant increase in the intrinsic stiffness of the ankle dorsiflexors in spastic multiple sclerosis subjects and observed an insignificant increase in the hemiplegics [Sinkjær and Magnussen, 1994]. These findings are consistent with physiological, morphometrical, and histochemical investigations demonstrating changes of the muscle fibers, which are specific to the spastic muscle [Dietz et al., 1986; Edström, 1970]. The prolonged twitch contraction times in the spastic muscles [Dietz and Berger, 1984] are consistent with increased force production as demonstrated in potentiated muscles [Burke et al., 1976; Sinkjær et al., 1992]. If the muscles were relatively immobilized, the subjects would probably be particularly susceptible to this type of potentiation.

Although the reason for the pathological changes in the mechanical properties of the contractile elements of the spastic muscles as well as alternations of the connective tissue (e.g. in the tendon) is still speculative, the marked increase in passive and intrinsic stiffness reported by several authors suggests that a peripheral non-reflex mediated input can importantly contribute to spastic muscle tone.

Reflex mediated mechanical muscle responses in the active muscle, the stretch reflex, make a large contribution to the total mechanical stretch response in able-bodied subjects [Allum and Mauritz, 1984; Sinkjær et al., 1988; Toft et al., 1991]. Rack et al., [1984] have shown that during a maintained muscle contraction in spastic hemiplegic persons, the mechanically measured stretch reflex is within the normal range of the reflex stiffness in able-bodied subjects, but in the upper end of the normal range. In moderately spastic multiple sclerosis subjects, the reflex mediated stiffness in the ankle plantar flexors was unchanged compared with control subjects [Sinkjær et al., 1993]. In spinal cord injured (SCI) subjects, a system identification method that separated non-reflex and reflex contributions [Kearney et al., 1994] showed increased non-reflex stiffness as well as increased reflex stiffness in the passive and weakly contracted ankle extensors [Mirbagheli et al., 1998]. The entire above subject groups had clinical signs of spasticity when measured by the Ashwort scale [Ashby et al., 1987].

The lack of pronounced increases in the muscle tone (reflex mediated stiffness), which was found in the active spastic muscle above [Rack et al., 1984; Sinkjær et al., 1993; Sinkjær and Magnussen, 1994], may also be due to too small stretches. Only at higher stretch velocities and when using larger amplitudes as in the clinical bedside examination, the increased stiffness might express itself. Powers et al. [1988] used stretches that are comparable with the stretches used in the clinical situation, yet they did not find increased total muscle responses in spastic elbow muscles.

Increased muscle tone could be caused by an increase in the non-reflex properties (the passive and intrinsic muscle components), but also to other mechanisms. In the situations described above, the subject was asked to maintain a constant contraction, and this might introduce a situation in which the able-bodied subjects set the stretch reflex in a facilitated state. It is, however, more inhibited in the clinical situation, in which the subject is asked to relax. This leads to the hypothesis that the spastic subjects are unable to inhibit the mechanically strong stretch reflex due to an impaired (descending) control in the relaxed "clinical" situation. The increased stretch reflex in the relaxed spastic muscle and at weak precontractions can be caused by reduced postsynaptic and presynaptic inhibitions, and/or changes in postactivation depression [Nielsen et al., 1995]. These are all inhibitory mechanisms, which are believed to be important to make the muscle relax in able-bodied subjects. As the muscle in able-bodied subjects is made increasingly active, these inhibitions are removed, and the reflex stiffness expresses itself fully, as it has already done in the spastic subject's relaxed "uninhibited" muscle.

EMG measured stretch reflex responses. Several possible pathways might be involved in explaining the threshold change of the stretch reflex without changing the gain such as absent reciprocal inhibition [Crone, 1993; Crone et al., 1994], a changed intrinsic regulation of transmitter release from the Ia afferents in spastic subjects [Nielsen et al., 1995], changes in γ-motoneuron activity [Matthews, 1959], and changes in the activity in descending motor pathways of the brainstem [Feldman and Orlowsky, 1972] that affect the postsynaptic inhibition [Matthews, 1959]. Since the stretch reflex is much less sensitive to presynaptic inhibition than the H-reflex [Morita et al., 1998], it is less clear if a decreased presynaptic inhibition [Delwaide, 1973; Faist et al., 1994; Stein, 1995] can explain a shift in threshold.

Muscle and cutaneous reflexes are highly modulated during locomotion in an adaptive manner within each phase of the step cycle [Crenna and Frigo, 1987; Duysens et al., 1990]. This modulation is often lost or seriously reduced in subjects with spasticity. To get a good understanding of how increased muscle tone relates to more functional motor tasks, it becomes, therefore, important also to investigate the "non-reflex muscle component" together with the spinal/central integration of afferent inputs during more functional motor tasks such as walking.

The increased passive stiffness and intrinsic muscle stiffness found in sitting spastic subjects are also present during walking. Based on indirect force measurements of Achilles tendon in hemiparetic subjects, Berger et al. [1984b] demonstrated that the non-reflex stiffness was increased during walking. They suggested that spastic hemiparetic subjects could develop a larger muscle tension during walking at a lower level of the neural drive compared to able-bodied control subjects. This was seen as a benefit since it facilitates the subject to support body weight during the stance phase of walking in spite of the inability to activate the soleus muscle. This might be correct, but it should be remembered that a major part of the increase in non-reflex stiffness is caused by an increased passive stiffness, which will impair dorsiflexion in swing [Sinkjær et al., 1996a and b] This becomes even more prominent in spastic subjects because they have a decreased voluntary drive to the ankle dorsiflexors. In addition, spastic subjects often cocontract their muscles during walking [Knuttsons and Richards, 1979], which further increases the non-reflex stiffness.

The reflex modulation that takes place during walking in able-bodied subjects [Capaday and Stein, 1986] is often lacking in spastic subjects [Fung et al., 1990; Yang et al., 1991; Sinkjær et al., 1995, 1996a and b]. The impaired reflex modulation has been interpreted to increase the muscle stiffness because of a disrupted, supraspinal control of the stretch reflex [Fung and Barbeau, 1994; Capaday, 1995].

Phasic Response to External Perturbation - Spasms. In addition to the increased muscle stiffness in persons with injuries of CNS very strong firing of the muscles has been observed. These sudden muscle contractions are often triggered by some peripheral input (e.g., touching the skin at the leg, moving the leg passively, moving the foot passively, transferring). The tetanic contraction of muscles leading typically to simultaneous bilateral extension has been documented [Kralj and Bajd, 1989]. In most paraplegic and tetraplegic subjects both legs (hips, knees, plantar flexion) will extend generating a painful and fatiguing pattern. The movement can be so strong that it "catapults" the body from the chair. This spasm is obviously centrally mediated and peripherally triggered. Experiments with standing of paraplegic subjects showed that these bilateral spasms are enhanced in low thoracic lesion (T11-T12), yet not so common in higher thoracic and incomplete cervical lesion subjects.

In children with cerebral paralysis, it was found that during a period of minutes or longer they developed strong tonus of extensor muscles (e.g., hip extensors, knee extensors). The extension can be so strong that it sometimes prevents a child from sitting in the chair or prevents his/her walking with assistive systems. Some of the children are treated by a dorsal root rizotomy that is the dorsal roots innervating the extensors in the legs are cut. This leads to unrepairable denervation of leg extensors, which is not necessarily positive. Pharmaceutical treatments can decrease to some extent the spasm, yet they interfere with some other behavior and are not always effective. The prolonged extension suggests that a higher central input that inhibits the extension is missing. Many connections are changed or missing after CNS injury developing very individual behavior; thus it is very difficult to generalize the motor changes, but spasms occur because the input of the higher CNS centers is missing to the part of the spinal cord below the lesion.

In most subjects with paraplegia the spasm can be eliminated by a simple manipulation: strong stretching of the one of the muscles that is contracted (e.g., Gastrocnemius m. and Soleus m.) would stop the spasm. It has been noted in paraplegic subjects that when treated with functional electrical stimulation to stand, the first standing trial is accompanied with spasm. Loading of the toes, adjusting the amount of electrical charge that is delivered, and over all pushing the hips forward, that is stretching the calf muscles, will stop the firing. When a subject stretches his leg extensors by going into a so-called "C" posture during the first stand; the spasms are not likely to repeat in standings to follow during the same session. Extension spasms do not occur during walking, however, clonus, that is a repetitive flexion-extension movement at the ankle joint with the frequency of about 2 to 5 Hz, does. The clonus is the consequence of previously described changes of the reflex response to peripheral input.

Joint contractures reduce the range of movement; thus, compromise the FES activated functional movements [Perry, 1981]. Our own experimental studies have been faced with a change in the musculo-skeletal system, which results in an inability for functional movement [Popović et al., 1991d]. The term functional contracture has been introduced to describe this change. It relates to the lack of performance because one joint movement restricts the movement of the neighboring joint. This is caused by increased tonus of muscles and shortening of the biarticular muscle-tendon systems. A clinical measurement of the range of joint movement does not include the testing of this behavior.

Osteoporosis [Lukert, 1982], normally found in SCI subjects, may compromise the use of legs for support and may lead to stress fractures [Rafil *et al.*, 1982] if used inappropriately. In the literature, there are some speculations that patterned electrical therapy can decrease osteoporosis [Phillips *et al.*, 1984], but other results with chronic subjects have been negative [Leeds *et al.*, 1990]. It might still be possible to prevent osteoporosis with chronic stimulation, if applied immediately after the onset of injury.

Energy efficiency of walking

Energy cost of paraplegic walking assisted by available orthoses or neuroprostheses, which restrict lower limbs to most rudimentary mechanical function and the propulsive forces are generated by the musculature of the upper body and extremities is intrinsically very high. The energy requirements of paraplegic walking using long leg braces and crutches have been studied in the past by various researchers. The pioneering study by Gordon [1956] showed that energy consumption when ambulating in a swing-through fashion is at least 3.5 times, sometime as high as 5.5 to 8 times of the basal requirements of the subjects who participated in the study. A study by Huang and associates [1979] showed that paraplegics consumed three times greater oxygen during walking than when they were at rest. A study by Chantraine and associates [1984] showed that when paraplegics are allowed to ambulate at their comfortable speed the energy consumption was lower in subjects who used their long leg braces regularly than in those who used braces sporadically. It was directly related to the level of spinal cord lesion. However, the gait velocity was directly related to brace use, *i.e.*, the velocity was higher in subjects with longer periods of regular use; and inversely related to the level of lesion, *i.e.*, walking velocity was slower in subjects with higher level lesions. Merkel and associates [1984] studied energy expenditure of paraplegics standing and walking using two types of KAFOs (Scott-Craig KAFO and Single Stopped long leg KAFO). They found that the energy cost of paraplegic locomotion with either variety of orthoses is about 5 to 12.8 times that of normal locomotion [Blessey, 1978]. Miller and associates [1984] measured energy requirements of paraplegic locomotion during negotiating turns, stairs and ramps using the same two varieties of KAFOs. They found that the energy consumption of paraplegic locomotion during negotiations architectural barriers was approximately the same as the one measured in able-bodied walkers (control group), yet the energy cost was as much as 15 times more than that of controls.

Waters and coworkers [1988a and b, 1992, 1994] provided a comprehensive analysis of the efficiency of walking (e.g., energy cost, energy rate, heart rate, blood

Table 4.3: Measures of the walking efficiency as function of the LEMS (lower extremity muscle score). Adapted from Waters *et al.*, 1994, with permission.

	LEMS 0 - 40 %	LEMS 40 - 60 %	LEMS 60 - 90 %
O$_2$ RATE [ml/ kg min]	15.2±3.4	13.2±1.6	14.6±3.0
O$_2$ RATE INCREASE	158±1114	110±60	49±35
O$_2$ COST [ml/ kg m]	0.76±0.61	0.51±0.25	15.2±3.4
VELOCITY [m / min]	30.5±15.6	31.4±11.4	57.5±12.3

pressure) as function of the measurable preserved functioning. They suggest that the classification on the lower extremity muscle score (described in Chapter 3) is highly correlated with velocity, cadence, oxygen (metabolic energy) cost and rate, axial peak loading of the legs and the ambulatory motor score. The study that included 36 paraplegic subjects [Waters et al., 1994] shows that there is a high correlation (Table 4.3) between the lower extremity muscle score (LEMS) and the energy efficiency.

All of the above mentioned studies concluded that paraplegics with high or mid thoracic level lesion are probably incompatible for walking. In all studies, subjects walked using a form of KAFO, and there was no trunk support provided during walking, therefore, energy was also utilized to maintain the upright posture. Nene and Patrick [1989] studied the energy cost of locomotion for thoracic level paraplegics using the ParaWalker, which gives adequate support to the trunk and provides better stability than KAFOs. They found that the energy consumption with the ParaWalker was about 3.5 times the resting level of the subjects. The energy cost was 4.9 times more than that of normal walking; this was in contrast to the findings for paraplegics with thoracic level lesion reported in the previous studies. They deduced that the efficiency of the ParaWalker lies in the intrinsic stability provided by the orthosis. Surface electrical stimulation of stance side Gluteal muscles helped to reduce the energy cost of locomotion by approximately 6.5 percent to 8 percent in the rather small study group of 5 subjects. In a study comparing energy requirements of ambulation using the RGO alone and hybrid RGO, Hirokawa et al., [1990] found approximately 16 percent reduction in the energy cost throughout the full range of walking speeds when RGO was combined with electrical stimulation of the thigh muscles. They concluded that at slow speeds the energy cost of ambulation using RGO was less than that using KAFOs. Winchester and associates [1993] examined the energy cost of ambulation using a standard RGO and using a modified RGO, i.e., Isocentric RGO. They found that with the standard RGO subjects' oxygen uptake was 14.2 ml/(kg min) (mean) and the mean velocity was 12.7 m/min; with the Isocentric RGO the oxygen uptake was 13.0 ml/(kg min) (mean), and the mean velocity was 13.5 m/min (the differences were statistically not significant).

Marsolais and Edwards [1988] reported energy requirements of walking using FES alone and compared those to using KAFOs in only 3 subjects. During FES walking energy consumption was about 59 to 75 percent of maximal aerobic power of the subjects. There was no increase in energy consumption when the walking speed was increased. The energy cost equaled that of KAFOs. At speeds approaching 25 m/min FES walking energy consumption was similar to that of KAFOs. They inferred that at speeds between 25 m/min and 36 m/min.

The ability to measure the efficiency by hart rate or some related measurable could be important, since measuring oxygen consumption is difficult and cumbersome. In the past it has been shown that it was possible to establish walking performance of subjects by monitoring speed and heart rate [Stallard et al., 1978; Stallard and Rose, 1980]. MacGregor [1979,1981] described a method of combining these two parameters to produce a single index called the Physiological Cost Index (PCI). The PCI is a measure of the cardiovascular stress, but it is not directly related to the metabolic energy consumption. Nene and Jennings [1992] measured the PCI of paraplegic locomotion using the ORLAU ParaWalker. In a study group of 16 subjects mean PCI was 3.11 heart beats per meter (b/m). It ranged from 1.47 b/m to 4.76 b/m. Bowker and associates [1992] reported a mean PCI value of 5.04 b/m for a group of

28 RGO users. Their subject group consisted of subjects with paraplegia due to varied pathology.

A paraplegic should be able to use the orthosis completely independently. This includes doffing and donning; transfers, *i.e.,* standing up, walking and sitting down again. The subject must also be able to negotiate commonly encountered architectural barriers such as gentle slopes, curbs, steps, *etc.* Transfers in and out of wheelchairs, cars and other means of transport are also essential for everyday life of a paraplegic. All presently available KAFOs can be donned, and doffed by the subjects independently.

Rosman and Spira [1974] surveyed the use of orthoses (KAFO) in 51 paraplegic subjects after their discharge from the hospital for 16 years in total. They used four groups based on the level of lesion (T1-T6, T7-T11, T12-L1, and L2-L5). The over all conclusion is that most subjects with the lesion above T11 abandon the use of an orthosis even for standing, some subjects occasionally use them for standing and only exceptionally for walking, and that about one third of the L2-L5 subjects use the assistance for walking.

Subjects with severe spasticity and contractures have some difficulty in doffing and donning the ParaWalker and the RGO [Moore and Stallard, 1991; Solomonow *et al.,* 1989]. The RGO had knee joints with automatic knee locks, which caused difficulty for some subjects. These have been modified and the newer generation of RGO has ratchet knee joints [Solomonow *et al.,* 1989]. The HGO users need to extend and lock their knees before they are able to stand up. A special assistive device can be made for individuals who have difficulty with locking their knees.

The other major factor, which can hamper independence, is the ability to perform toilet functions while using the orthosis. Use of either the ParaWalker or RGO certainly causes major problems in this area. Use of KAFOs, due to hips being unconstrained, does not cause serious inconveniences.

Any walking system used for paraplegic walking must have a very high level of reliability, but at the same time in case of any unforeseeable failure the user must not come to any physical harm. All mechanical systems currently in use are fairly robust and safe. Stand alone FES systems fail to provide any mechanical safety in the case of failure of electronic components during walking. With percutaneously implanted electrodes the rate of electrode failure is high thereby necessitating re-implantation of the electrodes. Additionally, the electrode insertion sites acting as portals for entry for infecting organisms remain a risk.

Technical and technological issues relate to the NP-neuromuscular interface and the biocompatibility of a NP. The NP-neuromuscular interface is realized with electrodes. Currently, several types of electrodes are in use or under development. The least invasive is transcutaneous electrical stimulation with surface electrodes, while other techniques use percutaneous or implanted electrodes. Percutaneous or implanted electrodes are applied to muscles, close to the motor point, to the nerve directly. The use of other types of electrodes is in its developmental phase. The use of implanted electrodes and stimulators; that is totally implanted neuroprostheses is progressively being used in many more subjects. The efficiency of the energy transfer between an implant and the external unit has to be improved, specially for NP that use rather sophisticated microcontroller, implanted sensors with amplifiers, and multichannel devices. An interface device that can be adapted for various users allowing them to control the NP is most probably the critical issue. The technology of using the brain interface is very appealing, yet it is in its infancy. Plausible use of implanted brain interface is another plausible command link, however, it is rather invasive, and at this stage does not fulfil the cost to benefit ratio.

The practicality of the system relates to the cosmesis, ease of donning and doffing, safety and reliability. These elements determine how easy a system could be accepted by potential candidates for using it, and over all the difference that the device is bringing in the quality of life of users.

The control issues being essential for improving the functioning of the NP are discussed in Chapter 5.

4.4 Artificial Legs

An artificial extremity is a morphological and functional replacement of a human limb [Muilenburg and Wilsson Jr, 1996]. Artificial extremity compensates for the disability caused by amputation of a limb or its part. The differences between the upper and lower extremity prostheses come from the dissimilarity in functions, which they have, to replace and/or compensate. An artificial leg should support the body weight (standing) and mainly perform so-called cyclic movement (e.g., walking, running). The arm prosthesis needs to endow with extremely complicated goal-directed movement (manipulation) in order to allow hand grasp. The states of the art of the leg, arm, and hand prostheses are presented to indicate what novelties are needed for improved function.

4.4.1 The Lower-Limb Prosthesis

An amputation results in a disabling condition. With modern prostheses and treatment methods, when the musculature is good, the circulation is adequate, and there is an absence of excessive scarring, however, the unilateral amputees can do many of the things, which they could before amputation. The objective of this section is to describe lower-limb prostheses available to users, including persons who have had a knee disarticulation, hip-disarticulation, or hemipelvectomy.

During the past few years the International Standards Organization (ISO) for prosthetics and orthotics has developed a standard method of describing amputations and prostheses that is being adapted worldwide. They adopted the term "transfemoral" in place of "above-knee" to identify an amputation between the knee and hip joint. This term has been selected to avoid confusion with disarticulation at the hip and amputations through the pelvis. The term

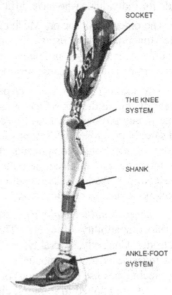

Fig. 4.101: Four main components of a transfemoral prosthesis (C-Leg® System): the socket, the knee, the shank, and the ankle-foot complex (www.ottobock.com)

"transtibial" instead of "below-knee" describing an amputation below the knee joint has been adopted accordingly. The ISO is also planning to adopt the term "stump" referring to that part of the limb that is left after amputation.

The lower-limb prosthesis has to duplicate the behavior of the missing portion of the leg. The biomechanical requirements for a lower-limb prosthesis have been summarized by Wagner and Catranis [1954] and refined by Radcliffe [1980].

The prosthesis must support the body weight of the amputee in a manner similar to the normal limb during the stance phase of level walking, on slopes, soft or rough terrain. This implies that the prosthesis provides for "stability" during weight bearing. The stability in this context refers to prevention from sudden or uncontrolled flexion of the knee during weight bearing. It is obvious that an "unstable" knee in the prosthesis can lead to dangerous situations and possible injury for the amputee.

The support of the body weight has to ensure that undesirable pressures of the amputation stump are excluded or that gait abnormalities due to painful contact between the stump and socket are prevented. The analysis of biomechanical factors, which influence the shaping, fitting, and alignment of the socket is a problem of itself. If the fitting has been accomplished in a manner, which allows the amputee to manipulate and control prosthesis in an active and comfortable manner, the socket and stump can be treated as one single body.

The third requirement placed upon the prosthesis is that it duplicates as closely as possible the kinematics and dynamics of normal gait. The amputee should be able to walk with an essentially normal appearance over a useful range of walking speeds associated with typical activities for normal persons of similar age. The latter requirement has received a great deal of attention in recent years, and fully integrated systems, so-called self-contained, active, transfemoral prosthesis, are being incorporated into modern rehabilitation. The self-contained principle implies that the artificial leg contains the energy source, actuator, controller, and sensors.

The prostheses cannot be unambiguously classified into passive and active ones. Such solutions as the polycentric knee mechanism [Cappozzo et al., 1980], the polycentric knee mechanism with hydraulic valve [Radcliffe, 1980], or the transfemoral prosthesis with friction type brake [Aoyama, 1980] satisfy some of the above performance requirements. Logically controlled transfemoral with the hydraulic valve represents a further bridge between purely passive and fully controllable assistive devices [Turajlić and Drakulić, 1981; James, 1983]. All o f the abo ve mentioned prostheses satisfy the stance phase requirements as well as the minimum power consumption principle. However, the amputee is not able to flex/extend the knee in the stance phase once it has been flexed. Extension in the swing phase requires additional metabolic energy. Gait asymmetry has to be minimized.

4.4.2 Transfemoral Prosthesis

The transfemoral prosthesis has four major parts: the socket, the knee system, the shank, and the foot-ankle system. A variety of sockets, knees, shanks, feet, and ankles are available and can be combined to produce prosthesis that meets the needs of each individual amputee.

Figure 4.101 shows an example of the transfemoral prosthesis with an advanced ankle-foot complex, hydraulic actuator at the knee joint capable of controlling the knee position throughout the walking cycle, and an endoskeletal shank (3C100 C-Leg® System, Otto Bock Orthopedic Industry, Germany).

The Socket

The socket is the basis for the connection between the user and the prosthesis. It always provides the means of transferring the weight of the amputee to the ground by way of the rest of the prosthesis. The shape of the socket is critical to comfort and function. The socket must not restrict circulation, yet it cannot be loose. Most sockets for above-knee prostheses cover the entire stump. There are several designs available to take maximum advantage of the muscles in the stump of the individual amputee for control of the prosthesis and for transferring the weight of the amputee to the floor.

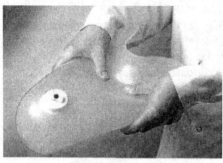

Fig.4.102: Flexible suction type socket for a transfemoral prosthesis

Most sockets are made of a rigid plastic, but some amputees prefer a flexible socket supported by a rigid frame because comfort during walking and sitting seems to be improved.

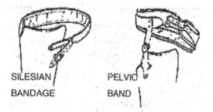

Fig. 4.103: Systems for fixing of a "loose" socket to the stump

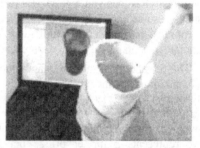

Fig. 4.104: CAD of the socket with the TracerCAD system (http://www.tracercad.com)

For most subjects, the prosthesis can be held in place by "suction" or a vacuum, provided by a close fit between stump and socket (Figure 4.102).

This is known as a suction socket. Nothing is worn between the stump and socket. When circulation is marginal or precarious, a looser fit should be provided. A loose fit requires use of soft, yet stable interface to fill in the "loose" contact. This is done with "socks" of wool worn over the stump. In such a case, it is necessary to add a system that will hold the socket in place (e.g., a Silesian Bandage, Figure 4.103).

To design a socket needs a lot of attention, and in many cases remains only the skill of a prosthetist. The stump of the leg changes its form (e.g., gaining or loosing weight, muscle atrophy) throughout the lifelong application of the prosthesis. Therefore, it is necessary to facilitate fast and adequate manufacturing of a socket.

Computer Aided Design (CAD), or as it was originally called Computer Aided Socket Design (CASD), is a technique, which uses computerized three-dimensional image of the stump and numerical machines to automatically fabricate the socket.

The first phase for automatic fabrication of the socket relates to creating a three-dimensional image of the stump. Since the stump is unique for each user, and because of the individual biomechanical features (e.g., aligning of the thigh vs. the pelvis, Figure 4.104), it is essential to include expert knowledge gained through experience in automatic design of the sockets.

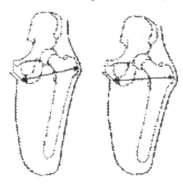

Fig. 4.105: Two similar, yet biomechanically different stumps.

TracerCAD® system (Figure 4.104) has introduced an example of direct and interactive expert intervention system, and it allows taking precise measurements with instantaneous and lifelike images of the process by using a "pen". The "pen" allows a prosthetist to mimic a touch with the stump that imitates the natural sweep of the fingers. The advantage of the system is that it enables clinical modifications directly on the subject. The method must include skeletal fit technology, not only the three-dimensional surface image. The example (Figure 4.105) shows two stumps having the same distance between the Anterior-Medial aspect of the Ramus and the Greater Trochanter, illustrated by the arrow, but different orientations; the long axis of the stump ensures that the force is transmitted in a direction which will not cause hip pain and possible injury.

The Knee System

The above-knee amputee needs a stable support while walking; thus, the prosthesis must have a knee joint that will allow only controlled buckling as he rolls over the artificial foot during the stance phase of walking. The same knee joint has to provide flexion during the swing phase to allow ground clearance and natural-like movement of the leg. Most prostheses, by engineering terms of automatic control, are under-powered systems. This means that at least one degree of freedom in the system does not have the actuation capabilities to control the movement at all times.

The simplest way to achieve walking with an under-powered prosthesis is to use mechanical friction about a bolt that connects the socket (the thigh) and the shank. The bolt must be located behind the line determined by the ground reaction force at all times during the stance phase of walking. If the axis of the knee rotation comes in front of the line of the ground reaction, the knee joint becomes unstable and a locking mechanism is instrumental.

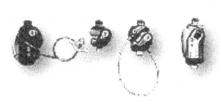

Fig. 4.106: Single-axis knee joint mechanism with a friction mechanism and a mechanical lock in fully extent position (http://www.Ottobock.com)

The mechanical friction system, which may be a simple adjustable braking mechanism, is needed to keep the shank from swinging forward too fast as the user swings the artificial leg. The principal limitation of a single-axis, constant friction design of the knee system is that appearance of walking is "normal" at only one speed of walking for a given setting of friction; hence, the amputee must be careful while walking, especially if walking on uneven surfaces.

A great deal of effort has been spent over the years developing knee systems which overcome the limitations of the single-axis, constant friction knee. Many designs have been somewhat successful, yet the constant friction knee system is still in use (Figure 4.106). The second level of complexity in knee systems is the use of a weight-actuated brake with constant friction. Two bolts are used at the knee so that when one pivots about the other when the amputee is standing, the force of the body weight engages a brake that keeps the knee from buckling.

To allow the amputee to vary his speed of walking, a number of hydraulic devices are available. In the simplest system, the piston is attached to a pivot in the thigh section of the prosthesis behind the knee bolt, and the cylinder is attached to a pivot in the shank (Figure 4.107). Because of the way oil acts when forced through a small hole, the amount of resistance required for a given velocity of walking is provided automatically.

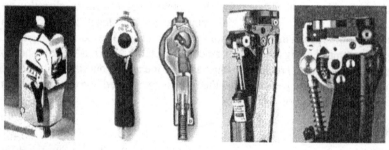

Fig. 4.107: Single-axis mechanisms for the knee joint assembly. 3R45 Modular Knee Joint, 3R80 Modular Rotary Hydraulic Knee Joint, 140 degree Flexion ESK Superior Knee Stabilization and Pneumatic Swing Phase Control (from the left to the right respectively) (http://www.Ottobock.com and http://www.endolite.com)

3R45 Modular Knee Joint is an ultralight, low profile, hydraulic single axis knee. It allows a wide range of flexion and extension resistance giving a higher subject activity level. Swing phase resistances are independently adjustable. The 3R80 Modular Rotary Hydraulic Knee Joint is the rotary hydraulic device that is responsive to the cadence of walking. It allows up to 135 degrees of flexion and adjustable resistance to flexion and extension during the swing. The new Endolite Stabilized Knee (140 degree Flexion ESK) incorporates many enhanced features: independent control of swing and stance, 140 degrees of knee flexion, high load capacity, rapid and reliable fitting. This knee can be equipped with various hydraulic and pneumatic actuators offered by Endolite. The novelty in the design of actuators is servo PSPC (Pneumatic Swing Phase Control), which allows variable knee joint angular velocity; hence, adaptation to the speed of walking within limits.

To provide better control of the transfemoral prosthesis during standing and the stance phase of walking, mechanical linkages between the socket and shank that provide a moving center of rotation have been introduced (Figure 4.108). Such designs are known as polycentric knees. Used originally for the knee-disarticulation case,

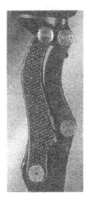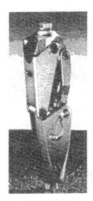

Fig 4.108: Polycentric knee mechanisms for the knee. Four-bar linkages provide movement of the center of rotation with respect to the thigh and shank following closely the movement of the center of rotation in the biological counterpart. The 3R60 EBS Knee, Otto Bock Industries, Inc. (left) and the Slim Profile 4-Bar Knee Disarticulation, Blatchford, Endolite (right) (http://www.Ottobock.com and http://www.endolite.com)

polycentric knees are now also used in prostheses for higher levels, especially when stability at heel strike is desirable. The swing phase control may be either mechanical friction or hydraulic resistance. The one limitation of the polycentric design is that the range of motion about the knee may be restricted to some degree, but not enough for it to be objectionable to most users. The 3R60 EBS Knee has unique new polycentric features imitating the human knee by providing up to 15 degrees of cushioned stance flexion.

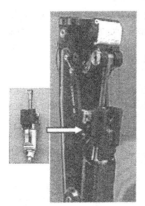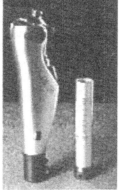

Fig. 4.109: The IP+ (http://www.endolite.com) (left) and 3C knee joint (http://www.Ottobock.com) (right) systems allow microcomputer intelligent control of leg behavior during walking.

Two hydraulic cylinders, one to influence the stance flexion, the other to control the swing phase, offer a more natural walking. The controlled knee buckling during the stance phase is especially effective for walking on uneven terrain. This polycentric knee allows flexion up to 150 degrees. The Slim Profile 4-Bar Knee Disarticulation can be equipped with different hydraulic or a pneumatic actuator providing great flexibility in providing a subject with the preferred solution for him/her. The linkages limit the knee flexion to 125 degrees. Complex carbon fiber composite used for the links ensures smooth profiles, lightweight, and durability.

The Intelligent Prosthesis Plus (IP+) automatically adjusts the swing of the knee to match the individual amputee's walking speeds. This control ensures better walking symmetry, and as shown in clinical tests involves reduced cognitive and cardiopulmonary stress. T he most complex knee systems of those available are those which control both the swing and stance phase with a single hydraulic cylinder (Figure 4.109).

The 3C100 C-Leg System represents the first and only commercially available microprocessor controlled hydraulic knee with swing and stance phase regulation (Figure 4.109). The operation of the system includes sensors detecting the loading of the leg and rotation in the knee joint. The program stored in the self-contained microcomputer uses sensory information and a sequence of logic operations, similar to reflexes in the natural control to provide control of both swing and stance. The 3C-knee joint can be combined with a variety of shank and foot assemblies. The same system permits the velocity of walking to be varied at will, being appreciated by many active amputees.

The Ankle-Foot Complex

The ankle-foot complex has to provide shock absorption at the heel strike, provide stability and rolling over the sole during the stance of walking, allow adaptation for uneven terrain and small obstacles, and possibly store the energy during the loading phase, which it will return to the leg during the push-off phase of the stance. The ankle joint has to allow some medial and lateral rotation, as well as eversion and inversion.

Artificial feet currently available can be divided into two classes: articulated, and non-articulated. Most of the non-articulated feet are available with toes molded in to provide a very realistic appearance. Articulated feet have moving joints generally requiring maintenance and are heavier than most of the non-articulated feet. Articulated feet may have one or more joints. The single-axis foot (one-joint) provides for ankle action that is controlled by two rubber bumpers, either of which can be changed to permit more or less motion as needed. It is often used to assist in keeping the knee stable. A multi-axis foot is often recommended for people who have to walk on uneven surfaces because it allows some motion about all three axes of the ankle. The simplest type of non-articulated foot is the SACH (solid ankle-cushion heel) foot. The keel is rigid.

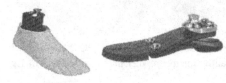

Fig. 4.110: The K2 Sensation (left) and Allurion (right), low profile multi-axial feet. (http:// www.flexfoot.com)

Ankle action is provided by the soft rubber heel, which compresses under load during the early part of the stance phase of walking. The rubber heel wedges are available in three densities: soft, medium, and hard.

The SAFE (solid ankle-flexible-endoskeletal) foot has the same action as the SACH plus the ability for the sole to conform to slightly irregular surfaces and thus makes it easier for the amputee to walk over uneven terrain. Feet of this type make walking easier because of the flexibility, and they are sometimes called "flexible keel" feet.

In recent years, there has been a proliferation of new designs for artificial feet (Figure 4.110). Most are capable of absorbing energy in a "flexible" keel during the "rollover" part of the stance phase of walking and springing back immediately to provide push-off, or assistance in getting the toe off of the ground to start the swing phase of walking. These designs are often called "dynamic response" feet.

Most of the systems used today are multi-axis feet with a limited range of movement. The ankle joint is not powered. The researchers have investigated the ankle joint articulation, but both the control and power requirements came as arguments against the usage of these assistive systems. A realization of an articulated ankle joint was with the coupled ankle-knee joint movement within transfemoral prosthesis (The WLR-7, Waseda leg, Japan).

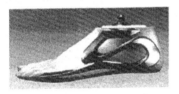
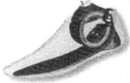

Fig. 4.111: The 1D25 Dynamic Plus Foot (left) and C-foot (right) fully articulated systems (http://www.Ottobok.com) providing shock absorption and storing of energy.

The K2 Sensation foot (Figure 4.110, left) provides multi-axial range of motion cushioning each step while helping to maintain control over barriers as raps or small obstacles like curbs. The full-length toes level, a flexible keel, and an integrated multi-axial design offer a smooth transition from heel strike to toe off that is absent in some other feet. This means added comfort and relief for those that may be struggling with dysvascular complications. The Allurion, low profile, dynamic response from Flexfoot (Figure 4.110, right) is designed for the amputees with long stump of knee units. The compact design of the Allurion provides all the function that an active amputee would expect. A carbon fiber is used for strength and durability, and it can be integrated with transtibial or transfemoral prosthesis through a titanium male pyramid, being standard today. The Carbon Active Heel provides shock absorption for the overall health and comfort. This heel harnesses heel strike energy and transfers that energy into the foot module enabling forward progression, which ensures decreased metabolic energy cost and rate for walking.

The 1D25 Dynamic Plus Foot (Figure 4.111, left) is designed for amputees who want a highly functional foot. It offers increased greater mobility to the amputee. The improved S-shaped spring offers enhanced physiological rollover during stance phase of walking. The stored energy returns to the forefoot at toe-off, therefore, further improving the initiation of swing phase. The 1C40 C-Walk Foot (Figure 4.111, right) provides true comfort. A carbon fiber

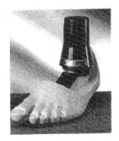

Fig. 4.112: The Endolite Multiflex Foot and Ankle (http://www.endolite.com)

foot combines comfort with dynamic response and multi-axial rotation. The C-element cushions the foot for a comfortable heel strike. The stored energy is released to facilitate a smooth rollover to mid-stance. As the fore foot loading increases, the C-spring element loads again along with the base spring. This energy is returned at toe-off to assist in initiating swing phase.

The Endolite "Muliflex" concept provides a unique foot and ankle combination capable of excellent performance (Figure 4.112). Torsional movement (medial and lateral rotations), inversion and eversion of the ankle give comfort and control customized to suit the individual's requirements. The walking performance is enhanced by careful design of the toe break. The break is reinforced with a polymer strip. A keel manufactured from a new lightweight, long fiber composite material has been incorporated. The foot design provides increased heel cushioning. The Multiflex ankle-foot complex provides "natural"-like rollover during the initial and mid-stance phases, a facilitated push-off due to the energy stored in the foot. All features of the Multiflex concept lead to decreased cardio-vascular stress, and metabolic energy cost and rate. The system can be directly integrated with a standardized endoskeletal shank.

The Shank

The primary purpose of the shank is to transfer the vertical loads caused by the weight of the amputee to the foot and onto the floor (Figure 4.113). Two types of shank systems are available: 1) the Crustacean or exoskeletal, which transfers the forces through the outside walls of the hollow shank which is shaped like a leg; 2) and the or pylon, or endoskeletal, where the forces are carried through a central structure, usually a tube, and the esthetics of provided by a foam covering.

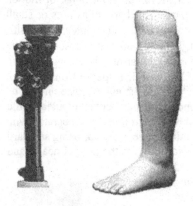

Fig. 4.113: The central, endoskeletal (left) and the Crustacean, or exoskeletal (right) shanks connected to the knee joint system.

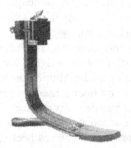

Fig. 4.114: Modular design of ankle-foot system (K2 Sensation) including the titanium pyramide for connecting it with the pylon (http://www.flexfoot.com)

Each design has advantages and disadvantages. The endoskeletal systems offer the most life-like appearance and "feel", but require more care to maintain. The crustacean design is suitable for heavy duty. Most endoskeletal parts are designed for moderate or light duty, but heavy-duty systems are available.

Another advantage of some of the endoskeletal systems is that knee units of great complexity can be introduced as the amputee becomes more proficient or his functional needs change.

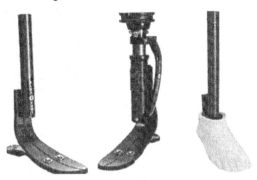

Fig. 4.115: Three different types of Flexfoot pylons (http://www.flexfoot.com)

The skeletal part of the prosthesis replacing the shank is designed as a rather rigid skeleton, or a flexible structure. The flexible solution of the skeletal part allows the user not only to walk and stand safely, but also to participate in sports and other intensive bipedal activities (e.g., dancing, hoping). The rigid skeleton, more frequently used, provides weight bearing and stability.

The Flexfoot support for the pylon promotes whole body comfort by providing lightweight, high strength, non-corrosive, exceptional energy storage and return system for support of the body (Figure 4.114). This construction minimizes the additional weight to the limb and offers maximum durability (Figure 4.115). Faster walk with less efforts is provided allowing lively, energy efficient functions.

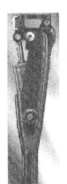 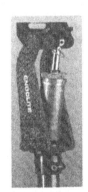 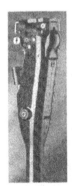

Fig. 4.116: The Uniaxail Knee Chassis (left), the 160 Hi-Activity Chasis, and the 160 Universal Shin Range pylon-knee mechanism housing (http://www.endolite.com)

The Stanceflex Uniaxial Knee Chasis (SFEUK) integrates the housing for the hydraulic or pneumatic actuator with the pylon (Figure 4.116). The construction allows 115 degrees of flexion and is primarily used with a CaTech hydraulic device that controls stance flexion. The whole structure absorbs the heel impact; it is energy efficient because it can give the energy back that was stored during loading of the leg.

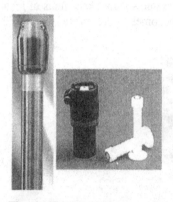

Fig. 4.117: The TT pylon and the demountable torque absorber (http://www. endolite.com)

The 160 HI-activity (Figure 4.116) chassis is a tough, long life, low maintenance pylon-knee actuator housing. It provides 120 degrees of knee flexion and is frequently applied with a CaTech cylinder that gives good swinging control. This uniaxial device includes super strong needle roller bearings for better support of high stresses. The 160 Universal Shin Range (Figure 4.116) is an integrated shank and knee-actuator housing for the transfemoral prosthesis. The system allows 130 degrees of knee flexion and is typically used with IP+ actuator. The endoskeletal structure is very convenient for use of both continuous and discontinuous cosmesis.

The TT pylon incorporates a vertical shock pylon and torque absorber in one compact package (Figure 4.117). A maximum movement of 1.5 cm ensures smooth vertical deceleration at heel strike and an improved push-off with any foot system. This is possible because of the high performance spring that is made in three grades to meet individual needs of amputees. Torsional resilience is controlled by a thermo-plastic torsion rod, available in three grades (firm, medium, and easy). The maximum rotation is 30 degrees in both medial and lateral directions. The amount of rotation is determined by external torque applied to the knee, while the foot is loaded during stance. This feature is extremely valuable for sports requiring twisting of the body (e.g., tennis, golf).

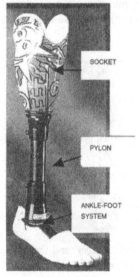

Fig. 4.118: The Endolite Below Knee System composed of three components: the suction type socket, the pylon and the foot-ankle system (http://www/endolite.com)

The demountable torque absorber allows up to 45 degrees of rotation in either direction (medial and lateral) from the neutral position. The rotation is resisted by an advanced plastic torsion element, which can be charged to give a stiffer or softer response to loading. The device contributes to the comfort of the prosthesis by limiting shear forces transmitted to the stump.

4.4.3 Transtibial Prosthesis

The basic difference between transfemoral and transtibial prostheses is that the later does not have any joints (Figure 4.118).

The transtibial prosthesis consists of three major components: the socket, the pylon, and the ankle-foot system (Figure 4.118). No transtibial prosthesis includes a mechanism to replicate the ankle joint, but does include elastic visco-elastic elements to absorb energy at heel impact, to store energy during the loading phase, "give back" energy during the push off, and to allow limited dorsi- and plantar flexion. The transtibial prosthesis allows limited inversion-eversion and medial-lateral rotation of the shank during the stance phase of walking.

The ankle-foot and socket considerations for the transfemoral prosthesis hold for the transtibial prosthesis.

The prosthesis for the subject with Syme's amputation is similar to the below-knee prosthesis except that the socket also serves as the shank (Figure 4.113, right). Because of the short space between the end of the stump and the floor, a special type of foot, usually a modification of one of the popular designs, has to be used. The prosthesis has the shape of the stump; hence, no other provision for suspension is necessary.

Two types of sockets are in general use: the plastic socket with an expandable liner and the plastic socket with a medial opening. Both types were designed for easy entry, yet they take advantage of the shape of the stump to provide suspension.

4.4.4 Hip-Disarticulation and Hemipelvectomy Prosthesis

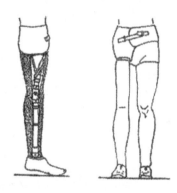

Fig. 4.119: Sketch of the hemipelectomy prosthesis.

Most of the components designed for above-knee prostheses are suitable for amputees who have lost function about the hip due to amputation just below the hip joint, at the hip joint (hip-disarticulation), or hemipelvectomy (when half of the pelvis has been removed). To provide good control of the leg, the artificial hip joint is placed on the front of the socket rather than opposite the anatomical hip joint; an arrangement that provides better control of the prosthesis (Figure 4.119).

For these prostheses, the socket is either made of laminated plastic or a thermoplastic, and the construction is usually modular that is, pylon or endoskeletal, because this type of construction results in a relatively lightweight prosthesis.

The hemipelvectomy prosthesis presents an added problem to the prosthetist because there is no ichial bone present to aid in weight bearing.

All of the instructions presented about use of the above-knee prosthesis apply equally to the hip-disarticulation and hemipelvectomy prostheses.

4.4.5 Preparatory Prosthesis

Fitting prosthesis to the stump as soon after surgery as possible helps to combat edema. A preparatory prosthesis is frequently used for several weeks or months until the stump has stabilized before the "permanent" or definitive prosthesis is provided.

The socket of the preparatory prosthesis may be made of either plaster-of-Paris or a plastic material and is attached to an artificial foot by a lightweight tube or strut, a pylon. When indicated, a suction socket is used. Most pylons are designed so that the alignment of the foot with respect to the socket can be changed when it is needed.

A belt about the waist is usually used to help keep the preparatory prosthesis on the stump properly. At least one prosthetic sock is worn between the socket and stump to provide for ventilation and general comfort. Prosthetic socks are used to prevent skin abrasion and to provide ventilation.

Regardless of the functions provided by the most sophisticated, mechanical devices, the most important factors in the usefulness of an artificial leg are fitting of the socket and alignment of the various parts with respect to the body and to each other. Fitting and alignments are difficult procedures that require a great deal of skill on the part of the prosthetist and a great deal of cooperation on the part of the amputee. During fitting and alignment of the first prosthesis, it is necessary to train the amputee in the basic principles of walking. The fitting affects alignment and *vice versa*, both affect comfort and function.

4.5 Artificial Hands and Arms

Pointing, reaching, and grasping allow humans to function independently and do many things that make them productive and enjoy many tasks of everyday life. Humans position the hand for all of the function by using the body and arm. Here we only discuss the arm. The shoulder joint provides for three degrees of freedom (flexion and extension, adduction and abduction, and medial and lateral rotation of the humerus), the elbow and forearm carry two degrees of freedom (flexion and extension, and pronation and supination of the forearm), and the wrist allows two degrees of freedom (dorsal and volar flexion, and radial and ulnar deviation). These seven possible rotations allow a human to bring the hand in the desired position and orient it in the appropriate direction. Total arm prosthesis would be a system with minimum six degrees of freedom and the grasping device. It will interface the trunk at the level "above" the shoulder. There is no total arm prosthesis available at this time. *Transhumeral prosthesis* is a replacement of the portion of the upper arm, the elbow, lower-arm, wrist, and the hand. It needs to functionally replace the positioning system of the elbow and wrist, in addition to allowing the grasping. Movement of the shoulder joint (e.g., moving the trunk and scapula) also helps the positioning of the hand. *The hand prosthesis* is a system that replaces a portion of the forearm, the wrist, and the hand. We will not discuss partial hand and finger prostheses.

4.5.1 Transhumeral Prosthesis

Transhumeral prosthesis interfaces the stump via a socket. Designing a socket follows the principles described in Section 4.4.1. The transhumeral prosthesis has to provide positioning of the hand and grasping, transport of the item grasped, and its eventual utilization. Grasping and positioning of the hand should not be separated, because there is a strong interaction between the type of the grasp and the approach trajectory that is the path of hand moving between the initial position and the target. In addition, once the object is grasped, the transport of the object is highly dependent on the object (e.g., cup of coffee, spoon, and fork).

The Elbow Joint

The artificial elbow joint should provide two degrees of freedom. One degree of freedom corresponds to the numeral rotation, while the other is for the forearm flexion and extension (Figure 4.120). The three joints to the right in Figure 4.120 are for endoskeletal designs, while the left one is for exoskeletal applications.

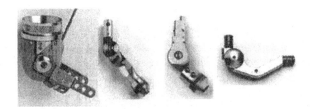

Fig. 4.120: Exoskeletal elbow mechanism (left), and endoskeletal mechanisms (right) for transhumeral prostheses (http://www.hosmer.com)

Both degrees of freedom should be powered and independently controlled. The body power or artificial actuators can drive the rotations.

The hinge for exoskeletal constructions can be realized by using different modules (Figure 4.121). Different constructions allow polycentric features, outside locking, or even flexible joints.

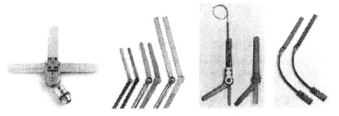

Fig. 4.121: The elbow joint components for assembling arm prostheses from left to right respectively: flexion abduction joint, single axis, outside locking and flexible hinges (http://www.hosmer.com)

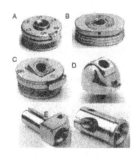

Fig. 4.122: The joints for articulation of the wrist: A) Quick Change Wrist, B) Oval Constant Friction Wrist, C) Flexion Friction Wrist, D) Sierra Wrist Flexion Unit, and E) Endoskeletal Wrists (http://www.hosmer.com)

The Wrist Joint

The wrist joint is to provide the correct orientation of the hand, assuming that the elbow and shoulder are able to bring the hand adequately close to the object to be grasped or handled. Two different construction are available: one-degree-of-freedom joint allowing pronation and supination (Figure 4.122, top panels), or two degrees of freedom allowing flexion and extension as well as pronation and supination (Figure 4.122, middle panels). Independent control of both joints is required for operation. Either artificial actuators or the body can power both degrees of freedom over the cables. The bottom panel (Figure 4.122) shows the endoskeletal wrist joints.

4.5.2 Artificial Hand

The split hook is a strong, lightweight, simple, functional, and reliable grasping device. It has functional shapes (narrow tips, flat gripping surface, specialized tool-holding grips), durability, and simplicity. Voluntary opening is as a control mechanism for most hooks so that the hook opens when the user activates it, and a spring closes it. Much of their simplicity is due to the fact that they have only one degree of freedom. Studies have been done to determine the useful acceptance of prostheses. The hook lacks cosmetic appeal, and it is difficult to stabilize some objects due to the shape and sometime insufficient force of the hook.

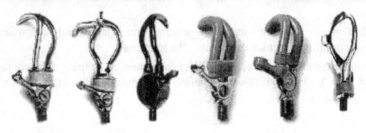

Fig. 4.123: Examples of commercially available hooks used for artificial arms from left to right respectively: Adult and LIO Adult Hook, Sierra Two Load Hook, Small Adult Hook, Child Hook and Contour Hook (http://www.hosmer.com)

The principle of operation is the force between the members opposed. The hooks are categorized as having a side opposition occurring transverse to the palm (Figure 4.123). They are structured so that a finer side opposition is available for precision grasping at the tips. The hooks do not have the surface area necessary for palm opposition, and their ability to pick up larger and irregularly shaped objects is limited. The contourhook (Hosmer Dorrance, CA) provides two neoprene covered curved fingers that can apply side opposition very much like the human thumb to the side of index finger. The Utah Split hook uses an improved design over standard split hook. The device has wider gripping surfaces than normal, and a special interlocking knife grip. The outside surface of the tips is urethane-rubber coated for increased friction. The side opposition is similar to the Hosmer Dorrance devices. The interlocking knife grip of the Utah hook allows the amputee to hold an object in opposition between the base of the two hooks. All hooks described can be opened volitionally, but they close by action of the spring with a predefined grasping force.

Artificial hands have a thumb and four fingers, although not all four are functional. They are covered with life-like cosmetic gloves that improve their appearance yet diminish their versatility. Most artificial hands have only one degree of freedom that can be driven by an electrical motor or a cable (body-power). Bilateral amputees do rarely use artificial hands because hooks are so much more functional. The mechanical hands are bulkier than the hooks. Without feedback, other than visual and auditory, amputees find them difficult to use. It is interesting, however, that many years after a multifunctional artificial hand [Rakić, 1964] has been clinically tested, this method has not been commercialized.

Several mechanical hands are presented in Figure 4.124. Dorrance Hand has a voluntary opening and includes the movable thumb, index, and middle fingers with adjustable closing force. The ring and little fingers do not move. The ARPL (Hosmer

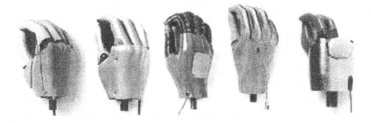

Fig. 4.124: Examples of commercially available mechanical hands from left to right respectively: Dorrance Hand, APRL Hand, Becker Imperial Hand, Becker Plylite Hand, and Mechanical Child Hand (http://www.hosmer.com)

Dorrance Corporation, CA) has voluntary closing and has two passive fingers as Dorrance Hand. The thumb can be pre-positioned in one of two positions, thus permitting the handling of a variety of objects. The ARPL is self-locking in any position. Becker Imperial and Becker Plylite Hands have similar functions to the Dorrance Hand, but a different construction (Hosmer Dorrance Corporation, CA).

The Mechanical Child Hand is designed for children between two and seven years of age (Figure 4.124, right). This device has two fingers and a thumb that articulates at the metacarpophalangeal joints. The nonfunctional ring and fifth fingers are passively mobile. The hand uses a voluntary opening four-bar linkage mechanism for adjusting the opening size. The fingers lock in a closed position.

Commercially available electric hands have a thumb and two fingers. The ring and fifth fingers are created by an inner glove, which covers and protects the mechanical and electronic parts. The Steeper Electric Hand (Hugh Steeper Ltd.) manufactures the hand in four different sizes. The movement of the thumb is in the plane parallel to the planes of movement of the index and middle fingers (opposition). The fingers are moved using a worm nut, being a self-locking mechanism.

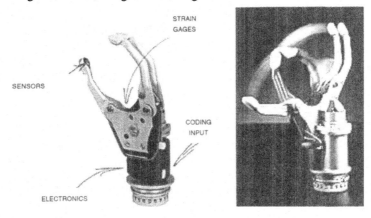

Fig. 4.125: The Sensor Hand (http://www.ottobock.com)

Otto Bock is for many years the leader in the field of myoelectric electric hands. Providing optimum subject care requires the meeting of different objectives, some of which are diametrically opposed. The demands for high functionality, durability, low susceptibility, high grip speed, and high grip power must be balanced with the desire for low weight, low power consumption, and an attractive appearance. Otto Bock Sensor Hand securely grasps any object, although it is a fragile and liquid–filled container (Figure 4.125). There is no need to keep a constant watch on the objects in the hand since the automatic grasping feature senses when an object is about to slip and makes necessary adjustments. The Flexi-Grip function gives the amputee a natural look and flexible grip. The hand is controlled by volitional contraction of muscles that are touching the socket. The electrodes are built into the socket. This hand is used with the passive wrist rotation with ratchet mechanism or optional friction wrist. The sensors in the Sensor Hand have been developed in co-operation with the Schweizerishe Unfall Versicheriung Anstalt (SUVA).

The Sensor Hand senses the change in the center of gravity and readjusts its grip automatically. The hand closes at maximum speed and grips an object with the least amount of force (10 N). When the contact of fingers and the object are sensed, the control changes to grip force control and increases the force to its maximum (100 N). Two programs can be executed: 1) controlling the opening speed by the strength of the muscle signal (contraction) in addition to controlling the closing speed based on a decrease in muscle tension, and 2) controlling both speed by the strength of the muscle contraction.

Electrohand 2000 is a children system (Figure 4.126). This system has a different mechanical design compared with the Sensor Hand and it is meant for children from 18 months to 13 years of age (five sizes). The device has minimal weight (light metal construction); natural appearance with balanced proportions, integrated with the myoelectric control, and miniaturized drive unit. Maximum force can be up to 55 N, and the mass with the cosmetic glove is less than 130 grams. The basic difference is the new type of grip motion, which ensures better visual contact of the process of grasping.

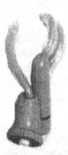

Fig 4.126: The Electrohand children system (http://www.ottobock.com)

4.5.3 Activity Specific Artificial "Hand"

This prosthetic option is designed specifically for activities in which the use of a passive, body-powered, electrically powered, or hybrid prosthesis would place unacceptable limitations on function or durability. Often this type of prosthesis is recreational in nature, but prostheses have been designed for such activities as art and work-related tasks.

Most common are the prostheses designed for fishing, swimming, golfing, hunting, bicycle riding, and work in the field. The real disadvantage to this prosthetic option is that its specificity limits what other activities can be performed outside of its intended use. Hayden & Preston System (HPS) are highly specialized in specific, artificial "hands" (Texas Assistive Devices, LLC, http://www.tgn.net/~pbetts/, is manufacturer and distributor of the HPS). The devices are modular and specially

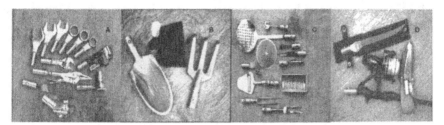

Fig. 4.127: Activity specific HPS terminal devices for artificial arm/hand systems: A) tools, B) gardening, C) cooking, D) hunting and fishing (Hayden & Preston Company, http://www/TAD.com)

designed to allow active life. The HPS is the only interchangeable prosthetic tool system in the world today that features a terminal device with a pitch adjustment of 45° including 360° rotation.

The universal push button quick insert-release terminal device is capable of utilizing a wide selection of custom designed and crafted tools and implements. Because of the unique design of the HPS, it allows the user to perform jobs, chores, and duties that he or she would not be able to perform otherwise. However, what exactly makes the HPS the product of choice can be easily seen from Figure 4.127. Although the HPS is relatively new, it has been introduced in everyday life due to positive feedback from many healthcare providers.

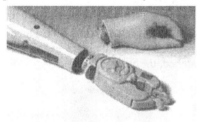

Fig. 4.128: The Electrogreifer. Terminal device designed by Otto Bock (http://www.otto bock.com)

Another commercially available device is the Otto Bock Electrogreifer (Figure 4.128). This device has more adjustable power and gripping surface than other grippers do. This device is especially suitable for persons engaged in skilled trades. The device is combined with the precision Dynamic Mode Control (DMC) significantly extending functional capabilities. DMC allows proportional control of both grip speed and grip force. The Greifer facilitates everyday life for work and hobby activities.

4.5.4 Passive Arm-hand Prosthesis

The simplest solution for replacing an amputated arm and hand is to provide a cosmetic duplication of the contralateral natural counterpart (Figure 4.129). This replacement of what was lost from amputation or congenital deficiency is similar in appearance to the non-affected arm and hand, but it does not carry adequate function. There are many amputees who prefer these simple systems, because they are very good by their subjective measures in performing all the tasks with their unaffected hand; hence, using the prosthesis does not improve their functioning and quality of life. These types of prostheses are often lighter than other prosthetic options and require minimal maintenance because they have very few moving parts. However, they do not allow performing activities that require bilateral grasping. A cosmetic prosthesis is called a passive prosthesis because it is non-functional in sense of the ability to grasp objects.

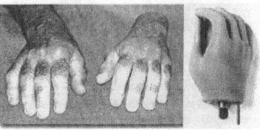

Fig. 4.129: Human hand (left), passive hand prosthesis with the silicon cosmetic glove (middle), and Hosmer Dorrance passive prosthesis (right) (http://www.hosmer.com)

Cosmetic restoration is achieved using the following materials: rigid polyvinyl chloride (PVC), flexible latex, or silicone rubber (Figure 4.130). Latex covering is the most common material utilized for cosmetic restorations. Thin latex material comes in pre-made sizes called gloves to fit over most available prosthetic hands. A glove is most often provided in a solid color that can be enhanced by custom painted details (e.g., nails and age spots). Partial hand restorations can be made with this material and often utilize a zipper in the palmar surface to allow the subject to easily don and doff, but still have the stability and confidence that the prosthesis is firmly attached. The advantages to this material are the lightweight and price, yet the disadvantage is that latex easily stains permanently. Rigid PVC covering is used on individuals with amputations or deficiencies above the wrist. A comprehensive line of rigid PVC gloves (e.g., Hosmer Dorrance Corporation, Campbell, CA) in a variety of colors and sizes is advantageous compared with latex because, if scratched, the color is retained.

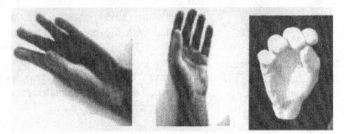

Fig. 4.130: Cosmetic covers for the hand and arm prostheses made of latex (left and middle) and silicone rubber (right) (http://www.hosmer.com)

Silicone rubber covering has recently been refined for upper extremity applications, and it provides the most realistic and long-lasting solution (Figure 4.130). Silicone allows the duplication of texture, size, and shape; it does not stain and lasts between three to five years. Silicone is heavier than latex and suitable only with endoskeletal prostheses.

4.5.5 Body-powered Prosthesis

Gross body movement controls a body-powered prosthesis, sometimes called a conventional prosthesis. The movement of the shoulder, upper-arm, or chest is

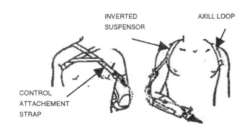

Fig. 4.131: Trans-Radial Figure 8 Harness.

captured by a harness system (Figures 4.131 and 4.132), which is attached to a cable that is connected to a terminal device (hook or hand).

For some levels of amputation or deficiency, an elbow system can be added to provide the amputee additional function. An amputee must possess at least one or more of the following gross body movements: glenohumeral flexion, scapular abduction or adduction, shoulder depression and elevation, and chest expansion in order to control body-powered prosthesis. In addition, sufficient residual limb length and sufficient musculature must exist. A body-powered prosthesis has a simple design; it is highly durable and can be used for tasks that involve water and dust and in other potentially hazardous environments.

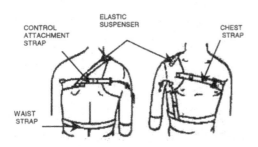

Fig 4.132: Shoulder disarticulation with chest strap.

There are two types of controls for body-powered hands and hooks, voluntary opening and voluntary closing: voluntary opening gives the subject grasping control even when he/she is relaxed. The tradeoff for this is limited grip force, often less than 30 Newton. Voluntary closing allows the subject to have substantially greater grip force, often over 150 Newton, but does not allow the subject to relax without losing grasp.

Many amputees who wear a body-powered prosthesis develop increased control due a phenomenon called extended proprioception. Extended proprioception gives the wearer feedback as to the position of the terminal device. The subject will know whether the hook is open or closed by how much pressure the harness is exerting on his or her shoulder area without having to visually inspect the operation. The maintenance is related to broken control cables, replacement harnesses, and realignment of terminal devices, which are very economical. An important element is that since there are no motors, the operation is silent. The most common complaint of amputees using body-powered prosthesis is the uncomfortable and restrictive control harness. The harness must capture the movement of the shoulder and suspend the prosthesis; thus, a tight harness is required sometimes leading to a restricted range of motion and the functional envelope.

The functional envelope, also called workspace, is the area in space where the subject can control the prosthesis. The workspace, when wearing a body-powered prosthesis, is often limited to a position directly in front of them from waist level to mouth level. It is very difficult to control the prosthesis out to the side, down by the feet, and above the head. Some amputees do not like the cosmetic appearance of the hook and control cables, and they request a "natural-like" part of the body replacement.

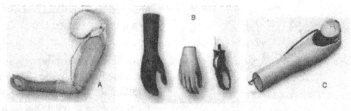

Fig. 4.133: An example of a Body-Powered Prosthesis. A) The complete system, B) Gripper with the cosmetic cover, C) powered elbow joint. (http://www.ottobock.com)

An example of the body-powered prostheses (Figure 4.133) includes a triple control system. This makes it possible to bend and extend the arm in the elbow joint in addition to hand function. Transmission of the motion by means of own power is well accepted by the users. The prosthesis can include various grippers, but it is most frequently used with the system hand that is manufactured in both voluntarily open (VO) and voluntarily close (VC) modalities. The hand and the silicone cosmetic cover are available in 18 sizes.

4.5.6 Electrically Powered Prosthesis

Electrically powered prosthesis uses electrical power to provide function. The electrical power is applied via motors located in the terminal device (hand or hook), wrist, and elbow (Figure 4.134). The grip force of the hand can be in excess of 100 Newton.

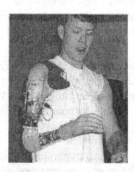

Fig. 4.134: The electrically powered artificial arm (http://www.armdynamics.com)

Command signals are generated either by voluntary contraction of muscles, so-called myoelectric control, or by using switches of different kinds. For applications that are more complex, both command signals are used for different operations (e.g., control of several degrees of freedom).

Myoelectric control is a very popular command method. It relies on the ability of the amputee to generate voluntary contraction of a muscle that he or she would normally use for the same function before the disability, or some other synergistic muscle at his/her subconscious level. Muscle contraction can be registered by recording of the electrical activity of muscles. The electric activity, so-called electromyogram (EMG), can be recorded accurately if the appropriate technology is used. EMG is a small voltage that has to be carefully extracted from "electrical noise". Using transducers, called electrodes, that contact the surface of the skin or are implanted under the skin, the EMG signal can be recorded, amplified, and then processed in real-time.

Many people prefer this type of control because it only requires the wearer to contract his muscles. This eliminates the need for a tight, often uncomfortable control harness. Another advantage of a myoelectric prosthesis is that because it does not require a control cable or harness, a cosmetic skin can be applied in either latex or silicone, greatly enhancing the cosmetic restoration.

The amputee can also operate the prosthesis over his head, down by his feet, and out to his side, all being almost impossible with a body-powered prosthesis. A myoelectrically controlled prosthesis also eliminates the suspension harness by using one of two suspension techniques: skeletal/soft tissue lock or suction.

A skeletal/soft tissue lock is a technique that involves designing the socket in such a way that it compresses in areas around the elbow or wrist to provide suspension. Suction suspension is achieved by fabricating the socket with a valve. Once the subject has donned the socket, the valve creates negative pressure inside the socket, providing adequate suspension.

The electrically powered prosthesis uses batteries, which require a certain amount of maintenance (charging, discharging, eventual disposal, and replacement). The electrically powered prosthesis is heavier than other prosthetic options. When properly fit and fabricated, electrically powered prostheses require no more maintenance than other prosthetic options. However, logistic support is required for longevity, leading to much higher costs.

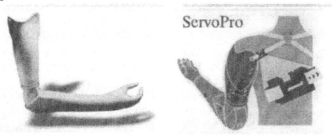

Fig. 4.135: The Utah Arm 2 (left), and ServoPro control system for amputees with the shoulder disarticulation or other severe bilateral disability (right).

Several companies produce quality myoelectric controllers, electric hands, wrists, and electric elbows. Motion Control from Utah offers the Utah Arm 2 for the transhumeral amputees (Figure 4.135). The Utah arm and hand system for transhumeral amputees allows sensitive control of elbow, hand, and wrist (optional) using only two muscles. The exclusive myoelectric system of Motion Control eliminates cables, letting the amputee move the arm and hand slowly or quickly in any position, ultimately leading to a more natural response with less effort. From forequarter to shoulder disarticulation, the mobility and fine-tuning of the Utah Arm allow any subject to achieve maximum function. Many amputees learn very fast to control the system. The Utah Arm, combined with its high performance hand control, supplies the wearer with superior cosmetic appearance. Smooth exterior hand covers provide natural look. For rugged tasks, the hand can be changed to another hand or terminal device. The optional electrically driven wrist joint allows hand pronation and supination. Proportional or on-off myoelectric controls are both available based on the subject's request and abilities.

The ServoPro is an exclusive feature of the Utah Arm (Figure 4.135). This system is designed for amputees with shoulder disarticulation, interscapulothorasic, or brachial plexus injuries. The ServoPro eliminates the electrodes normally required to operate the Utah Arm. The system may be the only option, which can provide functional control of both elbow and hand. The ServoPro is based on a harness, but instead of cables, electronic components are pushed and pulled to generate command signals that will control the electrically powered prosthesis. The ServoPro requires much smaller excursion of movement and less effort compared with body-powered cables in equivalent mechanical systems. The servo control is accurate, and it uses feedback from sensors in the elbow and hand.

4.5.7 Hybrid Prosthesis

The hybrid prosthesis often utilizes a body-powered elbow and a myoelectrically controlled terminal device - hook or hand (Figure 4.136). If desired by the wearer, a myoelectrically controlled wrist and a cosmetic restoration of the forearm and hand may also be included. Another type of hybrid prosthesis combines an electrically powered elbow with a body-powered hook or hand. While shoulder disarticulation level amputations or deficiencies have been fit with hybrid prostheses, these cases should be carefully considered because of the amount of gross body movement needed to operate this type of prosthesis and the EMG signal interference created during such movement.

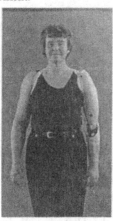

Fig. 4.136: The Hybrid transhumeral (Ergo Arm) prosthesis (http://www.ottobock.com)

There are several unique advantages to a hybrid prosthesis. Most important is the ability to simultaneously control elbow flexion and extension while opening or closing the electric hand/hook or while rotating the wrist. The other prosthetic options generally require the wearer to control one function at a time (flex the elbow, lock the elbow, open or close the terminal device). The hybrid prosthesis weighs less and is less expensive than a similar prosthesis with an electrically powered elbow and hand. The same disadvantages apply for the hybrid and the prosthetic options, which it incorporates.

The Ergo arm (Otto Bock) belongs to the group of hybrid prostheses (Figure 4.136). It uses the new 12K44 Elbow system (Figure 4.133), which can be unlocked or locked in any position, even under loads up to 250 N. A slight pull on the cable, lowers the forearm gradually. Releasing the cable immediately locks the elbow in that position. For normal locking or unlocking, the cable has to be pulled stronger. The elbow is designed to support myoelectric hand; there is a container for the battery and connectors for the cables coming from the sensor electrodes above the elbow and the wrist/hand system. When the prosthetic arm is extended, the system stores the energy to facilitate flexion. The arm swings smoothly while walking. Subject-adjustable counterbalance makes the arm feel lighter, even with an electric wrist and terminal device.

4.5.8 Artificial Extremities - Summary

The artificial leg is a morphological and functional replacement of the natural counterpart. The leg should provide the following functions during level walking: balance and support during the stance phase, and rotation around the hip joint in the knee-flexed position during the swing. The stance phase starts with the heel strike. The heel strike is an impact to the body; large forces are transmitted through the leg. It is important to allow absorption of at least a portion of energy, thereby, minimize the forces acting at the stump and the hip. This will be best achieved by allowing the knee buckling after the heel strike and using a shock absorbing material at the heel and in the pylon. The knee-buckle happening in parallel with the progression of the center of the body mass brings the foot in the horizontal position (foot-flat). The progression of the center of mass will raise the heel, in parallel with straitening of the knee. In the final phase of the stance, push-off requires energy, which is in nature generated with powerful ankle and toe extensor muscles. The swing phase is a process where the knee is flexing and then extending to the almost full extension. The flexion and extension may require energy from actuators (muscles) for some speeds of progression.

The transtibial prostheses described above provide most of the functions. The pylon is capable of absorbing energy, artificial foot can store energy, which will be released during the push-off phase, and flexibility of the ankle-foot system allows the transition from heel strike to foot-flat. The subjects can adjust their muscular activity at the hip and knee joints to compensate for imperfection of the biomechanics of the transtibial prosthesis. Therefore, many amputees can run, play sports, hop, dance, and do almost all, what they would be able to do if being able-bodied.

The transfemoral prosthesis with microcomputer control of the knee joint controlling both the stance and swing phase can do much; yet because of no power in the knee joint, the walking has to be adapted, and asymmetry will occur ultimately leading to increased metabolic energy cost and rate and cardiovascular stress. Integrating the most advanced pylon and torsion absorber could impose instability of the knee, leading to an unsafe feeling while walking; thus, transfemoral prosthesis in most cases incorporates somewhat stiffer pylon and ankle-foot system.

The application of prostheses starts to be more complex when subjects are to walk stairs, slope, and uneven terrain. Walking downstairs and down the slope requires the controlled flexion of the knee joint, and the flexion is totally dependent on the environmental conditions. James *et al.,* [1991] introduced a microcomputer control of the hydraulic system effecting stiffness in both flexion and extension from free to lock states. C-leg from Otto Bock, Germany is the first microprocessor-controlled knee joint which incorporates some of these features. Electronic sensors supply basic data for stance-phase stability and stance-phase control. This is the closest approximation to natural gait where subjects no longer have to think about walking. Walking upstairs and up slopes requires a powered knee joint, which is still not commercially available, neither developed for experimental purposes to the satisfaction of researchers, clinical, and over all potential users. Powered transfemoral prostheses have been suggested [Popović and Schwirtlich, 1988; Popović *et al.,* 1991b], but the technology and control have not been adequate.

There are two applications where the powered leg will make the difference: hip disarticulation and bilateral amputees. In both cases, amputees are not able to generate movement of the thigh that is required to drive the under-powered system; hence, the externally powered knee joint will compensate for lack of power by the user.

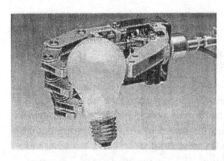

Fig. 4.137: The Southampton hand. The five-finger, multifunctional artificial hand (http://www.soton.ac.uk)

Prosthetics is an obviously emotive issue, as the absence of a limb, either by amputation or by congenital defect, is a highly visible "disability" Despite this prejudice, many of those with congenital defects do not consider themselves disabled, or in need of a prosthesis, due to their existing ability to adapt to the surrounding environment or tasks. Others, including the majority of amputees, often wish to regain at least some of the functionality, or more simply the appearance lost with the limb, by the use of a prosthesis. However, the potential use of functional prostheses, or cybernetic system involving an interface between man and machine, is also sometimes viewed as unnatural or unappealing. Consequently, to issue such as anthropomorphism becomes as critical in prosthesis design as the size, weight, and power consumption of the device. The current commercial hand prostheses have extremely limited performance compared with the able-bodied arm and hand.

The Southampton Artificial Hand has been in existence for several decades, and is based upon the original hypothesis for the development of a hierarchically controlled, myoelectric prosthesis. The mechanics of the Southampton hand has undergone several stages, however, the main hypothesis remained the same (Figure 4.137). Vast quantities of information are utilized to form a stable and comfortable grip in able-bodied humans. The grip is constantly adjusted to prevent the slip, deforming or crushing of the object, and incorrect orientation (e.g., spilling the content of a container). In all systems described above the grasping force is pre-selected based on experience, and rarely voluntarily adjusted based on visual feedback. The philosophy behind the development of the Southampton hand is to come with the adaptive, mechanical structure that uses sensors and intelligent control to generate optimum grip. The basis of the control is a finite state of modeling and use of synergistic model of movement of fingers and the thumb [Chappell and Kyberd, 1991; Kyberd and Chappell, 1994]. The hand has five functioning digits and four degrees of freedom. The index finger acts independently from the other three fingers, which move in tandem. The other two degrees of freedom are in the thumb. Slip transducers are built in the pads of the fingers.

The Utah/MIT, hand built in the early eighties, [Jacobsen et al., 1982, 1989] has four fingers, each having four degrees of freedom (Figure 4.138). Control of 16 degrees of freedom is performed at a "high" level in a powerful computer. The movements are generated by cables very much alike the tendons applied in a human hand. The Stanford/JPL hand was built to be able to exert arbitrary forces or impress arbitrary small motions on the grasped object when the joints are allowed to move, and to be able to "freeze" the object by locking all joints [Salisbury, 1985; Salisbury and Craig, 1982]. A three-fingered solution, each finger having three links, has been designed. Tendon-like driving of joints was incorporated, and a powerful computer was controlling the operation of this dexterous robot hand. The Belgrade/USC hand with its five mechanically coupled fingers (Figure 4.139) and three degrees of freedom uses a somewhat different concept of grasping [Rakić, 1989; Tomović et al., 1987].

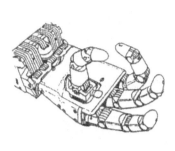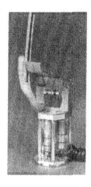

Fig. 4.138: The Utah/MIT hand (left) and the Belgrade/USC hand (right) developed for intelligent robotics.

The security of grasping benefits from maximizing the contact surface or number of contact points. The double rocker mechanism allows the adaptation of three joints at each finger (Figure 4.138). The Belgrade/USC hand is powered with three electrical motors housed in the hand, and sensory feedback is provided by slip and pressure sensors built in the finger pads. The original version of the Belgrade hand was built about 35 years ago [Rakić, 1965; Tomović and Boni, 1962] and provided excellent five finger articulation using only one DC motor, myoelectric control, and included sensory feedback, yet was not transferred to rehabilitation of amputees mostly because of the logistic support.

There is an obvious discrepancy between the concepts and the state of the art of prosthesis used in everyday life. One should bare in mind that more than 50 percent of amputees decide not to use the prosthesis at all and that the majority of prosthetic users prefer a hook to the artificial hand. There are several reasons, but among them, we would rank the cost/benefit reason to be the most important. The quality of life with the very sophisticated dexterous hand is not that much different compared with simple systems; thus, in order to improve the situation, the research has to provide better systems by greatly improving the interface, allow control of the system at subconscious level, improve the reliability and safety, and make it more human-like.

5. External Control of Movement

> "The difference between the hand of a man and the hand of a monkey lies not so much in the movement which the arrangements of muscles, bones and joints make possible, but in the purposive volitional movement which under ordinary circumstances the animal habitually exercise."
>
> Frederick Wood-Jones [1920]

Control is present in all domains of human activities and life processes. In spite of the extreme diversity of control tasks, a few basic features are common to all of them. Control always implies: 1) an object, the plant, which may be hard, soft, biological, or mechanical, whose behavior can be modified by change of the input; 2) the set of allowed input comprising at least two options; and 3) an optimization criterion. If any element is missing, control is not realizable [Tomović et al., 1995]. Any kind of control, mechanical or biological, has at its disposal a limited set of control input determined by the constraints inherent to the nature of the plant. Applying control beyond the limits set by constraints may be even disastrous. The concept of optimization is essential for the understanding of control. A dynamical system may change its states in a continuous way (e.g., the arm can reach a target in an infinite number of trajectories, the legs can move at many ways during the swing, yet providing the same speed of the walking and the same stride length). Without an optimization criterion, all trajectories of a dynamical system are equivalent. The term trajectory has a broad meaning; it refers to the way the system coordinates variations in the course of transition from the current to the next state. An optimization criterion assigns a value to each transition trajectory or to a subset of trajectories so that they can be arranged in the order of preference. In some cases, the trajectories of the dynamical system may be well ordered so that a single solution is best. Such a trajectory is called the optimal solution. Instances, where optimal solutions of control tasks exist or can be analytically determined, are relatively rare, yet the term is often used rather loosely in every day life.

Once the control task has been fixed, its solution, whether heuristic, computed, or analytical, must be determined. The development of optimization procedures appropriate for different classes of control problems is the main concern of control theory. What the phrase "solution of the control problem" means, is easily understood from the definition of control. Solution procedures for the control task must be able to assign value tags, numerical or not, to the allowed set of transition trajectories of the plant so that they can be partially or fully ordered. The controller then enforces the plant to follow the desired course. It goes without saying that different optimization criteria will induce different ordering relations of control input. This fact is crucial for the understanding of dynamical processes. All potential transition trajectories are equivalent. Only under the impact of an optimization criterion, some of the otherwise equivalent plant responses are becoming privileged. Without control, the systems, mechanical or biological, are free to evolve along any of the feasible courses.

5.1 Overview of Control Systems for Movement

The human musculoskeletal (mechanical) system being controlled is referred to as the plant. The configuration of the system at any instant in time comprises *the plant states*. Components that power the system (plant) are called *the actuators* (e.g., muscles). The signals driving the actuators are *the controls* (e.g., bursts of pulses carrying electrical charge to intact motoneurons generated by central nervous system or neuroprosthesis). *The controller* is the system, which generates the controls. The time histories of the plant states in response to the control signals is referred to as the system *trajectory* (e.g., the joint-angle time histories) [Tashman and Zajac, 1992].

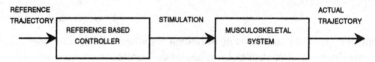

Fig. 5.1: The organization of an open-loop (reference-based) control system.

Open-loop controllers can be designed to function without knowledge of the actual plant trajectory as shown in Figure 5.1. Open-loop controller delivers command signals based on precomputed sequences; thus, if there is any perturbation or imperfection in the model or trajectory, an error will occur. An open-loop controller, also termed reference-based controller aim to ensure that the system follows the desired, so called reference trajectory. In the case of NP precomputed sequences are patterns of stimulation for the appropriate muscles and/or command signals for the orthosis actuators. Muscle stimulation patterns are heuristically determined (humans expertise) or computer generated by simulating movement. It is necessary to use a model of the plant characterized by the individualized set of parameters and the trajectory defined in the state space. Computer algorithms are used to find stimulation patterns, which will generate movement along the desired trajectory, believed to fulfill the motor task requirements. These algorithms use inverse dynamics to calculate stimulation patterns from an inverse of the musculo-skeletal system model and a set of trajectories known to accomplish the desired motor task.

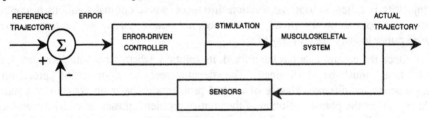

Fig. 5.2: The organization of a closed-loop (error-driven) control system.

Regardless of design method and implementation, the performance of any open-loop control system will probably be inadequate, since disturbances will cause performance to deviate significantly and lead to catastrophic behavior. A disturbance is any unexpected condition or event encountered by the plant. An externally controlled movement is likely to encounter such disturbances (e.g., walking over uneven terrain, spasm, fatiguing of muscles). Even in the absence of disturbances, open-loop control will probably be inadequate, since musculoskeletal properties can not be perfectly modeled even if they are perfectly understood.

To correct for disturbances and musculoskeletal modeling errors, a *closed-loop controller* with ongoing knowledge of the effects of the disturbance must be designed. Sensors (e.g., joint-angle sensors, contact force sensors) provide signals from which the current state of the system can be estimated, and fed back to the controller (Figure 5.2). Closed-loop controllers are error driven; they respond to the trajectory error, which is determined by comparing the actual and the desired trajectories. The term error-driven is used to describe that the input signal to the controller is the error. Closed loop control systems are suited to tasks where the desired trajectories are constant or slowly changing (e.g., control of posture).

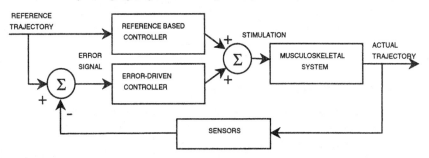

Fig. 5.3 The organization of an reference-based feedback control system.

To control tasks where trajectories change rapidly, yet predictably (e.g., walking, reaching), reference and error driven control are applied in parallel (Figure 5.3). Such control utilizes open-loop to generate an approximate trajectory, and a feedback to correct for errors resulting from disturbances and modeling errors. If the body deviates too far from the desired trajectory the stored controls would interfere with the feedback controller. This situation arises because the reference-based controller functions independently from the feedback controller and cannot adjust its stored stimulation patterns during the task.

Model-based controllers (Figure 5.4) are more robust; they utilize sensors and a dynamic model of the system to continuously recalculate the "desired" trajectory in order to accomplish the task. For example, during walking, if the body is following the desired path, the model-based controller generates the same muscle stimulation pattern as a reference-based controller designed with inverse dynamics. If the body deviates from the desired path, the model-based controller calculates a new path and generates a new muscle stimulation pattern which, according to the dynamic model, should maintain or restore stable walking. The complexity and computational requirements of model-based control continue to limit its application to simple problems.

In principle, closed-loop control has many advantages for NP compared to the application of open-loop systems. A closed-loop control system can automatically compensate for small disturbances and consequent trajectory errors. Closed-loop control regulates system behavior more precisely than open-loop control, for example, by smoothing the movement during walking and reducing the amount of stimulation [Marsolais and Edwards, 1988]. Such regulation may then result in efficient NP-controlled walking systems, since over stimulation and excessive torque production may be responsible for the high energy cost observed during NP tasks [Marsolais and Kobetič, 1987]. For example, a closed-loop system with both position and force feedback could be designed to provide stiffness control, being very important for grasping. Stiffness control specifies not only the desired position for a joint, but also the amount of force required to move the joint from that position. Stiffness control may be energetically inefficient because of cocontraction of muscles, yet it may reject disturbances and regulate limb interaction with the environment well enough [Crago et al., 1991; Hogan, 1984, 1985]. The feedback can also be used to detect potential falls in walking systems, thereby either act to compensate and correct the condition, or shift to a "safety" mode program that will reduce the chances of injury.

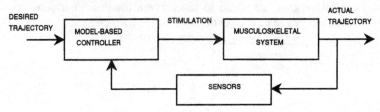

Fig. 5.4: The organization of the model-based control system.

The benefits of closed-loop control over the open-loop control are clear, yet one should keep in mind that the muscles act with delay, and in many applications the delay in generating the force is comparable with the duration of the movement. Closed-loop control systems require sensors and they are more complex to design and implement compared to open-loop controllers. Improper design can lead to instability, resulting in unpredictable and potentially dangerous performance. Controllers for "simple" (single-input, single-output) systems can be designed without a detailed knowledge of the plant.

A *dynamic model* is a set of equations that emulate the behavior of the physical system. Dynamic models specify how the current states of the system (e.g., body trajectories) depend on the past (e.g., the prior body trajectories and muscle forces). The inputs to a dynamic model of a human motor task are the muscle stimulation patterns, and the outputs are the computed body trajectories.

$$\dot{X} = f(X,U)$$
$$Y = g(X,U)$$

The differential equations can be written using a so-called Cauchy form. The left side of the first equation comprises first derivatives of the state variables (vector X). The left side of the second equation, vector Y comprises the output variables. The right sides of equations are nonlinear function f and g describing the plant dynamics. Vector U consists of the control variables.

A dynamic model of a human limb comprises three parts as described later. Muscle dynamics are specified by a set of differential and constraint equations that describe how neural stimulation patterns produce force in biological actuators [Zajac, 1989]. Muscle force to joint torque conversion is specified by a set of algebraic equations based on musculoskeletal geometry (*i.e.*, the physical arrangement of bones and joints and the attachment points of muscles and tendons to the skeleton). Finally, joint torques produce movement of the limb segments and the external objects connected to the body as dictated by segmental dynamics, which are specified by another set of differential and constraint equations (sometimes these equations are referred to as the equations of movement of the system).

Dynamic models are required because the movement of multi segmental systems, such as the human body, is so complex that even the qualitative effects of muscle forces cannot be predicted without the use of such models [Tashman et al., 1995]. For example, each muscle in general acts to cause an angular acceleration of every joint in the body because of the dynamic coupling of forces acting on one segment to accelerate another due to the articulations among the segments. Consider the equations of movement (or segmental dynamics) describing the movement of the body segments during standing-and walking [Khang and Zajac 1989 a and b; Yamaguchi and Zajac, 1990]. There are n equations, where n equals the number of degrees of freedom (DOF) of the system. The number of DOF is equal to the number of coordinates required to fully specify the position and orientation of all the segments of the body and all the objects touching the body, as determined by the number of segments and objects and the nature of the connections (joints) among the segments and objects [Kane and Levinson, 1985]. The n equations can be represented in vector form:

$$\ddot{\theta} = A^{-1}(\theta)[M_a + M_{in}(\theta,\dot{\theta}) + M_g(\theta)]$$

where, θ is the vector of joint angles, M_a, M_{in}, and M_g are the active, inertial and gravity force based torque respectively, and A^{-1} is the inverse matrix of the system. The muscle torque contribution is a vector of the torques produced by muscles spanning the joints. These torques are multiplied by A^{-1}, an inverse of the system matrix $A_{n \times n}$. A is time variable, it depends on the inertial properties of the system, but also from the positions of the system components, which vary during the movement (e.g., trigonometric functions of joint angles). When A^{-1} has only diagonal elements, then a muscle would cause angular acceleration of only the joint it spans. A^{-1} is generally a full matrix with significant off-diagonal terms, and therefore, muscles induce angular acceleration of many (sometime all) joints of the body. Biarticular muscles (muscles crossing two joints) could accelerate a joint they span in a direction opposite to their torque at the corresponding joints. The net direction of the angular acceleration of each joint is the direction resulting from all the torque. The net direction depends on body posture, body morphometry, and the relative magnitude of the two or more joint torques acting simultaneously.

Dynamic coupling can also alter the apparent action of a muscle crossing a single joint, if the joint has more than one DOF. For example, as it is described in Chapter 1, muscles crossing ball-and socket joints (three DOF) can generate an angular acceleration in a direction different from the direction of the muscle torque [e.g., Mansour and Pereira, 1987]. Thus, the precise action of a muscle in a multijoint, multi-DOF system is not always obvious, and can change during a task as the angles of the joint change.

Inverting the dynamic model to determine the muscle stimulation pattern that will produce a desired action is called inverse dynamics, since the inputs and outputs are reversed (the Russian literature dealing with Mechanics, Theory of Mechanisms, and Robotics terms the procedure of determining the forces and torque from the given trajectory the direct problem). The result of the simulation is the stimulation pattern that should theoretically drive muscles, thereby the system along the desired trajectory in the absence of disturbances. Some degree of modeling error is unavoidable, since dynamic models can never perfectly represent musculoskeletal systems, and the trajectory of the actual musculoskeletal system will differ from the one predicted by the model.

Developing a reference-based controller with inverse dynamics is not straightforward, because the controller equations cannot be determined merely by "flipping around" the dynamic model, since musculoskeletal geometry is generally noninvertible. That is, muscle forces are not uniquely determined from joint torque, though muscle forces uniquely specify joint-torque. When, for example, the human lower limb had only one muscle pulling in each direction at each joint, then the muscle forces required to produce a specified set of joint torque would be unique. However, different muscle force combinations can meet the required joint torque. The task of distributing a net joint torque among all the muscles crossing the joint is referred to as the muscle redundancy, or muscle force distribution problem.

One solution to the muscle redundancy problem is to replace all the muscles contributing to movement by a single, so called equivalent muscle [Bouisset, 1973]. Because muscle strength and endurance is limited (particularly for NP muscle), this approach is unfeasible. A commonly used method is to use static optimization, which requires that a construction is specified. The cost function is necessary for optimization. The cost function is a measure of the performance of a system. Minimizing (or maximizing) the cost function one selects the optimal solution (trajectory), therefore secures the best performance. The cost function can include any of the physical quantities being part of the process (e.g., time, energy, force, torque, jerk, fatigue, muscle activation, non-physiological loading, number of muscles used for the task, tracking error, and any combination of those) [Crowninshield and Brand, 1981a and b; Pederson *et al.*, 1987; Khang and Zajac, 1989a].

To obtain a solution that guarantees optimality over the entire task, dynamic optimization must be used, where a performance criterion applicable to the entire task is minimized. Using a dynamic model of the whole system, including a model of the biological actuator dynamics, a dynamic optimization algorithm finds the muscle stimulation pattern that provides the best performance. Although methods to solve dynamic optimization problems are few, and computations needed to find a solution many, dynamic optimization is conceptually very powerful and has been used to study lower limb tasks, including walking [Davy and Audu, 1987; Hatze, 1976; Oğuztöreli *et al.*, 1994; Popović *et al.*, 1999b].

Dynamic optimization can assist in the design of reference-based controllers. Muscle stimulation patterns providing the best performance, as determined by the dynamic optimization algorithm, would be stored in the controller before implementation of the NP system. These stimulation patterns should provide smooth, efficient movement, since they would have been designed to account for the dynamic interactions of the musculoskeletal components. Error-driven closed-loop control would still have to be implemented to compensate for modeling errors and disturbances.

Dynamic optimization can provide the basis to design a model-based optimal controller. An optimal controller is like a continually updated reference based controller. If sensors indicate significant deviations from the desired trajectory, the controller solves a dynamic optimization problem to determine a new path, which will bring the body from its current position back to the desired trajectory, while maintaining balance and stability. The future muscle stimulation pattern is computed based on the newly determined path. This scheme requires many dynamic optimizations and other computations at speeds beyond current software and hardware capabilities.

5.1.1 Modeling of the Musculoskeletal System

The human limb is generally modeled as a set of rigid limb segments, whose movements relative to each other are defined by the joint articulations (*i.e.*, skeletal geometry and ligamentous constraints). The interaction of external forces (e.g., gravity) and environmental constraints (e.g., ground, object) with the body segments also has to be modeled. The modeled segments and how they interact with the environment together define the body segmental dynamics. Human-generated power is provided to the segments via an assumed set of biological actuators, which generate forces that act on the segments (musculo-tendon dynamics). How much force an actuator generates depends on the relative position and movement of the segments, which is defined by musculoskeletal geometry. The direction of each musculo-tendon force relative to the segments (again defined by musculoskeletal geometry) affects the direction the segments will accelerate due to that force. The musculoskeletal system thus consists of three major elements: body segmental dynamics, musculoskeletal geometry, and biological actuator dynamics.

The complexity of a body-segment dynamical model depends on the number and types of body segments, the joints connecting the segments, and the interaction among the segments and the environment. A rather complex model is required to analyze movement. However, a complex model complicates the control system design process that good solutions are difficult or impossible to find. The predictive quality of a model depends not only on model complexity, but also on the accuracy with which model parameters (e.g., lengths, masses, and moments of inertia) and structure (e.g., of the joints) can be determined.

A distinction can be made between attempts to deal with an essentially complete system and reduced models. The problem is getting simplified by reducing the number of degrees of freedom in the model by, for example, treating the motion in only one plane at a time, or reducing the number of links in the model. Consequently, attempts to analyze multi-joint structures are often characterized by a search for ways of reducing the number of degrees of freedom to a manageable level. The dynamics of motion confined to a plane is much simpler than that in three dimensions. Fortunately, locomotion can often be decomposed into a dominant component in the sagittal plane with much smaller components in the frontal and horizontal planes. The reduction in complexity is usually achieved by both confining the model to a plane and using a small number of links, which implies that flexible or many jointed elements such as the vertebrate spine must be greatly simplified [Yamaguchi and Zajac, 1990]. Some decisions on how complex the model should be are simple; others are not. For instance, lower limb body segments can be assumed rigid during standing and walking, since bone deformations within a segment are small compared to intersegmental movement. More controversial is the decision on how many segments should be assumed (especially for the trunk and the foot), or how many DOF should be assumed for each joint. For example, models have ranged from a 1-segment, 1-DOF [Jaeger, 1986] to a 17-segment, 44-DOF model [Hatze, 1980]. These decisions on model complexity have important implications to the design of NP control systems.

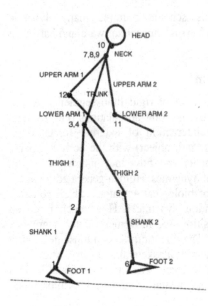

Fig. 5.5: The 13 segmental model of the human in the sagittal plane. The system has 12 hinge type joints.

Two-dimensional models have been used to study standing and walking. For example, a one-segment presenting the whole body [Jaeger, 1986], and a three-segment (head/arms/trunk, one thigh, and one shank) [e.g., Zajac and Gordon, 1989] model have been used to study sagittal plane standing and to design NP systems when both feet are assumed to be flat and stationary on the floor. However, additional segments may be required to adequately model NP-controlled standing and walking. For example, arm movements are significant during NP-controlled standing [Khang, 1988]. During walking, the pelvis may need to be modeled separately from the trunk [Hatze, 1977; Townsend and Seireg, 1973; Yamaguchi, 1990], and the foot may need to be modeled as multiple segments [Yamaguchi, 1990].

The ways of managing complexity may be summarized as follows: 1) reducing the number of degrees of freedom analytically by finding approximations and constraints, and by designing systems with the minimum number of joints (e.g., 12 degrees of freedom are usually used to describe a 13-segment body model) as shown in Figure 5.5; and 2) decomposing a complex problem into several simpler ones by, for example, separating the control of quantities that do not interact significantly.

To model human limbs Stepanenko and Vukobratović [1976] investigated a Newton-Euler approach to dynamics, instead of the somewhat more traditional Lagrangian approach. For efficiency, Orin and colleagues [1979] revised this work for the legs of walking robots. They improved the efficiency by writing the forces and moments in the local link reference frames instead of the inertial frame. They also noticed the sequential nature of calculations from one link to the next, and speculated that an efficient recursive formulation might exist. Armstrong et al., [1979] and Luh et al., [1980] improved the computing efficiency and presented an algorithm that

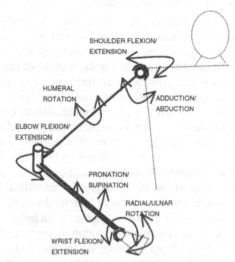

Fig. 5.6: The three dimensional model of the human arm. Seven degrees of freedom are included (three at the shoulder, one at the elbow, one at the forearm, and two at the wrist joint.

resolves the complexity. This was accomplished by setting up the calculations in an iterative (recursive) manner and by expressing the velocities and accelerations of the links in the local link frames. Koozekanani et al., [1983] applied the recursive free body approach to estimate net joint torque associated with observed human postural motion.

Three-dimensional simulation models have also received considerable attention for both walking and reaching (Figure 5.6). Huston et al., [1976, 1978] developed a general approach for studying a human body model using equations based on d'Alembert's principle. Onyshko and Winter [1980] developed a seven link planar model. Equations of motion formulated using Lagrangian mechanics, consist of a 7x7 matrix of anthropometric constants and segment angles, a vector of the angular accelerations and a vector containing the torques acting on the segments. Hatze [1980] used the traditional Lagrangian approach to define a mathematical model of the total human musculoskeletal system. The model comprised a linked mechanical and musculo-mechanical set of ordinary first-order differential equations, which describe the dynamics of the segment model and muscle model respectively. Hatze [1980] also reported a simulation of a planar long-jump take-off with seventeen segments, driven by 46 myoactuators and controlled by a controller subsystem. Zheng and Shen [1990] studied the impact problem and they showed that an impact, acting on a biped, subjects each link of the system to an instantaneous velocity change. Thus, an impact may cause large internal impulsive forces in the body.

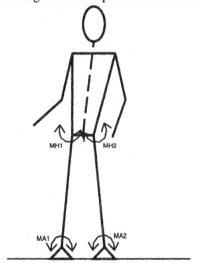

Fig. 5.7: Four degree of freedom model in the coronal plane to analyze standing. The net joint torque MA1, MA2, MH1, and MH2 contribute to the posture in the coronal plane.

Marshall et al., [1985] used a general Newtonian approach to simulate an N-segment open chain model of the human body. The model simulated planar movement using data for joint torques and initial absolute angular displacements and velocities for each body segment. These values are used to solve the direct dynamics problem, expressed in the form of n simultaneous linear equations, to yield angular accelerations. Zajac with collaborators [Khang and Zajac 1989a and b; Zajac, 1989] developed a planar computer model to investigate paraplegic standing induced by FES. The objective of the study by Yamaguchi and Zajac [1990] was to determine a minimal set of muscles that could approximate able-bodied gait trajectories without requiring either higher levels of force or precise control of muscle activation. They suggested that gait was more sensitive to changes in the on/off timing of the muscle stimulus than to its amplitude. The process of adjusting the muscle set and the admissible activation levels was critically dependent upon accurately understanding the effect of each muscle on the dynamic response of the system. The existing biomechanical models are very difficult to customize and hard to work with, due to their complexity.

Most NP systems would require control of movement in all three planes, not just in the sagittal plane. For example, coronal (Figure 5.7) as well as sagittal plane control (Figure 5.5) at the hip is probably required for postural stability [Abass and Chizeck, 1991]. Of the ten types of joint movement suggested as the most important to normal walking [Yamaguchi, 1990], only half are in the sagittal plane: hip flexion/extension, knee flexion/ extension, ankle plantar/dorsiflexion, foot rotation about the metatarsals, and sacral-pelvic flexion/extension. Three are in the frontal plane: hip abduction/ adduction, ankle inversion/ eversion, and sacral-pelvic lateral bending. Least significant are transverse plane rotations (e.g., hip external/internal rotation and axial trunk rotation). Frontal plane movement at the ankle, hip, and sacral-pelvic joints to keep the body center of mass over the stance foot is needed to reduce muscular effort and energy consumption [Yamaguchi, 1990]. Models with only one-DOF sagittal-plane hip joints cause the fore-aft ground reaction force to be poorly predicted during the single-support phase of walking, because multiple-DOF hips reduce the mechanical coupling between the swing and stance legs [Pandy and Berme, 1988]. Also, paraplegic NP-generated walking will probably not induce normal walking movement. Low-level thoracic SCI individuals will probably take advantage of trunk muscles under voluntary control to generate a rotational pelvic region in order to assist in the initiation of swing, as observed when they use non-NP orthotic walking aids (e.g., the RGO). These movements can only be analyzed with a three-dimensional (3-D) model.

During the swing phase of walking, or during the reaching the system forms an open kinematic chain, since only one end of the system contacts the ground (the shoulder in the case of reaching). The number of net joint-torque then equals the number of degrees of freedom, and the system is determinate. This means that the trajectory of the body segments uniquely determines the net torque acting at the joints. However, contact of the other foot or a crutch, or hand with the object during grasping makes the system a closed kinematic chain, and the number of degrees of freedom becomes less than the number of net joint torque and joint forces. Thus, segmental trajectories no longer uniquely determine the net joint torque, and the system is indeterminate. Many different combinations of joint torque can therefore be selected, and finding a reference-based controller is difficult or impossible [e.g., Onyshko and Winter, 1980].

When the muscles contract they pull on the segments (produce force) to the segments that they are attached. These internal forces for the system result with the joint reaction forces and net joint torque. For frictionless, rotary joints, the muscle forces have a net effect on body segmental movement that can be expressed by the net joint torque [Zajac and Gordon, 1989]. The conversion of a muscle force to a joint torque, in such cases, is dictated by musculoskeletal geometry and is conceptually straightforward. In reality, muscles are not straight lines and joints are not hinges. Muscles and tendons attach over a wide area and wrap around or slide over bone, making determination of "the line of force" almost impossible. Joints exhibit rolling and sliding movement (e.g., the knee), proscribing the use of fixed joint centers, or precluding the use of joint torque [Yamaguchi and Zajac, 1990]. Much anthropometric data have been collected that can be used to specify muscle lines of action and musculoskeletal geometry [Yamaguchi, 2000].

5.1.2 Modeling of the Musculotendonal Systems

Biological actuators as described in Chapters 1 and 2, consist of contractile muscle fibers and connect tissue and tendon. They have important dynamic characteristics inherent to their ability to develop force, including time delays, nonlinear elasticity, and nonlinear dependencies on the current muscle state (e.g., length and velocity of the muscle fibers) and past muscle states (e.g., history of the shortening/lengthening and activation of the muscle fibers). Two fundamental classes of mathematical models of actuators, based on normally innervated muscle, but with widely varying complexity, have been developed; macroscopic models, and microscopic models [Winters and Stark, 1987; Zahalak, 1990; Zajac, 1989].

Macroscopic models are not necessarily derived from the actual microscopic biophysical and biochemical mechanisms responsible for muscular contraction, though the Hill macroscopic model [Hill, 1938] had long been considered consistent with such mechanisms [Zahalak, 1990]. Instead, these phenomenological models attempt to describe the observed mechanical input-output behavior of muscle with comparatively simple ordinary differential equations [e.g., Winters, 1990], and thus require less computational effort and fewer parameters than the microscopic models.

Microscopic models are derived from the biophysical and biochemical molecular mechanisms of sarcomere force production [e.g., the cross-bridge and sliding filament models of contraction, Hodgkin and Huxley, 1945]. These microscopic models of sarcomere contraction have many parameters, which, for human tissue, are now unmeasurable and difficult to estimate, and require that partial differential equations be solved. Since partial differential equations require much more computation to solve than ordinary differential equations, microscopic models will probably not be used to design NP control systems. However, the "distribution-moment" model, which is a mathematical approximation to the cross-bridge model [e.g., Zahalak, 1992], offers hope in relating macroscopic to microscopic properties, and its computational efficiency may be sufficient to be employed in models of multi muscle motor control.

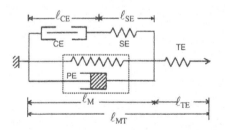

Fig. 5.8: Structure of the musculotendonal model (based on the Hill visco-elastic model). The abbreviations are: CE - contractile element, SE - series elastic element, PE - parallel viscoelastic element, TE - tendonal elastic element, ℓ - length, M - muscle, T - tendon.

Models of muscle under neural pulse stimulation (e.g., models of a normally innervated motor unit, or of a NP-excited muscle), whether developed from microscopic or macroscopic properties, have similar fundamental input-output properties; that is, they all recognize that muscle is basically a second-order low-pass filter. Muscle stimulation (neural excitation or NP) is considered to be pulse-like, with varying frequency. These pulses initiate a chemical reaction, which stimulates the contractile elements within the muscle, producing muscle force. Both macroscopic and microscopic models divide this process into two phases: activation dynamics (the chemical process associated with stimulation-contraction coupling) and contraction dynamics (the generation of force by activated contractile elements). Each of the two phases acts as a low-pass filter, with the output responding slower and more smoothly than the input. Though all models treat muscle as a low-pass filter, the complexity of the equations used to describe the filter varies greatly.

Only macroscopic models have been used to model NP-excited muscle (Figure 5.8). Though Hill-based models have been used to study design issues related to NP-controlled standing and walking [Khang and Zajac, 1989a; Yamaguchi and Zajac, 1990], simpler models may suffice and are particularly attractive for control-system design. Two such models use a nonlinear static recruitment curve (isometric force versus pulse-duration curve) to describe how much muscle tissue is being excited by the electrode pulses, followed by second-order linear dynamics, which models the basic filtering property of muscle [Bernotas et al., 1986; Durfee and MacLean, 1989]. The simulated isometric (or near-isometric) force trajectories to a train of pulses computed from these models compared well with the actual trajectories developed by the electrically stimulated cat muscles. The performance of these models during movement may not be as good, however, since the models do not account for the dependence of force on muscle fiber length and velocity.

A significant weakness in the application of all muscle models to NP systems is their failure to account for muscle fatigue. Muscle force output of electrically stimulated muscle has been shown to decrease due to fatigue. This effect becomes more significant as the duration and intensity of the stimulation increases [Levin and Mizrahi, 1999; Mizrahi et al., 1994; Mizrahi, 1997]. Since NP systems for standing and walking may involve stimulation for long periods of time, models of muscle fatigue must be developed.

Three-factor Muscle Model. Several studies that originated from the design of a single joint controller use a multiplicative model of a muscle as shown in Figure 5.9 [Crago, 1992; Veltink et al., 1992; Shue and Crago, 1998; Shue et al., 1995; Durfee, 1992; Popović et al., 1999b].

The nonlinear model of muscle dynamics used for joint angle control is a modified version of the Hill model, with many elements that have been contributed by Winters [1990]. Active muscle force depends on three factors: neural activation, muscle length and velocity of shortening or lengthening [Veltink et al., 1992; Shue et al., 1995]. The model is formulated as a function of joint angle and angular velocity, rather than muscle length and velocity. The joint angle-dependent moment arm determines the relations between velocity and angular velocity.

The three-factor model is given by:

$$M_a = A(u)M(\varphi)M_o(\dot{\varphi})$$

where M_a is the active torque generated by the muscle contraction, $A(u)$ is the dependence of torque on the level of evoked muscle activity u (depends on the stimulus amplitude, pulse width and stimulus frequency), M is the dependence on the angle φ and M_0 is the dependence on the angular velocity. The parameter u is normalized to the range $0 \leq u \leq 1$ and the function g has the value of 1 under isometric conditions. According to the literature [Veltink et al., 1992], the muscle model described can predict the muscle torque with 85-90% accuracy during simultaneous, independent, pseudo-random variations of recruitment, angle and angular velocity.

Figure 5.9 presents a loaded joint where one muscle is active. The torque generated by the active muscle and the torque contributed by passive elastic properties of antagonistic muscle and other passive tissues of joint sum to produce the total torque that acts on the load and produce movement. The information about the movement (position and velocity) is fed back to the muscle. The muscle response to electrical stimulation was approximated by a second order, critically damped, low pass filter with a delay [Bajzek and Jaeger, 1987; Baratta and Solomonow, 1990; Chizeck et al., 1988, 1991; Shue and Crago, 1998]. Thus, the activation dynamics was assumed to be expressed by:

$$\frac{A(j\omega)}{U(j\omega)} = \frac{\omega_p^2}{\omega^2 + 2j\xi\omega_p + \omega_p^2} e^{-j\omega\tau_d}$$

where $A(j\omega)$ is the Fourier transform of the muscle's contractile activity, $U(j\omega)$ is the Fourier transform of the muscle's electrical activity, ω_p is muscle's natural (pole) frequency ($\approx$ 1-3 Hz), τ_d is the excitation-contraction (and other) delays of the muscle ($\approx$ 20-50 ms). The nonlinear model of muscle dynamics used is a modified, discrete time version of Hill's model [Hill, 1938].

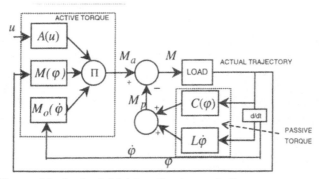

Fig. 5.9: The model of a loaded joint; active torque (a three-component multiplicative model) and the two component passive torque generate a movement. The passive torque is caused by the stretch. Functions M, M_0, c and the parameter L are described in text, u is the neural input, and φ the joint angle. Adapted from Popović et al., 1999 © IEEE.

The nonlinear function torque vs. joint angle is approximated by a quadratic curve, $M = a_0 + a_1\varphi + a_2\varphi^2$. The torque generated can not be negative for any angle; thus:

$$M(\varphi) = Mh(t), \quad h(t) = \begin{cases} 0, t < 0 \\ 1, t \geq 0 \end{cases}$$

Coefficients a_0, a_1, and a_2 define the shape of the torque-angle curve. The nonlinear curve relating torque vs. angular velocity of the joint is approximated by:

$$M_0 = K_0\left(\frac{c_{1V}}{\dot{\varphi}} + c_{0V}\right) \qquad M_0(\dot{\varphi}) = \begin{cases} c_{2V} = Const. & \wedge c_{2V} \leq M_0 \\ M_0 & \wedge 0 \leq M_0 \leq c_{2V} \\ 0 & \wedge M_0 \leq 0 \end{cases}$$

where K, c_{0V}, c_{1V} and c_{0V} are the coefficients determining the properties of the muscle.

5.1.3 Identification of Model Parameters

The identification of the model parameters is essential for the design of analytical controllers for assistive systems to restore movement of humans with sensory-motor disability. The complexity of the methods that have to be used to identify the parameters depends on the model of the plant that has been adopted. If, for example, the body is modeled as a single rigid body (e.g., inverted pendulum for analyzing standing, Figure 5.10) and the actuator is assumed to have a quadratic form, which is a function of the angle θ, then the movement is described with the following equation:

$$J_A \ddot{\theta} = M - mgL \sin\theta \quad \wedge \quad M = a_o + a_1\theta + a_2\theta^2$$

The parameters of the system are: J_A - axial moment of inertia for the axis perpendicular to the sagittal plane passing through the point A (ankle joint), distance $L=AC$ (C is the center of mass), m - the mass of the body, and actuator parameters a_0, a_1, and a_2. The system identification relates to a procedure, which will allow to determine the parameters by measuring the input and output, that is the angle θ and the torque M. When the model has many segments, and they are driven by a set of redundant actuators, then the identification becomes a very difficult problem. The complexity is contributed by the fact that many input and output variables can not be measured with sufficient accuracy with the non-invasive techniques.

There are two types of somewhat different physical variables to be identified: dynamic parameters of the skeletal system (e.g., inertia, length, position of the center of mass, distances between the centers of rotation) and parameters of the musculo-tendonal systems. Very large studies provide average data about the skeletal properties [e.g., Drillis and Contini, 1966; Zatsiorsky et al., 1984; Winter, 1990, 1991], but they can not be used for individual real-time control, yet it is very helpful in simulating the behavior of the system, because the small differences do not make much of differences.

Models of muscle have been identified "off line," using a sets of collected input and output data. The muscle model identification problem can be categorized by the following factors: 1) time domain: continuous-time or discrete-time models; 2) input types: stimulus period (SP), *i.e.*, pulse frequency modulation, pulse width (PW) modulation, or combinations of these; 3) model outputs: e.g., muscle torque or force, muscle length or position; 4) loading conditions: isometric or non-isometric loads, load transitions; and 5) model type: linear models, nonlinear Hill-type models, other nonlinear models;

Most of early experimental work in muscle model identification concerned linear, constant parameter, continuous-time dynamic models under isometric loading conditions. Mannard and Stein [1973] developed a second-order, constant parameter, continuous-time linear system model of isometric cat muscle, in which the pulse frequency was the modulated input signal. Sampled values of this input and the output (muscle force) were used to compute the linear system response model, using spectral density analysis methods. Frequency domain parameters (*i.e.*, gain, zeros and poles of the linear model or equivalently, the damping ratio and natural frequency) were identified.

Baratta and Solomonow [1990] considered muscle model identification of data obtained through nerve stimulation of cat hind limb muscles under isometric conditions. They also fit transfer function parameters of a second-order continuous-time linear system model, but using least-squares methods. Bobet *et al.*, [1993] identified linear second-order continuous-time models with time-varying parameters, using nonlinear optimization methods. Continuous-time Hill-type models of electrically stimulated muscles have been developed and used in numerous FES applications [e.g., Durfee and Palmer, 1994; Franken *et al.*, 1993, 1995; Yamaguchi and Zajac, 1990].

Although muscle forces or joint positions are inherently continuous-time signals, the electrical stimulation input signals, such as pulse duration (width) (PW), the pulse amplitude, or interpulse interval can be thought of as pulse-by pulse parameters. When the pulse stimulus frequency is constant, then the muscle stimulus signal can be represented as a discrete-time signal. If the force or position output signal is sampled, then a discrete-time dynamic system model of the stimulated muscle can be obtained. An advantage of this approach is that computationally simple recursive least square identification methods can be used to obtain real-time parameter identification. Bernotas *et al.*, [1986, 1997] applied these techniques to obtain a discrete-time second-order linear model of electrically stimulated cat muscle under isometric conditions. This was applied to adaptive control of cat muscle [Lan *et al.*, 1991] in both isometric and non-isometric situations. Allin and Inbar [1986a and b] carried out similar work in the human upper extremity, using a third-order model to include load properties.

Chia *et al.* [1991] extended this idea, to include the simultaneous identification of the nonlinear recruitment property of muscle in combination with the linear dynamics. A Hammerstein representation of the nonlinear system (*i.e.*, the nonlinearity precedes the linear dynamics), with a polynomial approximation of the recruitment nonlinearity, was used. Experimental evaluations were obtained under isometric loading conditions, using the Quadriceps m. of paraplegic subjects, with muscle stimulation provided via percutaneous intramuscular electrodes.

When the muscle is not under isometric loading conditions, it is significantly more difficult to obtain an identified discrete-time input-output model of the system, because of the interaction of muscle activation, force-velocity and length-tension phenomena. Two classes of input-output models were developed and tested by Shue *et al.* [1995] for cat soleus muscle. These models included the effects of joint angle (or muscle length) and velocity upon the output torque (or force) that is generated by the electrically stimulated muscle, as well as the effects of activation dynamics. The two models that were comparatively evaluated under different non-isometric loading conditions were as follows: a three-factor (activation dynamics, torque-velocity, and torque-angle) uncoupled Hill-type model, and a two-factor (activation dynamics and torque-angle) coupled nonlinear model, in which the activation dynamics model depends upon velocity.

Franken *et al.* [1993, 1995] identified the dynamics of the paraplegic knee joint, when freely swinging, using a parameterized analytical model. Scheiner *et al.* [1993] used measurements taken without muscle stimulation to obtain a model of the knee joint and shank dynamics. This passive model was then used, along with PW and force data taken during surface stimulation, to fit parameters of a model of the Quadriceps muscle. Their time-invariant model represented the stimulated muscle as a static nonlinearity in series with a linear system. It was fit using batch-identification methods. The work presented by Chizeck *et al.* [1999] differs because it considers muscle stimulation that involves combinations of PW and SP (*i.e.*, pulse frequency) modulation. A recursive-identification method was used, which allows for the fitting of time varying model parameters.

Methods are described for estimating the inertia, viscosity, and stiffness of the lower leg around the knee and the whole leg around the hip that are applicable even for the humans who are very spastic [Stein et al., 1996]. These procedures comprise several tests. A "pull test" in which the segment of the body is slowly moved throughout its range of motion while measuring angles and torque to determine passive stiffness. A "pendulum test" in which the segment of the body is moved against gravity and then released to move freely, while again measuring angles and torque. By limiting the extent of the movement and choosing the direction of the initial excursion of the segment, spasticity can be almost eliminated. Stein and coworkers compared their results from nine subjects with the literature data; the results report substantial differences between the estimated and literature data for both lower and whole leg.

Chizeck et al. [1999] presented the identification of electrically stimulated muscle model parameters, in real-time, when both the PW and SP are modulated and the identification of electrically stimulated muscle model parameters under different loading conditions, including isometric and non-isometric constant loading, and in the presence of load transitions.

Chizeck and coworkers use the following methodology: At each discrete-time k, the output torque (force) is $y(k)$ and $u(k)$ represents the PW stimulation input (constant pulse frequency). Let $\phi(k)$ be the measured knee angle (the muscle length) and let $V(k)$ be the angular velocity of the joint (the shortening velocity of the muscle). The discrete-time nonlinear models of muscle dynamics, which assumes that the output is result of the product of three uncoupled factors (activation, torque-angle and torque-angular velocity has the following form:

$$A(k) = T_V(k)[a_1 A(k-1) + a_2 A(k-2)] + bu(k-h)$$

$$T_a = 1 + d\phi(k)$$

$$T_V(k) = 1 - cV(k)$$

$$y(k) = A(k) T_a(k)$$

The parameter h represents an inherent time delay in the activation dynamics. The above model can be extended to include both SP and PW modulation using the following idea. First, a small "stimulus period minimum increment" is selected (e.g., 5 ms). All input interpulse intervals are constrained to be integer multiples of this increment. That is, SP modulation is quantized. For the input stimulus signals, if there is no pulse during a specific interval then u is set to zero; if there is a pulse, then it is set to the normalized PW value.

The output signal (muscle torque or force, or length or angle) is then sampled using this short sampling period. That is, the output is sampled at this fast time scale, corresponding to the SP minimum increment. The input and sampled output values at this fast time scale are then translated into discrete-time signals at a slow time scale (specifically, with a time step size that is a fixed-integer multiple of the SP minimum increment). Parameters for the discrete-time model are then fit, using this slow time scale. Chizeck and coworkers did not fit the model at the fast time scale, because this would require many "b" parameters, in order to capture the system dynamic response.

The use of more parameters in the model tends to decrease the accuracy that can be achieved, and increases the computational complexity of the parameter identification algorithm. The latter is of concern for real-time implementations.

In converting the input and output signals from the fast time scale to the slow one, it is impossible to discard data points so as to obtain a longer sampling interval. For example, if a stimulation (muscle input) signal at the 5 ms time scale were converted into one at a 20 ms time scale by discarding all but every fourth sample, the effect of an input signal that consisted of the first three points in each successive set of four will be completely lost. A causal (e.g., triangular) filter is applicable to resolve this problem.

Experiments were conducted on five male subjects and one female subject, each having complete lower extremity paralysis due to spinal cord injury [Chizeck *et al.*, 1999]. Three types of experiments were performed: 1) *passive trials*, during which leg motion was measured in the absence of stimulation. In pendulum trials, the leg was released with zero initial angular knee velocity from a fixed angle. In pull/release trials, the knee was slowly extended, by having the experimenter lift it with minimal acceleration, and then it was released. The knee angles (and pulling force, when present) were recorded; 2) *freely swinging leg trials*, the leg was allowed to swing freely at the knee joint (during electrical stimulation of the quadriceps muscle group), against gravity and inertial loads. The flexion/extension of the knee was measured using an externally mounted goniometer. Two uno-axial accelerometers were placed 10 cm apart on the long axis of the shank, to provide information about the angular acceleration; and 3) swing-to-stop trials then obtained knee joint velocity, the leg was allowed to swing freely during stimulation until a barrier was reached. Thus, the system encountered a fairly abrupt load transition. The aim was to loosely approximate the kind of load transition seen at heel strike during walking. The knee angle was measured by a goniometer. A restraining strap was attached to ankle of test leg to prevent full extension of knee under stimulation. A load cell was placed in series with this strap, so as to measure the contact torque of the leg when the mechanical constraint (and the load cell) was encountered. The stop angle was defined to be the knee angle at which the load cell measured the contact force.

A microprocessor-controlled stimulator was used to generate a specific "pattern" of stimulation PW's and SP's for each trial. For each type of loading, and for the various types of electrical stimulation input sequences, the measured sensor data was used to fit parameters of the muscle model. When non-isometric loads are involved, the knee torque generated by the electrically stimulated Quadriceps muscle cannot be directly measured (unlike the isometric case). Consequently, the identification of parameters for the model involves several steps.

Identification of the Parameters for Controlling the Elbow Joint - An Example

Popović M *et al.* [1994] applied similar methods to identify active and passive parameters of the elbow joint in order to simulate flexion/extension movement. She implemented the model of the joint described and presented in Figure 5.9. The results of simulation are integrated in the actuator level of a hierarchical hybrid controller. The mechanical model of the elbow joint suitable for analysis of reaching, pointing, tracking and other manipulation functions without grasping is a double spatial pendulum with only one degree of freedom, that is elbow flexion/extension. All muscles responsible for elbow movement were reduced to only a pair of muscles (flexor and extensor). One reason was essential for this simplification: one channel of stimulation was assumed to operate *per* flexor and extensor muscles.

Three groups of parameters are required: 1) geometrical and inertial properties; 2) biomechanical characteristics of neuro- musculo- skeletal "actuators" generating or participating in arm joint movements; and 3) recruitment of the actuator. Five volunteer tetraplegic subjects with spinal cord injury at the cervical level (C4/C6) resulting in lost or diminished reaching, absence of strongly manifested spasms, and preserved lower motor neurons.

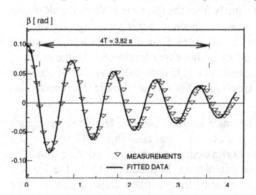

Fig. 5.10: The pendulum test for identifying moment of inertia, viscosity and elasticity of the joint. The triangles are experimental data, the full line the curve fitted using the equation of motion. Adapted from Popović M *et al.*, 1994, with permission.

The measurements comprised three tests: the pull, pendulum and electrically elicited motion. The inertial properties with respect to the rotation axis were determined using a pendulum test. The limb was pulled from the neutral position and then released while the joint angle was measured. The relationship between the period of oscillation and inertial properties was used to determine the moments of inertia.

Small oscillation of the limb has been analyzed in order to minimize effects of spasms, joint stiffness and other non-relevant effects (friction, air resistance, *etc.*). The neutral position for the forearm was vertical under the elbow, while the upper arm was fixed in the position of 30 degrees behind the vertical. The neutral position for the arm as a whole was vertical under the shoulder, while the human was slightly leaning towards this arm. The amplitude of oscillations was kept at below 0.1 radian. The equation of movement follows the law of rotation:

$$J_O \ddot{\beta} + B\dot{\beta} + K\beta = -mgd \sin\beta$$

where J_O is the moment of inertia about the horizontal axes, B and K parameters determining the viscosity and stiffness of the joint, m is the mass, d the distance from the center of the mass to the axes of rotation, g gravitational acceleration, and β the angle between the long axes of the segment to vertical. For small oscillations muscles will not be activated (confirmed with EMG recordings), and the angular velocity will be small enough; hence the axial moment of inertia could also be determined by simple formula:

$$J_O = \frac{mgdT^2}{4\pi^2}$$

where T is the period of oscillation (Figure 5.11).

The moment of inertia and parameters B (viscosity) and K (elasticity) have also been calculated by fitting the model to the experimental data (Figure 5.11). The fitting is done by using the above motion equation.

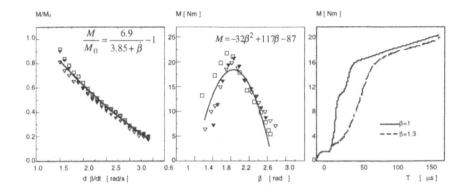

Fig 5.11: The experimental recordings (squares and triangles) and lines (results of the fitting) in a C4 tetraplegic subject (left and middle panels). See text for details. Adapted from Popović M *et al.*, 1994, with permission.

Fig 5.12: The recruitment curve for the elbow extensor muscle. Adapted from Popović M *et al.*, 1994, with permission.

During a "pull test" [Stein *et al.*, 1996] the measurements have been done during pulling the forearm in flexion and extension. A dynamometer was used for the force recordings, while the angles were measured with flexible goniometers. The relationship is nonlinear, and it was fitted by a quadratic equation:

$$M = c_2 \beta^2 + c_1 \beta + c_0$$

The least square method (LSM) was used to fit the experimental data (Figure 5.11 right panel). The pull test was done with different velocities, thus the joint torque *vs.* angular velocity data was generated (Figure 5.11 left panel). The data was used to fit the nonlinear model:

$$\frac{M_V}{M_0} = \frac{c_{1V}}{\dot{\beta}} + c_{0V}$$

which corresponds to the Hill muscle model [Hill, 1938].

Recruitment of a muscle was estimated by applying controlled bursts of stimulation while simultaneously measuring the angular changes and measuring the force generated for different joint angular velocities. This analysis was applicable for the elbow extensor muscles, yet it was very difficult to assess the effects of stimulation to flexor muscles because they have been in all cases partly innervated; thus, voluntary contraction was mixed with the externally elicited. A typical result is shown in Figure 5.12. The stimulation of the extensor muscles changed during the recording session because of the fast occurring muscle fatigue.

5.1.4 Control Methods for Movement of a Single Joint

Wilhere *et al.* [1985] designed and evaluated a digital closed-loop controller for the regulation of muscle force by recruitment modulation. Both the stimulator output and the muscle have been modeled as discrete time processes. A digital controller aims to cancel the plant dynamics. The controller was tested using animal model; the performance was judged on the basis of stability, linearity, reproducibility of response, and ability to respond to imperfection of the model and external disturbances. A block diagram of the system is shown in Figure 5.13.

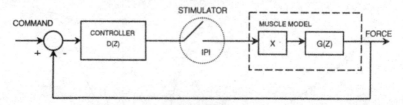

Fig. 5.13: A block diagram of the digital closed-loop control system for the regulation of muscle force via recruitment modulation. D(Z) is a discrete model of the controller, G(Z) a discrete model of the muscle. Adapted from Wilhere et al., 1985 © IEEE.

The primary components are: a digital controller with Z-domain transfer function $D(Z)$, a stimulator modeled as a sampler, and a muscle modeled as a memoryless nonlinearity X in cascade with a linear-time system with transfer function $G(Z)$.

The controller modulated the pulse duration; the interpulse interval (IPI) and amplitude of pulsed have been considered constant. The discrete model of the muscle and the controller transfer functions are:

$$G(z) = \frac{g_1 z + g_0}{(z + g_2)(z + g_3)}$$

$$D(z) = \frac{(a_1 z - a_0)(z + g_2)(z + g_3)}{(z - 1)(z - b_0)(g_1 z + g_0)}$$

Parameters g_i, a_i, and b_0, $i=1,2$ are unique for the system analyzed, and they have to be identified, which makes the use of this model complex.

The implementation of the system to control a single muscle in an isolated animal preparation showed advantages compared to the open-loop control (Figure 5.14).

Crago et al., (1988) studied the implementation of a closed-loop control for functional electrical stimulation of a single muscle in acute animal preparations (Figure 5.15). The interpulse interval and pulse duration have been both regulated to provide adequate recruitment and temporal summation of the muscle fibers. The force (feedback) was measured with a strain gauge based transducer attached to the end of the tendon. The main conclusions from the study are that it is feasible

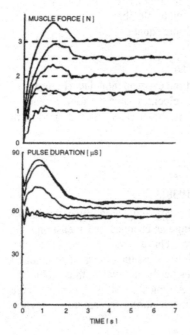

Fig 5.14: Step responses for four amplitudes of command signals. Adapted from Wilhere et al., 1985 © IEEE.

to design a controller that can apply a single command signal, which by regulating the pulse duration and the interpulse interval would provide linear input-output relation [Crago *et al.*, 1986b].

Bernotas *et al.*, [1987] continued to use the discrete time model of a muscle and developed an adaptive control, that allowed the system to operate at different loads, that is to adapt to the change of dynamic constraints in a wide range of forces. They used the second order deterministic autoregressive moving average (DARMA) model of the muscle [Bernotas *et al.*, 1986]. A direct, minimum prediction error, one-step ahead adaptive controller was implemented and tested in animal experiments [Goodwin and Sin, 1984]. Direct adaptive control means that the controller parameters are estimated on-line from the input and output observations. The system performance was confirmed by studying the step, staircase and sinusoidal input; excellent reproducibility, stability, robustness and tracking of the desired input were obtained.

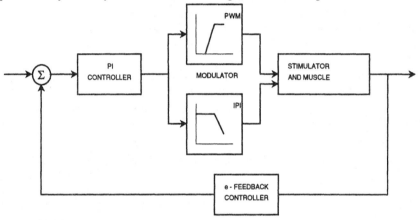

Fig. 5.15: Block diagram of the force modulation and closed-loop, force feedback control system. The error signal *e* is the difference between the desired (command) level and the actual measured force. PI stays for proportional-integral controller, PWM - pulse width (duration) modulation, IPI - interpulse interval. Adapted from Crago *et al.*, 1986 © IEEE.

Peterson and Chizeck [1987] tested the use of a discrete time control with the aim to optimize the force for a given trajectory of a linear second-order external load. The linear quadratic regulator theory has been applied to a system of two muscles (agonist and antagonist); the pulse amplitude and interpulse interval have been constant, the regulator varied the pulse duration on only one muscle, the other was considered only as a visco-elastic (no contractile elements) opponent for generating the net joint torque. The simulation studies showed that the system is very sensitive to the model, as well as the tuning parameters.

Zhou *et al.* [1987, 1997] used a computer-controlled, two-channel electronic stimulator capable of manipulating skeletal muscles within a very wide rang of action potential firing rates and motor-unit recruitment controls. The aim of the study was to optimize the stimulation paradigm, and to develop a strategy that would work in different muscles no matter what their structure is. The basis of the research was that the muscle force could be controlled within first 50 percent of the range by modulating the "recruitment", and be expanded up to the range of 100 percent by increasing the firing rate (the biological basis for this work can be found in Chapter 2).

Zhou et al. [1987, 1997b] assumed that the force is more or less linearly related to the increase of the pulse duration (recruitment), yet nonlinear behavior is characteristic for the variation of the firing rate. This strategy has been selected to match the physiological contraction mechanisms reducing the problems of muscle fatigue. The firing rate was varied up to 600 pulses per second, and the pulse duration was increased up to 100 µs; experiments have been performed in cat muscles using bipolar cuff electrodes placed on the sciatic nerve.

Baratta et al., [1998] evaluated the strategy of combining the recruitment and firing rate within the force feedback to control a single muscle. Adaptive controller was used in isolated animal preparation and the control performances were much improved compared to the open-loop system (Figure 5.16). The authors suggest that the development of sensory feedback techniques, such as selective recordings from nerves, could provide the required sensory signal directly from the muscle controlled. Zhou et al. [1997a and b] evaluated the more complex problem of controlling the joint by simultaneously stimulating both the flexor and extensor muscles, yet using a combined recruitment and firing rate control paradigm. One of the most important issues deals with the level of cocontraction that is contributing to position and force control, yet not leading to muscle fatigue. The stiffness control [Hogan, 1984] has been used in many studies leading to optimal control.

Allin and Inbar [1986a and b] developed several controller schemes for the human elbow and wrist movement and tested them on able-bodied subjects. Among the more successful of these schemes were a third order feed-forward controller and a model reference adaptive controller. The parameters have to be chosen on the basis of parameterized muscle models through an empirical determination. Hartwell et al. [1991] developed a model reference controller for the knee joint of paraplegic subjects. The model deals with the unloaded leg (swing phase) under electric stimulation. The model consists of a nonlinear part followed by linear dynamics described by deterministic autoregressive moving average (ARMA) models. The models have been used for the design of the adaptive controller. The results showed that the control rate constraint was overcame and smoothly changing signal generated. The authors report that such signals could prevent the occurrence of spastic reflexes. The

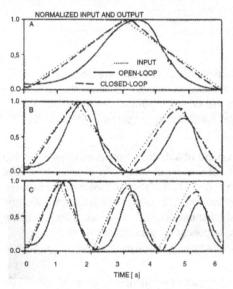

Fig. 5.16: Panels A, B, and C show sample input, open-loop and closed-loop signals when applying force feedback recruitment control of a muscle (isometric conditions). Adapted from Baratta et al., 1998 © IEEE.

model has to be expanded to include the stance phase of walking.

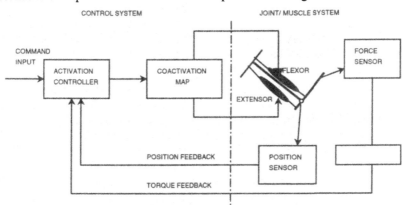

Fig. 5.17: The closed-loop control system for controlling a single joint activated by a single coactivation map. The controller uses one of the three described strategies. The joint/muscle system comprises inertial, viscosity, passive and active components of skeleto-musculo-tendonal components. Adapted from Lan et al., 1991 © IEEE.

Lan et al. [1991] tested three feedback control algorithms of varying complexity for controlling three different tasks during electrical stimulation of muscles. Two controllers use stimulus pulse duration modulation to grade muscle force (the fixed parameter and first order pulse duration control system, and the adaptive controller).

The third controller varies stimulus pulse duration and interpulse intervals. The three tasks tested with the listed control schemes were isometric torque control, unloaded position tracking and control of transitions between isometric and unloaded conditions.

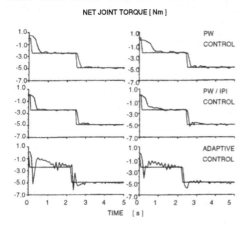

Fig. 5.18: Results obtained under isometric conditions by the three controllers: PW - pulse width (duration), IPI - interpulse interval. Straight lines are the desired net joint torques. See text for details. Adapted from Lan et al., 1991 © IEEE.

All experiments have been done in animal models by analyzing the ankle joint movement and stimulating the flexor and extensor muscles (Figure 5.17). The simplest pulse duration controller demonstrated robustness, the combined recruitment and firing rate operated better for isometric and transition tasks, but was problematic when the joint was unloaded. The adaptive controller was not better, as if it was expected (Figure 5.18). Abrupt changes in the system (e.g., recruitment nonlinearity, loading transition) limit the performance of the adaptive controller.

Lan and Crago [1994] presented results of an optimal control of antagonistic muscles applied for single joint arm movement. The optimization was based on minimizing the effort. A hierarchical model has been developed based on the equilibrium position theory (as described in Chapter 2). For point-to-point movements, the model provides prediction on movement trajectory, equilibrium trajectory, muscle control inputs, and joint stiffness by the level of cocontraction.

The movement trajectory captures the bell shaped profiles of angular velocity, sigmoidal joint movement trajectory, as well as a triphasic burst pattern of muscle control inputs typical for able-bodied subjects. The results show that fast arm movements involve explicit planning for equilibrium trajectory and joint stiffness, if the effort has to be minimized. For slow movements the joint stiffness is less important, yet the equilibrium planning remains the key issue. The model is sensitive to system parameters (musculotendonal and recruitment characteristics) since they affect the correlation between the movement and equilibrium trajectory.

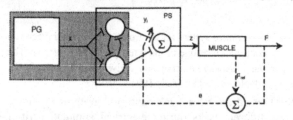

Fig. 5.19: Pattern generator (PG)/pattern shaper (PS) adaptive control system scheme. The muscle input z generates the muscle force F, which should track the reference force F_{ref}. The error signal e adapts the summation weights on the signal from the internal unit y_j. Adapted from Abbas and Triolo, 1997 © IEEE.

Abbas and Triolo [1997] experimentally evaluated feed-forward control that utilizes artificial neural network techniques to generate isometric muscle contractions to track the reference force. The evaluation has been done with intramuscular electrodes to stimulate the Quadriceps m. of paraplegics. This works closely follows the work of Abbas and Chizeck [1995] where two sequential artificial neural networks have been suggested to mimic the generation of walking based on the principle of a central pattern generator (see Chapter 2). The first neural network is the central pattern generator, and the second one is modulating the phasic input from the rhythm generator (Figure 5.19).

The actual controller applied to control the knee net joint torque by stimulating the knee extensors (isometric conditions) is a simplified version of the originally developed system. A periodic signal (basic rhythm) was assumed; thus only one neural network was used as a feed-forward control system. The real-time calculation *de facto* only applies for adaptation, since the non-perturbed activity can be stored in form of a look-up table (off-line calculations). The neural networks learn, thereby the performance was improved after few trials, and remained good enough during the later experiments. The learning (adaptation) is a process, which requires some time and few repetitions (Figure 5.20). The feed-forward in this case operates with a neural network instead of the traditional proportional-integral-derivative adaptive controller.

A strategy of stimulating different portions of a muscle with different stimulation channels has been introduced by Petrofsky and Phillips [1985]. Stimulation of the lower and upper part of the quadriceps muscle with two channels and three electrodes allows the reduction of the stimulation frequency reducing the problems with the fatigue that is induced by the continuous relatively high frequency stimulation of muscles. Brown et al., [1999] used distributed and interleaved stimulation of portions of the muscles to generate a near equal tension contribution. The modeling allows to calculate the stimulation regimes; thus to optimize the stimulation.

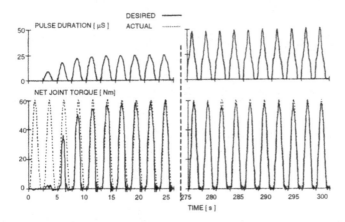

Fig 5.20: Input and output traces at the beginning (0 to 25 seconds, left panels) and end of the stimulation session (275 to 300 seconds, right). The top panels are the pulse duration, the bottom panels the net joint torque. The error at the beginning is the consequence of the "untrained" network. Adapted from Abbas and Triolo, 1997 © IEEE.

Riess and Abbas [1999] evaluated the performance of an adaptive feed-forward controller and its ability to automatically develop and customize stimulation patterns for use in functional electrical stimulation systems. Results from previously described pattern generator/pattern shaper controller in isometric contractions have been extended to isotonic conditions. This study required considering muscle length vs. both tension and force-velocity properties, in addition to the limb dynamics. The performance of the adaptive controller was compared with that of a proportional-derivative feedback controller, and better tracking has been documented. The experiments were done with freely swinging legs using a special apparatus, which holds subjects above the ground. The system does not consider walking, since the ground reaction forces and closed kinematic chains are not discussed.

Optimal control for multi-joint systems - An example

An example how inverse dynamics can be used to determine the stimulation pattern is included to demonstrate the complexity of the problem. The method presented uses dynamic programming to resolve the redundant system; it optimizes the performance of the system by minimizing the cocontraction of agonist and antagonist muscles and minimize the tracking error from the desired joint trajectories [Popović et al., 1999]. The model used for this analysis is a greatly simplified and reduced planar model of bipedal walking. The model considers the whole body, yet the simulation explicitly analyzes the ipsilateral leg coupled with the remaining parts of the body and the environment. The remaining parts of the body (arms, head, trunk and the contralateral leg) are replaced by the interface force and joint torque acting at the hip using the method of D'Alembert. The movement of the hip is also included in the simulation as an input. The ipsilateral leg comprises two rigid segments connected with hinge joints. The ground reaction force acts at the sole of during the stance phase

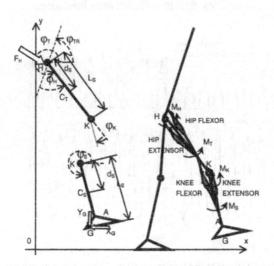

Fig. 5.21: The dynamic model for synthesizing the stimulation patterns for walking. The notations are: S - the shank segment (including the foot); T- the thigh segment; C_S, C_T- the center of the mass of the shank and thigh segments; H- the hip joint; K - the knee joint; G - the point of ground contact; d_S, d_T - distances of the proximal joint to the centers of the masses; L_S, L_T - lengths of the shank and thigh F_H - force acting at the hip joint; X_G, Y_G - horizontal and vertical components of the ground reaction force; M_S, M_T - total torque acting at the shank and thigh segments; M_K, M_H - joint torque at the knee and hip joints; φ_S, φ_T- angles of the shank and thigh vs. the horizontal axis (Ox); φ_K, φ_H- angles of the knee and hip joint; φ_{TR}- angle of the trunk vs. the horizontal axis (Ox).

of the walking cycle, and its acting point shifts its position along the sole of the foot during the stance phase.

The double pendulum representing the leg (Figure 5.21) allows the knee and hip to flex and extend within typical physiological range of movement. Two pairs of monoarticular muscles acting around the hip and knee joints (Figure 5.21) drive the leg. Biarticular muscles would add to the net joint torque, but they are ignored at this stage [Herzog and Keurs, 1988].

The model treats the hip acceleration, angle of the trunk vs. the horizontal, and ground reaction forces as input to the simulation, so they should remain unchanged; thus, the assumption is that human would volitionally compensate for the tracking errors. The model does not include active ankle and phalangeal joints, which would reflect the walking with ankle-foot orthoses.

The following system of differential Equations (5.1 - 5.2) describes the dynamics:

$$A_1 \ddot{\phi}_S + A_2 \ddot{\phi}_T \cos(\phi_T - \phi_S) + A_3 \dot{\phi}_T^2 \sin(\phi_T - \phi_S) - A_4 \ddot{x}_H \sin\phi_S$$
$$- A_5 (\ddot{y}_H + g)\cos\phi_S - X_G L_S \sin\phi_S + Y_G L_S \cos\phi_S = M_S \quad (5.1)$$

$$B_1 \ddot{\phi}_T + B_2 \ddot{\phi}_S \cos(\phi_T - \phi_S) + B_3 \dot{\phi}_S^2 \sin(\phi_T - \phi_S) - B_4 \ddot{x}_H \sin\phi_T$$
$$- B_5 (\ddot{y}_H + g)\cos\phi_T - X_G L_T \sin\phi_T + Y_G L_T \cos\phi_T = M_T \quad (5.2)$$

$$A_1 = J_{C_S} + m_S d_S^2, \quad B_1 = J_{C_T} + m_S L_T^2 + m_T d_T^2$$

$$A_2 = m_S d_S L_T, \quad B_2 = A_2, \quad A_3 = -A_2, \quad B_3 = B_2$$

$$A_4 = m_S d_S, \quad B_4 = m_S L_T + m_T d_T, \quad A_5 = -A_4, \quad B_5 = -B_4$$

The notations are shown in Figure 5.21; other terms are m_S, m_T, J_{CS}, and J_{CT} the inertia parameters of the shank and thigh, and g is the gravitational acceleration. The relations between the net moments acting at the segments and the net joint torque are defined with Equation 5.3:

$$M_S = -M_K, \quad M_T = M_K + M_H$$
$$M_K = M_K^f - M_K^e - M_K^r, \quad M_H = M_H^f - M_H^e - M_H^r \quad (5.3)$$

Flexion of a joint is defined to be the positive direction for angular changes; hence, the flexor torque is assumed to be positive. Index f is for the equivalent flexor muscle, and index e for the equivalent extensor muscle. The contribution of passive tissue crossing the joints was included by a "resistive" torque (index r), which will be described below in Equations 5.10 and 5.11. The difference in the signs of the extension and flexion components of joint torque arises from the definition of the reference frame.

The muscle model [Wilkie, 1950] used for simulation of flexor and extensor equivalent muscles follows the original work of Hill [1938]. As shown in Figure 5.9 the active joint torque depends on the product of three factors: the neural activation inputs, the length and the velocity of the muscle. The knee and hip joint angles $\varphi_K = \varphi_T - \varphi_S$ and $\varphi_H = \varphi_T - \varphi_{TR} - \pi$, and their derivatives are related to the length and the velocity of the shortening of muscles. This leads to the following Equations 5.4-5.7:

$$M_K^f = (c_{12}\phi_K^2 + c_{11}\phi_K + c_{10}) g_K^f(\dot{\phi}_K) u_1 \quad (5.4)$$

$$M_K^e = (c_{22}\phi_K^2 + c_{21}\phi_K + c_{20}) g_K^e(\dot{\phi}_K) u_2 \quad (5.5)$$

$$M_H^f = (c_{32}\phi_H^2 + c_{31}\phi_H + c_{30}) g_H^f(\dot{\phi}_H) u_3 \quad (5.6)$$

$$M_H^e = (c_{42}\phi_H^2 + c_{41}\phi_H + c_{40}) g_H^e(\dot{\phi}_H) u_4 \quad (5.7)$$

The coefficients c_{ij} ($j=0,1,2$; $i=1,2,3,4$) in Equations (5.4-5.7) determine the best second order polynomial fit through the experimental data recorded in able-bodied or SCI subjects, and are user specific. The quadratic polynomial was selected as the simplest adequate fitting curve. The procedure for determination of the parameters is described in the next section [Stein et al., 1996]. Note that each of the quantities is non-negative. The normalized joint torque vs. joint angular velocities in Equations 5.4-5.7 are determined by:

$$g_K^e(\dot{\phi}_K) = \begin{cases} 0, \dot{\phi}_K < -1/c_{23} \\ 1+c_{23}\dot{\phi}_K, -1/c_{23} \leq \dot{\phi}_K < (c_{24}-1)/c_{23} \\ c_{24}, (c_{24}-1)/c_{23} \leq \dot{\phi}_K \end{cases} \qquad (5.8)$$

$$g_K^f(\dot{\phi}_K) = \begin{cases} c_{14}, \dot{\phi}_K < (1-c_{14})/c_{13} \\ 1-c_{13}\dot{\phi}_K, (1-c_{14})/c_{13} \leq \dot{\phi}_K < 1/c_{13} \\ 0, 1/c_{13} \leq \dot{\phi}_K \end{cases} \qquad (5.9)$$

The equations for the hip joint have the same form but the coefficients c_{13}, c_{14}, c_{23} and c_{24}, should be replaced with c_{33}, c_{34}, c_{43} and c_{44} respectively, and index K with H. The coefficients c_{ij} ($i=1,2,3,4$; $j=3,4$) determine the slope and saturation level of the linearized torque vs. velocity of the muscle shortening. These coefficients were determined using the method described in [Popović et al., 1994].

The control inputs u_i ($i=1,2,3,4$) are variables constrained between 0 and 1, and give the level of activation of each of the equivalent muscles, and their determination is the purpose of simulation. This example intentionally uses only the levels of activation to simplify the explanation. A complete model would include the activation dynamics (as shown in the previous example).

$$M_K^r = d_{11}(\phi_K - \phi_{K0}) + d_{12}\dot{\phi}_K + d_{13}e^{d_{14}\phi_K} - d_{15}e^{d_{16}\phi_K} \qquad (5.10)$$

$$M_H^r = d_{31}(\phi_H - \phi_{H0}) + d_{32}\dot{\phi}_H + d_{33}e^{d_{34}\phi_H} - d_{35}e^{d_{36}\phi_H} \qquad (5.11)$$

Equations 5.10-5.11 show the nonlinear resistive torque, which depend on both the joint angle and its angular velocity. The two first terms in Equations 5.10 and 5.11 are the contributions of passive tissues crossing the joints (dissipative properties of joints) reduced to first order functions. The other terms are the nonlinear components of the resistive torque around the terminal positions, and are modeled as double exponential curves [Stein et al., 1996]. The determination of the resistive torque is complex in humans with paraplegia. The parameters d_{ij} ($i=1,3$; $j=1,2,3,4,5,6$) were determined from the experimental data. The angles φ_{K0}, φ_{H0} are the neutral positions for the knee and hip joints where the net moments are zero. Lengths and inertial parameters depicted in Figure 5.10 have been determined using the procedure described in Stein et al., [1996] for each individual subject (Table 5.1).

The input file for the simulation was prepared using the processed data consisting of the angle of the trunk vs. the horizontal, the hip and knee joint angles, the hip acceleration and the ground reaction forces. Data were recorded from an able-bodied subject walked on a powered treadmill wearing ankle-foot orthoses. The sensors were: four force sensing resistors built into the insole of the shoe, flexible goniometers at the leg joints, and a pendulum potentiometer at the trunk [Medri et al., 1994]. The data were captured at 100 Hz. The original kinematic and dynamic recordings were low-pass filtered at 5 Hz [Winter, 1990]. The components of the hip acceleration were calculated using the kinematic data. Two sets of surface electrodes recorded the EMG activities of the quadriceps and hamstring muscles. The EMG was amplified, rectified and integrated at intervals of 10 ms.

Table 5.1: Biomechanical parameters of an able-bodied and one paraplegic subject used for simulation [Popović et al., 1999].

	SHANK (S)		THIGH (T)	
	ABLE-BODIED SUBJECT	PARAPLEGIC SUBJECT	ABLE-BODIED SUBJECT	PARAPLEGIC SUBJECT
J_C [kgm^2]	0.23	0.21	0.19	0.18
L [m]	0.51	0.54	0.42	0.44
d [m]	0.24	0.26	0.18	0.19
m [kg]	4.5	3.2	8.1	7.2

The mathematical model for simulation was derived in state space. The vector of state variables is $x=(x_1, x_2, x_3, x_4)$ where

$$x_1 = \phi_S, x_2 = \dot{\phi}_S, x_3 = \phi_T, x_4 = \dot{\phi}_T$$

State variables in this system are constrained by the limited physiological range of motion to:

$$0 \leq \phi_K \leq \pi/2 \qquad -\pi/4 \leq \phi_H \leq 3\pi/8 \qquad 2\pi/5 \leq \phi_{TR} \leq 3\pi/5$$

implying the constraints to the state variables $a \leq x_1 \leq b$, $c \leq x_1 \leq d$, where $a=1.15\pi$, $c=0.65\pi$ and $b=d=1.975\pi$.

By solving the system (5.1-1.2) with respect to $\dot{x}_2$ and $\dot{x}_4$, we can describe the dynamics of the leg controlled by two muscle equivalents at the hip and the knee:

$$\dot{x}_1 = x_2, \quad \dot{x}_2 = P_2 + \sum_{j=1}^{4} G_{2j} u_j$$
$$\dot{x}_1 = x_2, \quad \dot{x}_2 = P_2 + \sum_{j=1}^{4} G_{2j} u_j \qquad (5.12)$$

The terms P_2, P_4, G_{2j}, G_{4j} (j=1,2,3,4) are nonlinear functions obtained as the result of a series of elementary transformations of the system (5.1-5.11) [Oğuztöreli et al., 1994]. In order to choose an admissible control $u=u(t)$ in such a way that the actual trajectory $X=X(t)$ will be as close as possible to the desired trajectory $Z=Z(t)$ and constraining the activation levels of muscles it is necessary to introduce the cost function (5.13).

The discrete form of Equation (5.12) can be obtained after introducing $h=(T-t_0)/n$, $t_n=t_0+nh$ (N=0,1,..,N) where N is a sufficiently large integer and T is the stride cycle. Further, for any $x=x(t)$ we put $x(t_n)=x_n$. Then, using the approximation

$$\dot{x}(t_n) = \dot{x}_n \approx (x_{n+1} - x_n)/h$$

the motion can be described in the form:

$$x_{1,n+2} \approx y_{1,n} + h^2 \sum_{j=1}^{4} G_{2j,n} u_{j,n}$$

$$x_{3,n+2} \approx y_{3,n} + h^2 \sum_{j=1}^{4} G_{4j,n} u_{j,n}$$

$$y_{1,n} = x_{1,n} + 2h\, x_{2,n} + h^2 P_{2,n}$$

$$y_{3,n} = x_{3,n} + 2h\, x_{4,n} + h^2 P_{4,n}$$

and, after manipulation and rearrangement:

$$x_{1,n+1} \approx x_{1,n} + h\, x_{2,n}$$

$$x_{2,n+1} \approx x_{2,n} + h[\, P_{2,n} + \sum_{j=1}^{4} G_{2j,n} u_{j,n}\,]$$

$$x_{3,n+1} \approx x_{3,n} + h\, x_{4,n}$$

$$x_{4,n+1} \approx x_{4,n} + h[\, P_{4,n} + \sum_{j=1}^{4} G_{4j,n} u_{j,n}\,]$$

$$x_{i,N} = x_{i0} \quad (i=1,2,3,4)$$

Considering the limitations in the maximum activity of muscles, the set

$$\Omega = \{ (u_1, u_2, u_3, u_4): 0 \le u_k \le 1\ (k=1,2,3,4) \}$$

will be designated as the control region. The motion of the leg is determined by the angles $\varphi_S = x_1$ and $\varphi_T = x_3$. Accordingly, $X(t)=(x_1(t), x_3(t))$, $t_0 \le t \le t_0 + T$, is the trajectory called admissible if the state variables are within the physiological range of movement. Let $Z(t)=(z_1(t), z_3(t))$ be the desired trajectory of the functional movement. The assumption is that the initial conditions are:

$$x_{1,0} = z_{1,0},\ x_{1,N} = z_{1,N},\ x_{3,0} = z_{3,0},\ x_{3,N} = z_{3,N}$$

In order to choose an admissible control $u=u(t)$ the following cost function was assumed used:

$$R(u) = \int_{t_0}^{t_0+T} \{ [\, x_1(t) - z_1(t)\,]^2 + [\, x_3(t) - z_3(t)\,]^2$$

$$+ \lambda_1 [\, u_1^2(t) + u_2^2(t)\,] + \lambda_2 [\, u_3^2(t) + u_4^2(t)\,]\, \} dt. \tag{5.13}$$

This cost function imposes that the overlap of agonist and antagonist activity is minimized, yet in the same time the total activity of two muscle pairs was not optimized. The values of λ_1, λ_2 can be varied between 0 and 1, and in the simulation presented they were both set at the value 1.

A discrete form of the cost function is:

$$R(u) = h [\, \sum_{n=0}^{N-2} r_n(X_n, u_n) + r_{N-1}(X_{N-1}, u_{N-1})\,]$$

where the terms r_n, r_{N-1} are determined by:

$$r_n(X_n,u_n) = \lambda_1[u_{1,n}^2+u_{2,n}^2] + \lambda_2[u_{3,n}^2+u_{4,n}^2] + (x_{1,n}-z_{1,n})^2 + (x_{3,n}-z_{3,n})^2 +$$
$$(y_{1,n}-z_{1,n+2}+h^2\sum_{j=1}^{4}G_{2j,n}u_{j,n})^2 + (y_{3,n}-z_{3,n+2}+h^2\sum_{j=1}^{4}G_{4j,n}u_{j,n})^2, \quad (n=0,1,...,N-2)$$

and

$$r_{N-1}(X_{N-1},u_{N-1}) = \lambda_1[u_{1,N-1}^2+u_{2,N-1}^2] + \lambda_2[u_{3,N-1}^2+u_{4,N-1}^2]$$

The optimization is now reduced to the system of equations:

$$\frac{\partial r_n(X_n,u_n)}{\partial u_{k,n}} = 0 \quad (k=1,2,3,4) \qquad \bar{u}_{j,n}^{-0} = \begin{cases} 0, & \bar{u}_{j,n} < 0 \\ \bar{u}_{j,n}, & 0 \leq \bar{u}_{j,n} \leq 1 \\ 1, & \bar{u}_{j,n} > 1 \end{cases}$$

The optimal trajectory is:

$$\bar{x}_{1,n}^{-0} = \begin{cases} a, & \bar{x}_{1,n} < a \\ \bar{x}_{1,n}, & a \leq \bar{x}_{1,n} \leq b \\ b, & \bar{x}_{1,n} > b \end{cases} \qquad \bar{x}_{3,n}^{-0} = \begin{cases} c, & \bar{x}_{3,n} < c \\ \bar{x}_{3,n}, & c \leq \bar{x}_{3,n} \leq d \\ d, & \bar{x}_{3,n} > d \end{cases}$$

$$\bar{x}_{2,n}^{-0} = \bar{x}_{2,n}, \quad \bar{x}_{4,n}^{-0} = \bar{x}_{4,n}$$

Further details can be found in Popović et al., [1991d, 1995].

The simulation of the walking of an able-bodied human and a subject with SCI at the thoracic level are presented. The data for both simulations (Figure 5.22) are from the normal walking of an able-bodied subject. She walked wearing ankle-foot orthoses (limited plantar flexion to 5 degrees and dorsiflexion to 8 degrees). The stride length varied between Δ = 0.88 m and Δ= 1.08 m, with a cycle T between 1.24 and 1.35 seconds.

The body and parameters determining the relationships in equations 5.1-5.11 are summarized in Tables 5.1 and 5.2. The neutral angles were $\varphi_{K0}=0.5$, $\varphi_{H0}=0$.

The left panels in Figure 5.23 show the recorded (desired) joint angles superimposed on the results of simulation for the able-bodied subject. The right

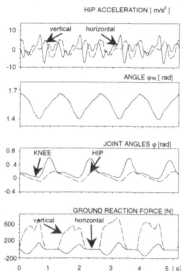

Fig. 5.22: Trajectory used for determining of the patterns for muscle activation required for driving muscles in both, an able-bodied and a paraplegic subject. From Popović et al., 1999b © IEEE.

panels show the results for the paraplegic subject. The measure of the quality of tracking is the difference between the desired angles φ_K, φ_H and the calculated values φ_{K^*}, φ_{H^*}. The mean absolute errors in radians have been defined as:

$$e_K = \sum_{i=1}^{n}\left|\varphi_{Ki} - \varphi_{Ki}^*\right|/n \quad e_H = \sum_{i=1}^{n}\left|\varphi_{Hi} - \varphi_{Hi}^*\right|/n$$

These errors have been calculated for the whole sequence of walking (230 consecutive strides) with the sampling interval of 10 ms. The magnitude of errors are $e_K=0.0124$, $e_H=0.083$ radian, with the standard deviations $\sigma_K=0.0104$, $\sigma_H=0.065$ radian. The maximum absolute errors were $e_{Kmax}=0.06$, $e_{Hmax}=0.13$ radian. The tracking errors for the subject with paraplegia (Figure 5.12) reached $e_K=0.0364$, $e_H=0.156$ radian, the standard deviations were $\sigma_K=0.0516$, $\sigma_H=0.161$, and the maximum errors $e_{Kmax}=0.177$, $e_{Hmax}=0.293$ radian.

The simulation output is a set of discrete activation values for four muscle groups (Figure 5.24). Left panels are for the able-bodied subject, while the right for the paraplegic person. The activation levels for the able-bodied subject never reach

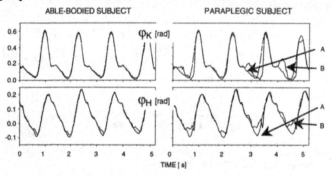

Fig. 5.23: (A) Desired (input) and (B) calculated knee and hip joint angles are superimposed for the able-bodied (left) and paraplegic (right) subjects. Four consecutive, non-identical strides are presented. The error between the desired and estimated joint angles is discussed in the text. Adapted from Popović et al., 1999b © IEEE.

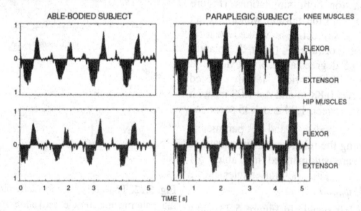

Fig. 5.24: The calculated activity ($0<u<1$) of the knee and hip flexor and extensor muscles for an able-bodied (left) and paraplegic (right) subjects (level walking). The model (Figure 5.10) has been customized by using individual parameters (Table 5.2), yet the same trajectory (Figure 5.11) for both subjects. Adapted from Popović et al., 1999b © IEEE.

maximum ($u=1$), yet the activation for the paraplegic subject saturates, suggesting that the muscles are not strong enough. The antagonist muscle activity is deliberately presented inverted, pointing down in Figure 5.24 to display that the effects are opposing the actions of the agonist muscles.

Table 5.2: Biomechanical parameters determining the actuators' properties of four musculo-tendonal systems (active and passive properties) of two joints for able-bodied subject (upper part) and paraplegic subject - complete lesion T_{10} (lower part). [Popović et al., 1999b].

$c_{10}=61.6$	$c_{11}=1.54$	$c_{12}=-9.24$	$c_{13}=0.06$	$c_{14}=1.2$	
$c_{20}=56.45$	$c_{21}=368.67$	$c_{22}=-128.77$	$c_{23}=0.04$	$c_{24}=1.5$	
$c_{30}=206$	$c_{31}=76$	$c_{32}=54$	$c_{33}=0.05$	$c_{34}=1.2$	
$c_{40}=158.4$	$c_{41}=114.84$	$c_{42}=-52.8$	$c_{43}=0.04$	$c_{44}=1.5$	
$d_{11}=9$	$d_{12}=0.5$	$d_{13}=0.002$	$d_{14}=5.02$	$d_{15}=50.61$	$d_{16}=-29.32$
$d_{31}=10$	$d_{32}=0.6$	$d_{33}=0.84$	$d_{34}=2.5$	$d_{35}=0.05$	$d_{36}=-14.99$
$c_{10}=28$	$c_{11}=0.7$	$c_{12}=-4.2$	$c_{13}=0.1$	$c_{14}=1.4$	
$c_{20}=43.2$	$c_{21}=282.15$	$c_{22}=-98.55$	$c_{23}=0.3$	$c_{24}=1.2$	
$c_{30}=167.37$	$c_{31}=61.75$	$c_{32}=-43.87$	$c_{33}=0.05$	$c_{34}=1.4$	
$c_{40}=108$	$c_{41}=78.3$	$c_{42}=-36$	$c_{43}=0.06$	$c_{44}=1.2$	
$d_{11}=17$	$d_{12}=0.6$	$d_{13}=0.005$	$d_{14}=5.048$	$d_{15}=98.57$	$d_{16}=-28.56$
$d_{31}=16$	$d_{32}=0.7$	$d_{33}=1.67$	$d_{34}=2.5$	$d_{35}=0.1$	$d_{36}=-15.04$

The maximum activation is assumed to be $u=1$, while the resting muscle is described with the activation value $u=0$. The simulation of the walking of a subject with paraplegia (lesion at T_{10} level) was done by using her body and muscle parameters (Tables 5.1 and 5.2), yet using the same trajectory as the one used for the able-bodied subject (Figure 5.22). The externally activated muscles in a paraplegic subject generate net joint torque that are smaller compared to the net joint torque generated volitionally by the able-bodied subject; thus, the electrical stimulation can not develop the net joint torque that are required to track the desired trajectory good enough. When the error accumulates, the simulation becomes unstable, and the computer comes with the error message indicating that the walking pattern is not achievable.

A weakness of this model is that it reduces walking to a planar system, and includes only four actuators per leg. The complexity of the optimization algorithm was the main reason to select this reduced model. The limitation of the analysis to only four muscle groups is still suitable for the design of an FES system which commonly only has four to six channels of stimulation for walking with ankle-foot orthoses.

Dynamic models allow body-segment trajectories to be determined from muscle stimulation patterns. This process is known as *simulation* or *forward dynamics* (in Russian literature this problem is called inverse problem of mechanics). Simulation provides a tool to evaluate the performance of different controller designs and predict the response of the controlled system to disturbances. Once a system has been selected, simulation can help predict its stability and behavior under various conditions (e.g., disturbances), and sensitivity of performance to parameter and modeling errors.

Linear control theory and reduced-order nonlinear models are frequently employed to simplify the control system design process. Since the dynamic model is simplified, the performance of the controller should always be tested with simulations based on the full, nonlinear model of the human motor task. In this way, fine-tuning of the feedback parameters can be made to give even better performance, or if performance is unsatisfactory, the control design can be discarded before hardware implementation.

Dynamic modeling and simulation can provide benefits beyond the design and testing of NP control systems. All elements of the model can be explored in great detail, revealing information about internal forces and movements, which cannot be directly measured from the human body. Simulation provides a faster, cheaper alternative to hardware implementation and initial testing of NP systems. The predictive capability of the simulated control system, however, depends on the accuracy of the musculoskeletal model.

5.2 Hybrid Hierarchical Control Systems

Hybrid means, in general, heterogeneous in nature or composition. The term "hybrid systems" is understood to describe systems with behavior defined by entities or processes of distinct characteristics. The hybrid systems of interest here are dynamic systems where the behavior is determined by interacting continuous and discrete dynamics. These systems typically contain variables or signals that take values from a continuous set (e.g., the set of real numbers) and also variables that take values from a discrete, typically finite set (e.g., the set of symbols {a, b, c}). These continuous or discrete-valued variables or signals depend on independent variables such as time, which may also be continuous or discrete; some of the variables may also be discrete-event driven in an asynchronous manner [Antsaklis and Nerode, 1998].

There are many examples of hybrid systems. In the control area, a very well-known instance of a hybrid system is when a continuous-time linear time-invariant plant described by linear differential equations (which involve continuous valued variables that depend on continuous time) is controlled by a discrete-time linear time-invariant plant described by linear difference equations (which involve continuous-valued variables that depend on discrete time). These types of systems are typically studied in courses under the name of sampled data systems or digital control systems; digital control systems may of course include more general types of systems such as time-varying and nonlinear plants and controllers. If one also considers quantization of the continuous-valued variables or signals, then the hybrid systems contain not only continuous valued variables that are driven by continuous and discrete times, but also discrete-valued signals as well. Note that recent studies of digital control systems in the hybrid system literature typically involve nonlinear plants and controllers. Another familiar example of a hybrid control system is a switching system where the dynamic behavior of interest can be adequately described by a finite (small) number of dynamical models, *i.e.*, typically sets of differential or difference equations, together with a set of rules for switching among these models. These switching rules are described by logic expressions or a discrete-event system with a finite automaton or a Petri net representation. Another existing area, which has recently been brought under the hybrid systems framework, is the study of properties (e.g., stability) of dynamical systems described by differential equations with discontinuities present.

There are several reasons for using hybrid models to represent the movement. Reducing complexity was and still is an important reason for dealing with hybrid systems. This is accomplished in hybrid systems by incorporating models of dynamic processes at different levels of abstraction. For another example, in order to avoid dealing directly with a set of nonlinear equations, one may choose to work with sets of simpler equations (e.g., linear) and switch among these simpler models. This is a rather common approach in modeling physical phenomena. In control, switching among simple dynamical systems has been used successfully in practice for many decades. Recent efforts in hybrid systems research along these lines typically concentrate on the analysis of the dynamic behaviors and aim to design controllers with guaranteed stability and performance. The advent of digital machines has made hybrid systems very common indeed.

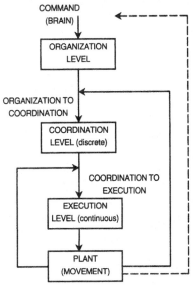

Fig. 5.25: The organization of a hierarchical, hybrid control system for restoring movement.

Hybrid control systems typically arise from the interaction of discrete planning algorithms and continuous processes, and, as such, they provide the basic framework and methodology for the analysis and synthesis of autonomous and intelligent systems, *i.e.*, planning to move the hand and grasp an object. Hybrid control systems contain two distinct types of components, subsystems with continuous dynamics and subsystems with discrete-event dynamics that interact with each other.

Another important way in which hybrid systems arise is from the hierarchical organization of complex control systems (Figure 5.25). In these systems, a hierarchical organization helps to manage the complexity, and higher levels in the hierarchy require less detailed models (discrete abstractions) of the functioning of the lower levels, necessitating the interaction of discrete and continuous components. The study of hybrid control systems is essential in designing sequential supervisory controllers for continuous systems, and it is central in designing intelligent control systems with a high degree of autonomy.

There are analogies between certain current approaches to hybrid control and digital control system methodologies. Specifically, in digital control one could carry the control design in the continuous-time domain, then approximate or emulate the controller by a discrete controller and implement it using an interface consisting of a sampler and a hold device (A/D and D/A, respectively). Alternatively, one could obtain first a discrete model of the plant taken together with the interface and then carry the controller design in the discrete domain. In hybrid systems, in a manner analogous to the latter case, one may obtain a discrete-event model of the plant together with the interface using automata or Petri nets; the controller is then designed using DES supervisor methodologies. Approaches analogous to the former also exist. The optimization methodologies are also used in hybrid control synthesis that includes convex optimization and game theoretic approaches. A detail description on hybrid systems may be found in a series of lecture notes [Grossman et al., 1993; Antsaklis et al., 1995; Alur et al., 1996; Antsaklis et al., 1998; Morse, 1996].

Switched Systems. The prototypical example of a switched system is

$$\dot{x}(t) = f_i(x(t)), \quad i \in Q \equiv \{1,2,..,N\}$$

where $x(t) \in R^n$ and the following switching rules apply: each f_i is globally Lipschitz continuous, and the is are picked in such a way that there are finite switches in finite time. The switched systems of interest have variable structure, i.e., they are multi-modal. The particular "i" at any given time should be chosen by some "higher" process, such as a human operator (supervised) or be a function of time or state (or both), in which case the system is autonomous. The movement control belongs to operator controlled (supervised) systems with automatic operation at lower levels. An equivalent discrete system to the model is described with a difference equation:

$$x[k+1] = f_i(x[k+1]), \quad i \in q \equiv \{1,...,N\}$$

where $x[k] \in R^n$. Here, the additional assumption for f_i is that they are globally continuous in the Lipschitz sense. These equations can be thought of as the "continuous" portion of the dynamics of hybrid systems combining difference equations and finite automata.

A *continuous switched system* is a system with the additional constraint that the switched subsystems agree at the switching time. More specifically, consider the defined model and assume that at times t_j, $j = 1, 2, 3,..$, there is a switch from f_{kj-1} to f_{kj}. Then, the requirement is $f_{kj-1}(x(t_j), t_j) = f_{kj}(x(t_j),t_j)$ in order to fulfil the continuity law over time.

Hybrid systems inherently combine logical and continuous processes, usually coupled finite automata and differential equations. Thus, the continuous dynamics are modeled by a differential equation:

$$\dot{x}(t) = \xi(t), \quad t \geq 0$$

where $x(t)$ is the continuous component of the state taking values in some subset of a Euclidean space. $\xi(t)$ is a controlled vector field that depends on x(t) and the aforementioned logical or finite dynamics. Two categories of switched systems are of interest: autonomous switching where the vector field $\xi(\cdot)$ changes discontinuously when the state $x(\cdot)$ hits certain boundaries, and controlled switching where $\xi(\cdot)$ changes abruptly in the response to a control command, possibly with an associated cost.

A (continuous-time) autonomous hybrid system may be defined as follows:

$$\dot{x}(t) = f(x(t),q(t))$$

$$q(t) = v(x(t),q(t^-))$$

where $x(t) \in R^n$, $q(t) \in Q \equiv \{1, .. , N\}$. Here, $f(\cdot,q) : R^n \to R^n$, $q \in Q$, each globally Lipschitz continuous represents the continuous dynamics, and v: $R^n \times Q \to Q$ is the finite state dynamics. Here, the notation t^- indicates that the finite state is piecewise continuous. Thus, starting at $[x_o, i]$, the continuous state trajectory $x(\cdot)$ evolves according to $x(t) = f(x,i)$. If $x(\cdot)$ hits some $(v(\cdot,i))^{-1}(j)$ at time t_i, then the state becomes $[x(t_i),j]$, from which the process continues.

Clearly, this is an instantiation of autonomous switching. Switching is a fixed function of time that could be taken care of by adding further state dimension. This definition is closely related to the so-called differential automata; it is a simplified view of the hybrid systems models [Branicki, 1998].

A continuous-time controlled hybrid system is

$$\dot{x}(t) = f(x(t), q(t), u(t))$$
$$q(t) = v(x(t), q(t^-), u(t))$$

where everything is as above except that $u(t) \in R^m$, with f and v modified appropriately.

Continuation Program for Hybrid Systems. The additional constraint of the continuous, switched system introduced above leads to a simpler class of systems to consider. At the same time, it is not overly restrictive since many switching systems naturally satisfy this constraint. Indeed they may even arise from the discontinuous logic present in hybrid systems. These can result in discontinuous control input, which, after passing through a dynamical system (e.g., actuator dynamics), yields switching controls at the plant level that preserves continuity in the derivative.

More generally, we may approximate the finite dynamics of a hybrid system by considering singular perturbations that are "continuations" of them:

$$\dot{x} = f(x, z)$$
$$\varepsilon \dot{z} = [v(x, z) - z]$$

This is a linear interpolation of the dynamics, although others are possible, including appending states so that the continuations of the discrete transitions are well defined.

The hybrid hierarchical control could be implemented for standing, walking, reaching, and grasping neuroprostheses. The control should have three levels [Tomović et al., 1995; Prochazka, 1993; Loeb et al., 1999]. It has to support both the parallel and hierarchical communication pathways as it is suggested in Sections 5.3 to 5.5. The top, decision level of the controller is to remain entirely biological. The coordination level, the interface between the decision and the execution of control commands could be understood as interface between the command signals and actuators, and its main role is the distribution of the command. This level should maximize from implementing natural like synergies; in this way it the preserved and externally controlled parts of the system could maximize their effects. The synergistic coordination reduces the problems of actuator and degrees of freedom redundancy. The actuator control level drives musculo-tendonal systems; thus, it should be customized to the eventual user. This actuation would work the best if it applies model-based control.

5.2.1 Nonanalytical Methods for Coordination of Movement

Nonanalytical Control (NAC) of movement is a symbolic technique, which uses non-numerical tools and relies on non-parametric models of human body and movement trajectories [Tomović et al., 1995]. Non-numerical tools are the identification techniques, which in most cases rely on heuristics. The non-parametric models use the set theory and symbols in a multidimensional phase space instead of differential equations of movement, optimization and numerical simulations [Tomović et al., 1995]. NAC inherently deals with the following problems of movement control: 1) redundancy, nonlinearity, and time variability of the plant; 2) redundancy of plausible trajectories; and 3) the significance of the preference criteria based on the task. NAC models have hierarchical and hybrid structure; they resemble to the biological counterpart described in Chapter 1. Non-numerical identification techniques are used at all levels of the hierarchical structure and each of the levels is reduced to a black box; the complexity of both the model and uncertainty of trajectories are included and represented with symbols. Nonanalytical methods have been developed to eliminate the extremely complex modeling, parameter identification, and numerical operations for real-time applications.

The simplest non-numerical model of movement is based on a finite state description of the process [Tomović and McGhee, 1968; Tomovićet al., 1991]. The quadrupedal locomotion of a robot has been described by the states of the legs (e.g., on the ground, off the ground). The joint states have been originally reduced to: free (loose), locked, flexion and extension [Tomović et al., 1981, 1982, 1990]. Finite state methods, initially used the so-called "on-off" control, then evolved into a rule-based control systems that use set theory to define the behavior based on the states and transitions between these states [Tomović, 1984 and 1991]. The states are descriptions of the movement using a multidimensional phase space (e.g., joint locked by cocontraction, agonist muscles activated and antagonistic muscles inhibited, full extension, joint flexion, heel contact, maximum angular velocity). The rules are logical relations (e.g., IF-THEN, AND, OR) that connect state variables and define transition between the states.

5.2.2 Rule-Based Control (RBC) Systems

Rule-Based Control (RBC) systems are based on heuristics and non-parametric mapping. The heuristic procedures consist of choosing methods, which seem promising, while allowing the possibility of changing to other if the first seems not to lead quickly enough to a solution. The RBC are able to learn from mistakes and their performance improves because they take into account the past errors.

The RBC uses the predicate calculus, which is an extension of the propositional. The propositional calculus is defined by two sets of rules: those of the syntax, governing the form of the statements that can be made in the language, and those governing the derivation of new statements from olds. To every legal statement, called a proposition, one of two plausible (Boolean) values *True* or *False* is assigned. The predicate calculus extends from the propositional calculus by introducing the concept of a variable. The basic relation in a RBC is a production rule. A production rule is a situation - action couple; *i.e.*, whenever a certain situation is encountered, given as the left side of the rule the action on the right side of the rule is to be executed. There are no a priori constraints on the forms of the situations or of the actions. A system based on production rules have three components: 1) the rule base, consisting of the set of production rules; 2) one or more data structures containing the known facts relevant to the domain of interest, possibly also some useful definitions; these are often called facts bases; and 3) the interpreter of these facts and rules, which is the mechanism that decides which rule to apply and initiates the corresponding action.

Each rule is an independent item of knowledge, containing all the conditions required for the application. The interpreter introduces relations between rules, a rule itself is ignorant to others; thus, RBC has modular structure. Because of the modularity RBC systems can be modified easily and the addition, deletion or modification of a rule does not affects the architectural structure of the program. An important feature of the RBC systems is the ability to look first at the established facts and to proceed forward (forward chaining) or to start from the aims, *i.e.,* from the action part of the rules (backward chaining). Neither method has shown clear advantage over the other as far as overall efficiency is concerned. The forward method has the advantage of providing better control over the order in which data are acquired. The backward method is better in that it enables the interpreter to get closer to the tasks it wishes to reach, as it can apply only those rules that are relevant to these tasks. It is, however, difficult to foresee in which order these rules will be applied.

The problem of knowledge representation is fundamental for the efficiency of the RBC systems. Only rarely can the knowledge concerning a particular field be out in terms of a single formalism. There are usually some items of a heuristic nature. There are procedural items in addition to heuristics. The knowledge built into RBC system often consists of "tricks of the trade" in addition to the type of knowledge, which is expressed explicitly.

5.2.3 Methods and Tools to Define Rules for RBC

The rules can be either heuristically defined through a procedure known as *handcrafting,* or automatically generated thorough a procedure known as *machine learning* or *pattern mapping and classification* (e.g., inductive learning, artificial neural networks, adaptive logic networks, fuzzy-logic networks, wavelet networks).

The handcrafted rules and states are defined by a human, based on his/her previous experience and intuition using the inductive procedures. The inductive procedures for defining rules rely entirely on the ability to represent and transfer human expertise in a form that can be used by a machine. The expertise required for designing of a set of rules (knowledge base) for real-time control is gained by analyzing the sensory patterns acquired while observing the process and the plant (e.g., able-bodied subjects, amputees or paraplegics walking at different speeds and under various conditions). The sensory patterns are coded (e.g., single threshold, multi threshold, timing, local *vs.* absolute minimum or maximum), and the rules define the relationship between sensory patterns and required motor activities. A set of sensors providing feedback signals has been so far arbitrarily determined (e.g., ground reaction force or pressure sensor, switch, goniometer, inclinometer, accelerometer, and proximity sensor); the choice is based on availability of sensors, reproducibility of the sensory recordings, and over all practicality of plausible day to day usage. Sensors that are functionally equivalent to those used in biological control systems are preferred. Increasing the number of sensors produces very fast growth of the number of control rules making the definition process time consuming and very difficult.

An example of handcrafted, rule-based control, which operates with supervisory input from the user, but no feedback, is the walking assisted with a multichannel stimulator described by Kobetič and Marsolais [1994]. The stimulator controls as many as 48 percutaneous electrodes in many muscles that are needed for bipedal walking of a paraplegic subject [Marsolais *et al.,* 1990]. The initial pattern of the stimulation sequence is a "copy" of an normalized sequence of EMG recordings from muscles of able-bodied humans when walking. Since the external activation of muscles does not result with the same net joint torque as if the muscles are driven by the central nervous system, and the walking of a paraplegic is assisted with a walker or crutches (quadrupedal walking) the resulting movement of legs differs from the desired one. The iterative procedure is used to correct for differences; the stimulation sequence is adjusted to correct the joint movement through a "trial and error" method. The result is a handcrafted, preprogrammed sequence of stimulation, which could be described as a decision tree. The compensatory movement to stabilize the system and correct for eventual errors comes from the movement of the upper body and arms acting over the walker or crutches. The results depend exclusively on experts' ability to express acquired knowledge explicitly in states and rules.

The hand-crafted rules have been applied for control of transfemoral prostheses [e.g., Aeyels et al., 1992, 1997; Bar et al., 1983; James et al., 1991; Popović et al., 1991b], hybrid assistive systems [e.g., Andrews et al., 1988; Phillips et al., 1988; Popović, 1991d; Popović and Schwirtlich 1988; Popović et al., 1990b, Jaspers et al., 1996], and grasping systems [Kilgore et al., 1989].

Strange and Hoffer [1999a and b] presented results of a long-term evaluation of the cuff electrodes implanted in the forelimb of a cat. They implemented a real time FES states controller that was designed to use sensory nerve cuff signals to control the timing of activation with FES of the Palmaris Longus (PalL) muscle during walking on the treadmill. This study involved three experiments: prediction of the timing of muscle activity in an open-loop configuration with no stimulation, prediction of the timing of muscle activity in a closed-loop configuration with stimulation of the muscle over natural EMG, and temporary paralysis of selected forelimb muscles coupled with the use of state controller and stimulation of the PalL. Strange and Hoffer used the recordings from the median and superficial radial nerves to detect the timing to start and stop stimulation of the PalL, which is an improvement of the technique suggested by Popović and coworkers [1993] who used the neural recordings to detect the instant

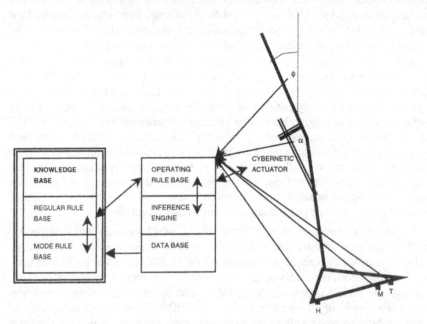

Fig. 5.26: Schema of the organization of the rule-based controller for the Belgrade transfemoral prostheses. See text for details.

to start the stimulation, yet the duration of the burst of stimulation was estimated on the duration of the previous stride.

One of the first successful applications of the RBC control for assistive technology was the Belgrade leg with the hydraulic actuator [Tomović *et al.*, 1978, Tomović *et al.*, 1982]. The motorized, externally powered version of the Belgrade leg [Popović and Schwirtlich, 1988] used the RBC system consisting of the following blocks: data base, inference engine, regular rule base, operating rule base, mode rule base [Popović *et al.*, 1991b].

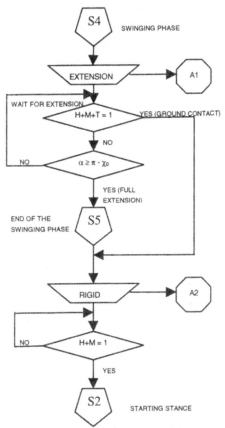

Fig. 5.27: The sequence of reflexes for the swing phase of the Belgrade transfemoral prosthesis. H, M, and T are switches at the heel metatarsal and toe zones of the sole of the foot (1 - closed switch, 0 – open), α is the knee angle, χ_0 the boundary threshold (Figure 5.26). A1 and A2 are the flexion/extension and damping control actuators at the knee joint. Adapted from Tomović *et al.*, 1981, with permission.

The regular rule base has two subsets of rules, regular and hazard rules. Regular rules are couples "situation - action" within a specific walking modality. Hazard rules deal with the conflict situations that are not included in walking sequences (e.g., hardware of the leg can not generate the appropriate movement, unexpected event during walking). The term *firing the rule* is used to describe the execution of a rule. Firing of the rule from the regular rule base is motor action, that is the change of the actuator state. The cybernetic actuator incorporates four states: locking, unlocking, extension and flexion of the knee joint.

The mode rule base comprises several subsets of rules, each corresponding to one modality of walking (e.g., walking up-stairs, walking up the slope, turning around, sitting down, quite standing, fast walking, slow walking). Firing of a rule from the mode base results with transferring of the appropriate subset of rules from the MRB to the RRB (Figure 5.26).

The data base consists from a set of user dependent thresholds and other parameters required for operation. The operating rules base uses the rules from regular rule base and delivers command signals via the inference engine. The sensory system includes three switches positioned at the heel (H), metatarsal (M) and toe (T) zones at the sole of the artificial foot, the joint angle transducer (α), and the vertical displacement sensor of the thigh (ϕ).

Table 5.3: Ipsilateral coded sensory input (IF part of rules) for ten rules (level walking) determined by a preferential network. See text for details. The rules are sequentially organized, *i.e.*, next rule is triggered only if the sensory input is recognized and the previous rule has been executed.

RULE No #	HIP	KNEE	ANKLE	TOE	HEEL	THIGH
1	0	1	0	-2	1	-1
2	0	1	1	-2	1	-1
3	-1	0	0	-2	1	-1
4	-1	-1	-1	1	0	-1
5	0	0	-1	1	-1	-1
6	1	1	0	0	-1	0
7	1	-1	1	-1	0	1
8	1	-1	-1	-2	-2	1
9	0	-1	1	-2	-2	1
10	0	0	0	-2	-2	1

Table 5.4: The execution (THEN) part of the ten rules determined by a preferential network for level walking. The abbreviations are: B – blocked state of the joint, L – loose (free) state of the joint, X – no action, F – flexion, E – extension. MAX TIME is the percentage of the previous walking gait cycle. If the sensory pattern does not match the next sequential expected combination, the change to different modality (network) occurs.

RULE No #	HIP	KNEE	ANKLE	MAX. TIME
1	B	L	X	5
2	B	B	X	9
3	E	E	X	11
4	E	B	X	25
5	E	B	X	41
6	F	L	E	58
7	F	F	F	65
8	L	L	F	83
9	E	E	X	88
10	L	E	X	93

After the user switches the system on, information of instantaneous position of the leg with respect the external reference frame is updated. The user has to bring the leg in the appropriate position by moving the stump and/or the trunk; the intention detection system will then initiate automatic control.

All rules are organized using the IF-THEN structures. The actual organization of the single rule will be explained using an example: the control of the leg during the swing phase of walking (Figure 5.27). This example shows that the operations are simple logical expressions; thus, very suitable for real-time applications. The rule has the following form:

IF:
- the knee angle φ is bigger than the threshold value φ_T,
- the knee angular velocity is negative,
- the toe force F_T and the heel force are smaller than the threshold F_0, and
- the previous movement was initial flexion

THEN:
- turn off the flexion motor unit,
- allow free state (brake mechanism is in the unlock state).

The threshold value is selected to correspond to the forces required to close the switch mounted at the heel and toe zones of the sole. The Belgrade transfemoral prosthesis comprises the total of 97 rules for 14 different modalities of walking [Popović et al., 1991b]. The program developed for the Belgrade active transfemoral prosthesis has been modified and adapted for an custom designed hydraulic actuator [James et al., 1991], now implemented for the Otto Bock commercial product called C-leg (described in Section 4.4).

The handcrafted rule based control has been developed and tested with partially powered hybrid assistive systems [Tomović et al., 1995]. The reasons for developing the automatic control have been to extend the inadequate FES generated step length and transform the slow, quasi static; FES generated ambulating into a dynamic process. The task to reproduce normal walking by hybrid assistive system is intentionally not mentioned, because at this point, such an ambition is not realistic. Two options have been considered: parallel operation of the biological and external control, and sequential operation of the biological and external control.

Mulder et al. [1980] analyzed rule–based control to minimize the quadriceps force while standing. The knee joint angle and angular velocities have been used to control the amplitude of stimulation pulses applied to the quadriceps muscle. The hand-crafted rules provided a reduced knee extension net joint torque if the knee joint and its angular velocity remained within the preset thresholds, but comprised alertness of the controller to increase the force and prevent collapsing when and if necessary. Mulder with coworkers [Mulder et al., 1992a and b] compared the performance between the open-loop control and rule-based control of standing with FES system used to stimulate bilateral quadriceps muscles. The rule based control allowed subjects to stand for 2.5 to 12 times longer, and the quadriceps forces have been decreased between 30 and 80 percent compared to open-loop (maximum) regime. In a parallel study, Veltink and Franken [1996] used the accelerometers to detect the changes at the knee joint angle and rule-based control while applying FES system for standing of paraplegic subjects. The use of accelerometer was proven superior to the application of goniometers, since they provide information that is preceding the change of the angular velocity and the knee joint angle. Jaspers et al., [1996] reported about positive effects of handcrafted rule-based control for a hybrid gait orthosis comprising an ARGO and FES systems.

In order to apply computer for defining rules, a formal model of locomotion has to be adopted. The model could be derived in several ways [Tomović et al., 1991]:

1) recording and analyzing movements and joint trajectories without interfering with the neuromuscular system. Such a modeling procedure is conveniently called the external approach; 2) integrating the computer input into the afferent paths of the motor control system so that the model is driven by natural sensory patterns. This is called the hybrid approach; 3) integrating both the computer input and output into corresponding paths of the neural network responsible for the motor act. Such modeling is quite close to what may be called computer grafting.

Popović [1993] defined the finite state model of walking using the following elements: sensors to monitor the hip, knee and ankle angular velocities, ground reaction forces, and displacements of the body segments from the vertical. The sensory information from the joint angles was used to code the joint states: flexion (F), extension (E), and no rotation (NR). These three states could be realized by four actuator states: loose (L), blocked (B), flexion (F) and extension (E) of the joint. A joint state is not identical to the actuator state (e.g., a joint can be locked by co-contraction of agonist and antagonistic muscle groups or with no muscle activation at some joint positions and adequate posture). The preferential neural network [Dujmović, 1991] was chosen to identify the significance of each of the sensors for the mapping and classification as well as to determine the rules. This technique provides both the control laws and the sensitivity analysis of the performance to the input. The sensitivity analysis is essential for minimizing the number of sensors and selecting their appropriate characteristics [Popović *et al.*, 1990b]. Preferential neural networks are a version of fuzzy logic network.

Ground reaction forces also have been coded: value 1 was associated with an increase of the force, -1 to the decrease, 0 to changes smaller then the arbitrary small threshold, and -2 for the force being zero. Sensors monitoring displacement from the vertical were coded to 1, when the angle is positive, and coded to −1, when the angle is negative. Tables 5.3 and 5.4 show both the IF and THEN "sides" of 10 rules for level walking. Different sets of rules have been determined for faster and slower gait, as well as for slope, stairs and other modalities of walking [Popović, 1993].

The results of the learning been tested in a single subject [Popović, 1993]. A subject with complete T10 traumatic spinal cord injury walked assisted with a six-channel surface stimulation system and the under elbow crutches using hand switches [Kralj and Bajd, 1989] and automatic control based on the preferential networks. The automatic control allowed the speed of walking of 0.73 m/s, compared to 0,31 m/s with hand control. The oxygen consumption was decreased for 30 percent, and the upper extremity forces decreased in average for 28 percent when automatic control was used. The automatic control was applicable for level, slope, and stairs walking.

5.2.4 Machine Learning for Determining of the Rules for RBC

Artificial neural networks (ANN) are inspired by biological nervous systems. The ANN is composed of many simple elements working in parallel, and the network function is determined largely by the connections between them [Haykin, 1993]. During the learning process to perform a particular function, the values of connections between elements are adjusted (Figure 5.28).

Multilayer Perceptron. Investigations of the multilayer perceptron (MLP) have been intensified since the formulation of the backpropagation (BP) learning algorithm [Rumelhart *et al.*, 1986]. It was found that this algorithm represents a simple and powerful tool for adjusting the connections between elements of the networks with

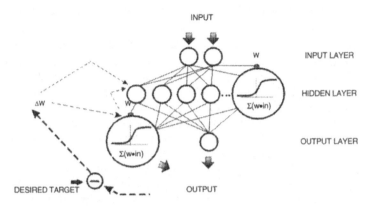

Fig. 5.28: A typical of a three-layer structure of the neural network. Courtesy of Dr. Francisco Sepulveda, Aalborg University, Denmark.

arbitrarily complex architecture. Typically, MLP consists of several layers of nonlinear processing nodes, called hidden layers with a linear output layer. The processing node takes as input only the output of the previous layer, which is combined as a weighted sum and then passed through a nonlinear processing function known as the activation function. This activation function is typically sigmoidal in shape. The MLP with three hidden layers can form arbitrarily complex decision regions and can separate the classes that are meshed together. It can form regions as complex as those formed using mixture distributions and nearest neighbor classifiers [Lippmann, 1987].

The MLP usually used has a single linear output node and single hidden layer with sigmoidal activation functions. The BP learning algorithm is a generalization of a gradient descent algorithm. It uses a gradient search technique to minimize a cost function equal to the sum square difference between the desired and estimated net output. Derivatives of error (called delta vectors) are calculated for the output layer of the network and then backpropagated through the network until delta vectors are available for each hidden layer of the network. The BP algorithm may lead to a local, rather than a global error minimum. If the local minimum found is not satisfactory, the use of several different sets of initial conditions or a network with more neurons can be tried.

Radial Basis Function Artificial Neural Network. Radial Basis Function (RBF) ANN [Chen et al., 1991] usually uses a single output node and a single hidden layer that contains as many neurons as are required to fit the function within the specifications of the error goals. The transformation from the input space to the hidden-unit space is nonlinear, whereas the transformation from the hidden-unit space to the output space is linear. A common learning algorithm for RBF networks is based on choosing randomly some data points as radial basis function centers and then using singular value decomposition to solve the weights of the network. An arbitrary selection of centers may not satisfy the requirement that centers should suitably sample the input domain. Furthermore, in order to achieve a given performance, an unnecessarily large RBF network may be required. Since a performance of an RBF network critically depends upon the centers chosen, an alternative learning procedure based on the orthogonal least squares (OLS) learning algorithm [Chen et al., 1991] is often used.

Adaptive Logic Network. An Adaptive Logic Network (ALN) can be considered a special type of the feedforward MLP in which the signals in the network are restricted to be Boolean (binary) after a layer of processing units that act on whatever other types of signals are present to produce Boolean values. ATREE versions 2.7 and earlier [Armstrong and Gescei, 1979] deal with binary numbers and with continuous quantities that are using fixed operators such as threshold units to encode real numbers as bit strings. The nodes of the ALN tree are two types: adaptive elements and leaves. Each adaptive element is a two-input logic gate, which can be any one of the following four Boolean functions: AND, OR, LEFT, and RIGHT, i.e., $g(x,y)=xy$, $x+y$, x, y respectively [Armstrong and Gescei, 1979]. The leaves are the nodes of the first layer of an ALN tree used to connect binary input from the encoder to the tree (Figure 5.29). The leaves of the tree are connected to input variables either in a one-to-one fashion (the disjoint case) or with a multiplicity of connections going to the same variable of the binary tree and its inverse.

In the ATREE Ver. 3.0 [Armstrong and Thomas, 1994], the logic trees containing AND and OR operators have been furnished with input operators in the form of linear threshold elements (LTEs). The logic gates (AND and OR) may have an arbitrary number of logical input, and produce a logical output. The LTE is the basic element of approximation, and it is very similar to the Perceptron developed in the 1950s. The direct consequence of the new ALN design is possibility to apply ALN directly to real values and thus define piecewise linear approximations of functions. This approach is not restricted to approximating functions, but can approximate relationships of more general types represented as sets of data points, which are important for pattern recognition applications.

Fuzzy Logic Networks. Fuzzy sets [Zadeh, 1965] represent the vagueness of everyday life. One of the biggest differences between conventional (crisp) and fuzzy sets is that every crisp set always has a unique membership function, whereas every fuzzy set has an infinite number of membership functions that may represent it. This is at once both a weakness and a strength; uniqueness is sacrificed, but this gives a concomitant gain terms of flexibility, enabling fuzzy models to be "adjusted" for maximum utility in a given situation. The question unresolved yet concerns the relationship of fuzziness to probability. The fuzzy models and the statistical models possess different kinds of information: 1) fuzzy memberships, which represent similarities of objects to imprecisely defined properties; and 2) probabilities, which convey information about relative frequencies. Moreover, interpretations about and decisions based on these values also depend on the actual numerical magnitudes assigned to particular objects and events.

The typical steps of a "fuzzy reasoning" consist of: 1) fuzzification: comparison of the input variables with the membership functions of the premise parts (the if-part of the rule is called the antecedent or premise) in order to obtain the membership values between 0 and 1; 2) weighing: applying specific fuzzy logic operators (e.g., "AND" operator - minimum, "OR" operator – maximum, *etc.*) on the membership values of the premise parts to get a single number between 0 and 1, *i.e.*, the firing strength of each rule; 3) generation: creation of the consequent (the then-part of the rule is called the consequent or conclusion) relative to each rule; and 4) defuzzification: aggregation of the consequent to produce the output.

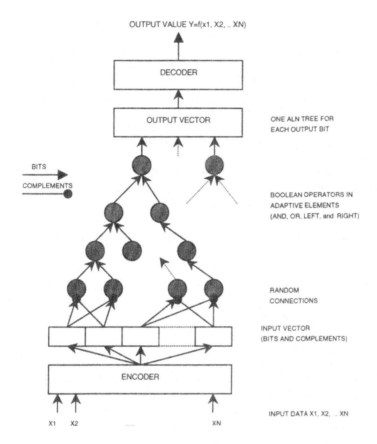

Fig. 5.29: The structure of ALN binary trees. The input data X1, X2, .. XN are encoded into a binary vector containing original bits and their complements. These elements are randomly connected to fixed elements (leaves) and adaptive elements (AND, OR, LEFT, RIGHT) of a three that changes during learning. The output of each tree is a single bit. Bits are combined to form an output vector which is then decoded to produce the output Y=f(x1, X2, .. , XN). Adapted from Kostov *et al.*, 1995 © IEEE.

Entropy Minimization Type of Inductive Learning Technique. An inductive learning (IL) method is based on an algorithm called "hierarchical mutual information classifier" [Sethi and Sarvarayudu, 1992]. An effective method of integrating results of a mutual information algorithm into a production rule formalism [Pitas *et al.*, 1992; Watanabe, 1985] is shown in Nikolić and Popović [1996, 1998]. While generating the decision tree, the algorithm performs a hierarchical partitioning of the domain multidimensional space. Each new node of the decision tree contains a rule based on a threshold of one of the input signals. Each new rule further subdivides the example set. The learning is finished when each terminal node contains members of only one class. An excellent feature of this algorithm is that it determines the threshold automatically based on the minimum entropy [Pitas *et al.*, 1992]. This minimum entropy method is equivalent to the determination of the maximum probability of recognizing a desired event (output) based on the information from input.

Combination of Neural Networks and Rule-Based Learning Techniques. The advantage of a rule-based learning method (e.g., IL method and fuzzy logic) compared with an ANN (e.g., MLP, ALN, RBF network) is that the rules determined are both explicit and comprehensible, whilst the rules used by the ANN are implicit within its structure and not easily comprehensible. There are methods which extract approximate classification rules from a trained ANN, and they help evaluating the learned knowledge [Narazaki et al., 1996]. Furthermore, ANN are computationally intensive. In view of the versatility of ANN and rule-based learning method, their combination exhibits many advantageous features like: 1) the parameters of the system have clear physical meanings, which they do not have in general ANN; 2) a network structure facilitates the computation of the gradient for parameters of the system; and 3) human linguistic descriptions or prior expert knowledge can be directly incorporated, for example, into fuzzy neural network structure. In contrast, the disadvantage is that the network structure requires a large number of term nodes, and there is no efficient process for reducing the complexity of combined neural network with rule-based method.

Adaptive Network based Fuzzy Inference System (ANFIS) is an example of an often used combination of FIS and ANN [Jang, 1993; Jonić et al., 1999]. The training procedure usually has two steps. In the first step is used subtractive clustering method for initial identification of a first-order Sugeno-type FIS [Chiu, 1994]. In the second step is used an adaptive-network with BP and least square algorithms for tuning of initially identified linear and nonlinear parameters of FIS respectively [Jang, 1993]. Adaptive-network corrects the rules determined by initial identification of FIS. The result is FIS, which corresponds to the minimum training error. An example where the combination of the minimum entropy IL and the RBF network is readily used is the estimation of the muscle activation [Jang 1993].

5.3 Control Methods to Restore Standing

Kralj and Bajd [1989] have suggested the open-loop, hand triggered control method to restore standing by stimulating bilaterally the knee extensors. This control allows paraplegic subjects who can control their balance when using hand supports (e.g., crutches, parallel bars) to stand for period of time determined by the posture, muscle fatigue, and muscle strength. The continuous, non-physiological stimulation is fatiguing; thus, it became obvious that the control has to be improved. The muscle fatigue occurs after only few minutes or less, yet there are subjects who could stand for much longer periods with continuous stimulation. This prolonged standing is possible because some paraplegics can stand in a posture that keeps their legs and trunk "locked" physiologically because the gravity force acts in a direction that is forcing the joints to rotate against the natural constraints imposed by ligaments and joint structure. This posture, however, can by no means withstand the external perturbations. When standing in this biomechanically secured posture, the stimulation can be turned-off because it does not contribute to the standing. Prolonged standing in this posture could cause joint and tissue damage.

The use of a floor reaction orthosis, which holds the ankle joint in a position that forces the knee joint to be ahead of the center of pressure, also uses an on-off method [Andrews, 1986]. A force sensor measures the pressure between the shank and the orthosis; when the force becomes zero, then the Quadriceps m. stimulation is turned-on to extend the knee joints, and once the force is positive again, the stimulation is turned off. The use of floor reaction orthosis and this sensory driven control allowed a selected number of paraplegics to stand for periods longer than one hour. This work led to the design of several control ideas implemented with hybrid assistive systems.

Kralj and Bajd [1989] proposed to prolong standing by generating a slow sway of the body with a low amplitude about the vertical line. This sway can be realized by using functional electrical stimulation if appropriate modulation of muscle activity and correct timing to switch from one to the other muscle group are available. In order to provide this control, cocontraction of agonist and antagonist muscles is required, because the stiffness control is the most important element for good postural control [e.g., Matjačič and Bajd, 1998a]. Cocontraction leads to faster muscle fatigue, yet if it is at low level, its contribution to fatigue is marginal. The major problems in the potential use of switching control are that the major knee extensors (Quadriceps m.) have to be active for prolonged periods of swaying, and the correct switching is rather difficult to achieve because of the muscular properties.

Khang and Zajac [1989a and b] used a linearized model of paraplegic standing, formulated about the vertical set point, to design an output feedback control law for unassisted standing in which the upper body forces were considered to be external disturbances. The model was able to maintain standing and recover when disturbed or from an initial position halfway between sitting and standing. The optimization technique used to determine the control law has been a computationally demanding procedure; thus, not suitable for real-time application. This technique is yet to be proved in clinical use with real-time functional electrical stimulation systems.

Donaldson and Yu [1998] proposed a controller for minimizing the handgrip reaction forces by referring them to the equivalent leg joint moments. The static equilibrium equations must be solved for the equivalent leg joint moments, and inverse models of the muscle recruitment curves are required to find the appropriate muscle stimulation levels. Ewins *et al.* [1988] used proportional-integral-derivative (PID) closed-loop knee controllers for FES standing up, and smoother trajectories were observed. Quintern *et al.* [1989] proposed a combination of a closed-loop PID and an open-loop feed-forward controller for paraplegic standing. The feed-forward control signal was either a simple ramp-up or was calculated using a model of standing. They suggested that more attention must be given to man-machine synchronization to improve the quality of FES movements.

The necessity of coordination between the artificial controller and the intact natural motor control has also been emphasized in a work by Hunt *et al.* [1997, 1998] and Munih *et al.* [1997] where they used linear quadratic Gaussian controller to restore unassisted standing in paraplegia. The "wobbler" [Donaldson *et al.*, 1997] system is used to support the body; it transforms the whole body to a single rigid inverted pendulum that can rotate around the ankle joints. The controller implemented was a two-level three nested structure (Figure 5.30].

Two parallel inner loops operate independently for each ankle joint; their sum connects to the outer loop that controls the position (angle). Due to the time constants involved, the inner loop has a much higher bandwidth that the outer loop. This provides the benefit that the uncertain effects of muscle nonlinearity and time variation are reduced. The inner loop controllers are based upon an empirically derived muscle model. The outer loop is then designed, taking into account both the inner closed-loop and the body dynamics. The optimal control theory is used for both loops. The

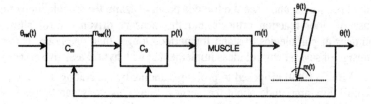

Fig. 5.30: Feedback control of unsupported standing. θ(t) is the measured ankle joint angle, m(t) is the measured ankle net joint torque, p(t) is the muscle stimulator output (variable pulse duration), θ$_{ref}$(t) and m$_{ref}$(t) are the references (desired joint angle and torque), and C$_θ$ and C$_m$ the position and force feedback controllers. Adapted from Hunt et al., 1997 © IEEE.

nonlinear muscle is described in Hammerstein form with a static input nonlinearity followed by a linear transfer function [Hunt et al., 1998]. The muscle model consists of a static recruitment nonlinearity, followed by a discrete-time linear transfer function. The output from the recruitment is the activation level, and the output from the muscle model is m(t), the control signal (torque).

Mulder et al. [1992a and b] used closed-loop on/off control based on a predetermined phase-plane switching curve of the desired knee velocity versus knee angle. A considerable improvement has been reported in decreasing the terminal velocity of the knee joint and the amount of stimulation, yet the sit-stand maneuver took longer, and more arm force was required.

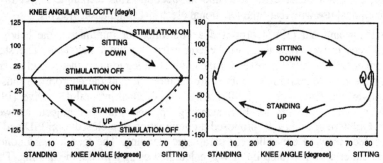

Fig. 5.31: Typical phase plot of the knee angle vs. knee angular velocity for able-bodied (right) and controller generated (left) standing up/sitting down. Note that only on and off regimes are used for external control. Adapted from Dolan et al., 1998 © IEEE.

Dolan et al. [1998] designed a switching curve controller for functional electrical stimulation assisted standing up and sitting down. A low-level, closed-loop controller has been applied. The rationale when designing the controller was to mimic the behavior found in able-bodied subjects by looking in the phase plane defined by the joint angle and joint angular velocities (Figure 5.31). The bang-bang control, i.e., the system that uses only on and off regimes, was selected. The primary objective of the switching curve controller was to control the terminations of the maneuvers, i.e., the locking of the knee joints while standing and the contact with the seat while sitting, to protect the joints and tissue from injuries.

Matjačić and Bajd [1998a] developed a model to control unsupported standing, i.e., no arm support assisted standing. The method is suitable for subjects who are able to generate the isometric and isokinetic torques around the lumbosacral joints (L5-S1).

They suggest that the control of stiffness of the appropriate joints is the key issue for successful standing. The results [Matjačić and Bajd, 1998] documented that with the increased stiffness of the ankle joints, paraplegics can balance in the sagittal plane and bring their center of mass in a position that ensures the so-called C-posture. The perturbations have been imposed in antero/posterior direction; the results show that the increased stiffness generated by a specially designed standing frame allows the recovery of posture with the abdominal and trunk muscles while no arm and hand intervention are needed. The study of Matjačić and Bajd is a well-documented confirmation of the results tested with the hybrid system based on the use of floor reaction orthosis [Andrews *et al.*, 1988]. The stiffness of the ankle joints has to be initially set to values in the range of about 20 Nm, while it can be decreased later to values between 6 to 10 Nm. The stiffness could be controlled by means of functional electrical stimulation (cocontraction of ankle dorsi- and plantar flexors).

This stiffness control scheme also applies to the control in the coronal plane (latero/medial control of balance). Matjačić *et al.* [2000] suggest that the coronal plane stability is controlled mostly at the hip joints. This line of thinking follows the literature analyzing postural adjustments after multiple direction perturbations (see Chapter 2). A de-coupling between the ankle and hip joints is very distinct with respect to the postural adjustments after perturbations imposed in an arbitrary direction. By increasing the stiffness at the hip joints it is possible to provide necessary stability in the coronal plane and allow humans to control the balance with their trunk movement.

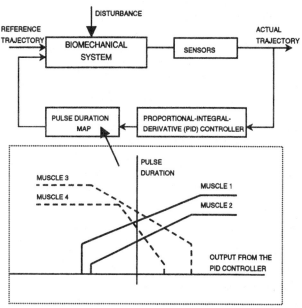

Fig. 5.32: The sketch of the closed-loop control system used to regulate posture in the coronal plane. Muscles 1 to 4 are the hip abductors and adductors on both legs. Adapted from Abbas and Chizeck, 1991 © IEEE.

Abbas and Chizeck [1991] analyzed the control of coronal plane hip angles and later applied the closed-loop control in real-time. The control system included sensors and a two-stage controller (Figure 5.32). The discrete time proportional-integral-derivative single-input, multiple output system was designed. The study concentrated on the ability of the feedback controller to compensate for perturbations in the coronal plane. The pulse duration map was designed which included the cocontraction of hip adductors and hip abductors resulting in the increased stiffness of the hip joints in the coronal plane.

A computer simulation was developed to demonstrate the feasibility of robust and self-adaptive control using reinforcement learning [Davoodi and Andrews, 1998]. The control algorithm has its origin in animal learning and is based on the commonsense notion that if an action is followed by a satisfactory outcome, then the tendency to produce that action should be reinforced. In able-bodied subjects, high knee net joint torque occurs at seat lift-off; this torque is progressively reduced resulting in knee angular velocities close to zero at full extension. Therefore, it was reasonable to develop neuroprostheses that would minimize the upper limb work and stress when standing up and improve the stimulation regime to match closer the behavior found in the able-bodied population.

Davoodi and Andrews demonstrated that the performance improved when analyzing the trajectory smoothness, knee end velocity, and the arm forces. The proportional-integral-derivative control was compared with the on/off phase plane switching technique. The amount of manual tuning required to optimize the fuzzy controller precluded its practical application. Davoodi and Andrews also analyzed the feasibility of determining the parameters of the fuzzy logic controller by using a genetic algorithm optimization method. However, the large number of trials before convergence to the optimal solution (n>600) and computational overhead of the present algorithms makes them unsuitable for on-line tuning. This experience led to the development of a self-adaptive scheme that uses reinforcement learning to tune the parameters of the fuzzy logic controllers (Figure 5.33).

The learning algorithms are a combination of a procedure introduced by Suton [1988], known as the temporal difference procedure, and the reinforcement learning procedure [Barto et al., 1989]. The combined algorithms can address the goal directed sequential decision making problems, traditionally solved by dynamic programming but do not require the model of the environment. The formal convergence proofs have only been obtained for the finite, stationary Markovian decision process [Suton, 1988]. Although most physical processes cannot strictly meet the formal conditions for applying these techniques, many researchers have been successful in applying them [Salatian et al., 1997; Gillapelli, 1995].

Due to the changes in the body such as muscle fatigue, the problem posed here is not stationary. Further, the control actions and states are considered as continuous variables, *i.e.*, they can assume infinite number of values. The main objective, however, was to evaluate the performance of the reinforcement learning and temporal difference in the presence of these violations of the formal conditions.

It was shown [Davoodi and Andrews, 1997] that the reinforcement learning was able to compensate for weak arm forces by identifying the system very quickly and raising the stimulation intensity just high enough to allow the maneuver to be successfully completed. In the experiment to minimize arm forces, the fuzzy logic algorithm learned to increase the stimulus intensity to the hip and knee extensor muscles in order to reduce the arm forces, resulting in shorter and faster maneuvers.

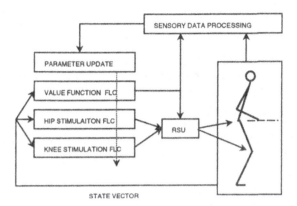

Fig. 5.33: Structure of the learning system. Fuzzy Logic Controls (FLC) are used to represent the knee and hip joint controllers (pulse duration). Random search unit (RSU) provides the exploration of the action selection. Adapted from Davoodi and Andrews, 1998 © IEEE

Patient driven control of FES-supported standing-up has been studied with a rather complex model [Riener and Fuhr, 1998]. A three-segmental model consisting of the shanks, thighs, and upper body describes the human body. Nine muscle groups are included inducing torques about the ankle, knee, and hip joints. Each group has its own activation and contraction dynamics. The input to each muscle group is the continuous time signal of the modulated pulse duration (width) and pulse frequency as provided by an electronic stimulator. Muscle activation is computed considering the effect of spatial and temporal summation by a nonlinear recruitment curve, a nonlinear activation-frequency relationship, and a linear second order calcium dynamics [Riener and Fuhr, 1998].

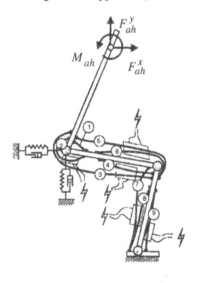

Fig 5.34: Three-segmental model with nine muscle groups. All muscle groups (except #1) have been activated in experiments. The visco-elastic elements represent body-seat interaction. The two forces and one torque at the shoulders represent the actions of the upper body. Adapted from Riener and Fuhr, 1998 © IEEE.

A fatigue model was incorporated, which also takes into consideration the recovery of the muscle force. An additional constant time delay was included, which is responsible for finite conduction velocities in the membrane system and delays from the chemical reactions involved. The torque from a single muscle group is calculated from its moment arm and the muscle force, depending on maximum isometric muscle force, muscle activation, force-length, and force-velocity relations.

In the body-segmental dynamics (Figure 5.35) the net joint torque is the sum of active, passive elastic, and passive viscous joint torques. The active joint torque is the sum of the joint torques produced by all muscle groups. Passive muscle properties have been separated from the active muscle properties, and are assigned to the joints in order to keep the number of muscle parameters lower. Passive elastic properties are modeled by double exponential equations, which account for the influence of the adjacent joint angles. Passive viscous joint moments are modeled by linear damping functions. Equations of motion with three degrees of freedom describe the segmental dynamics of the body as well as the interaction with the environment (shoulder forces and seat interaction).

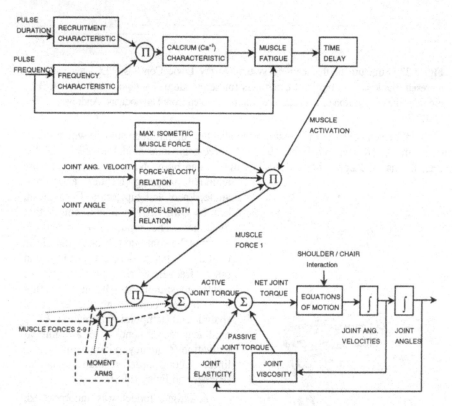

Fig. 5.35: The model of the stimulated plant comprises an activation (top), muscle structure (middle) and body segmental dynamics (bottom). Each of the nine muscles has its own activation and contraction dynamics. The joint angles are the ankle (φ_A), knee (φ_K), and hip (φ_H) joint angles. Adapted from Riener and Fuhr, 1998 © IEEE.

The subject-driven motion reinforcement control accounts for voluntary upper body effort, but does not require the recording of hand reactions. It is assumed that the subject can provide sufficient arm force and is capable of controlling both the position and orientation of the trunk with his/her intact upper body. The control is aiming to reduce the upper body efforts while standing up. Actual joint positions and velocities are used as feedback signals into the inverse dynamic model, which predicts the stimulation pulse duration needed for the movement.

This complex model shows, that it is feasible to simulate biomechanics, and it is possible after sufficient fitting of data to provide reasonable tracking of computer generated and experimentally recorded trajectories; yet its practical value for real-time implementation is very limited.

5.4 Controlling Neuroprosthesis for Walking

The existing NP systems for standing and walking are described in Chapter 4. The simplest ones, from a technical point of view, are single and dual channel stimulation systems. These systems are only suitable for hemiparetic subjects who can perform limited walking while partly supported with their upper extremities over crutches or canes. The NP in these humans is used to activate one or two muscle groups [Kralj and Bajd, 1989]. A multichannel system with a minimum of four channels of functional electrical stimulation is required for walking of a paraplegic subject with a complete motor lesion of the legs, yet preserved innervation and balance control. Appropriate bilateral stimulation of the quadriceps muscles locks the knees during standing. Stimulating the common peroneal nerve on the ipsilateral side, while switching-off the quadriceps stimulation on that side, produces a flexion of the leg. This flexion combined with adequate movement of the upper body and the use of the upper extremities for support allows ground clearance and is considered as the swing phase of the gait cycle. Hand or foot switches can provide the flexion-extension alternation needed for a slow forward or backward progression. Sufficient arm strength must be available to provide balance in parallel bars (clinical application) and with a rolling walker or crutches (daily use of FES). The use of more channels can enhance the posture, and somewhat improve the walking, but the walking speed, ability to negotiate obstacles, the range that can be covered while walking, and energy efficiency are still very low.

Multichannel percutaneous systems for walking of paraplegic subjects have been suggested and tested in clinical environment. These systems used exclusively a preprogrammed sequence that can be classified as a rudimentary form of a rule-based control. The hand held interface is used to select the mode, *i.e.*, the sequence that will be executed, and in some cases even to trigger each stride once the subject decides that he/she wants to continue to walk [Kobetič and Marsolais, 1994]. The use of technology for cochlear implants uses the same preprogrammed control method [Davis *et al.*, 1997] as well as the method that applies spinal roots electrodes [Rushton *et al.*, 1990].

The use of hybrid system[1] is more complicated since the controller has to deal with both the mechanical and biological system. The use of orthosis in parallel with the skeletal system facilitates the mounting of sensors and provides some safety features, yet it has not reached the stage of effectively assisting the life of paraplegic subjects.

5.4.1 Analytical Methods to Control Walking

The practical success of using functional electrical stimulation is still seriously limited because of the inadequate control. The control methods developed for robots and other complex large systems are still difficult to apply mostly because of the

---

[1] The term "hybrid control system" applies to control, while the term "hybrid assistive system" to a combination of FES and an external orthosis.

occurrence of muscle potentiation and fatigue [Mizrahi et al., 1997; Giat et al., 1996; Franken et al., 1993], inadequate timing of applied stimulation [Yamaguchi and Zajac, 1989], variability in response of stimulated muscle [Trnkotzy, 1978], muscle spasms [Stefanovska et al., 1989], poor selectivity and electrical accessibility of muscles that generate gait propulsion; and sensitivity to external disturbances.

As described earlier it is possible to control a single joint movement and provide smooth and reproducible patterns (Section 5.1). However, the coordination of multiple joints, which are dynamically coupled requires more sophisticated technology and body of knowledge than available today. The parameters for the cyclic stimulation patterns required for walking need to be chosen and optimized for each individual subject and situation. These parameters, once selected, have to be continuously adapted to compensate for external disturbances and system performance deterioration. The problem becomes even more difficult when both legs are at the ground (closed kinematic chain) because of the undeterministic biomechanical structure.

Therefore, most of the control studies analyzed the methods that are applicable only to the swing phase of the gait cycle. Several methods to derive stimulation patterns for cyclic leg movement have been reported (e.g., McNeal et al., 1989]. The trial-and-error method has been applied to determine the appropriate stimulation pattern of the Hamstrings m. and the Quadriceps m. in order to control the position of the lower leg in a cyclic motion (trajectory error minimization). The resulting stimulation sequence was applied in open loop. The initial responses of the lower leg matched the desired trajectory very well. However, the response significantly deteriorated owing to fatigue when the stimulation patterns were applied for several minutes.

Yamaguchi and Zajac [1989] computed the stimulation sequences on the basis of a biomechanical simulation model to restore unassisted paraplegic gait. The stimulation sequences were derived using dynamic programming and a trial-and-error adjusting method. Minimizing a cost function, supposedly related to minimal energy consumption of the stimulated muscles, optimized the stimulation sequence. The resulting suboptimal set of stimulation patterns yielded a step motion in their computer model; this procedure was not validated experimentally, and the effect of fatigue was also not accounted for.

Stanič et al. [1978] and Vodovnik et al. [1981] derived open-loop multichannel stimulation patterns for the correction of hemiplegic gait, successfully preventing several abnormalities. The stimulation patterns were synchronized with the heel-on event, detected by a foot switch. No strategy was included to adapt the stimulation patterns when fatigue occurred.

Hausdorff and Durfee [1991] demonstrated the use of an open-loop feed-forward position controller for the knee joint in able-bodied humans, stimulating the Quadriceps m. and Hamstrings m.. They concluded that it was beneficial to account for the non-linear length dependence of stimulated muscle output. Muscle fatigue was still not compensated for. The stimulation pulse duration for the Quadriceps m. and Hamstrings m. was computed on-line. The stimulation amplitude and frequency were kept constant. A reference knee angle signal needed to be tracked; the tracking performance of this position controller was not good enough.

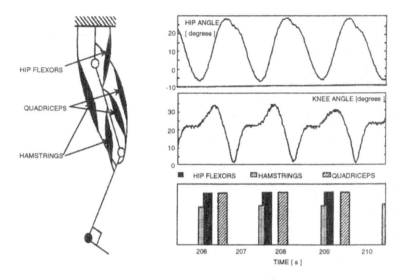

Fig. 5.36: The model of swinging leg in the sagittal plane with three prime movers comprising both mono- and bi-articular muscles (left). The hip angle, knee angle, and stimulation sequence obtained by using cycle to cycle proportional-integral-derivative controller. Adapted from Franken et al., 1995 © IEEE.

Veltink et al. [1990] experimentally tested this cycle-to-cycle concept in able-bodied subjects in the control of a cyclic lower leg movement with Quadriceps m. stimulation. The objective was that the lower leg should reach a certain maximal knee angle of each swing cycle. The open-loop burst duration was adapted in each cycle on the basis of the error between the desired and actually obtained maximal knee angle in previous cycles, successfully maintaining the desired objective.

Franken et al. [1995] experimentally investigated the control of the swing phase of paraplegic gait by cyclically stimulating the hip flexors, Hamstrings m. and Quadriceps m. The initial stimulation patterns were experimentally optimized to obtain the desired movement. The swing phase was parameterized on the level of the cycle. The leg for the swing phase of the gait cycle was assumed as a double pendulum (Figure 5.36, left) moving in the sagittal plane.

To derive the required stimulation patterns for the hip flexors, Hamstrings m. and Quadriceps m., a nominal walking pattern has been selected. The minimum foot-clearance in the forward swing (Figure 5.37) has been selected as the most important element (prevention of the stumbling). To ensure subsequent heel-contact phase, the knee extension with activated quadriceps was desired at the end of the forward swing.

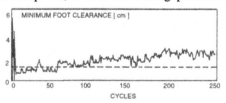

Fig. 5.37: The minimum foot clearance obtained by the use of cycle to cycle proportional-integral-derivative controller for swing phase of the leg (250 cycles). Adapted from Franken et al., 1995 © IEEE.

A discrete-time proportional-integral-derivative controller was chosen to adjust the duration of the hip flexor stimulation. The controller computed the new stimulation burst duration at the end of each swing cycle to be used in the next stride; the time step of the PID controller did not instantaneously account for disturbances during a swing cycle.

The gain, poles, and zeros of the combined system and controller determine the time-characteristics of a (linear) closed-loop system. The PID controller was tuned to an experimentally identified model of the total system on the level of a cycle and performed very well (Figure 5.36, right). Model characteristics were obtained from a passive swing of the leg using the methods described in Section 5.2.

The PID controller could not adapt fast enough for the effect of potentiation at the initial part of the experiments; thus the error was relatively high, yet it decreased and became positive leading to a safe walking pattern (Figure 5.37). Boom et al. [1993] reported that the effect of potentiation on the mechanical output of intermittently stimulated muscle has a significantly smaller time constant than the effect of fatigue. The controller could thus have been tuned to react faster. Its initial output (hip flexor burst duration) could also have been smaller. However, Quadriceps stimulation at the end of the forward swing to obtain knee extension also contributed to a higher hip angle range. This was not compensated for by the PID controller, which only adapted the hip flexor stimulation.

The control space for hip flexor stimulation was determined by the mechanical output of the hip flexor muscles. The stimulation frequency employed in the study [Franken et al., 1995] for the hip flexors was significantly higher than that used in the FES-induced paraplegic standing and walking feasibility studies. Whereas a typical stimulation frequency between 20 and 30 Hz has appeared sufficient to generate movement [Kralj and Bajd, 1989], the hip flexors were stimulated at 50 Hz. This was chosen to ensure a reasonable control space, in terms of burst duration, in case of muscle fatigue. Hamstrings and Quadriceps were stimulated at 25 Hz comparable with other published studies. The recruitment modulation appeared insufficient as the control parameter. The parameterization of FES-induced paraplegic gait on the level of a cycle facilitates adaptation of the applied stimulation from cycle to cycle based on the estimated deviation between the desired and actually obtained functional objectives.

5.4.2 Nonanalytical Techniques to Determine Walking Synergies

Following the work of Michie and Chambers [1968], Kirkwood et al. [1989] proposed to use the inductive learning (IL) technique for the upper level controller for FES-aided walking of subjects with incomplete spinal cord injury. The walking schema to be copied was obtained by recording sensory states when paraplegic subjects walked assisted with a two-channel FES system and a hand-switch. The automatic control of the same system used sensory data acquired from traditional transducers in real-time, and the motor commands have been reduced to the action of the switch (on-off). Heller et al. [1993] evaluated in parallel rule-base inductive learning and a connectionist (neural network) machine learning technique to reconstruct muscle activation patterns from kinematic data measured during normal walking at several speeds. Heller et al. [1993] showed that it is possible to use both techniques and that the prediction of timing is accurate, yet the integrated value of the activation bursts (analog to rectified, integrated EMG) is less accurate. The neural network gives a quasi-continuous output, whereas the rule-based IL gives selected number of discrete levels. The advantage of IL is that the rules are explicit and comprehensible, whilst the rules used by the neural network were implicit within its structure and not very difficult to comprehend.

Tong and Granat [1999] used a three-layer structure artificial neural network to clone the expertise of walking with hand-switches. They used a system with 10 force and pressure sensors (FSR transducers mounted in the shoe insoles and strain gauges mounted in the crutches). Another set included 13 sensors (goniometers over hip and knee joints, accelerometers on the mid line of the anterior aspect of the thigh and tibial tuberosity on shank, inclinometer on thigh, shank and crutch and heel and toe switches. The kinematic sensors were also *virtual* sensors derived from motion analysis system [Tong and Granat, 1998]. The results from one incomplete paraplegic subject indicate that only three sensors can provide the accuracy similar to the accuracy when all sensors are used. The selection of the three sensors that gave the best results followed tedious trial and error method. The accuracy was defined as the ratio of correct points and total number of samples expressed in percent.

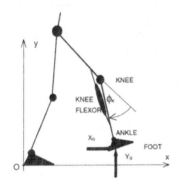

Fig. 5.38: The diagram showing the data used for determining the rules by means of machine learning.

In a study analyzing the applicability of ANFIS (see Section 5.2) to movement control, the muscle timing is estimated using minimum entropy IL, and the level of muscle activation is estimated using RBF network with OLS learning algorithm [Jonić and Popović, 1997]. The RBF network estimates the muscle activation level very well because it gives a "continuous" output. Hence, the rules designed with the IL method correct the muscle timing estimated by means of an RBF network. The parameters of RBF network were calculated based only on data from the input and output training sets which fall in the interval in which a muscle was estimated to be active using the IL method.

Jonić and Popović [1997] presented the use of RBF ANN for the design of the rule-based controller. The objective of the study was to define mapping between the activation pattern of a muscle, and the knee joint angle using only preceding sensory data (Figure 5.38). An RBF network with OLS training algorithm was selected for the pattern matching because of the following characteristics: 1) fast training; 2) good generalization; and 3) simple application because it requires only the spread constant to be assumed, while all other parameters are selected automatically.

The data used for training and testing of the network were prepared from walking simulation of a fully customized model of a human body assisted with FES [Popović *et al.*, 1999b]. The sampling rate for all data was 100 Hz. The input for the network is the following sensory data: knee joint angle, horizontal ground reaction force, and vertical ground reaction force. The desired output from the network is: muscle activity of the knee flexors and the knee joint angle as predicted by the network.

During the training phase, the number of the nodes and parameters of the network have been tuned using the input and desired output of the system, called the examples in a supervised machine learning procedure. In order to test the generalization of the network the input was divided into data to be used for training and data to be used for

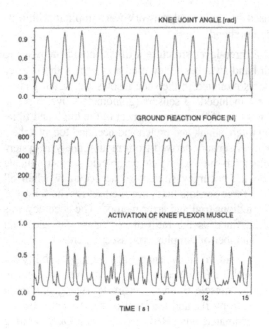

Fig. 5.39: An example of data used for machine learning. The top two panels are the input data (processed experimental data describing kinematics and dynamics of walking). The output is the result of simulation using optimal control and customized biomechanical model. The activation is normalized to tetanic activity.

testing. The matching between the predicted and desired data was used for assessing the performance of the obtained network.

The data shown in Figure 5.39 include twelve strides of level walking. An example of input (Figure 5.39, top and middle panels) used for machine learning was obtained from recordings of kinematics and dynamics of an able-bodied subject walking on the slope with ankle joints constrained with ankle-foot orthoses. The output was (Figure 5.39, bottom) obtained by calculating the required knee flexor activity, using a customized biomechanical model by optimizing the activation levels of both the flexor and extensor muscles in addition to minimizing the tracking error [Popović et al., 1999b]. The data used for testing have been generated using the same set-up and methods, yet the data have not been applied for determining the rules. The kinematics of walking is different in amplitude of joint angles, and ground reaction forces and activation of the knee flexor muscles changed accordingly. The cross-correlation (K) between the desired output and the predicted output by the network has been selected as a measure of the generalization:

$$K = \frac{\sum_{i=1}^{r} s(i) s_{des}(i)}{\sqrt{\sum_{i=1}^{r} s^2(i)} \sqrt{\sum_{i=1}^{r} s_{des}^2(i)}}$$

where $s_{des}(i)$ and $s(i)$ are the ith sample of the desired output and the network generated output, and r is the number of samples.

Note the differences in joint range of the original and predicted signals for the sequence not used for the training (Figure 5.40, right bottom panel). The desired output (full line) and predicted output (dashed line) are superimposed.

The coherence in patterns and the timing between the joint angle are good, but the predicted output does not go over the value of 0.9 radian, although the desired joint angles reach 1.2 radian. This discrepancy is because the training set included only small joint angle range; the network never used the joint angle bigger than 0.9 radian during the training; hence, it cannot predict bigger values. The network cannot provide an equivalent to what is called analytical extrapolation of data. The results obtained from the network are acceptable because they do not prevent the gait cycle from being finalized in correct timing. The smaller knee flexion does not interfere with the ground clearance.

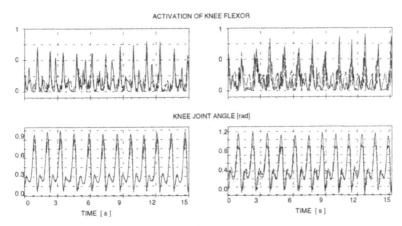

Fig. 5.40: The network predicted (full line) and original (dashed line) normalized muscle activity of the knee joint flexor and the knee joint angles for level walking (12 strides) are superimposed. The original signals are recordings of the knee joint and simulated activity using the methods described in Popović et al., [1999b]. Left panels show data used for training, and right the data used only for testing of the generalization.

The network used for this study had the following structure. The spread constant for the RBF network predicting muscle activity was 112. The spread constant was selected to maximize the matching between input and output data, and it followed the trial and error procedure. The spread constant for the RBF network predicting the joint angle was 28. For both output variables, the network had 792 nodes in the hidden layer, and the number of training epochs was one. The cross-correlation between the desired and network generated muscle activity for the data used for training was 0.94, and it was decreased to 0.89 when applied to the set of data which was not used for the training. The cross-correlation between the desired and the network generated knee joint angle using the data previously used for the training was 0.99, and dropped down to 0.94 when applied to data previously not shown to the network. The timing error was within 50 milliseconds for both the training and testing series.

Kostov et al. [1995] used ALN for real-time control of walking subjects with incomplete spinal cord injury that limited their ability to walk. All of the subjects were able to stand and walk very slowly and for only a limited distance with great difficulty even when assisted with FES. The sensory signals used for ALN have been recorded from two types of transducers: force sensing resistors (Interlink Inc., CA) positioned under the medial metatarsal and heel areas of both feet, and flexible goniometers (Penny and Giles Ltd., UK) across the hip, knee, and ankle joints. The FES system used in the subjects operated with switches; thus, the task was to define rules based on sensory information that will replace the hand-controlled switches. The signals from

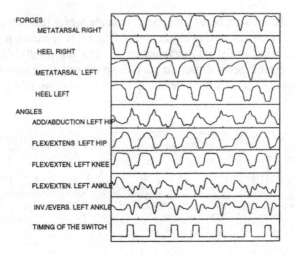

Fig. 5.41: An example of training signals recorded in an incomplete tetraplegic subject walking assisted with stimulation and the rolling walker. The bottom trace is the output signal; the ALN aims to learn the timing using the sensory input from the sensors. Adapted from Kostov *et al.*, 1995, with permission.

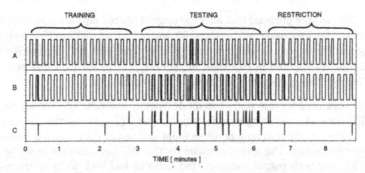

Fig. 5.42: The ALN determined mapping (B) of the timing of manual switch (A). The bottom panel (C) shows the error, positive pulses are delays and the negative proceeding of the estimated signals vs. the original signals. The total presented sequence is about 8 minutes; first sequence shows the mapping of data used for training, second the sequence used only for testing of the generalization, and third the testing data, yet when the restriction rules are applied. See text for details. Adapted from Stein *et al.*, 1992, with permission.

transducers were amplified, low-pass filtered at 25 Hz, sampled at 50 Hz by a 12-bit A/D converter, and processed using a PC based computer.

A dual-pass, fourth order, zero phase shift Butterworth filter also filtered the obtained digital signals. The output for learning is the data shown at the bottom panel in Figure 5.41, being a binary signal (on-off).

The ALN (Figure 5.29) used for the synthesis of rules for control of walking contained 2048 leaves and 2048 adaptive elements [Kostov *et al.*, 1994, 1995], a maximum of 20 presentations of the input to the learning algorithm and seven voters

(ALN trees per each bit in the output vector). The relative error of the output was limited to 6 percent. The learning can be improved significantly by adding samples from the past to the input formed from the current samples, as suggested by Lan *et al.* [1994]. Kostov [1995] introduced the term *restriction rules* for additional logical conditions that can eliminate errors that occur because of the discrete nature of signals. The restriction rule is a predefined minimal duration of the output value; it is an analog to the hysteresis function in systems where the noise can cause switching type oscillations of the output.

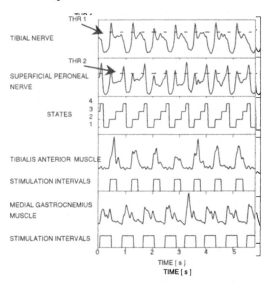

Fig. 5.43: Thresholds (THR 1 and THR 2) were set to code the input signal (real-rime processed neural recordings from the Tibial nerve and Superficial Peroneal nerve to two states (low and high). The ALN has been used to predict timing of muscle activity of the ankle joint extensor (Medial Gastrocnemius m.) and flexor (Tibialis Anterior m.) during the treadmill walking of a cat. Adapted from Popović *et al.*, 1993 © IEEE.

ALN have been used for several other control problems. Popović *et al.* [1993] used ALN to determine the timing for switching on and off ankle extensor and flexor muscles in a walking cat. Cuff electrodes have been implemented to superficial peroneal and tibial nerves; recordings have been amplified, rectified, and BIN integrated in real-time. In parallel the EMG activities from the Tibialis Anterior m. and Triceps Surae muscles have been recorded as shown in Figure 4.65. Using the ALN, the thresholds have been estimated; thus, timing for turning on and off the stimulation to drive the ankle joint determined. The experiments in several chronic cats showed that ALN generalized the input/output well enough to provide active ankle movement, although the muscles have been temporarily cut out from natural control by anaesthetizing the sciatic nerve. The ALN provided a four-state output as shown in Figure 5.43. The application of ALN for predicting the timing to control foot-drop stimulator and other sensory data from neural recordings is described in Chapter 4.

The ANN is widely used for analyzing electrophysiological signals such as electromyogram EMG, electrocardiogram (ECG), and electroencephalogram (EEG). Graupe and Kordylewski [1995] developed a so-called "patient responsive controller" for a walking NP. The controller uses ANN for recognition of time series (TS) of EMG signals recorded from the muscles that are voluntarily controlled. The ANN also controls the levels in the onset of muscle fatigue by analyzing response-EMG signals from stimulated sites. Initially, Graupe [1989] suggested EMG control for FES walking, yet without the use of the ANN techniques. The ANN that uses EMG for real-time control must continually modify its weight vectors, given that it changes its properties with time and environmental conditions.

Sepulveda *et al.* [1993, 1997, and 1998] originally developed, and later improved a version of ANN to control walking. The model that they used is displayed in Figure 5.44. The input for the model consisted of hip, knee, and ankle angles and vertical ground reaction forces. The output signal corresponded to the electrical activity of five leg muscles that are instrumental for walking, although other muscles could improve the walking by controlling coronal plane movement. The model was trained to yield values equivalent to the linear envelope of electromyography (EMG). They used a three layer structure, all neurons from a layer were connected to all elements in the subsequent level, a sigmoidal neuronal transfer function with outputs ranging from zero to 1 was used, and the output for all networks corresponded to EMG linear envelope values. Many changes were made on the basic network structure attempting to match the natural behavior closely.

A standard generalized back-propagation algorithm simulated learning in the networks with pattern learning (e.g., IL). The task was to evaluate the need for explicit temporal connections within the various network elements. The networks were trained using able-bodied walking data for the right leg, whereas the evaluation of network performance was done by use of clinical data from the literature [Vaughan *et al.*, 1992]. The gait cycle was divided in 20 (twenty) frames. Thus, each data set presented to the networks represented a 5 percent progression in the gait cycle. To accelerate network training, all training data were normalized between 0.2 and 0.8. The normalization of EMG data was done according to maximum and minimum values including all muscles, whereas normalization of joint angles and vertical ground reaction forces followed maxima and minima for each individual curve.

All synaptic weights were initially randomized between -0.5 and 0.5. The learning tolerance was set to 0.1. The learning rate was variable between 1.0 and 0.05, obeying a linear relationship between the learning rate and the number of units that yield an output greater than the tolerance. To keep the network output away from unwanted energy minima, the learning rate was reset to 2.0 whenever 1,000 (one thousand) iterations went by without change in the number of neurons with unacceptable output. This was found to work better than the traditional synaptic weight resetting technique since the jump produced by the technique used here is rather small. It takes the network away from the unwanted minimum without wasting all the learning already effected.

About 66 percent of data was used for training (able-bodied humans walking) and to evaluate the ability of the networks to generalize within the normal domain. The remaining data ($\approx$ 33 percent) were used to test the generalization on the data that have not been used for the training. The remaining data were collected in a human with motor and sensory disability. The network responses were compared with actual data by means of mean square error estimates; the values were calculated for each network, for both the swing and stance phases, and for the complete gait cycle. The study was done in a subject who was 32 years old, 11 years with a Brown Sequard lesion, C5/C6

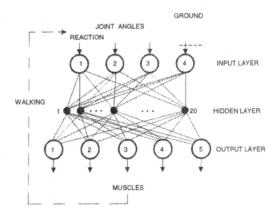

Fig 5.44: Scheme of the artificial neural network used for control of walking. The actual number and type of inputs may vary (e.g., more input from ground reaction force sensors, or more kinematic data). All units from a layer are connected to all units in the subsequent level. Courtesy of Dr. Francisco Sepulveda, Aalborg University, Denmark.

level, Frankel grade D. The results of the study have been applied in a testing session making the subject to ambulate in the parallel bars in the clinical setting.

Most of the positive aspects of this work result from the characteristics of the artificial neural networks. The control scheme is computationally very simple and flexible. In fact, the very same neural network algorithm can be used with any number of stimulation channels and biomechanical sensors by the mere addition or subtraction of neurons in the network. Also, as long as network input and output data are normalized to fall into the (0.0, 1.0) domain, any signal processing can be done. This is the main advantage of neural algorithms (which extract implicit rules from any data) as compared with rigid systems with a fixed set of rules. Thus, although the results presented here apply only to the test subject, the control system can be easily adapted to any clinical situation. Automatic on-line learning was later added to the above system [Sepulveda *et al.*, 1998].

To meet the requirement of pattern modification without changing all previously learned information while continuing with normal operation, the binary adaptive resonance theory neural network structure has been implemented. The learning of this type of ANN belongs to the so-called unsupervised training, yet Graupe and Kordylewski [1995] used it in a supervised mode. The basis of using the muscles that are above the lesion and not included in the movement execution is that there are muscles that undergo unique patterns of activity just before the subject is to move the leg. Because of the near-Gaussian nature of the above lesion, the surface EMG signals and their piecewise stationarity, an autoregressive model could be used:

$$y_k = \sum_{i=1}^{n} a_i y_{k-1} + w_k$$

where y_k is the recorded signal at discrete time k, a_i are autoregressive parameters, w_k are the white noise residuals, and n is the order of model. The ANN [Carpenter and Grossberg, 1991] has been used for determining the autoregressive parameters and white noise residuals. This rather intriguing method has yet not been presented in practical NP for restoring movement.

Ng and Chizeck [1997] applied fuzzy model identification methods to construct an identifier of five discrete events that occur in a cyclic process (e.g., level walking) as shown in Figure 5.45. The events correspond to changes in the stimulation patterns required to restore walking of paraplegic subjects.

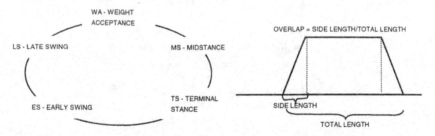

Fig. 5.45: The five cyclic event of walking. Adapted from Ng and Chizeck, 1997 © IEEE.

Fig. 5.46: The definition of the overlap for fuzzification. Adapted from Ng and Chizeck, 1997 © IEEE.

In fuzzy system identification, input is applied to the system, and the resulting output is measured. These input/output (I/O) pairs of data are used to estimate a fuzzy model of the system. Consider a k-input single-output system, as described by a set of relational equations whose solutions form the fuzzy model

$$y(t) = u_1(t) \circ u_2(t) \circ ... \circ u_k(t) \circ R$$

where $u_k(t)$ is the vector of fuzzy memberships of input variable i of a k-input system at time t, $y(t)$ is the vector of fuzzy memberships of output y at time t, R is the relational matrix, and $\circ$ is a fuzzy composition operator (max-min or max-product).

Since the system is dynamic, the vector u should include past input and present input. The input and output are normalized to the range [0, 1]. The R matrix represents a rule base, which maps each possible combination of fuzzy input to a fuzzy output. The larger the element in the matrix R, the stronger the correspondence between that particular set of fuzzy input and output. Ng and Chizeck [1997] used six inputs: joint angles and angular velocities of the hip, knee, and ankle of one leg. The universes of discourse for the three angles contain five reference sets each. All input references for each fuzzy model were limited to having the same shape and size.

The overlapping shapes (Figure 5.46) were restricted to be all trapezoidal or triangular (except for the reference sets at either end of each input universe of discourse where abrupt transitions between memberships from zero to one are included). The identification has been evaluated using the recordings from the walking of three incomplete paraplegic subjects. The paraplegic subjects walked with the preprogrammed pattern using the 48 stimulation site system with percutaneous electrodes [Kobetič and Marsolais, 1994]. The first stride was used to identify the states, while the remaining strides were used to test the performance of the network (Figure 5.47).

The sampling interval for the recordings was 16 ms, and a hysteresis of 48 ms (similar to restriction rules described earlier) was added. To test whether the use of a fuzzy rule base was a good choice for this application, a comparison of the classification achieved using a fuzzy rule base (with varying amounts of fuzziness) and that achieved by using a look-up table was performed. The varying of the fuzziness

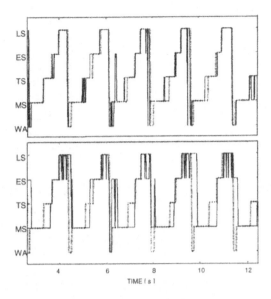

Fig. 5.47: Plot of predicted (full line) *vs.* actual events (dashed line) for a paraplegic subject walking assisted with NP and a walker. The abbreviations are: LS – late swing, ES – early swing, TS – terminal stance, MS – mid stance, WA – weight acceptance. The top graph used a fuzzy rule-base, the bottom graph use a non-fuzzy rule-base. Adapted from Ng and Chizeck, 1997 © IEEE.

was done by changing the overlap (Figure 5.46) between the adjacent reference sets of each universe of discourse. The greater the amount of overlap between the membership functions, the fuzzier the system. If there is no overlap, the fuzzy system is reduced to a look-up table. For three subjects, the detection performance was analyzed using trapezoidal reference sets with 0 to 50 percent. The 50 percent overlap reduces the trapezoidal form to a triangle; thus, to its maximum. Figure 5.48 shows the percentage of correctly predicted time steps for various degrees of overlap. The results were found using the Wilcoxon signed ranks test (based on detection percentages in 16 ms time slices). Figure 5.48 shows that the correct prediction of the event, at correct time, occurs in more than 60 percent, yet when the two phases behind and ahead are also counted in reaches to about 90 percent.

Van der Spek and coworkers [van der Spek *et al.*, 1996] used a similar method to control the leg during the swing phase of a walking paraplegic subject. The neurofuzzy control strategy for control of cyclic leg movement was specified by three swing phase objectives: hip angle range, foot clearance, and knee extension. The hip angle range relates to the behavior found in able-bodied subjects when walking, where the hip joint excursions determine the dynamics; the movement has to be generated by stimulating hip flexor muscles. The foot clearance is secured with the adequate knee flexion during the hip flexion; this is to be achieved by stimulating the hamstrings just before the onset of the swing. The knee extension is the final phase of the swing; and it has to be assisted if necessary by stimulating the quadriceps. The neurofuzzy controller has been designed following the design of a PID controller [Franken *et al.*, 1995] using a so-called cycle-to-cycle method. The results show that neurofuzzy control can

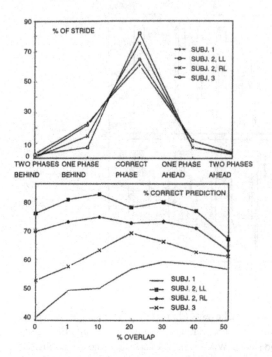

Fig. 5.48: The predicted phases relative to the actual phases of walking for three subjects (top) and comparison of performance when various overlaps between reference sets were used (bottom). Adapted from Ng and Chizeck, 1997 © IEEE.

compensate for changes in the muscle response because of the muscle fatigue, yet all the experiments were done in artificial conditions, not in a walking paraplegic.

Feedback Error Learning (FEL) [Kawato et al., 1987] uses machine mapping to replace the estimation of parameters within the feedback loop in a closed-loop control scheme. FEL is a feed-forward neural network structure which, when trained, "learns" the inverse dynamics of the controlled plant. This method is based on contemporary physiological studies of the human cortex [Miyamoto et al., 1988; Kawato, 1990].

The total control effort u applied to the plant is the sum of the feedback control output and network control output. The ideal configuration of the neural network would correspond to the inverse mathematical model of the system's plant. The network is given the information of the desired position and its derivatives, and it will calculate the control effort necessary to make the output of the system follow the desired trajectory. If there are no events perturbing the system, the error will be zero.

The configuration of the neural network should represent the inverse dynamics of the system once the training is completed. It is convenient to use a total energy of the system as the basis for the neural network application, because only the variables and their first derivatives are used in explicit form [Kalanović, 1996; Kalanović and Tseng, 1996].

Figure 5.49 depicts the FEL strategy. The system input and output are labeled θ_d and θ. The proportional-derivative (PD) feedback controller is included to provide stability during training of the neural network [Nordgren and Meckl, 1993; Rao et al., 1994; Szabo et al., 1994]. Enclosed in the dashed rectangle is an FEL controller, putting out the necessary control signal, based on the desired input. The training of the FEL controller is facilitated by changing the synaptic weights based on the output from a PD controller. The learning rule used is based on the Hebbian learning scheme, and Kawato, Furukawa, and Suzuki [1987] proposed it in the following form:

$$w_{i\ new} = w_{i\ old} + u_{PD} A \eta\ \Delta t$$

where $w_{i\ new}$ is the new value of the synaptic weight, $w_{i\ old}$ is the old value, u_{PD} is the output from the PD controller, A is the network functional associated with weight w_i, η is the learning rate, and Δt is the integration step used in the computer simulation. The learning rate is included to control the rate of growth of the synaptic weights. The learning rule [Kawato, 1990] is based on the assumption of slow growth of the synaptic weights. The weights are initialized at zero, and the learning rates adjusted so the growths of the weights are uniform.

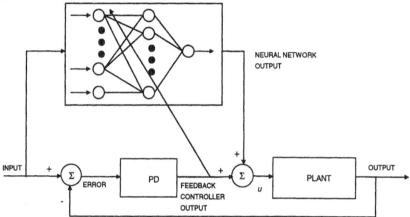

Fig. 5.49: Principle of Feedback Error Learning (FEL) control system. PD stays for proportional-derivative regulator. Adapted from Kalanović *et al.*, 2000 © IEEE.

This causes the weights to reach their final value at the same point in time, causing the error to approach zero. Subsequently, the learning as a function of error will level off, and the training of the neural network will be completed. However, if the growth of the weights is not homogeneous, it will result in an unbounded growth of the weights. The diagonal line (Figure 5.49) pointing upwards symbolizes the learning. After the total energy is calculated, the time derivative is taken and divided by the desired velocity. The losses are calculated by multiplying the desired velocity by the appropriate weight, and then added to the control signal. Finally, the control effort from the FEL controller is added to the PD control effort.

In essence, the output of the feedback controller is an indication of the miss-match between the dynamics of the plant and the inverse-dynamics model obtained by the neural network. If the true inverse-dynamic model has been learned, the neural network alone will provide the necessary control signal to achieve the desired trajectory [Szabo *et al.*, 1994]. During the initial training period, the control signal generated by the neural network is small compared with the signal from the PD controller. As the number of learning trials increases, however, the signal from the neural network will be more dominant. If the weights in the network are converging to the "true" system parameters, the network output will finally be the total control effort. At this point, the training is completed.

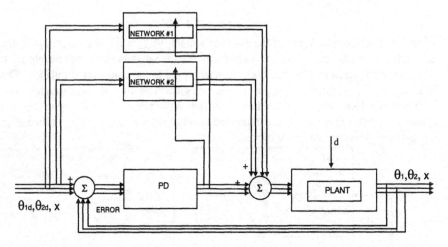

Fig. 5.50: The FEL control configuration for the transfemoral powered prosthesis. The input are the desired knee (θ_{1d}) and hip (θ_{2d}) angles and the acceleration of the hip (x). Adapted from Kalanović et al., 2000 © IEEE.

Kalanović et al. [2000] used FEL to design control of a transfemoral prosthesis. The initial phase of using FEL neural networks was to train it in accordance with the principle of modular training (each joint movement separately). The trajectory was sinusoidal function; the learning rates were adjusted so that the convergence speeds of the weights have been approximately uniform. The initial values of the synaptic weights were all zero. The training time was set to 1000 runs for both the shank and the thigh. A PD controller was used in a feedback configuration (Figure 5.50). The only criterion used to select the gains of the controller was the stability of the system. Any other set of values that satisfies this condition would lead to satisfactory training results as verified in other experiments (not shown here).

The application of feedback error learning was suitable to identify the inverse dynamic model within 1000 repetitions of training. The error was reduced to about zero after the training was completed; the control performance of the FEL neural network improved during the training, and that network took gradually over as a main controller instead of the feedback. The generalization of the FEL was proved by comparing the values of the weights obtained by the training with the "true" values that have been calculated from the mathematical model (Table 5.5). For details see Kalanović et al. [2000]. Once the networks have been trained, they could control different movement than the ones used for training. FEL can adapt to disturbances: simulation showed that the weights would converge although the networks do not match the new plant that comprises the disturbances. However, some of the weights would converge to new values compared with the undisturbed system.

Qi et al. [1999] developed a neurofuzzy controller for selective stimulation using a multipolar electrode. The neurofuzzy controller uses similar structure as described by Kawato [1990]. The study is of specific interest since the variability of the anatomy of peripheral nerves is great, and an adaptive and self tuning procedure could greatly increase the applicability of multipolar selective stimulation of large nerves (described in Section 4.3). Chang et al. [1997] applied an almost identical procedure to the methods described by Kawato et al. [1987] for the control of the stimulation of the quadriceps muscle in paraplegic subjects aiming to control the knee joint position. A multilayer feed-forward time-delay neural network was used and trained as an inverse model of FES induced quadriceps-lower leg system for direct feed-forward control. The Nguyen and Widrow [1990] method was used to initialize the neural connection weights. The method has been tested in one paraplegic subject and suggested further improvement in the algorithm.

Table 5.5: The FEL determined weights and the true values of system parameters

Value	Weight 1 HIP [Nm]	Weight 2 KNEE [Nm]	Weight 3 HIP [kgm^2]	Weight 4 KNEE [kgm^2]	Weight 5 HIP [Ns/m]	Weight 6 KNEE [Ns/m]
"True"	42.289	16.267	.8789	.2277	20.000	10.000
FEL	41.700	16.030	.900	.226	19.980	9.950

Abbas and Chizeck [1995] suggested a different method of using neural network control for functional electrical stimulation aiming to control movement. In the simulation study, they evaluated two sequential networks, one operating as a rhythm generator (analog to the central pattern generator discussed in details in Chapter 2), the second modulating the output from the first and generating functional movement. The model included nonlinear recruitment, linear dynamics, and multiplicative nonlinear torque-angle and torque-velocity scaling factors (as described in Section 5.1). The study analyzed only a single joint; results suggest that this may be suitable for the control of FES systems, yet there was no continuation of this study.

5.4.3 Hierarchical Hybrid Control of Walking

The method called the hierarchical, hybrid control [Lima and Saridis, 1999] carries similarities with natural control of movement as described in Chapter 2. The organization of the controller for restoring the walking is presented in Figure 5.51.

Coordination level. The production rule control (PRC) system is applicable for the coordination level of control. This level deals with the following: 1) the strategy how to employ the resources available, and 2) the methodology how to maximize the efficiency of the resources.

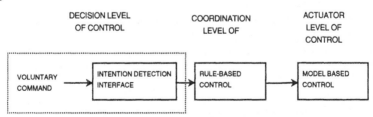

Fig. 5.51: Hierarchical hybrid controller for FES to restore locomotion.

The control uses sensory information, joint state, and actuator state data as input and generates control actions by using the knowledge representation concerning which actions are appropriate in which circumstances [Tomović et al., 1995]. The PRC system for the coordination level of walking comprises several elements (Figure 5.52). The regular rule base contains "regular" rules grouped into sets. These rules are expressed as situation-action pairs, relevant within a specific gait mode, and they execute (fire) when the expected sensory patterns are recognized. The regular rules are firing in a well-defined sequence. The maximum and minimum times are parts of the sequential operation of the rules; *i.e.*, if the next state of the system is not achieved during the defined time, the hazard situation or change of modality will be recognized.

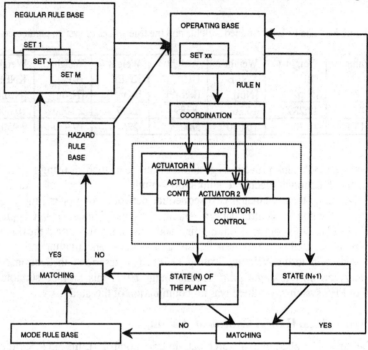

Fig. 5.52: The organisation of the production rule system operating at the coordination level of a hierarchical, hybrid controller for walking.

The hazard states are the conflict situations, *i.e.*, the sensory and system states that are unexpected within the specific mode of movement. The conflict situations occur due to the uncertainty of the available sensory information and/or hardware limitations, in addition to unexpected gait events. The hazard rules result in the safety "behavior", which is attempting to minimize the eventual catastrophic consequences of the hazard (e.g., falling, obstacles, non-physiological loading). The hazard rules are part of the mode rule base, but they are called if regular rules are not achieving the expected result [Popović *et al.*, 1991b].

The mode rule base [Popović and Sinkjær, 2000] comprises two parts: external and internal mode rules (Figure 5.54).

The external mode rules are expressed as situation-action pairs dealing with environmental recognition and adaptation. Environmental recognition depends on the environmental pattern, and the current relevant activity and state of the system. The internal mode rules are expressed as situation-action pairs dealing with adaptation within the specific gait mode (terrain slope angle, gait speed, and the like).

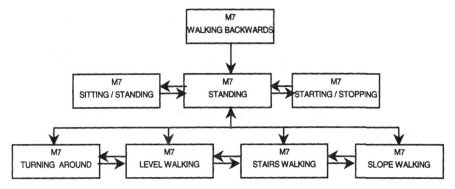

Fig. 5.53: Example of the organisation of the mode rule base. Each of the blocks contains the set of regular reflexes to be used within this activity. Internal mode rules take care of the adaptation within one mode (Figure 5.54)

One example of a mode rule base is shown in Figure 5.53. The arrows indicate possible transitions between different modes, suggesting that some transitions are not allowed. These transitions may be allowed as well, but the real-time control necessitates restrictions on the size of the operating rule base. The organization of rules appropriate for the level walking is shown in Figure 5.54. There are four classes of rules: internal mode, external mode, regular and hazard. Two classes exist within the mode rule base, and two within the regular rule base.

INTERNAL MODE RULES	WALKING INITIATION WALKING TERMINATION SPEED ADAPTATION
EXTERNAL MODE RULES	TRANSITION TO OTHER MODES OF WALKING
REGULAR RULES	PUSH-OFF INITIAL FLEXION TERMINAL FLEXION INITIAL EXTENSION TERMINAL EXTENSION HEEL-CONTACT KNEE BOUNCE HEEL-OFF
HAZARD RULES	OBSTACLE SENSOR FAILURE ACTUATOR FAILURE "UNKNOWN" STATE

Fig. 5.54: Set of rules for level walking.

The operating rule is hosting a subset from the regular rule base. The regular rules appropriate for one mode of walking are transferred based on the recognition of the intention or change of modality. Once the change of mode or intention is recognized, the content of the operating rule base changes (Figure 5.52).

The actual organization of a single rule is illustrated by an example. Each of the rules is organized using *IF-THEN* structures, as described earlier.

Actuator Level: Customized, Model Based Control. The lower, actuator control level is responsible for executing the decisions from the coordination level. Executing commands in sense of artificial reflexes means that electrical stimulation has to be delivered to a group of muscles that are controlling a joint. Single joint control is achieved through a coordinate action of several muscles acting at the neighboring segments (monoarticular muscles) or non-neighboring bone segments (biarticular muscles). The muscle actions result in joint torque, and this torque depends on several factors: neural activation of different muscles contributing to the torque, muscle length of these muscles vs. their length in resting state, and their velocity of shortening or lengthening [Huston *et al.*, 1976].

According to the literature [e.g., Jonić *et al.*, 1999], the muscle model can predict the muscle torque with 85-90% accuracy during simultaneous, independent, pseudo-random variations of recruitment, angle and angular velocity if the parameters of model are known with sufficient accuracy. A model that has been investigated in detail is a three-component multiplicative model: 1) activation dynamics; 2) muscle forces *vs.* muscle length characteristic; and 3) muscle force *vs.* velocity of shortening characteristic.

There is no method yet to determine *in situ* the individual muscle characteristics. By using the two muscle model (agonistic and antagonistic) a simplified model of the joint will be produced. This model will include the same three components, and they can be measured in a clinical setting by relatively simple, non-invasive assessment session [Stein *et al.*, 1996; Chizeck *et al.*, 1999]. A second order, critically damped, low-pass filter with a delay can approximate the activation [Veltink *et al.*, 1992; Bajzek and Jaeger, 1987; Baratta and Solomonow, 1990; Shue and Crago, 1998]. A parabolic function is a good approximation of the joint torque vs. the joint angle [e.g., Stein *et al.*, 1996], and a hyperbolic function is a good approximation of a model for normalized joint torque vs. joint angular velocity (Figure 5.55). These models have been developed heuristically using the experimental procedure described in Popović M *et al.* [1994].

The left panel (Figure 5.55) shows a joint torque *vs.* joint angle for the knee extensor muscles. A large zone was determined in a clinical study that included 12 humans with a complete lesion between the T6 and T10 levels. In some cases the maximum torque is only about 40 Nm, while for other humans the joint torque reaches over 140 Nm. The isometric joint torque has been measured after at least four week of extensive exercise of the quadriceps muscles, and the measurements were averaged from three sessions to minimize day-to-day variation and effects of muscle fatigue. Figure 5.55 shows a normalized joint torque vs. joint angular velocity assessed in the same 12 subjects. When the fitted curve is steep (e.g., in about 70 percent of the subjects tested), then generating desired functional movements becomes very difficult or even impossible.

The joint torque depends on the amount of electrical charge delivered to the muscle and the muscle properties (e.g., number of motor units, number of fast and slow twitching fibers, muscle fatigue). The joint torque also depends on the electrodes applied for stimulation. Figure 5.55 (right panel) shows the joint torque vs. the electrical charge for the surface electrodes applied over the quadriceps muscles. Monophasic, compensated, constant current pulses have been delivered *via* 5 cm x 10 cm carbon rubber electrodes with conductive gel. The isometric joint torque has been measured on different days and averaged for all 12 subjects from three sessions. The large zones have been determined suggesting great variability among the paraplegic population.

The last figure is included to illustrate that it is essential to know with certain level of accuracy the properties of the joint and actuators, since the variability among paraplegics is very large. It is feasible to estimate only the parameters at the joint level, not at the individual musculo-tendonal level, however, this is applicable for designing a controller [e.g., Chizeck *et al.*, 1999]. Soft tissue, passive stretching of antagonistic muscles, and ligaments introduce nonlinearities, which must be included in the model, if the goal is to end the research with a working apparatus [Popović *et al.*, 1999].

Although this neuro-muscular model is very complex, it is only the great simplification of the biological counterpart. The model does not include multiple muscles that are acting at the same joint; it actually combines them in a single

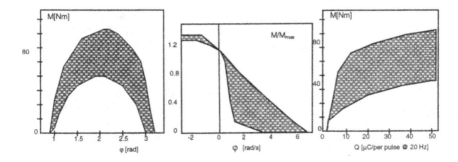

Fig. 5.55: The nonlinear properties of the knee joint extensor actuator. The data comprise results from 12 paraplegics. See text for details.

equivalent flexor or extensor muscle. The reason behind this simplification is that it is not feasible to determine individual features of each muscle, yet it is possible to estimate their total net effect at the level of the joint. A method that can simplify the estimation of parameters with accuracy is the feedback error learning, which uses fuzzy-logic networks to "learn" feedback for closed-loop control at the level of a single joint [Kawato, 1990].

5.5 Controlling Neuroprostheses for Grasping and Reaching

The goal directed movement, such as the reaching and grasping, can follow an infinite number of trajectories, yet able-bodied humans single out a solution that is almost unique for all of them. This solution is task dependent and suboptimal using the terminology of automatics; it is based on the musculo-skeletal substrate, experience and acquired skills, and the environment (e.g., muscle strength or disease, unknown complex tracking, obstacle between the initial and final position of the hand, precision of grasping). A suboptimal performance is adequate in the widest possible range of circumstances; rather than the optimal for constrained conditions. The multi-joint, multi-actuator biological systems such as the arm-hand system cannot be externally controlled using only state space methods and conventional techniques developed for machine and robots [Tomović et al., 1995]. In order to be effective, external control of movement has to be integrated with the preserved biological mechanisms. The external and biological control work in parallel contributing to the same task when NP is used to restore movement (e.g., control the elbow movement by stimulating the elbow extensor muscles of a human who retained voluntary flexion of the elbow).

5.5.1 Control Methods to Restore Grasping

Functional electrical stimulation is used in open-loop mode to provide grasp and release for tetraplegic subjects [Kilgore and Peckham, 1993b]. A key issue for implementation of the open loop NP is the synthesis of the grasp stimulus map, which is the relationship between the input control signal (volitionally controlled) and the output stimulus to each electrode.

The procedure for synthesizing the grasp involved determining the command input to the stimulus output relationship, or grasp parameters. This involved four phases: electrode profiling, selection of grasp configuration, initial grasp parameter set-up, and

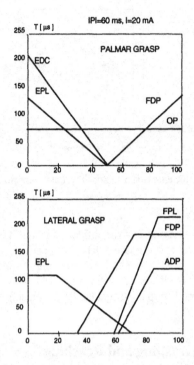

Fig. 5.56 The diagram of the stimulation profiles for four muscles providing the palmar and lateral grasp in a tetraplegic subject using the percutaneous intramuscular electrodes and a version of the Freehand system. The horizontal axis shows the position of the proportional interface controlled by the user: 0 - hand open, 100 - hand closed. The abbreviations used for muscles are described in text.

parameter modification [Kilgore et al., 1989]. Electrode profiling is a procedure of determining the output characteristics of each electrode/muscle combination. The threshold, selectivity, direction, and length dependence are determined for each electrode that is implanted (percutaneous, intramuscular electrodes). Two grasp configurations have been selected, the palmar and lateral, since humans can do most of the daily activities by using only them, but also because it is almost impossible to control the pinch grasp effectively.

The muscles, which are typically instrumented with electrodes, are the following: 1) finger flexors Flexor Digitorum Profundus (FDP), Flexor Digitorum Superficialis (FDS); 2) finger extensors - Extensor Digitorum Communis (ECD), Extensor Indicus Proprius (EIP); 3) thumb flexors - Adductor Pollicis (ADP), Flexor Pollicis Brevis (FPB), Flexor Pollicis Longus (FPL); 4) thumb extensors - Extensor Pollicis Longus (EPL), Extensor Pollicis Brevis (EPB), and 5) thumb Abductors - Abductor Pollicis Brevis (ABPB), Opponens Pollicis (OP).

Depending of the injury some of the muscles, which are required, are not innervated; thus, they cannot be stimulated. In addition stimulation of some muscles at levels that generate adequate force is spreading to neighboring muscles, which may be counterproductive. An example of the stimulation profiles that have been determined to work well enough for several years is shown in Figure 5.56. The user controls a linear transducer (e.g., Hall effect sensor, potentiometer, optical encoder) with his/her preserved movement functions (e.g., contralateral shoulder movement, ipsilateral wrist position) from 0 to 100, where 0 reflects the hand open, and 100 hand closed (Figure 5.56). The switch has been included to select between two profiles, *i.e.*, to select the palmar or lateral grasp.

Kilgore and Peckham [1993a] developed an automatic procedure, which will compensate for the influence of the electrode-position dependent recruitment properties on the grasp output. A method called the external grasp synthesis procedure (GSP) has been developed. The GSP uses an external moment of model of the hand, which describes the interaction between the active moments produced by electrical stimulation, the passive joint moments, and the total joint moment an angle. The GSP was used to develop the stimulus map for many subjects, and it allows iterative improvements (Figure 5.57).

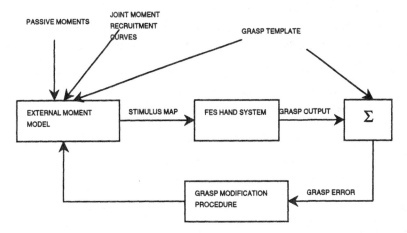

Fig. 5.57: The method of grasp stimulus synthesis called the external moment grasp synthesis procedure. Adapted from Kilgore and Peckham, 1993a © IEEE.

External moment model (EMM) describes the interaction between the active moments produced by electrical stimulation, the passive moments and the total joint position and moment output. It is called the external moment model because it incorporates only the externally measurable active and passive moments about the joints of the hand with no assumptions regarding the forces developed on each tendon and ligament. It assumed that the active moments produced by each electrode/muscle combination could be summed with the passive moments to predict the total moment. The joint angle was predicted as the angle at which the sum of moments was zero. The objective of EMM is to find the combination of stimulus levels to each electrodes which minimizes the difference between the desired grasp output and the predicted grasp output, *i.e.*, minimizes the grasp error. This objective states as follows:

$$\Phi = G^T \cdot E$$

where Φ is the objective function to be minimized, E is the vector of grasp error terms, and G is the vector of grasp error term gains. The error vector term E is the grasp error values for each moment component of the grasp output (e.g., thumb extension/flexion, index finger extension/flexion). The gain vector G indicates the relative importance of each moment component to the overall grasp output. Each error term is calculated as the difference between the desired grasp output and the predicted grasp output for each moment component. The predicted grasp output is the sum of the passive moment and the active moments produced by each electrode. This can be stated in the general case for a single moment component as follows:

$$M_{pred} = M_{pas}(\theta_1,...,\theta_n) + M_{E1}(PW,\theta_1,...,\theta_n) + ... + M_{En}(PW,\theta_1,...,\theta_n)$$

The PW is the duration (pulse width) of the stimulation pulse, M_{pred} is the predicted total joint moment, M_{pas} the passive joint moment and M_{En} the active joint moment produced by electrode n, and θ_n the joint angle component n. The passive moment is a function of the angles of each joint, while the active moment is obtained by using the recruitment curves. The stimulus values, which are minimizing the objective function Φ, can be found by searching all combinations of pulse-width values for each electrode, yet using the peace-wise linear recruitment. The singular value decomposition has been suggested for the optimization when peace-wise linearization is applied for the recruitment curves.

The solution for a single command signal-pulse width pair is achieved by searching through the possible combinations of linear segments until a valid solution is found. The least-squares solution has been found at 21 points along the grasp input/output relationship (5 percent increment of command). The resulting output of the EMM is a set of 21 pulse-duration for each electrode.

This method is an effective computerized version of forming the opposition space when grasping. The synergistic control of muscle contributing to prehension and closing grasping pattern is essential to generate adequate stiffness, smoothness, and secure grasp.

The model has a preference for a solution with a low level of cocontraction. In some cases, however, it may be advantageous to increase the stiffness of the hand. A cocontraction constraint can be added to the EMM that requires the solution to be above a certain level of cocontraction. The error term (constraint) has been included in the EMM in the following form:

$$E_{CC} = CC - \{|M_{pas}| + |M_{E1}| + .. + |M_{En}|\}$$

where E_{CC} is the cocontraction error term, CC is the cocontraction level; other terms are described above. The GSP was implemented and tested with several tetraplegic individuals. An improvement from the previously developed and used semi-automatic method of synthesizing the grasp [Kilgore et al., 1989] has been documented. The levels of stimulation have been decreased, ultimately leading to less muscle fatigue, and more muscle could be integrated providing better functionality [Kilgore and Peckham, 1993b].

Crago with coworkers [Crago et al., 1991] suggested to use feedback to control the hand grasp opening and contact force during stimulation of paralyzed muscles. A fixed parameter, discrete time, first order feedback system has been used to regulate FES in hand muscles. The stiffness of the grasp is kept constant by linearly combining force and feedback signals. A single continuous command signal can control the size of the grasp opening prior to object acquisition and both the aperture and force after the contact. A feedback control system employing a combination of force and position feedback can provide the regulation of grasp under full range of mechanical loading conditions.

A block diagram (Figure 5.58) shows the principle for the design of the controller. The input-output relationship is given by $E = K_C(P_C - P) - F$, where K_C is the regulated stiffness, P_C is the reference position input command, E is the error driving the activation controller, F is the force generated (force sensor), and P actual position (position sensor). Under ideal conditions the error would be zero.

The coactivation map (Figure 5.59) shows the required overlap for safe and smooth operation of the control system. The map is serving to avoid over stimulation and under stimulation that are potentially dangerous and certainly ineffective, as well as to control the degree of coactivation.

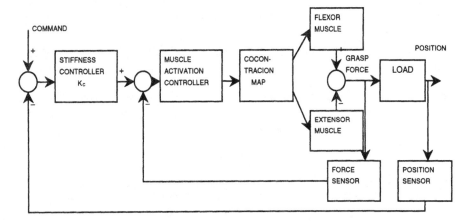

Fig. 5.58: Block diagram of the grasp controller that uses position and force feedback to regulate the prehension and contact force. Adapted from Crago *et al.*, 1991 © IEEE.

The main role of the cocontraction map is to establish different gains for the following three operating regimes: single muscle extension, coactivation, and single muscle flexion. The map has been determined somewhat arbitrarily, since there are no objective criteria or measures defined yet.

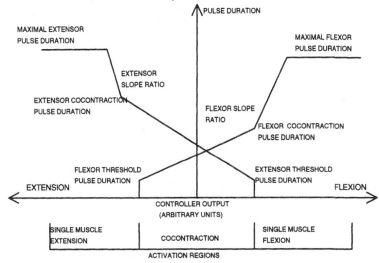

Fig. 5.59: Cocontraction mapping scheme for control of two antagonist muscles. The maps determine the stimulus pulse duration for each muscle as a function of the activation controller output. The overlap between the outputs for the two muscles determines the degree of coactivation. Adapted from Crago *et al.*, 1991 © IEEE.

The system provides isometric functioning with excellent reproducibility, it has proven to be robust to perturbations (joint angle and controller gain). The system is applicable for the control of a single joint. The controller has been tested for functional tests in a tetraplegic subject who already received a version of the Freehand system, and it showed improved performance by leading to less fatigue, safer grasp, and minimized grasping force. However, the position and force feedback require that the system is instrumented with sensors; thus, the system has not still yet reached clinical or home usage.

Lemay et al. [1993] presented the tuning methodology for the closed-loop control of a single joint. The methods have been tested in animal experiments, and then combined with the open-loop control system for grasping in tetraplegic subjects. The subjects' commands have been used to tune the parameters of the closed loop controller, i.e., the user was a teacher, while the computer was the student. Once the parameters have been tuned, the computer could operate the systems without the user's intervention.

Prochazka et al. [1997] presented an open loop system that allows the user to enhance his/her tenodesis by applying electrical stimulation to finger flexors and extensors via surface electrodes. The open-loop controller uses the signal from a position sensor to start the stimulation of either an opening or hand closing combination of synergistic muscles. The system included audio feedback to help the user during the training phase to know if the device was delivering electrical pulses to the appropriate muscles and how strong the stimulation was. The user could select to turn off the audio feedback at any time during and/or after the usage. The stimulator provided control of the amplitude, while keeping the pulse duration and frequency constant.

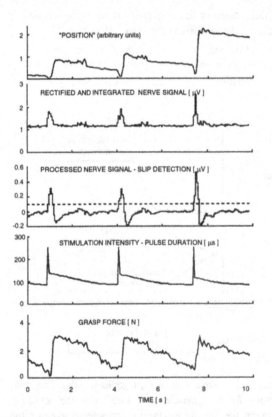

Fig. 5.60: The slip detection algorithm used for control of the stimulation applied for providing the safe grasp with minimal level of stimulation. The subject who uses the modified version of the Freehand system holds a testing object. The experimentator pushes the object; the controller detects the slip, increases the stimulation intensity and provides firm grasp (in real-time). Adapted from Haugland et al., 1999, with permission.

The use of a natural sensors to provide a signal that could serve for control has been investigated in Aalborg, Denmark [Haugland et al., 1999] as described in Chapter 4 (Figure 5.60). The sensory information is processed to allow detection of the change of the force or slippage; thus, the algorithm built into the grasping system is constantly decreasing the level of stimulation up to the detection of the slip of the held object. Once the system detects the neural activity the signal is generated to increase the stimulation intensity as shown in the section on Neuroprosthesis (4.3). There is an artifact "checker" that eliminates false neural activity, thus safe and secure operation is guarantied. The measurements showed that the average grasp force during a meal of a tetraplegic subject, who uses the system, is decreased for 40 percent compared with open loop control.

Scott *et al.* [1996] developed he myoelectric control for bilateral use of Freehand systems. They suggested using the recordings from sternocleido-mastoid muscle with surface electrodes. A differential pair of electrodes has been placed over the muscles close to the sternum in order to reduce the amount of muscle movement under the skin during the turning. The signals were amplified and band-pass filtered between 15 and 150 Hz. The RMS value of the signal was assessed in 50 millisecond windows. The subjects have been shown a monitor, and the task was to control the objects on the screen by generating a distinct EMG pattern at the sternocleido-mastoid muscles. The maximum EMG activity has been used to normalize the recordings. Three-state command was proposed for the control based on detection of left and right zero, weak and strong EMG. The commands were issued while the head position was maintained and, subsequently, a strong co-contraction was made. It was possible to decide whether a right or left and even bilateral command was generated. The three desired states have been clearly discernible; different levels of activity were detectable using RMS compared with the background. The initial findings have been proved in five able-bodied and two tetraplegic subjects [Scott *et al.*, 1996]. This interface is somewhat controversial, and seven of twelve tetraplegic subjects, who participated in the evaluation of a different grasping system, have tried to use this control, yet they were not able to use it reliably (Popović, unpublished results).

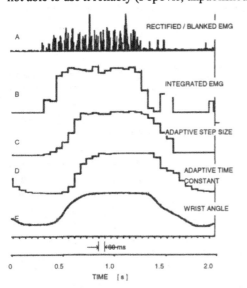

Fig. 5.61: An example of the myoelectric control signals from wrist extensor muscles during stimulation in parallel with the wrist joint angle. The range of the wrist movement was between 20 and 40 degrees. Adapted from Hart *et al.*, 1998 © IEEE.

Hart *et al.* [1998] compared different interfaces that could provide a proportional continuous signal to control the grasping from open to close position. The study included wrist joint angle, contralateral shoulder positioned joystick, and the wrist myoelectric signals (MES). The MES was obtained from three surface electrodes (bipolar recordings) placed over the wrist extensor muscles. The proportional signals were determined based upon the amplitude of the MES (Figure 5.61). It was necessary to use blanking circuit to minimize the stimulation artifacts (Figure 5.61, A). Since the stimulation frequency used 60 ms interpulse interval, the actual period for collecting EMG data was 35 ms (between the pulses). The original signal saw amplified, filtered (300 Hz to 1 kHz), and BIN integrated.

Two other processing technique have been tested: adaptive time constant filter (Figure 5.61, C) and adaptive step size (slew rate limiting) filter as shown in panel D, Figure 5.61 [Park and Meek, 1995]. The consistence of the EMG signals was compared with the wrist joint angle transducer (Figure 5.61, E), and adequate timing and amplitude correlation can be observed.

The study of the EMG controlled system [Saxena et al., 1995] tested the applicability of EMG recordings as a control signal to enhance tenodesis by FES. Six complete tetraplegic subjects with a lesion at C5/C6 were selected among the twelve potential volunteers, since they had preserved voluntary wrist movements (extension and weak flexion), voluntary elbow movement, and acceptable passive range of movement of fingers, yet no grasping ability. The control signal was obtained by using three surface, disposable, self-adhering electrodes positioned over the wrist extensor muscles. The recordings were real-time amplified, rectified, and BIN integrated (10 ms). The obtained signal depended upon the placement of the electrodes and skin to electrode impedance, yet the day-to-day sessions showed a reproducible pattern of EMG recordings. The threshold method that has been used allowed switching on and off the stimulation. During 30-minute long sessions of continuous use of the hand, the peak of the integrated rectified EMG signal (RMS ≈ 100 µV) dropped for almost 60 percent compared with its maximal value (RMS ≈ 250 µV) at the beginning of the session which follows the results of Lenman et al. [1989]. This required the tuning of the system during its use. The tetraplegic SCI subjects were asked to perform a set of typical daily activities used for the evaluation of the shoulder control in the multichannel implanted NP [Wijman et al., 1990]. Ten activities were studied, and the final score of each task, both with and without the assistive system, was defined from the interview, video recordings done during the sessions, and patient files that have been taken during the testing. It was found that grasping was improved for most of the activities, hence this device improved the quality of daily living in a selected group of tetraplegic subjects.

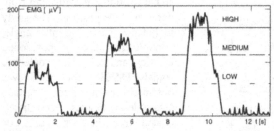

Fig. 5.62: The three-threshold control method to grade the strength of the grasp. Data shown is recorded during the use of the EMG controlled FES system. Subject can switch from a lower to higher level just by volitionally increasing the EMG, yet the algorithm required to turn the stimulation off before the stimulation could be switched to the lower intensity. Adapted from Saxena et al., 1995, with permission.

The described control operates using binary output (on-off); there is no gradation of the stimulation generated force. It was feasible to grade the strength of the stimulation using the recordings and multi-threshold triggering, hence the performance could be improved (Figure 5.62). However, subjects who participated in the study, preferred the single threshold device, because of the simplicity of the application. It was possible to stimulate motor nerves with variable pulse width using a multi-threshold control strategy, but it required fine-tuning of the gain of the device and thresholds. The experiments showed not to be practical at this point, because the subjects had great difficulties in selecting the appropriate EMG levels and maintaining those; pronation and supination or manipulating heavier objects deteriorated the distinction between levels of EMG.

Meek and Fetherston (1992) analyzed the methods to maximize the EMG signals recorded with surface electrodes to allow control of a multifunctional transhumeral prosthesis. The processing is a two-phase procedure: myoelectric processing and pattern recognition of the multi EMG signals. For prosthesis control, the EMG signal is detected from the surface of the skin through the use of stainless steel electrodes without any skin preparation.

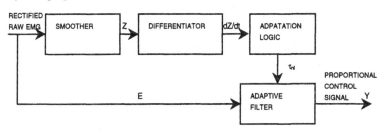

Fig. 5.63: Adaptive filter signal flow. Adapted from Meek and Fetherston, 1992, with permission

This requires very high performance preamplifiers with high common mode rejection ratio and high input impedance to be positioned as close as possible to the electrodes. An EMG signal is stochastic, yet its amplitude is correlated with the force generated by the muscle. The best use of the EMG recordings would be after processing if a signal is obtained that is proportional with the muscle force. A possible method to obtain the signal, which is reproducible and proportional to the muscle force, is to use adaptive filtering technique [Meek and Fetherston, 1992]. The adaptive filter has to be designed according to the rate of change of the EMG signal. The rate of change of the EMG signal relates to the rate of change of the muscle contraction. This rate can be determined by the derivative of the smoothed signal. When the signal is changing rapidly (high amplitude of the derivative) during rapid movement, the time constant is low, allowing fast response but with more noise. When the signal is steady (derivative amplitude is low) during slow, precise movement, the time constant is high, allowing a high signal to noise ratio, yet slow response (Figure 5.63).

The adaptive filter can be realized with two filters operating in parallel. The derivative of the output of one filter with a time constant τ_z is used to control the time constant τ_{nl} of the other filter. Several parameters can be adjusted to control the response of the filter: the time constant τ_z on the parallel filter; the maximum and minimum time constant of the adaptive filter τ_1 and τ_s respectively; and the gain "a" of the adaptation logic. The relationship for the adaptation logic and the rise time, signal to noise ratio, and squared error can be defined as:

$$\tau_{nl} = \frac{\tau_1 - \tau_2}{a\dot{Z}^2 + 1}$$

$$E = \tau_{nl}\dot{Y} + Y , \; E = \tau_z \dot{Z} + Z$$

where τ_{nl} is the adaptive time constant, τ_1 is the maximum time constant of the adaptive filter, τ_2 is the minimum time constant of the adaptive filter, Z is the smoothed EMG signal, E is the rectified unsmoothed EMG signal, Y is the output (control) signal, a is the gain, and τ_z is the time of the parallel filter.

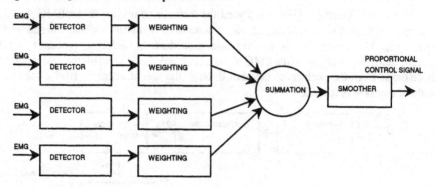

Fig. 5.64: The schema of the signal flow through the spatial filter. See text for details. Adapted from Meek and Fetherston, 1992, with permission.

Spatial filtering is the use of multiple sensors (differential electrode pairs) to pre-whiten the EMG spectrum. Pre-whitening increases the randomness of the signal; thus, making the signal spectrum whiter. It is postulated that limited spatial sampling produces a low frequency artifact and that by combining the signals of several sensors, more of the total muscle is monitored, and the low frequency artifact disappears.

The process is a weighted least-squares estimate filtering [Meek et al., 1990]. Each sensor channel is weighted by a constant, and all the channels are summed, forming one signal, which is then smoothed by a low pass filter (Figure 5.64). The weighting of each channel is defined by the eigenvalues and the eigenvectors determined from a time-series of EMG data by the following procedure: 1) time series of four channels of EMG data are collected for a constant isometric contraction of a muscle; 2) the eigenvalues and eigenvectors for each channel are computed for these data; 3) the eigenvectors transform each channel to create four new channels to maximize the independence; and 4) each of the new channels is weighted according to the eigenvalues and summed, producing a single signal that is then smoothed. In other words, each channel contributes to the summation according to its eigenvalue. A channel with no difference in eigenvalues is essentially ignored.

5.5.2 Control Methods to Restore Elbow and Wrist Movement

Methods to control the whole arm and assist manipulation (reaching) in humans lacking voluntary shoulder, elbow, and wrist movement control received lately more attention [Crago et al., 1998; Grill and Peckham, 1998; Lemay and Crago, 1997; Smith et al., 1996]. All NP from the Case Western Reserve University, Cleveland, OH, for restoring arm movement are expanded versions of the Freehand grasping system, and they all use the same basic strategy used for the grasping. Additional channels to control the wrist, elbow, and eventually the shoulder movement aim to provide control to subjects who could benefit from FES assisted grasping, yet their working space is limited, and grasping is therefore not effective.

Lan et al. [1994] presented the use of artificial neural network (ANN) to generate muscle stimulation patterns for the control of elbow movement. They compared three different types of ANN. The study was limited to the control of a single joint movement. The stimulation patterns to be classified and matched have been obtained from optimal control analysis of movement. Simple feed-forward ANN, feed-forward with recurrent feedback, and feed-forward with recurrent feedback and input time delays have been compared. The recurrent feedback improves the convergence and the time delay the accuracy, *i.e.*, the generalization. This result follows the expectations; since the movement is a dynamic process, thus the prehistory is affecting the behavior (inertia), and the feedback plays a significant role when optimization criteria are applied [Jonić *et al.*, 1999]. Lan *et al.* [1994] were the first to conclude that basically all machine learning techniques are applicable, yet some will guaranty better generalization, some will be relatively simple to apply, and the speed of convergence will be different.

Wrist control [Lemay *et al.*, 1997] was evaluated in two individuals with tetraplegia. In most cases subjects with spinal cord lesion at C5 have their primary wrist movers (Extensor Carpi Radialis Brevis and Longus (ECRB and ECRL) and the Flexor Carpi Radialis (FCR) m.) denervated. Surgical intervention (Chapter 4), *i.e.*, tendon transfer of the Brachioradialis m. into the ECRB, can restore limited voluntary control of extension that is sufficiently strong to overcome wrist flexion due to the stimulation of the finger and thumb flexor muscles. The extension strength can be augmented by transferring the paralyzed (innervated) Extensor Carpi Ulnaris (ECU) m. and stimulating it [Adamczyk *et al.*, 1996]. This result imposed analyzing methods to control the position of the wrist by means of FES. Lemay and coworkers investigated one open-loop and two closed-loop controllers. The open-loop control system used coactivation, *i.e.*, increased stiffness, to stabilize position against disturbances in the flexion or extension direction while the two closed-loop controllers did not use any coactivation. The open-loop controller was investigated, since it does not require any sensors; thus, it is the simplest one for application. The level of stimulation of extensor muscles is about 20 percent of the maximum. One of the closed-loop methods used position and moment feedback to regulate the stiffness of the wrist, with the equilibrium point at neutral [Lemay *et al.*, 1993]. The control system was synthesized by applying methods developed by Crago *et al.* [1991] and Lan *et al.* [1991], described earlier in this Chapter. The second closed-loop controller was a proportional-integral-derivative position controller using only position feedback. In theory, this controller can reject static torque disturbances as long as there is sufficient strength. The conclusions from the study are that the stiffness closed-loop controller works best among the three systems tested; it requires less stimulation than the open-loop controller and provides better posture of the wrist.

Miller *et al.* [1989] investigated the possibility to stimulate the Triceps Brachii m. in order to restore elbow extension in C5 tetraplegic subjects who have preserved shoulder movement and elbow flexion. The control system included three input signals (flexion/extension and adduction/abduction of the upper arm, and elbow flexion/extension) and one output signal (stimulator activating elbow extensor *via* an intramuscular percutaneous electrode). Both the sensory and motor parts of the NP are at the same arm. Recruitment modulation was used to regulate the level of activation by varying the duration of the stimulus pulse. The off-line experiments provided the look-up table; different loads in the hand have been included. Two tetraplegic subjects participated in the testing. The results suggest that stimulation of elbow extensor is beneficial and functional. Subjects quickly learned to control the elbow flexion strength; thereby, compensated the externally driven extension to ensure desired movement or posture. The system was shown to be highly complex for daily tuning and setting in operation; the cost to benefit ratio from using it was not adequate.

Crago et al. [1998] evaluated a portable, hand grasp/elbow extension neuroprosthesis in two persons with C6 level tetraplegia (complete lesions). Both subjects initially received an implantable stimulator for restoring grasping, and later one or two intramuscular electrodes have been added for stimulation of the Triceps Brachii muscle. The block diagram of the controller is shown in Figure 5.65. The system has a three component command interface: a switch, a gravity sensor, and a joint angle sensor. The switch and the joint angle sensor are used for turning the system on and off, select between the lateral and palmar grasps, and proportionally control the grasping. The gravity sensor is used to turn on and off the stimulation of the elbow extensor muscles. In order to eliminate the so-called "bouncing" problem with the switch, the controller includes a hysteresis function for the gravity sensor. Once the subject volitionally raises his/her upper arm above the shoulder line, the stimulator delivers bursts of electrical impulses to the Triceps Brachii m. of the same arm contributing to the elbow extension. The user controls the elbow angle by volitionally contracting the non-paralyzed Biceps Brachii muscle. This regime of cocontraction increases the stiffness of the elbow joint, but it leads to faster fatigue of both the externally stimulated extensors and volitionally controlled flexor muscles.

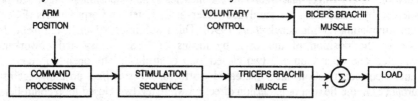

Fig. 5.65: The block diagram of the control scheme for NP assisted elbow extension. The arm position determines the signal picked up by the accelerometer. The elbow flexor (Biceps Brachii m.) is considered functional. Adapted from Grill and Peckham, 1998 © IEEE.

Grill and Peckham [1998] combined the grasping and elbow extension NP using the micromachined silicon accelerometer to measure the magnitude of the component of the gravitational acceleration. High frequency acceleration signals have been low-pass filtered, by using a second order filter with a cut-off frequency of 4.8 Hz. The sensor was placed over the ulna near the elbow joints so that its sensitive axis was along the gravitational direction acting about the elbow joint. This placement minimizes the effects of pronation/supination on sensor output. A desktop computer was used to control the elbow stimulation. Two subjects participated in the study, and the commands were tabulated so that a look-up table could be used to select the pattern of stimulation to be delivered to the elbow extensor muscles. Maximum elbow extension torque exceeded 4 Nm, being sufficient for most tasks as mentioned earlier. Many of the results have been employed by Crago et al. [1998] with a portable, microcomputer based stimulator.

The evaluation showed that both subjects could develop the elbow net joint torque larger than 4.5 Nm, being large enough for most of the daily activity. One of the subjects, prior to the implantation of the elbow extension NP, received a tendon transfer for elbow extension, yet the net joint torque was still only about 1.5 Nm (4 Nm is required for independent functioning, [Crago et al., 1998]). The overall success rate at the far and near locations/orientations was very large (>96 percent) compared with 49 (subject #1) and 6 (subjects #2) percent without the stimulation. The domains of the workspace where the performance was the worst are the far, ipsilateral, and above the head parts of the desirable workspace. Subjects with the grasp/elbow system benefited in general because of the larger number of functions that they can independently perform; thus the over all quality of life. Other tasks that would benefit from elbow extension are pushing objects at low heights, weight shifts, transfers, and wheelchair propulsion. These function, however, require different command interface and control.

Smith *et al.* [1996] presented the case study for three C4 tetraplegic subjects who used the implanted (percutaneous intramuscular electrodes) system to enhance reaching and grasping. The following muscles have been stimulated: Pectoralis Major (upper arm adduction), Latissimus dorsi and Triceps Brachii m. (elbow flexion and extension respectively), Extensor Carpi Ulnaris (forearm supination), Adductor Pollicis (thumb adduction), Abductor Pollicis Brevis (thumb abduction), Flexor Pollicis Longus (thumb flexion), Extensor Pollicis Longus (thumb extension), Extensor Digitorum Communis (fingers extension), and Flexor Digitorum Superficialis and Profundus (fingers flexion). The Latissimus Dorsi muscle was transposed to provide elbow flexion, and Extensor Carpi Ulnaris tendon transfer was performed to allow external control of supination. A 48 channel programmable stimulator was used: pulse amplitude I = 20 mA, frequency f = 17 pulses per second, and pulse duration in the range of T = 0 - 200 µs. The control input is the contralateral shoulder position, and the stimulation follows the preprogrammed sequence.

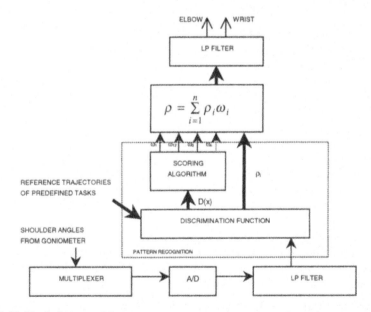

Fig 5.66: Block diagram of the synergistic control of the elbow and wrist joints based on the pattern recognition and state space model of movement. Adapted from Aghili and Haghpanahi, 1995, with permission.

Aghili and Haghpanahi [1996] analyzed methods to control a transhumeral prosthesis with emphasis on the extended proprioception [Simpson, 1974].

The basis for their controller was that the shoulder, elbow, and wrist joints display synergistic behavior in the state space formed by the relative joint angles and that these synergies are task specific. The hypothesis was that it would be possible to control the elbow joint in real-time by using the kinematics of the shoulder joint and a pattern recognition technique. All experiments have been performed in able-bodied subjects. The control system requires that the synergies for the set of predefined tasks, determined within the limited workspace are stored and that this information is supplemented in real-time with the data from the goniometer at the shoulder joint measuring the flexion/extension, abduction/adduction, and humeral rotation of the upper arm (Figure 5.66).

The system was evaluated by comparing the recorded arm trajectories of humans while they moved the arm and the computer generated trajectories. The tracking error was less than 15 percent; the errors were bigger at the wrist joint than in the elbow. This result was expected since the synergy between the shoulder and elbow is stronger compared with the synergy between the shoulder and wrist joints. The wrist joint is used to orient the hand during the prehension phase and change the position of the object once it has been grasped, while the elbow joint contributed mostly with manipulation and bringing the wrist and hand into a desired position.

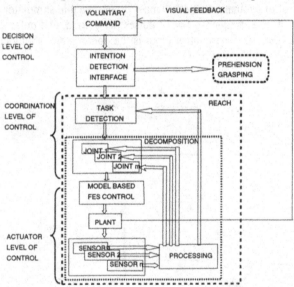

Fig. 5.67: Diagram of a three-level controller for elbow/grasp neuroprosthesis. The coordination level uses rule-based control; rules correspond to synergies found in able-bodied subjects. The lower actuator level uses customized model that reflects specifics of the neuro-musculo-skeletal system of the user.

Popović M *et al.* [1993] suggested a method that is based on extended physiological propriception [Simpson, 1974] and between synergies of joints, being applicable to both implantable and surface stimulation systems. The control follows the findings that the movement of the neighboring segments is "connected" by synergies. The synergies allow to plan the functional movement based on the trajectory of the most distal segment, while the cognitive (volitional) control is only applied to the most proximal segment [Latash, 1993]. The adopted control for reaching restoration follows this method.

The Belgrade Grasping/reaching System (BGS) uses four channels of FES to assist grasping and two channels to control elbow joint movement. The hierarchical hybrid control structure has been applied (Figure 5.67).

The controller for elbow NP has a three level hierarchical structure (Figure 5.67). The top level is voluntary; the user transmits commands to the coordination by using the appropriate interface (push button switch keyboard). The external control comprises two levels: the coordination uses the off-line prepared rules and distributes the controls to the actuator level. The actuator control is model-based, sensory driven, and fully customized to the user [Popović *et al.*, 1994; Popović *et al.*, 1995]. The synergistic control of the elbow NP was initially based on the scaling law between the flexion/extension (FE) at the shoulder and elbow joints determined in able-bodied humans [Popović M *et al.*, 1993; Popović M and Popović, 1994, 1995 and 2000].

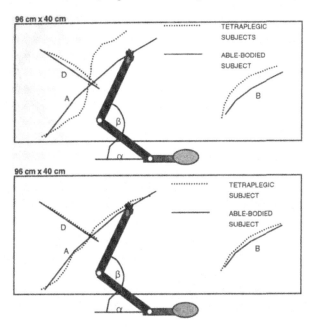

Fig. 5.68: Three volitional movements (A, B, and D) of able-bodied subjects (full line) and the same three movements achieved with the reaching NP (dashed line) using the scaling law (top panel) and IL determined synergies (bottom panel). α and β are the FE of the shoulder and elbow joints. Adapted from Popović M and Popović, 2000.

Clinical trials with the Belgrade Grasping/reaching System (BGS) suggested that the scaling law is not well suited for some domains of the working space, and that this control leads to errors in the positioning of the hand [Popović *et al.*, 1998]. An example of errors can be seen when analyzing the discrepancy between the desired paths (three movement: A, B, and D) shown with full lines and the actual trajectories generated by a tetraplegic subject when using the elbow NP with the scaling control shown with dashed lines (Figure 5.68, upper panel).

The reason for the mismatch is that the scaling law comprises that the elbow and shoulder velocity profiles have the simultaneous peaks. It has been determined, however, that there are: 1) movement when FE velocity *vs.* time at one joint has two peaks, while the velocity profile of the other joints *vs.* time has a single peak; 2) movement when both FE velocities have one peak, and they are time shifted with respect to each other; and 3) a group where the bell-shaped velocity profiles *vs.* time have simultaneous peaks. The inductive learning (IL) was applied to capture the highly nonlinear synergy (IL is described earlier in this Chapter). The IL used a training set that has been prepared from kinematics recorded in able-bodied humans. Able-bodied humans were instrumented with joint motion sensors, and they performed the activities of daily living.

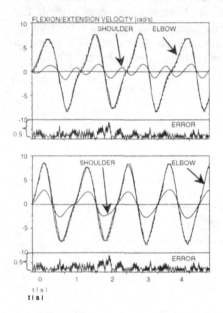

Fig. 5.69: Results of IL for determining the synergies between flexion/extension for two different movements. The desired and IL estimated FE velocities *vs.* time are superimposed, and their difference shown at the bottom.

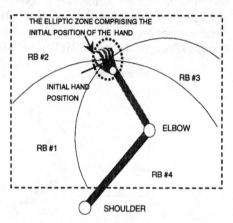

Fig. 5.70: The projection to the horizontal plane of the division of the workspace to four domains (zones). Domain is characterized with the applicability of the same set of rules for movement. The dashed line ellipse indicates the region that is considered as the initial position. The workspace division corresponds to 3D movement. Adapted from Popović and Popović, 2000.

The FE angles at the shoulder and elbow joints have been recorded and processed, and the angular velocities calculated. Figure 5.69 shows the calculated FE velocities at the shoulder joint from the recorded data, and two superimposed series: calculated FE velocities at the elbow joint from recordings and estimated FE velocities by IL [Popović and Popović, 2000a and b]. The matching between the original and estimated FE velocities was very good (Figure 5.69) even for movement groups 1) and 2); the difference between the desired and estimated trajectory, the error, has been extracted at the bottom of both panels. The mean error, *i.e.*, the mean difference between the recorded and IL estimated FE velocity, is 0.12 radian/s, with the maximum error of 0.48 radian/second for the example shown in Figure 5.69. The measures of the quality of learning with IL are the correlation coefficient K, and the time error delay t_{er} defined earlier in this chapter; the machine learning generalizes good enough based on these two objective values.

The novel control method has been tested using the modified BGS as an elbow NP. The interface for selecting the zone was a push button device. The subject was trained to press the appropriate button depending on the zone that he wanted to move the hand with the contralateral hand. Each button was associated with an off-line determined synergy.

The stimulation profiles delivered to motorneurons via electrodes have been determined based on off-line simulation of elbow joint FE. The simulation has been customized to the eventual user [Popović M *et al.*, 1994]. The sensors used are the flexion/extension goniometers at the elbow and shoulder joints.

Once the command signal was sent to the coordination level, the command signal to the electronic stimulator was the recalculated pulse duration based on the desired angular velocity at the shoulder joint; the elbow angular velocity is used as feedback for correcting the pulse width selected from the look-up table [Popović and Popović, 1998 a and b].

Figure 5.68, lower panel shows the reaching trajectory for the same three types of movement A, B, and D, when using the described controller. The subject, who participated in the presented experiments, has innervated paralyzed Triceps Brachii m. (grade 0) and non-functional Biceps Brachii m. (grade 1). The results are average from 30 trials after the subject was given the opportunity to practice in the laboratory setting for five days, each day for about 30 minutes. The repeated trials during the recording showed large variability in the tracking of the trajectory, yet not in reaching the final position. The differences in hand paths shown in Figure 5.68 are acceptable since tetraplegic subjects can compensate for small errors by moving the trunk for a few centimeters. The learning was performed well, and the generalization is very high ($K >$ 98 percent) for all cases presented, and similarly high for other cases analyzed. The timing error t_{er} for all data presented is zero.

The elbow and shoulder FE belong to different synergies for movement in various zones of the workspace [Popović and Popović, 2000b]. The rules learned for one domain of the workspace are not valid for other domains. Therefore, it is necessary to determine the rules for different domains. Figure 5.70 shows four zones within the workspace, each being "covered" with one set of rules. Each zone is characterized by a single synergy; the correlation between learned and recorded data within each of the zones was $K > 98$ percent. Margins between zones, indicated in Figure 5.70 are narrow bands (about 4.5±1.2 centimeters wide) when averaged over eight study subjects.

6. Epilogue

> "I am glad to say: There is work enough left for you to do"
> Rudolph Magnus [1926]

The Motivation

Never in history have there been so many people with sensory-motor disability, as today, and never has the individual lived as long as he or she does today. The literature data show that the long-term survival rates for persons with sensory-motor disability have steadily risen and, for some individuals, these rates now approach normal. There are many studies showing that activity is beneficial to the overall health of humans with disability, yet the number of practical assistive systems for effective restoration of movement is limited. The Authors strongly believe that the comprehensive development of clinical practice guidelines and better assistive systems are important milestone for the improved treatment of humans with disabilities; and therefore decided to write a book that is meant to serve these purposes. The book reviews different methods and suggests which are the alternative roots to resolve some complex problems that potentially would integrate the results from motor control studies and neural engineering.

The Message

Compared with other classes of dynamical systems, the sensory and motor systems supporting the execution of functional motions in humans, have three unique features: 1) they are highly redundant; 2) they are organized in a hierarchical structure, yet with many parallel channels; and 3) they are self-organized relying, among other things, on an extremely complex connectionism. In spite of the above complexity, the movements resulting from the action of sensory system, as a rule, are deterministic and they follow the preferred way of performing the intended motor task.

The book explains some of the above phenomenon taking a comprehensive approach; *i.e.*, it is discussing general findings from motor physiology, biomechanics, and automatic control. The book offers a plausible explanation as to how the self-organized systems are able to force otherwise uncontrollable system components to perform the desired movement, essentially, in a deterministic, non-stochastic way.

Where to Go?

The technology has spawned many different types of control system; each suited to a particular application. Over a much larger time scale, the biological organisms have evolved control systems to suit many of species and physiological functions. The two streams of development have converged in the area of motor control rehabilitation. The book proposes the integration of these two control strategies. In rehabilitation of movements the aim is to activate joints in a controlled way so as to restore as much motor function as possible in humans with motor disabilities. The control strategies implemented in most of rehabilitation devices have so far been fairly simple, and have been developed largely in relation to the design of machines rather than to the design of nervous systems. Recent neurophysiological data show that some of these strategies have converged, so as to be quite similar to those in analogous natural systems. The question now is, how general is this outcome? In artificial devices, should we always strive to mimic the relevant natural control system on the assumption that it has been optimized in the course of evolution, and could we always mimic nature, given that our abilities to reproduce components of the neuromuscular system are limited? The method that the Authors choose and believe is the one which holds the most promises integrates three methods, all incorporating as the condition *sine qua non* the quantitative assessment before and during the rehabilitation process (Figure 6.1).

Neuroregeneration of the central nervous system is a method that will eventually provide a cure. Although it is still only a perspective, it must be kept in mind as an emerging option; thus, it is very important to preserve as much as possible all resources so that they can be integrated when the time comes.

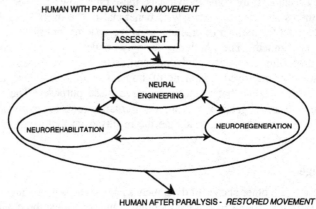

Fig. 6.1: The comprehensive model for effective restoration of movement.

Neurorehabilitation is a method that allows the preserved structures to find their best use if appropriately trained. The intensive, task dependent exercise is showing dramatic effects in handicapped humans (e.g., non-ambulating subjects can unassisted walk for some distances). The possible role of central motor programs that are existing at the level of spinal cord, although controversial, is an option that deserves more attention.

Neural engineering is where the ultimate successes at this stage must come. The development of new implantable devices that interface directly the central and peripheral nervous system allowing wireless communication with the outside world opens new horizons. The implanted technology and micromachining make dramatic impact and provide that has been difficult to imagine, yet the intelligent control that resembles to natural control is the link that would make this approach a viable, effective rehabilitation systems.

Assessment is necessary to objectively measure functional impairments and identify the biomechanical and neurophysiological changes caused by the injury or disease. This facilitates essential customization of a rehabilitation neuroprosthesis by providing the following: 1) identification of the "minimum muscle set" needed to provide functional movements; 2) identification of the output forces required to provide functional movements; and 3) assessment if the available muscles can generate the required muscle output.

The ultimate goal of the work in this field is to improve the quality of life of subjects with sensory-motor disability. There is no rule which technique will work the best; clinical studies and the feedback from the users are the only measure of the quality of the rehabilitation.

The belief is that only a comprehensive work that will maximize the usage of the knowledge of motor control and integrate the technology into the natural control systems is likely to be effective. This book follows that trust and provides a solid foundation for studying, doing research, developing, and applying assistive technology.

References

Abbas JJ, Chizeck HJ (1991) Feedback control of coronal plane hip angle in paraplegic subjects using functional neuromuscular stimulation. IEEE Trans Biomed Eng BME-38:687-698

Abbas JJ, Chizeck HJ (1995) Neural network control of functional neuromuscular stimulation systems: computer simulation studies. IEEE Trans Biomed Eng BME-42:1117-1127

Abbas JJ, Triolo RJ (1997) Experimental evaluation of an adaptive feedforward controller for use in functional neuromuscular stimulation systems. IEEE Trans Rehab Eng TRE-5:12-22

Abend W, Bizzi E, Morasso P (1982) Human arm trajectory formation. Brain 105 (Pt 2):331-48

Adamczyk MM, Crago PE (1996) Input-output nonlinearities and time delays increase tracking errors in hand grasp neuroprostheses. IEEE Trans Rehabil Eng TRE-4(4):271-279

Adler E, Tal E (1965) Relationship between physical disability and functional capacity in hemiplegic patients. Arch Phys Med 46:745

Aebischer P, Guénard V, Winn SR, Valentini RF, Galletti PM (1988) Blind-ended semipermeable guidance channels support peripheral nerve regeneration in the absence of a distal nerve stump. Brain Res 454(1-2):179-187

Aebischer P, Guénard V, Brace S (1989) Peripheral nerve regeneration through blind-ended semipermeable guidance channels: Effect of the molecular weight cutoff. J Neurosci 9:3590-3595

Aebischer P, Guénard V, Valentini RF (1990) The morphology of regenerating peripheral nerves is modulated by the surface microgeometry of polymeric guidance channels. Brain Res 531:211-218

Aeyels B, Peeraer L, Van der Sloten J, Van der Perre G (1992) Development of an above-knee prosthesis equipped with a microprocessor-controlled knee joint: first test results. J Biomed Eng 14:199-202

Aeyels B, van Petegem W, van der Sloten J, van der Perre G, Peeraer L (1997) An EMG-based finite state approach for a microcomputer controlled above-knee prosthesis. In: Proc 19th EMBS IEEE Conf, Chicago, pp 1315-1316

Aghili F, Haghpanahi M (1995) Use of a pattern recognition technique to cotnrol a multifunctional prosthesis. Med Biol Eng Comp 33:504-508

Aguayo AJ (1985) Axonoal regenration from injured neurons in the adult mammalilan central ervous system. In: Cotman CW (ed.) Synaptic plasticity. The Guilford Press, Ney York, pp 457-484

Aisen ML, Krebs H, Hogan N, McDowell F, Volpe BT (1997) The effect of robot-assisted therapy and rehabilitative training on motor recovery following stroke. Arch Neurol 54:443-446

Alaimo AM, Smith JL, Roy R, Edgerton VR (1984) Electromyographic activity of slow and fast ankle extensors following spinal cord transection. J Appl Physiol 56:1608-1613

Alexander GE, Crutcher MD (1990) Functional architecture of basal ganglia circuits: neural substrates of parallel processing. Trends Neurosci 13(7):266-271

Alexander GE, De Long M, Crutcher M (1992) Do cortical and basal ganglionic motor areas use motor programs to control movement? Behav and Brain Sci 15:656-665

Allin J, Inbar GF (1986a) FNS control schemes for the upper limb. IEEE Trans Biomed Eng BME-33:818-828

Allin J, Inbar GF (1986b) FNS parameter selection and upper limb characterization. IEEE Trans Biomed Eng BME-33:809-817

Allum JH, Mauritz KH (1984) Compensation for intrinsic muscle stiffness by short-latency reflexes in human triceps surae muscles. J Neurophysiol 52:797-818

Allum JH, Honegger F (1993) Synergies and strategies underlying normal and vestibulary deficient control of balance: implication for neuroprosthetic control. Prog Brain Res 97: 331-348

Allum JH, Honegger F, Schicks H (1993) Vestibular and proprioceptive modulation of postural synergies in normal subjects. J Vestib Res 3(1):59-85

Alstermark B, Lindstrom S, Lundberg A, Sybirska E (1981) Integration in descending motor pathways controlling the forelimb in the cat and ascending projection to the lateral reticular nucleus from C3-C4 propriospinal also projecting to forelimb motoneurones. Exp Brain Res 42(3-4):282-298

Alur R, Henzinger T, Sontag E (eds.) (1996) Hybrid Systems III-Verification and Control. (Lecture Notes in Computer Science, no 1066) Springer-Verlag, New York

Andersson O, Grillner S (1981) Peripheral control of the cat's step cycle. 1. Phase dependant effects of ramp-movements of the hip during fictive locomotion. Acta Physiol Scand 113: 89-101

André-Thomas A, Autgarden T (1966) Locomotion from pre- to postnatal life. Lavenham Suffolk Spastic Society

Andrews BJ, Bajd T (1984) Hybrid orthosis for paraplegics. In: Popović D (ed.) Advances in External Control of Human Extremities, ETAN (Suppl), pp 55-57

Andrews BJ (1986) A short leg hybrid FES orthosis for assisting locomotion in SCI subjects. In: Proc 2nd Vienna Int Workshop on Functional Electrostimulation, Vienna, pp 31-35

Andrews BJ, Baxendale RM, Barnett R, Phillips G, Paul J, Freeman P (1987) A hybrid orthosis for paraplegics incorporating feedback control. In: Popović D (ed.) Advances in External Control of Human Extremities IX, ETAN, Belgrade, pp 297-310

Andrews BJ, Baxendale RH, Barnett R, Philips GF, Yamazaki T, Paul JP, Freeman PA (1988) Hybrid FES orthosis incorporating closed loop control and sensory feedback. J Biomed Eng 10(2):189-195

Andrews BJ, Barnett RW, Philips GF, Kirkwood CA (1989) Rule-Based control of a hybrid FES orthosis for assisting paraplegic locomotion. Automedica 11:175-199

Annet J, Golby CW, Kay H (1958) The measurement of elements in an assembly task. The information output of the human motor system. Q J Exp Psychol 10:1-11

Antonsson EK, Mann RW (1985) The frequency content of gait (abstract). J Biomech 18:39

Antsaklis P, Kohn W, Nerode A, Sastry S (eds.) (1995) Hybrid Systems II. (Lecture Notes in Computer Science, no 999) Springer Verlag, New York

Antsaklis P, Kohn W, Lemmon M, Nerode A, Sastry S (eds.) (1998) Hybrid Systems V. (Lecture Notes in Computer Science) Springer Verlag, New York

Antsaklis PJ, Nerode A (1998) Hybrid control systems: An introductory discussion to the special issue. IEEE Autom Control AU-43:457-459

Aoyama F (1980) Lapoc System Leg. J Biomechanisms (Japan) pp 59-67

Arabi K, Sawan MA (1999) Electronic design of a multichannel programmable implant for neuromuscular electrical stimulation. IEEE Trans Rehabil Eng 7(2):204-214

Arbib MA (1980) Interacting schemas for motor control. In: Stelmach GE, Requin J (eds.) Tutorials in Motor Behavior. North-Holland, Amsterdam, pp 71-81

Arbib MA (1981) Perceptual structures and distributed motor control. In: Brooks VB (ed.) Handbook of Physiology - The Nervous System. (II Motor control) Am Phys Soc, Bethseda, pp 1449-1480

Arbib MA (1985) Schemas for the temporal control of behavior. Hum Neurobiol 4:63-72

Archibald SJ, Shefner J, Krarup C, Madison RD (1995) Monkey median nerve repaired by nerve graft or collagen nerve guide tube. J Neurosci 15(5 Pt 2):4109-4123

Armstrong DM (1988) The supraspinal control of mammalian locomotion. J Physiol (Lond) 405:1-37

Armstrong WW (1979) Recursive solution to the equations of motion of an n-link manipulator. In: Proc 5th World Congress on the Theory of Machines and Mechanisms, Montreal, pp 1343-1346

Armstrong WW, Gecsei J (1979) Adaptation Algorithms for Binary Tree Networks. IEEE Trans Syst Man Cybern SMC-9:276-285

Armstrong WW, Thomas MM (1994) Dendronic decisions Atree 3.0 beta release 1. ALN Theory. (A Practical Guide to Approximating Relations) Univ of Alberta, Edmonton

Aruin AS, Latash ML (1995) The role of motor action in anticipatory postural adjustments studied with self-induced and externally triggered perturbations. Exp Brain Res 106:291-300

Aruin AS, Hanke TA, Sarma A (1999) Step width feedback in the rehabilitation of stroke patients. In: Gantchev N, Gantchev G (eds.) From Basic Motor Control to Functional Recovery. Acad Publ House, Sofia, pp 458-462

Ashby P, Malis A, Hunter J (1987) The evaluation of "spasticity". Can J Neurol Sci 14:497-500

Ashe J, Taira M, Smyrnis N, Pellizzer G, Georgakopoulos T, Lurito JT, Georgopoulos AP (1993) Motor cortical activity preceding a memorized movement trajectory with an orthogonal bend. Exp Brain Res 95(1):118-130

Atkeson CG (1989) Learning arm kinematics and dynamics. Ann Rev Neurosci 12:157-183

Babinski L (1896) Sur le reflex cutand plantaire dans certaines affections organiques du systeme nerveux central. C R Soc Biol (Paris) 48:207-208

Bajd T, Bowman B (1982) Testing and modelling of spasticity. Biomed Eng 4:90-96

Bajd T, Kralj A, Turk R (1982) Standing-up of a healthy subject and a paraplegic patients. J Biomech 15:1-10

Bajd T, Kralj A, Turk R, Benko H, Sega J (1983) The use of a four channel electrical stimulator as an ambulatory aid for paraplegic patients. Phys Ther 63:1116-1120

Bajd T, Gregorič M, Vodovnik L, Benko H (1985) Electrical stimulation in treating spasticity resulting from spinal cord injury. Arch Phys Med Rehabil 66:515-517

Bajd T, Kralj A, Turk R, Benko H (1986) FES rehabilitative approach in incomplete SCI patients. In: Proc 9th Annu Conf Rehabil Eng Soc Am, pp 316-319

Bajd T, Kralj A, Turk R, Benko H, Sega J (1989) Use of functional electrical stimulation in the rehabilitation of patients with incomplete spinal cord injuries. J Biomed Eng 11:96-102

Bajzek TJ, Jaeger RJ (1987) Characterization and control of muscle response to electrical stimulation. Ann Biomed Eng 15:485-501

Baker JH (1983) Segmental necrosis in tenotomized muscle fibres. Muscle Nerve 6:29-39

Bar A, Ishai P, Meretsky P, Koren Y (1983) Adaptive microcomputer control of an artificial knee in level walking. J Biomed Eng 5:145-150

Baratta R, Ichie M, Hwang S, Solomonow M (1989) Method for studying muscle properties under orderly stimulated motor units with tripolar nerve cuff electrodes. J Biomed Eng 11:141-147

Baratta R, Solomonow M (1990) The dynamic response model of nine different skeletal muscles. IEEE Trans Biome Eng BME-37: 243-251

Baratta RV, Zhou BH, Solomonow M, D'Ambrosia RD (1998) Force feedback control of motor unit recruitment in isometric muscle. J Biomech 31(5):469-478

Barbeau H, Rossignol S (1987) Recovery of locomotion after chronic spinalization in the adult cat. Brain Res 412:84-95

Barbeau H, Rossignol S (1994) Enhancement of locomotor recovery following spinal cord injury. Curr Opin Neurol 7:517-524

Barbeau H, McCrea DA, O'Donovan DJ, Rossignol S, Grill WM, Lemay MA (1999) Tapping into spinal circuits to restore motor function. Brain Research Reviews 30:27-51

Bard G, Hirschberg GG (1965) Recovery of voluntary motion in upper extremity following hemiplegia. Arch Phys Med 46:345

Barde YA (1988) What, if anything, is a neurotrophic factor? Trends Neurosci 11:8 343-346

Barto AG, Sutton RS, Watkins CJCH (1989) Learning and sequential decision making. Univ Massachusetts, Amherst, COINS Tech Rep, pp 89-95

Basmajian JV (1976) The human bicycle, In: Komi PV (ed.), Biomechanics V-A, Univ Park Press, Baltimore, pp 254-258

Basmajian JV (1978) Muscles Alive, 4th edn. Williams and Wilkins, Baltimore

Bastian AJ, Martin TA, Keating JG, Thach WT (1996) Cerebellar ataxia: abnormal control of interaction torques across multiple joints. J Neurophysiol 76(1):492-509

Bauswein E, Kolb FP, Leimbeck B, Rubia FJ (1983) Simple and complex spike activity of cerebral Purkinje cells during active and passive movements in the awake monkey. J Physiol 339:379-394

Beasley W (1961) Quantitative muscle testing: Principles and application to research and clinical services. Arch Phys Med Rehabil 42:398-425

Beaubaton D, Grangetto A, Paillard J (1978) Contribution of positional and movement cues to visuo-motor reaching in split-brain monkey. In: Russell I, van Hoff MW, Berlichi G (eds.) Structure and Function of Cerebral Commissures. Univ Park Press, Baltimore, pp 371-384

Bélanger M, Patla AE (1984) Corrective responses to perturbation applied during walking in humans. Neurosci Lett 49(3):291-5

Beleckii VY, Gurfinkel VS, Paltsev YI (1967) Elements of control of voluntary movements. Biophys 12:154-161

Belikan T, Hollander HJ, Vossius G (1986) Microprocessor-controlled 8-channel stimulator with surface electrodes for FES of gait. In: Proc 2nd Vienna Int Workshop on Functional Electrostimulation, pp 71-73

Bennet DJ, Gorassini M, Prochazka A (1994) Catching a ball: contribution of intrinsic muscle stiffness, reflexes, and higher order responses. Can J Physiol Pharmacol 72(5):525-534

Bennett KM, Lemon RN (1996) Corticoneuronal contribution to the fractionation of muscle activity during precision grip in the monkey. J Neurophysiol 75:1826-1842

Berger W, Altenmüller E, Dietz V (1984a) Normal and impaired development of children's gait. Hum Neurobiol 3:163-170

Berger W, Horstmann G, Dietz V (1984b) Tension development and muscle activation in the leg during gait in spastic hemiparesis: Independence of muscle hypertonia and exaggerated stretch reflexes. J Neurol Neurosurg Psychiat 47:1029-1033

Bernotas LA, Crago PE, Chizeck HJ (1986) A discrete-time model of electrically stimulated muscle. IEEE Trans Biomed Eng BME-33:829-838

Bernotas LA, Crago PE, Chizeck HJ (1987) Adaptive control of electrically stimulated muscle. IEEE Trans Biomed Eng BME-34:140-147

Bernstein NA (1967) The Coordination and Regulation of Movements. Pergamon Press, London (original work in 1926-1935)

Bigland B, Lippold OGJ (1954) The relation between force, velocity, and integrated electrical activity in human muscles. J Physiol (Lond) 123:214

Bigland-Ritchie B, Jones DA, Woods JJ (1979) Excitation frequency and muscle fatigue: electrical responses during human voluntary and stimulated contractions. Exp Neurol 64(2):414-427

Bigland-Ritchie B, Woods JJ (1984) Changes in muscle contractile properties and neural control during human muscular fatigue. Muscle Nerve 7(9):691-699

Bijak M, Sauerman S, Schmutterer C, Lanmueller H, Unger E, Mayr W (1999) A modular PC-based system for easy setup of complex stimulation patterns. In: Proc 4nd Intern Conf IFESS, Sendai

Biryukova EV, Roby-Brami A, Mokthari M, Frolov AA (1998) Reconstruction of 7DOF human arm kinematics from Polhemus Fastrack recordings. J Biomech 31 (suppl 1): 84

Bizzi E, Dev P, Morasso P, Polit A (1978) Effect of load disturbances during centrally initiated movements. J Neurophysiol 41(3):542-556

Bizzi E, Accornero N, Chapple W, Hogan N (1984) Posture control and trajectory formation during arm movement. J Neurosci 4:2738-2744

Bizzi E, Mussa-Ivaldi S, Giszter F (1992) Does the nervous system use equilibrium-point control to guide single and multiple joint movements? Behav and Brain Sci 15:603-613

Black FO, Shupert CL, Horak FB, Nashner LM (1988) Abnormal postural control associated with peripheral vestibular disorders. Prog Brain Res 76:263-275

Blessey R (1978) Energy cost of normal walking. Orthop Clin North Am 9:356-358

Bobet J, Stein RB, Oğuztöreli MN (1993) A vlinear time varying model of force generation in skeletal muscle. IEEE Trans Biomed Eng BME-40:1000-1006

Bogataj U, Gros N, Maležič M, Kelih B, Kljajič M, Aćimović R (1989) Restoration of Gait During Two to Three Weeks of Therapy with Multichannel Electrical Stimulation. Phys Ther 69(5):319-327

Bohannon RW, Larkin PA (1985) Passive ankle dorsiflexion increases in patients after a regimen of tilt table-wedge board standing. A clinical report. Phys Ther 65(11):1676-1678

Bohannon RW (1989) Is the measurement of muscle strength appropriate in patients with brain lesions? (A special communication). Phys Ther 69(3):225-236

Boom HB, Mulder AJ, Veltink PH (1993) Fatigue during functional neuromuscular stimulation. Prog Brain Res 97:409-418

Borges G, Ferguson K, Kobetic R (1989) Development and operation of portable and laboratory electrical stimulation systems for walking in paraplegic subjects. IEEE Trans Biomed Eng BME-36(7):798-801

Bouisset S (1973) EMG and Muscle Force in Normal Motor Activities. In: Desmedt JE (ed.) New Developments in EMG and Clinical Neurophysiology. (vol 1), pp 547-583

Bouisset S, Zattara M (1981) A sequence of postural movements precedes voluntary movement. Neurosci Lett 22:263-270

Bouisset S, Do MC, Zattara M (1992) Posturo-kinetic capacity assessed in paraplegics and Parcinsonians. In: Woollacott M, Horak F (eds.) Posture and Gait: Control Mechanisms. Univ Oregon Books, pp 19-22

Boureslom NC (1967) Predictors of long-term recovery in cerebro-vascular disease. Arch Phys Med 48:415

Bower TGR (1972) Object perception in infants. Perception 1:15-30

Bowker P, Messenger N, Ogilvic C, Rowley DI (1992) Energetics of paraplegic walking. J Biomed Eng 14:344-350

Bowman B, Baker L (1985) Effects of waveform parameters on comfort during transcutaneous neuromuscular electrical stimulation. Ann Biomed Eng 13:59-74

Bowman RB, Erickson RC (1985) Acute and chronic implantation of coiled wire intraneural electrodes during cyclical electrical stimulation. Ann Biomed Eng 13:75-93

Brand RA, Gabel RH, Johnston RC, Crowninshield RD (1981) Instrumented walkway. Bull Prosthet Res BPR-10-35 18:282

Branicki MS, (1998) Multiple Liapunov Functions and other analysis tool for switched and hybrid systems. IEEE Trans Autom Control AU-43:475-482

Bregman BS, Kunkel-Bagden E, Reier PJ, Dai HN, McAtee M, Gao D (1993) Recovery of function after spinal cord injury: Mechanisms underlying transplant-mediated recovery of function after spinal cord injury in newborn and adult rats. Exp Neurol 123:3-16

Bregman DB, Du L, Li Y, Ribisi S, Warren SL (1994) Cytostellin distributes to nuclear regions enriched with splicing factors. J Cell Sci 107(Pt 3):387-396

Brindley GS, Polkey CE, Rushton DN (1978) Electrical splinting of the knee in paraplegia. Paraplegia 16:428-435

Brindley GS, Polkey CE, Rushton DN, Cardozo L (1986) Sacral anterior root stimulators for bladder control in paraplegia: the first 50 cases. J Neurol Neurosurg Psychiat 49:1104-1114

Brodmann K (1909) Vergleichende Lokalisationslehre der Grosshirnrinde in ibren Prinziplen dargestelit auf Grund des Zellenbaues. Barth, Leipzig

Bromstroom S (1966) Motor testing procedures in hemiplegia. J Am Phys Thet Ass 46:357

Brown MC, Holland M, Hopkins WG (1981) Motor nerve sprouting. Ann Rev Neurosci 4:17-42

Brown SH, Cooke JD (1984) Initial agonist burst duration depends on movement amplitude. Exp Brain Res 55:523-527

Brown TIH, Huang Y, Morgan FL, Proshke U, Wise A (1999) A new strategy for controlling the level of activation in artificially stimulated muscle. IEEE Trans Rehab Eng TRE-7:167-173

Brumfield RH, Champoux JA (1984) A biomechanical study of normal functional wrist motion. Clin Orthop 87:23

Brunnstrom F, Dennen M (1931) Round table on muscle testing. In: Proc Ann Conf Am Phys Ther Assoc Feder of Crippled and Disabled, New York, pp 1 –12

Bryson AE, Ho YC (1975) Applied Optimal Control. Wiley, New York

Buckett JR, Peckham PH, Thrope GB, Braswell SD, Keith MW (1988) A flexible, portable system for neuromuscular stimulation in the paralyzed upper extremity. IEEE Trans Biomed Eng BME-35:897-904

Bullock D, Grossberg S, Guenther FH (1993) A self-organizing neural model of motor equivalent reaching and tool use by a multijoint arm. J Cogn Neurosci 5:408-435

Bunge RP, Puckett WR, Becerra JL, Marcillo A, Quencer RM (1993) Observations on the pathology of human spinal cord injury. A review and classification of 22 new cases with details from a case of chronic cord compression with extensive focal demyelination. Adv Neurol 59:75-89

Bunge RP (1994) The role of the Schwann cell in trophic support and regeneration. J Neurol 242(1 Suppl 1):S19-S21

Bunnel S (1949) Tendon transfers in the hand and forearm. Am Acad Orthop Surg Instructional Course Lectures, No 6, Mosby, St. Louis

Burdett RG, Skrinar GS, Simon SR (1983) Comparison of mechanical work and metabolic energy consumption during normal gait. J Orthop Res 1:63

Burke RE, Levine DN, Tsairis P, Zajac FE (1973) Physiological types and histochemical profiles in motor units of the cat gastrocnemius. J Physiol (London) 234:723-748

Burke RE, Rudomin P, Zajac FE (1976) The effect of activation history on tension production by individual muscle units. Brain Res 109:515-529

Burke RE (1981) Motor units: anatomy, physiology, and functional organization. In: Brookhart JM, Mountcastle VB (eds.) Handbook of Physiology: The Nervous System. Am Phys Soc, Bethesda

Burnod Y, Grandgullaume P, Otto I, Ferraina S, Johnson PB, Caminiti R (1992) Visuomotor transformation underlying arm movements toward visual targets: a neural network model of cerebral cortical operations. J Neurosci 12:1435-1453

Burridge JH, Taylor PN, Hagan S, Swain ID (1997a) Experience of Clinical Use of the Odstock Dropped Foot Stimulator. Artif Organs 21(3):254-260

Burridge JH, Taylor PN, Hagan S, Wood DE, Swain ID (1997b) The effects of common peroneal stimulation on the effort and speed of walking: a randomized controlled trial with chronic hemiplegic patients. Clin Rehabil 11(3):201-210

Bütefisch C, Hummelsheim H, Denzler P, Mauritz KH (1995) Repetitive training of isolated movements improves the outcome of motor rehabilitation of the centrally paretic hand. J Neurol Sci 30(1):59-68

Cajal S Ramon y (1890) Sur l'origine et les ramifications des fibres nerveuses de la moelle embryoniaire. Anat Anx 5:85-95, 111-119

Cajal S Ramon y (1928) Degeneration and Regeneration of the Nervous System (May RM, translated and edited). (2 vols) Oxford Univ Press, New York

Calancie B, Needham-Shopshire B, Jacobs P, Willer K, Gregory Z, Green B (1994) Involuntary stepping after chronic spinal cord injury: Evidence for a central rhythm generator for locomotion in man. Brain 117:1143-1159

Caldwell CB, Wilson DJ, Braun RM (1969) Evaluation and treatment of the upper extremity in hemiplegic stroke patient. Clin Orthop 63:69

Cameron T, Loeb GE, Peck RA, Schulman JH, Strojnik P, Troyk PR (1997) Micromodular implants to provide electrical stimulation of paralyzed muscles and limbs. IEEE Trans Biomed Eng BME-44(9):781-790

Cameron T, Liinama T, Loeb GE, Richmond FJR (1998a) Long term biocompatibility of a miniature stimulator implanted in feline hind limb muscles. IEEE Trans Biomed Eng BME-45:1024-1035

Cameron T, Richmond FJR, Loeb GE (1998b) Effects of regional stimulation using a miniature stimulator implanted in feline posterior biceps femoris. IEEE Trans Biomed Eng BME-45:1036-1045

Capaday C, Stein RB (1986) Amplitude modulation of the soleus H-reflex in the human during walking and standing. J Neurosci 6:1308-1313

Capaday C (1995) The effect of baclofen on the stretch reflex parameters of the cat. Exp Brain Res 104:281-296

Cappozzo A (1991) The mechanics of human walking. In: Patla A (ed.) Adaptability of Human Gait. (Advances in Psychology, 78) North- Holland, Amsterdam, pp 167-186

Cappozzo A, Figure F, Leo T, Marchetti M (1978) Movements and mechanical energy changes in upper part of the human body during walking. In: Asmunssen E, Jorgensen K (eds.) Biomechanics VI-A. Univ Park Press, Baltimore, pp 272-279

Cappozzo A, Leo T, Cortesi S (1980) A Polycentric Knee-Ankle Mechanism for Above-Knee Prostheses. J Biomech 13:231-239

Carpenter GA, Grossberg S (1991) Pattern recognition by self-organizing neural network. MIT Press, Cambridge

Carpenter MG, Allum, JHJ, Honegger F (1999) Directional sensitivity of stretch reflexes and balance corrections for normal subjects in the roll and pitch planes. Exp Brain Res 129:93-113

Carter MC, Smith JL (1986a) Simultaneous control of two rhythmical behaviors. II Hindlimb walking with paw-shake response in spinal cat. J Neurophysiol 56(1):184-195

Carter MC, Smith JL (1986b) Simultaneous control of two rhythmical behaviors. I Locomotion with paw-shake response in normal cat. J Neurophysiol 56(1):171-183

Cavagna GA, Margaria R (1966) Mechanics of walking. J Appl Phys 21:271-278

Cavagna GA (1975) Force platforms as ergometers. J Appl Physiol 39:174

Chang GC, Luh JJ, Liao GD, Lai JS, Cheng CK, Kuo BL, Kuo TS (1997) A neuro-control system for the knee joint position control with quadriceps stimulation. IEEE Trans Rehabil Eng TRE-5:2-11

Chantraine A, Crielaard JM, Onkelinx A, Pirnay F (1984) Energy expenditure of ambulation in paraplegics: Effects of long term use of bracing. Paraplegia 22:173-181

Chappell PH, Kyberd PJ (1991) Prehensile control of a hand prothesis by a microcontroller. J Biomed Eng 13:363-369

Chen A, Xu XM, Kleitman N, Bunge MB (1996) Methylprednisolone administration improves axonal regeneration into Schwann cell grafts in transected adult rat thoracic spinal cord. Exp Neurol 138:261-276

Chen S, Cowan CFN, Grant PM (1991) Orthogonal least Squares learning Algorithm for Radial Basis Function Networks. IEEE Trans Neu Net NN-2:302-309

Cheng H, Cao Y, Olson L (1996) Spinal cord repair in adult paraplegic rats. Partial restoration of hindlimb function. Science 273:510-513

Cheng H, Fraidakis M, Blomback B, Lapchak P, Hoffer B, Olson L (1998) Characterization of a fibrin glue-GDNF slow-release preparation. Cell Transplant 7(1):53-61

Chia TL, Chow P, Chizeck HJ (1991) Recursive parameter identification of constrained systems: An application to electrically stimulated muscle. IEEE Trans Biomed Eng BME-42:212-223

Chiu DT, Lovelace RE, Yu LT, Wolff M, Stengel S, Middleton L, et al. (1988) Comparative electrophysiologic evaluation of nerve grafts and autogenous vein grafts as nerve conduits: an experimental study. J Reconstr Microsurg 4(4):303-309

Chiu S (1994) Fuzzy Model Identification Based on Cluster Estimation. J Intel Fuzzy Syst 2:111-122

Chizeck HJ, Crago PE, Kofman LS (1988) Robust closed-loop control of isometric muscle force using pulse width modulation. IEEE Trans Biome Eng BME-35:510-517

Chizeck HJ, Lan N, Sreeter-Palmiere L, Crago PE (1991) Feedback control of electrically stimulated muscle using simultaneous pulse width and stimulus period variation. IEEE Trans Biomed Eng BME-38:1224-1234

Chizeck HJ, Chang S, Stein RB, Scheiner A, Ferencz DC (1999) Identification of electrically stimulated quadriceps muscles in paraplegic subjects. IEEE Trans Biomed Eng BME-46(1):51-61

Close JR, Todd N (1959) The phasic activity of the muscle of the lower extremity and the effect of tendon transfer. J Bone Joint Surg 41-A:89-208

Cobb J, Claremont DJ (1995) Transducers for foot pressure measurement: survey of recent developments. Med Biol Eng Comp 33:4 525-32

Colbourne GR, Olney SY, Griffin MP (1993) Feedback of ankle joint angle and soleus EMG in rehabilitation of hemiplegic gait. Arch Phys Med Rehabil 74:1100-1106

Cole JD, Sedgwick EM (1992) The perceptions of force and of movement in a man without large myelinated sensory afferents below the neck. J Physiol (Lond) 449:503-515

Collins RD (1962) Illustrated Manual of Neurologic Diagnosis. Lippincott, Philadelphia

Comarr AF, Hutchinson RH, Bors E (1962) Extremity fractures of patients with spinal injury. Am J Surg 103:732-739

Conti P, Beaubaton D (1976) Utilisation des informations visuelles dans le controle du mouvement: etude de la precision des pointages chez l'homme. Le Travail Humain 39:19-32

Corlett JT, Patla AE, Williams JG (1985) Locomotor estimation of distance after visual scanning by children and adults. Perception 14(3):257-263

Coulombe RF (1984) Fiber optic sensors - catching up with the 1980s. Sensors 1(12):5-11

Crago PE, Peckham PH, Mortimer JT, Van der Meulen J (1974) The choice of pulse duration for chronic electrical stimulation via surface, nerve and intramuscular electrodes. Ann Biomed Eng 2:252-264

Crago PE, Peckham PH, Thrope GB (1980) Modulation of muscle force by recruitment during intramuscular stimulation. IEEE Trans Biomed Eng BME-27(12):679-684

Crago PE, Chizeck HJ, Neuman MR, Hambrecht FT (1986) Sensors for use with functional neuromuscular stimulation. IEEE Trans Biomed Eng BME-33(2):256-268

Crago PE, Nakai RJ, Chizeck HJ (1991) Feedback regulation of hand grasp opening and contact force during stimulation of paralyzed muscles. IEEE Trans Biomed Eng BME-38:17-28

Crago PE (1992) Muscle input-output model: The static dependence of force on length, recruitment and firing period. IEEE Trans Biomed Eng BME-39:871-874

Crago PE, Memberg WD, Usey MK, Keith MW, Kirsch RF, Chapman GJ, et al. (1998) An elbow extension neuroprosthesis for individuals with tetraplegia. IEEE Trans Rehabil Eng TRE-6(1):1-6

Crenna P, Frigo C (1987) Excitability of the soleus H-reflex arc during walking and stepping in man. Exp Brain Res 66:49-60

Crone C (1993) Reciprocal inhibition in man. PhD thesis, Lægeforeningens Forlag, Copenhagen

Crone C, Nielsen J, Petersen N, Ballegaard M, Hultborn H (1994) Disynaptic reciprocal inhibition of ankle extensors in spastic patients. Brain 117:1161-1168

Crowninshield RD, Brand RA (1981a) The prediction of forces in joint structures: distribution of intersegmental resultants. In: Miller DI (ed.) Exercise and Science Reviews. Franklin Institute Press, Boston

Crowninshield RD, Brand RA (1981b) A physiologically based criterion of muscle force prediction in locomotion. J Biomech 14:793-801

Cutkosky MR, Howe RD (1990) Human grasp choice and robotic grasp analysis, In: Venkataraman ST, Iberall T (eds.) Dextrous Robot Hands. Springer Verlag, New York, pp 5-31

Da Silva CF, Madison R, Dikkes P, Chiu TH, Sidman RL (1985) An in vivo model to quantify motor and sensory peripheral nerve regeneration using bioresorbable nerve guide tubes. Brain Res 342(2):307-315

Dai R, Stein RB, Andrews BJ, James KB, Wieler M (1996) Application of tilt sensors in functional electrical stimulation. IEEE Trans Rehabil Eng TRE-4(2):63-72

Daniels L, Williams M, Worthingham C (1956) Muscle Testing: Techniques of Manual Examination, 2nd ed. Saunders, Philadelphia, PA

Daniels L, Worthingham C (1972) Muscle Testing: Techniques of Manual Examination, 3rd edn. Saunders, Philadelphia, PA

Darian-Smith J, Kenins P (1980) Innervation density of mechanoreceptive fibers supplying glabrous skin of the monkey's index finger. J Physiol (Lond) 309:147-155

Dario P, Domenici C, Bardelli R, DeRossi D, Pinotti PC (1983) Piezoelectric polymers: new sensor materials for robotic applications. In: Proc 13th Int Symp Indust Robots, p 1434

Dario P, De Rossi D, Domenici C, Francesconi R (1984) Ferroelectric polymer tactile sensors with anthropomorphic features. In: Proc IEEE Int Conf Rob, Atlanta, pp 332-340

Davis LA, Gordon T, Hoffer JA, Jhamandas J, Stein RB (1978) Compound action potentials recorded from mammalian peripheral nerves following ligation or resuturing. J Physiol (Lond) 285:543-559

Davis R, Houdayer T, Andrews BJ, Emmons S, Patrick J (1997) Paraplegia: prolonged closed-loop standing with implanted nucleus FES-22 stimulator and Andrews' foot-ankle orthosis. Stereotact Funct Neurosurg 69:281-287

Davoodi R, Andrews BJ (1998) Computer simulation of FES standing up in paraplegia: A self-adaptive fuzzy controller with reinforcement learning. IEEE Trans Rehab Eng TRE-6:151-161

Davy DT, Audu ML (1987) A dynamic optimization technique for predicting muscle forces in the swing phase of gait. J Biomech 30:187-201

De Leon RD, Hodgson JA, Roy RR, Edgerton VR (1998) Full weight-bearing hindlimb standing following stand training in the adult spinal cat. J Neurophysiol 80:83-91

De Weerdt W, Crossley SM, Lincoln NB, Harrson MA (1989) Use of augmented sensory feedback to achieve symmetrical standing. Phys Ther 58:553-559

Delcomyn F (1980) Neural basis of rhythmic behavior in animals. Science 210:4469

Delcomyn F (1991a) Perturbation of the motor system in freely walking cockroaches. II. The timing of motor activity in leg muscles after amputation of a middle leg. J Exp Biol 156:503-517

Delcomyn F (1991b) Perturbation of the motor system in freely walking cockroaches. I. Rear leg amputation and the timing of motor activity in leg muscles. J Exp Biol 156:483-502

Delwaide PJ (1973) Human monosynaptic reflexes and presynaptic inhibition. An interpretation of spastic hyperreflexia. In: Desmedt JE (ed.) Developments in Electromyography and Clinical Neurophysiology. Karger, Basel, pp 508-522

Den Dunnen WF, Van der Lei B, Schakenraad JM, Blaauw EH, Stokroos I, Pennings AJ, Robinson PH (1993) Long-term evaluation of nerve regeneration in a biodegradable nerve guide. Microsurgery 14(8):508-515

Desmedt JE and Godaux E (1976) Ballistic contractions in man: Characteristics recruitment pattern of single motor units of the tibialis anterior muscle. J Physiol (Lond) 264:673-693

Desmedt JE, Godaux E (1979a) Recruitment patterns of single motor units in the human masseter muscle during brisk jaw clenching. Arch Oral Biol 24(2):171-178

Desmedt JE, Godaux E (1979b) Voluntary motor commands in human ballistic movements. Ann Neurol 5(5):415-421

Desmurget M, Pelisson D, Rossetti Y, Prablanc C (1998) From eye to hand: planning goal-directed movements. Neurosci and Biobehav Rev 22(6):761-788

Dettmann MA, Linder MT, Sepic SB (1987) Relationships among walking performance, postural stability, and functional assessments of the hemiplegic patient. Amer J Phys Med 66:77-90

Dickstein R, Hocherman S, Pillar T, Shaham R (1986) Stroke rehabilitation. Three exercise therapy approaches. Phys Ther 66(8):1233-1238

Diener HC, Bootz F, Dichgans J, Bruzek W (1983a) Variability of postural reflexes in humans. Exp Brain Res 52:423-428

Diener HC, Dichgans J, Mauritz KH (1983b) What distinguishes the different kinds of postural ataxia in patients with cerebellar diseases? Adv Otorhinolaringol 30:285-287

Diener HC, Dichgans J (1985) Postural ataxia in late atrophy of the cerebellar anterior lobe and its differential diagnosis. In: Black FO, Igarashi M (eds.) Vestibular and Visual Control of Posture and Locomotor Equilibrium, pp 282-289

Dietz V, Quintern J, Berger W (1981) Electrophysiological studies of gait in spasticity and rigidity. Evidence that altered mechanical properties contribute to hypertonia. Brain 104:431-449

Dietz V, Berger W (1984) Interlimb coordination of posture in patients with spastic paresis. Impaired function of spinal reflexes. Brain 107:965-978

Dietz V, Ketelsen U-P, Berger W, Quintern J (1986) Motor unit involvement in spastic paresis. Relationship between leg muscle activation and histochemistry. J Neurol Sci 75:89-103

Dietz V (1992) Human neuronal control of automatic functional movements: Interaction between central programs and afferent input. Physiol Rev 72:33-69

Dietz V, Colombo G, Jensen L (1994) Locomotor activity in spinal man. Lancet 344:1260-1263

Dietz V, Colombo G, Jensen L, Baumgartner L (1995) Locomotor capacity of spinal cord in paraplegic patients. Ann Neurol 37:574-582

Dietz V (1997) Neurophysiology of gait disorders: present and future applications. Electroencephalogra. Clin Neurophysiol 103:333-355

Dimitrijević MR, Nathan PW (1971) Studies of spasticity in man 5: dishabituation of the flexion reflex in spinal man. Brain 94:77-90

Dimitrijević MR, Prevec TS, Sherwood AM (1983) Somatosensory perception and cortical evoked potentials in establishing paraplegia. J Neurol Sci 60:253-265

Dimitrijević MR, Dimitrijević MM, Faganel J, Sherwood AM (1984) Suprasegmentally induced motor unit activity in paralysed muscles of patients with established spinal cord injury. Ann Neurol 16:216-221

Dimitrijević MR (1988) Head injuries and restorative neurology. Scand J Rehab Med (Suppl) 17:9-13

Dimitrijević MR, Gerasimenko Y, Pinter MM (1998) Evidence for a spinal central pattern generator in humans. Ann NY Acad Sci 860:360-376

Dinken H (1967) The evaluation of disability and treatment in hemiplegia. Arch Phys Med 28:263

Ditunno JF (1992) Functional assessment in CNS trauma. J Neurotrauma 9:S301-S305

Ditunno JF, Young W, Donovan WH, Creasey G (1994) The Int Standards Booklet for Neurological and Functional Classification of Spinal Cord Injury. Paraplegia 32:70-80

Dinnerstern AJ, Lowentahl M, Dexter M (1965) Evaluation of rating scale of ability in activities of daily living. Arch Phys Med 46:579

Dolan MJ, Andrews BJ, Veltink PH (1998) Switching curve controller for FES-assisted standing up and sitting down. IEEE Trans Rehab Eng TRE-6:167-170

Donaldson N (1986) A 24-output implantable stimulator for FES. In: Proc 2nd Vienna Int Workshop Functional Electrostimulation, Vienna, pp 197-200

Donaldson N, Munih M, Phillips GF, Perkins TA (1997) Apparatus and methods for studying artificial feedback-control of the plantar flexors in paraplegics without interference from the brain. Med Eng Phys 19:525-535

Donaldson N, Yu C (1998) A strategy used by paraplegics to stand up using FES. IEEE Trans Rehab Eng TRE-6:162-166

Doolabh VB, Hertl MC, Mackinnon SE (1996) The role of conduits in nerve repair: a review. Rev Neurosci 7(1):47-84

Dornay M, Uno Y, Kawato M, Suzuki R (1996) Minimum muscle tension change trajectories predicted by using a 17-muscle model of the monkey's arm. J Mot Behav 28:83-100

Douglas R, Larson PF, D'Ambrosia R, McCall RE (1983) The LSU Reciprocating Gait Orthosis. Orthopedics 6:34-39

Drew T (1988) Motor cortical cell discharge during voluntary gait modification. Brain Res 457(1):181-187

Drillis RN, Contini R (1966) Body segment parameters. Tech Report New York University 1106.03, New York

Dujmović J (1991) Preferential neural networks. In: Antognetti P, Milutinović V (eds.) Neural networks concepts, applications and implementations. (vol 2) Prentice Hall, pp 109-143

Dul J, Townsend MA, Shiavi R, Johnson GD (1984) Muscular synergism - I. On criteria for load sharing between synergistic muscles. J Biomech 17:663-673

Durfee WK, Mac Lean KE (1989) Methods of estimating the isometric recruitment curve of electrically stimulated muscle. IEEE Trans Biomed Eng BME-36:654-667

Durfee WK (1992) Model identification in neural prostheses system. In: Stein RB, Pechkam PH, Popović D (eds.) Neural Prostheses: Replacing motor function after disease or disability. Oxford Univ Press, New York, pp 58-87

Durfee WK, Palmer KI (1994) Estimation of force activation, force-length, and force-velocity properties in isolated electrically stimulated muscle. IEEE Trans Biomed Eng BME-41:205-216

Duysens J (1977) Reflex control of locomotion as revealed by stimulation of cutaneous afferents in spontaneously walking premammilary cats. J Neurophysiol 40:737-751

Duysens J, Pearson KG (1980) Inhibition of flexor burst generation by loading ankle extensor muscles in walking cats. Brain Res 187:321-332

Duysens J, Trippel M, Horstman GS, Dietz V (1990) Gating and reversal of reflexes in ankle muscles during human walking. Exp Brain Res 82:351-358

Easton TA (1972) On the normal use of reflexes. Am Sci 60(5):591-599

Edell DJ, Churchill JN, Gourley IM (1982) Biocompatibty of a silicon based peripheral nerve electrode. Biomater Med Devices Artif Organs 10(2):103-122

Edwards RG, Lippold PCJ (1956) The relation between force and integrated electrical activity in fatigued muscle. J Physiol (Lond) 132:677

Eidelberg E, Waldem JG, Nguyen LH (1981) Locomotor control in macaque monkeys. Brain 104:647-663

Eidelberg E, Yu J (1981) Effects of corticospinal lesions upon treadmill locomotion in the cat. Exp Brain Res 45:101-103

Eidelberg E, Nguyen H, Polich R, Waiden JG (1989) Transsynaptic degeneration of motoneurons caudal to spinal cord lesions. Brain Res Bull 22:39-45

Eklund G, Hagbarth KE, Hagglund JV, Wallin EU (1982a) Mechanical oscillations contributing to the segmentation of the reflex electromyogram response to stretching human muscles. J Physiol 326:65-78

Eklund G, Hagbarth KE, Hagglund JV, Wallin EU (1982b) The late reflex responses to muscle stretch: the resonance hypothesis versus the long-loop hypothesis. J Physiol (Lond) 306:79-90

Elbert T, Pantev C, Wienbruch M, Rockstroh B, Taub E (1995) Increased cortical representation of the fingers of the left hand in string players. Science 170:305-307

Elliott DH (1965) Structure and function of mammalian tendon. Biol Rev, Cambridge Philos Soc 40:392-421

Enoka RM (1983) Muscular control of a learned movement: The speed control system hypothesis. Exp Brain Res 51:135-145

Enoka RM (1988) Muscle strength and its development: new perspectives. Sports Med 6:146-168

Evarts EV (1976) Neurophysiological mechanisms in Parkinson's disease. In: Birkmayer W, Homykiewiez O (eds.) Advances in Parkinsonism: Biochemistry, Physiology, Treatment. 5th Int Symp on Parkinson's Disease, La Roche, Vienna, Basel, pp 37-54

Ewins DJ, Taylor PN, Crook SE, Lipczynski RT, Swain ID (1988) Practical low cost stand/sit system for mid-thoracic paraplegics. J Biomed Eng 10(2):184-8

Faist M, Mazavet D, Dietz V, Pierrot-Deseilligny E (1994) A quantitative assessment of presynaptic inhibition of Ia afferents in spastics: Differences in hemiplegics and paraplegics. Brain 117:1449-1455

Farrell M, Richards JG (1986) Analysis of the reliability and validity of the kinetic communicator exercise device. Med Sci Sports Exer 18:44-49
Feldman AG (1966) Functional tuning of nervous system with control of movement or maintenance of a steady posture. II Controllable parameters of the muscle. Biophys 11:565-578
Feldman AG, Orlovsky GN (1972) The influence of different descending systems on the tonic stretch reflex in the cat. Exp Neurol 37:481-494
Feldman AG (1979) Central and reflex mechanisms of motor control. Nauka, Moscow (in Russian)
Feldman AG, Latash ML (1982) Interaction of afferent and efferent signals underlying joint position sense: Empirical and theoretical approaches. J Mot Behav 14:174-193
Feldman AG (1986) Once more on the equilibrium-point hypothesis (lamda model) for motor control. J Mot Behav 18:17-54
Feldman AG, Adamovitch SV, Ostry DJ, Flanagan JR (1990a) The origin of electromyograms - Explanations based on the equilibrium point hypothesis. In: Winters JM, Woo SL-Y (eds.) Multiple Muscle Systems. Biomechanics and Movement Organization. Springer-Verlag, New York, pp 195-213
Feldman AG, Flanagan JR, Ostry DJ (1990b) Equilibrium vector spaces for the control of multi-muscle systems. Abstr Soc Neurosci 16:1088
Feng CJ, Mak AF (1997) Three-dimensional motion analysis of the voluntary elbow movement in subjects with spasticity. IEEE Trans Rehabil Eng 5(3):253-262
Fields RD, Le Beau JM, Longo FM, Ellisman MH (1989) Nerve regeneration through artificial tubular implants. Prog Neurobiol 33(2):87-134
Fisk J, Lackner JR, Dizio P (1993) Gravitoinertial force level influences arm movement control. J Neurophysiol 69:504-511
Fitts PM (1954) The information capacity of the human motor system in controlling the amplitude of movement. J Exp Psychol 47:381-391
Fitzpatrik RC, Burke D, Gandevia SC (1996) Loop gain reflexes controlling human standing measured with the use of postural and vestibular disturbances. J Neurophysiol 76(6):3994-4008
Flanagan JR, Wing AM (1993) Modulation of grip force with load force during point-to-point arm movements. Exp Brain Res 95:131-143
Flanagan JR, Wing AM (1997a) Effects of surface texture and grip force on the discrimination of hand-held loads. Percep Psychophys 59:111-118
Flanagan JR, Wing AM (1997b) The role of internal models in motion planning and control: Evidence from grip force adjustments during movements of hand-held loads. J Neurosci 17:1519-1528
Flash T (1987) The control of hand equilibrium trajectories in multijoint arm movements. Biol Cybern 57:257-274
Flash T (1990) The organization of human arm trajectory control. In: Winters J, Woo S (eds.) Multiple Muscle System. Biomechanics and Movement Organization. Springer-Verlag, pp 282-301
Flash T, Hogan N (1995) Optimization principles in motor control. In: Arbib M (ed) The Handbook of Brain Theory and Neural Networks. MIT Press, Cambridge, pp 682-685

Forssberg H (1979a) On integrative motor functions in the cat's spinal cord. Acta Physiol Scand Suppl 474:1-56
Forssberg H (1979b) Stumbling corrective reaction: a phase-dependent compensatory reaction during locomotion. J Neurophysiol 42(4):936-53
Forssberg H, Grillner S, Halbertsma J (1980a) The locomotion of the low spinal cat. I. Coordination with a hind limb. Acta Physiol Scand 108:283-295
Forssberg H, Grillner S, Halbertsma J, Rossignol S (1980b) The locomotion of the low spinal cat. II. Interlimb coordination. Acta Physiol Scand 108:283-295
Forssberg H, Svartengren G (1983) Hardwired locomotor network in cat revealed by a retained motor pattern to gastocnemius after muscle transposition. Neurosci Lett 41:283-288
Frankel HL, Hancock DO, Hyslop G, Melzak J, Michaelis LS, Ungar GH (1969) The value of postural reduction in the initial management of closed injuries of the spine with paraplegia and tetraplegia. Paraplegia 7(3):179-92
Franken HM, Veltink PFH, Tijsmans R, Nijmeijer H, Boom HBK (1993) Identification of passive knee joint and shankj dynamics in paraplegics using quadriceps stimulation. IEEE Trans Rehab Eng TRE-:154-164
Franken HM, Veltink PH, Tijsmans R, Nijmeijer H, Boom HBK (1995) Identification of quadriceps-shank dynamics using randomized interpulse interval stimulation. IEEE Trans Rehab Eng TRE-4:182-192
Freehafer AA, Kelly CM, Peckham PH (1987) Planning tendon transfers in tetraplegia: Cleveland technique. In: Hunter J, Schneider L, Mackin E (eds.) Tendon Surgery in the Hand. Mosby, St Louis
Frigo C, Rabuffetti M, Kerrigan DC, Deming LC, Pedotti A (1998) Functionally oriented and clinically feasible quantitative gait analysis method. Med Biol Eng Comp 36(2):179-185
Fugl-Meyer AR, Jääskö L, Leyman I, Olsson S, Steglind S (1975) The post-stroke hemiplegic patient. 1. a method for evaluation of physical performance. Scand J Rehabil Med 7(1):13-31
Fung J, Blunt R, Barbeau H (1990) The soleus H-reflex modulation pattern in spastic paretic subjects during standing and walking. In: Brandt TH, Pauluo W, Bleo W, Dieterich M, Krafczyk S, Straube A (eds.) Disorders of Posture and Gait. Thienne, New York, pp 398-401
Fung J, Barbeau H (1994) The effects of conditioning cutaneomuscular stimulation on the soleus H reflex in normal and spastic paretic subjects during walking and standing. J Neurophys 72(5):2090-2104
Gardiner PF, Lapointe MA (1988) Daily in vivo neuromuscular stimulation effects on immobilized rat hindlimb museles. J Appl Physiol 53:960-966
Gelfand IM, Gurfinkel VS, Fomin SV, Tsetlin ML (eds.) (1971) Models of the structural-functional organization of certain biological systems. MIT Press, Cambbridge
Gelfand IM, Latash ML (1998) On the problem of adequate language in motor control. Mot Contr 2(4):306-313
Gentilucci M, Castiello U, Corradini ML, Scarpa M, Umilta C, Rizzolatti G (1991) Influence of different types of grasping on the transport component of prehension movements. Neurophys 29:361-378

Gentilucci M, Chieffi S, Scarpa M, Castiello U (1992) Temporal coupling between transport and grasp components during prehension movements: Effects of visual perturbation. Behav Brain Res 47:71-82

Georgopoulos AP, Kalaska JF, Caminiti R, Massey JT (1982) On the relations between the direction of two-dimensional arm movements and cell discharge in primate motor cortex. J Neurosci 2:1527-1537

Georgopoulos AP, Kalaska JF, Crutcher JF, Caminiti R, Massey JT (1983a) The representation of movement direction in the motor cortex: Single cell and population studies. In: Edelman GM, Cowan WM, Gall WE (eds.) Dynamic aspects of neocortical function. John Wiley and Sons, New York, pp 501-524

Georgopoulos AP, Caminiti R, Kalaska JF, Massey JT (1983b) Spatial coding of movement: A hypothesis concerning the coding of movement direction by motor cortical populations. In: Massion J, Paillard J, Schultz W, Wiesendanger M (eds.) Neural Coding of Motor Performance. Springer-Verlag, Berlin, pp 327-336

Georgopoulos AP, Kalaska JF, Caminiti R, Massey JT (1983c) Interruption of motor cortical discharge subserving aimed arm movements. Exp Brain Res 49:327-340

Georgopoulos AP, Caminiti R, Kalaska JF (1984) Static spatial effects in motor cortex and area 5: quantitative relations in two dimensional space. Exp Brain Res 54:446-454

Georgopoulos AP, Kalaska JF, Caminiti R (1985) Relations between two-dimensional arm movements and single-cell discharge in motor cortex and area 5: Movement direction versus movement and point. Exp Brain Res (Suppl) 10:175-183

Georgopoulos AP (1986) On reaching. Ann Rev Neurosci 9:147-170

Georgopoulos AP, Kettner RE, Schwartz AB (1988) Primate motor cortex and free arm movements to visual targets in three-dimensional space. II. Coding of the direction of movement by a neuronal population. J Neurosci 8(8):2928-2937

Georgopoulos AP (1992) Behavioral neurophysiology of the motor cortex. J Lab Clin Med 124(6):766-774

Georgopoulos AP, Taira M, Lukashin A (1993) Cognitive neurophysiology of the motor cortex. Science 260:47-52

Georgopoulos AP (1995) Current issues in directional motor control. Trends Neurosci 18:506-510

Georgopoulos AP, Pellizzer G, Poliakov AV, Schieber MH (1999) Neural coding of finger and wrist movements. J Comput Neurosci 6(3):279-88

Geschwind N (1985) Mechanisms of change after brain lesions. In: Nottebohm F (ed.) Hope for a New Neurology. (vol 457) Ann NY Acad Sci, pp 1-11

Ghez C, Gordon J, Ghilardi MF, Christakos CN, Cooper SE (1990) Roles of proprioceptive input in the programming of arm trajectories. Cold Spring Harb Symp Quant Biol 55:837-847

Ghilardi M, Gordon J, Ghez C (1995) Learning a visuomotor transformation in a local area of work space produces directional biases in other areas. J Neurophysiol 73(6):2535-2539

Giat Y, Mizrahi J, Levy M (1996) Fatigue and recovery in paraplegic's quadriceps muscle when subjected to intermittent stimulation. J Biomechan Eng 118:357-366

Gielen CC, Houk JC (1984) Nonlinear viscosity of human wrist. J Neurophysiol 52:553-369

Gillapalli V (1995) Direct associative reinforcement learning methods for dynamic systems control. Neurocomp 9:271-292

Gillespie MJ, Stein RB (1983) The relationship between axon diameter, myelin thickness and conduction velocity during atrophy of mammalian peripheral nerves. Brain Res 259:41-56

Giszter SF, Mussa-Ivaldi FA, Bizzi E (1993) Convergent force fields organized in the froges' spinal cord. J Neurosci 13:467-491

Giuliani CA, Smith JL (1987) Stepping behaviors in chronic spinal cats with one hindlimb deafferented. J Neurosci 7:2537-2546

Glasby MA, Gschmeissner SG, Hitchcock RJ, Huang CL (1986) The dependence of nerve regeneration through muscle grafts in the rat on the availability and orientation of basement membrane. J Neurocytol 15(4):497-510

Goldfarb M, Durfee WK (1996) Design of a controlled-brake orthosis for FES-aided gait. IEEE Trans Rehab Eng TRE-4:13-24

Goldman JE (2000) Glial differentiation and lineages. J Neurosci Res 59(3):410-412

Goldspink DF, Goldspink G (1975) The role of passive stretch in retarding muscle atrophy. In: Nix WA, Vrbova G (eds.) Electrical Stimulation and Neuromuscular Disorders. Springer-Verlag, Berlin, pp 91-100

Goldspink DF (1977) The influence of immobilization and stretch on protein turnover of rat skeletal muscle. J Physiol (Lond) 264:267-282

Goldstein G (1957) Класическая Механика. Москва, Гостехиэдат

Gomi H, Kawato M (1996) Equilibrium-point control hypothesis examined by measured arm stiffness during multi-joint movement. Science 272:117-120

Goodale MA (1996) Visuomotor modules in the vertebrate brain. Can J Physiol Pharmacol 74:390-400

Goodwin C, Sin KS (1984) Adaptive filtering, prediction and control. Prentice Hall, Englewood Cliffs, NJ

Gordon EE (1956) Physiological approach to ambulation in paraplegia. JAMA 161:686-688

Gordon J, Ghez C (1984) EMG patterns in agonist muscles during isometric contraction in man: relations to response dynamics. Exp Brain Res 55:167-171

Gordon J, Ghilardi M, Cooper S, Ghez C (1994a) Accuracy of planar reaching movements. II. Systematic extent errors resulting from inertial anisotropy. Exp Brain Res 99:112-130

Gordon J, Ghilardi MF, Ghez C (1994b) Accuracy of planar reaching movements. I: Independence of direction and extended variability. Exp Brain Res 99:97-111

Gordon T, Hoffer JA, Jhamandas J, Stein RB (1980) Long-term effects of axotomy on neural activity during cat locomotion. J Physiol (Lond) 303:243-263

Gordon T, Gillespie J, Orozco R, Davis L (1991) Axotomy-induced changes in rabbit hindlimb nerves and the effects of chronic electrical stimulation. J Neurosci 11:2157-2169

Gordon T, Pattullo MC (1993) Plasticity of muscle fiber and motor unit types. Exerc Sport Sci Rev 21:331-362

Gordon T, Yang JF, Ayer K, Stein RB, Tyreman N (1993a) Recovery potential of muscle after partial denervation: a comparison between rats and humans. Brain Res Bull 30(3-4): 477-482

Gordon T, Patullo MC, Rafuse VF (1993b) Motor unit heterogeneity with respect to speed and fatiguability in cat muscles after chronic stimulation or paralysis. In: Sargeant AJ, Kernell D (eds.) Neuromuscular Fatigue. Elsevier Science Publishers, Amsterdam pp 63-66

Gordon T, Mao J (1994) Muscle atrophy and procedures for training after spinal cord injury. Phys Ther 74(1):50-65

Gossard J-P, Hultborn H (1991) On the organization of the spinal rhythm generation in locomotion. In: Wernig A (ed.) Plasticity of Motoneuronal Connections. Eisevier, Amsterdam

Gottlieb GL, Agarwal GC (1970) Filtering of electromyographic signals. Amer J Phys Med 49:142-146

Gračanin F, Prevec T, Trontelj J (1967) Evaluation of use of functional electronic peroneal brace in hemiparetic patients. In: Advances in External Control of Human Extremities III, ETAN, pp 198-210

Gračanin F, Kralj A, Reberšek S (1969) Advanced version of the Ljubljana functional electronic peroneal brace with walking rate controlled tetanization. In: Advances in External Control of Human Extremities, ETAN, pp 487-500

Granat MH, Nicol DJ, Baxendale RH, Andrews BJ (1991) Dishabituation of the flexion reflex in spinal cord-injured man and its application in the restoration of gait. Brain Res 559(2):344-346

Granat MH, Maxwell DJ, Ferguson ACB, Lees KR, Barbenel JC (1996) Peroneal Stimulator: Evaluation for the Correction of Spastic Drop Foot in Hemiplegia. Arch Phys Med Rehabil 77:19-24

Grandjean PA, Mortimer JT (1986) Recruitment properties of monopolar and bipolar epimysial electrodes. Ann Biomed Eng 14:53-66

Granit R (1970) The Basis of Motor Control. Academic Press, London

Graupe D, Kline WK (1975) Functional separation of EMG signals via ARMA identification methods for prosthesis control purposes. IEEE Trans System Man Cybern SMC-5:252-259

Graupe D, Kohn K (1988) A critical review of EMG-controlled electrical stimulation in paraplegics. CRC Crit Rev Biomed Eng 15:187-210

Graupe D (1989) EMG pattern analysis for patient-responsive control of FES in paraplegics for wakler-supported walking. IEEE Trans Biomed Eng BME-36-711-719

Graupe D, Kordylewski H (1995) Artificial neural network control of FES in paraplegics for patient responsive ambulation. IEEE Trans Biomed Eng BME-42:699-707

Graupe D, Kohn KH (1997) Transcutaneous functional neuromuscular stimulation of certain traumatic complete thoracic paraplegics for independent short-distance ambulation. Neurol Res 19:323-333

Greensmith L, Vrbová G (1997) Disturbances of neuromuscular interaction may contribute to muscle weakness in spinal muscular atrophy. Neuromuscul Disord 7(6-7):369-372

Gregor RJ, Abelew TA (1994) Tendon force measurements and movement control: a review. Med Sci Sports Exerc 26(11):1359-1372

Grill HJ, Peckham PH (1998) Functional neuromuscular stimulation for combined control of elbow extension and hand grasp in C5 and C6 quadriplegics. IEEE Trans Rehab Eng TRE-6:190-199

Grill WM, Mortimer JT (2000) Neural and connective tissue response to long-term implantation of multiple contact nerve cuff electrodes. J Biomed Mater Res 50(2):215-226

Grillner S (1975) Locomotion in vertebrates: Central mechanisms and reflex interaction Physiolog Rev 55:247-304

Grillner S, Zangger P (1975) How detailed is the central pattern generation for locomotion? Brain Res 288(2):367-71

Grillner S (1981) Control of locomotion in bipeds, tetrapods, and fish. In: Brookhart JE, Mountcastle VB, Brooks VB, Geiger SR (eds.) Handbook of Physiology. (sect 1, vol 2(2)) Am Phys Soc, Bethesda, pp 1127-1236

Grillner S, Zangger P (1984) The effect of dorsal root transection on the efferent motor pattern in the cat's hindlimb during locomotion. Acta Physiol Scand 120(3):393-405

Grillner S (1985) Neurobiological bases of rhythmic motor acts in vertebrates. Science 228:143-149

Grillner S, Dubuc R (1988) Control of locomotion in vertebrates: Spinal and supraspinal mechanisms. In: Waxmann SG (ed.) Advances in Neurology. (Functional Recovery in Neurological Disease, vol 47) Raven Press, New York, pp 425-453

Grossman RL, Nerode A, Ravn AP, Rischel H (eds.) (1993) Hybrid Systems. (Lecture Notes in Computer Science, no 736) Springer Verlag, New York

Gruner JA, Mason CP (1989) Nonlinear muscle recruitment during intramuscular and nerve stimulation. J Rehab Res Develop 26(2):1-16

Guenard V, Kleitman N, Morrissey TK, Bunge RP, Aebischer P (1992) Syngeneic Schwann cells derived from adult nerves seeded in semipermeable guidance channels enhance peripheral nerve regeneration. J Neurosci 12:3310-3320

Guest JD, Bunge RB (1995) Functional studies of human Schwann cells transplanted to the nude rat spinal cord. J Neurotrauma 12:427

Guest JD, Rao A, Olson L, Bunge MB, Bunge RP (1997) The ability of human Schwann cell grafts to promote regeneration in the transected nude rat spinal cord. Exp Neurol 148(2):502-522

Guest RS, Klose KJ, Needham-Shropshire BM, Jacobs PL (1997) Evaluation of a training program for persons with SCI paraplegia using the Parastep 1 ambulation system: part 4. Effect on physical self-concept and depression. Arch Phys Med Rehabil 78(8):804-807

Gurfinkel VS, Levik YS (1991) Perceptual and autonomic aspects of the posture body scheme. In: Paillard J (ed.) The Brain and Space. Oxford Univ Press, pp 147-162

Guttman L (1973) Spinal Cord Injuries: Comprehensive Management and Research. Blackwell Scientific Publications, Oxford

Guyton AC (1991) Textbook of Medical Physiology. Saunders WB, Philadelphia

Haggard P, Wing AM (1991) Remote responses to perturbations in human prehension. Neurosci Letters 122:103-108

Haggard P, Richardson J (1996) Spatial patterns in the control of human arm movement. J Exp Psychol Human Percept Perform 22:42-46

Hallet M, Shahani B, Young R (1975) EMG analysis of stereotyped voluntary movements in man. J Neurol Neurosurg Psychiatr 38:1154-1162

Hallet M, Marsden CD (1979) Ballistic flexion movements of the human thumb. J Physiol 294:33-50

Hallet M (1993) Physiology of basal ganglia disorders: an overview. Can J Neurol Sci 20:177-183

Hallet M, Cohen LG, Pascual-Leone J, Brasil-Neto J, Wasserman EM, Cammarota AN (1993) Plasticity of the human motor cortex. In: Thilman AF, Burke DJ, Rymer WZ (eds.) Spasticity: Mechanisms and Management. Springer-Verlag, Berlin

Hamrin E, Eklund G, Hillgren AK, Borges O, Hall J, Hellström O (1982) Muscle strength and balance in post-stroke patients. Ups J Med Sci 87(1):11-26

Handa Y, Hoshimiya H, Iguchi Y, Oda T (1989a) Development of percutaneous intramuscular electrode for multichannel FES system, IEEE Trans Biomed Eng, BME-36(7): 705-710

Handa Y, Ohkubo K, Hoshimiya N (1989b) A portable multi-channel functional electrical stimulation (FES) system for restoration of motor function of the paralyzed extremities. Automedica 11(1-3):221-232

Hanke KA (1999) Therapeutic uses of feedback. In: Nelson RM, Hayes KW, Corrier DP (eds.) Clinical electrotherapy, 3rd edn. Appleton and Lange, Stanford, pp 489-522

Hansen M, Kostov A, Haugland M, Sinkjær T (1998) Feature extraction in control of FES using afferent nerve signals in humans. Canadian J Physiol Pharmacol 76(2)

Hanson MA, Moore PJ, Nijhuis JG (1987) Chronic recording from the phrenic nerve in fetal sheep in utero. J Physiol (Lond) 394:4P

Harris CM, Wolpert DM (1998) Signal-dependent noise determines motor planning. Nature 394:780-784

Hart RL, Kilgore KL, Peckham PH (1998) A comparison between control methods for implanted FES hand-grasp systems. IEEE Trans Rehab Eng TRE-6:208-218

Hartwell MS, Oderkerk BJ, Sacher CA, Inbar GF (1991) The development of a model reference adaptive controller to control the knee joint of paraplegics IEEE Trans Autom Control AU-36:683-691

Hasan Z (1986) Optimized movement trajectories and joint stiffness in unperturbed, initially loaded movements. Biol Cybern 53:373-382

Hatze H (1976) The complete optimization of the human motion. Math Biosci 28:99-135

Hatze H (1977) A complete set of control equations for the human musculo-skeletal system. J Biomech 10:799-805

Hatze H, Buys JD (1977) Energy-optimal controls in the mamalian neuromuscular system. Biol Cybern 27:9-20

Hatze H (1980) Neuromusculoskeletal control systems modeling - a critical survey of recent developments. IEEE Trans Automat Control AC-25:375-385

Haugland M, Hoffer JA (1994a) Slip information provided by nerve cuff signals: application in closed-loop control of functional electrical stimulation. IEEE Trans Rehab Eng TRE-2(1):29-36

Haugland M, Hoffer JA (1994b) Artifact-free sensory nerve signals obtained from cuff electrodes during functional electrical stimulation of nearby muscles. IEEE Trans on Rehab Eng TRE-2:37-39

Haugland M, Lickel A, Riso R, Adamczyk MM, Keith M, Jensen IL et al. (1995) Restoration of lateral hand grasp using natural sensors. In: Proc of the 5th Vienna Int Workshop on FES, Vienna, pp 339-342

Haugland M, Sinkjær T (1995) Cutaneous whole nerve recordings used for correction of footdrop in hemiplegic man. IEEE Trans on Rehab Eng TRE-3:307-317

Haugland M (1996) A Flexible Method for Fabrication of Nerve Cuff Electrodes. In: Proc of the 18th Ann Int Conf IEEE EMBS, pp 964-965

Haugland MK (1997) A Miniature implantable nerve stimulator. In: Popović D (ed.) Proc 2nd Int Symp FES, Burnaby, pp 221-222

Haugland M, Lickel A, Haase J, Sinkjær T (1999) Control of FES thumb force using slip information obtained from the cutaneous electroneurogram in quadriplegic man. IEEE Trans Rehab Eng TRE-7(2):215-227

Haugland MK, Sinkjær T (2000a) Control with natural sensors. In: Winters JM, Crago PE (eds.) Biomechanics and Neural Control of Posture and Movement. Springer Verlag, New York, in print

Hausdorff JM, Durfee WK (1991) Open-loop position control of the knee joint using electrical stimulation of the quadriceps and hamstrings. Med Biol Eng 29(3):269-280

Hausler E, Lang H, Schreiner FJ (1980) Piezoelectric high polymer foils as physiological mechanic-electric energy converters. In: Proc IEEE Frontiers Eng Health Care Conf, pp 333-334

Haut RG, Little RW (1972) A constitutive equation for collagen fibres. J Biomech 5:423-430

Haykin S (1991) Adaptive Filter Theory, 2nd edn. Prentice Hall, pp 418-428

Haykin S (1993) Neural Networks. A Comprehensive Foundation, Macmillan College Publishing Company, New York

Heath CA, Rutkowski GE (1998) The development of bioartificial nerve grafts for peripheral nerve regeneration. Tibtech 16:163-168

Held R, Hein A (1963) Movement-produced stimulation in the development of visually guided behavior. J Comp Physiol Psychol 56:872-876

Heller B, Veltink PH, Rijkhoff NJM, Rutten WLC Andrews BJ (1993) Reconstructing muscle activation during normal walking: a comparison of symbolic and connectionist machine learning techniques. Biol Cybern 69:327-335

Herman R (1968) Reflexes and rheologic propertise of the spastic gastrocnemius-soleus muscle group. Arch Phys Med Rehabil 49:723-727

Hermens HJ, Baardman G, Franken HM, Veltink P, Boom HBK, Zilvold G (1994) Advances in hybrid systems. In: Proc 10th Cong ISEK, USA

Herzog W, derKeurs HEDJ (1988) Force-length relation of in vivo human rectus femoris muscles. P Flügens Arch 411:643-647

Hesse S, Bertelt C, Jahnke MT, Schaffrin A, Baake M, Maležič M, Mauritz KH (1995) Treadmill training with partial body weight support as compared to physiotherapy in non-ambulatory hemiparetic patients. Stroke 26:976-981

Hesse S, Helm B, Krajnik J, Gregoric M, Mauritz KH (1997) Treadmill training with partial body weight support: influence of body weight release on the gait of hemiparetic patients. J Neurol Rehab 11:15-20

Hesse S, Sarkodie-Gyan Th, Uhlenbrock D (1999) Development of an Advanced Mechanised Gait Trainer, Controlling Movement of the Centre of Mass, for Restoring Gait in Non-ambulant Subjects. Biomedizinische Technik, Heft 7(81):194-201

Heumann R (1994) Neurotrophin signalling. Current Opinion in Neurobiol 4:668-679

Hiebert GW, Gorassini MA, Jiang W, Prochazka A, Pearson KG (1994) Corrective responses to loss of ground support during walking. II. Comparison of intact and chronic spinal cats. J Neurophysiol 71(2):611-622

Hill TL (1938) The heat of shortening and the dynamic constants of muscle. Proc R Soc London Biol 126:135-195

Hines AE, Crago PE, Billian C (1995) Hand opening by electrical stimulation in patients with spastic hemiplegia. IEEE Trans Rehab Eng TRE-3:193-205

Hirokawa S, Grimm M, Le T, Solomonow M, Baratta R, Shoji M, D'Ambrosia RD (1990) Energy consumption in paraplegic ambulation using the reciprocating gait orthosis and electric stimulation of the thigh muscles. Arch Phys Med Rehabil 71:687-694

Hirokawa S, Matsumura K (1989) Biofeedbcak training system for temporal and distance factors. Med Bio Eng Comp 27:8-13

Hislop H, Perrine J (1967) The isokinetic concept of exercise. Phys Ther 47:114-117

Hodgkin AL, Huxley AF (1945) Resting and action potentials in single nerve fibers. J Physiology 247:276

Hoff B, Arbib M (1993) Models of trajectory formation and temporal interaction of reach and grasp. J Mot Behav 25:175-192

Hoffer JA, Stein RB, Gordon T (1979) Differential atrophy of sensory and motor fibers following section of cat peripheral nerves. Brain Res 178:347-361

Hoffer JA, Loeb GA (1980) Implantable electrical and mechanical interfaces with nerve and muscle. Ann Biomed Eng 8:351-360

Hoffer JA, Loeb GE, Pratt CA (1981) Single unit conduction velocities from averaged nerve cuff electrode records in freely moving cats. J Neurosc Meth 4:211-225

Hoffer JA, Sinkjær T (1986) A natural force sensor suitable for closed-loop control of functional neuromuscular stimulation. In: Proc 2nd Vienna Int Workshop on Functional Electrostimulation, Vienna, pp 47-50

Hoffer JA, Loeb GE, Marks WB, O'Donovan MJ, Pratt CA, Sugano N (1987) Cat hindlimb motoneurons during locomotion. I. Destination, axonal conduction velocity and recruitment threshold. J Neurophysiol 57:510-529

Hoffer JA (1988) Closed loop, implant sensor, functional electrical stimulation system for partial restoration of motor functions. United States Patent [19], Patent Number 4,750,499

Hoffer JA (1990) Techniques to record spinal cord, peripheral nerve and muscle activity in freely moving animals. In: Boulton AA, Baker GB, Vanderwolf CH (eds.) Neurophysiological Techniques: Applications to Neural Systems. (Neuromethods 15) Humana Press, Clifton, NY, pp 65-145

Hoffer JA, Stein RB, Haugland KK, Sinkjær T, Durfee WK, Schwartz AB, Loeb GE, Kantor C (1995) Neural signals for command control and feedback in functional electrical stimulation. J Rehabil 33(2):145-157

Hogan N (1984) An organization principle for a class of voluntary movements. J Neurosci 4:2745-2754

Hogan N (1985) The mechanics of multijoint posture and movement control. Biol Cybern 52:325-332

Hogan N, Flash T (1987) Moving gracefully: quantitative theories of motor coordination. Trends in Neurosci 10:170-174

Holle J, Frey M, Gruber H, Kern H, Stohr H, Thoma H (1984) Functional electrostimulation of paraplegics: Experimental investigations and first clinical experience with an implantable stimulation device. Orthopaedics 7:1145-1160

Hollerbach JM, Flash T (1982) Dynamic interactions between limb segments during planar arm movement. Biolog Cybern 44:67-77

Hollerbach JM, Moore SP, Atkeson CG (1986) Workspace effect in arm movement kinematics derived by joint interpolation. In: Ganchev G, Dimitrov B, Patev P (eds.) Motor Control, Plenum

Hollerbach JM, Atkeson CG (1987) Deducing planning variables from experimental arm trajectories: Pitfalls and possibilities. Biol Cybern 56:279-292

Hollins M, Rao S, Young F (1993) Perceptual dimensions of tactile surface texture: A multidimensional-scaling analysis. Percept Psychophys 54:697-705

Holmes G (1939) The cerebellum of man. Brain 62:1-30

Holzreiter S, Kastner J, Wagner P (1993) Motion measurement with high-speed video. J Biomed Eng 15:140-142

Horak FB, Nashner LM (1986) Central progrmming of postural movements: Adaptation to altered support surface configuarations. J Neurophys 55:1369-1381

Horak FB, Nashner LM, Diener HC (1990) Postural strategies associated with somatosensory and vestibular loss. Exp Brain Res 82:167-177

Horak FB, Diener HC (1994) Cerebellar control of postural scaling and central set in stance. J Neurophysiol 72:479-493

Horak FB, Macpherson JM (1995) Postural orientation and equilibrium. In: Rowell LB, Shepherd JT (eds.) Handbook of physiology. (vol 7), pp 255-292

Hoshimiya N, Naito N, Yajima M, Handa Y (1989) A Multichannel FES System for the Restoration of Motor Functions in High Spinal Cord Injury Patients: A Respiration-Controlled System for Multijoint Upper Extremity. IEEE Trans Biomed Eng BME-36:754-760

Houk JC (1979) Motor control processes: New data concerning motoservo mechanisms and a tentative model for stimulusresponse processing. In: Talbott RE, Humphrey DR (eds.) Posture and Movement. Raven Press, New York, pp 231-241

Hristić D, Vukobratović M, Stojiljković Z (1974) Development of Active Antropomorphic Exoskeletons. J Med and Biol Eng 12:66-80

Hristić D, Vukobratović M, Timotijević M (1981) New model of autonomuos Active Suit for distrophic patients. In: Advances in External Control of Human Extremities VII, ETAN, pp 33-42

Huang CT, Kuhlemeier KV, Moore NB, Fine PR (1979) Energy cost of ambulation in paraplegic patients using Craig-Scott braces. Arch Phys Med Rehabil 60:595-600

Hufschmidt A, Mauritz KH (1985) Chronic transformation of muscle in spasticity: A peripheral contribution to increased tone. J Neurol Neurosurg Psychiatry 48:676-685

Hukins DWL (1982) Biomechanical properties of collagen. In: Weiss JB, Jayson MIV (eds.) Collagen in Health and Disease. Churchill-Livingstone, Edinburgh, London, pp 49-72

Hukins DWL (1984) Collagen orientation. In: Hukins DWL (ed.) Connective Tissue Matrix. Macmillan, London, pp 211-240

Hunt KJ, Munih M, Donaldson N (1997) Feedback control of unsupported standing in paraplegia - Part I: Optimal control approach and Part II: Experimental Results. IEEE Trans Rehab Eng TRE-5:331-352

Hunt KJ, Munih M, Donaldson N, Bar FMD (1998) Identification of the Hammerstein hypothesis in the modeling of the electircally stimulated muscle. IEEE Trans Biomed Eng BME-45:998-1009

Hunter IW, Kearney RE (1982) Dynamics of human ankle stiffness: Variation with mean ankle torque. J Biomech 15:747-752

Huston RL, Passerello CE, Harlow MW (1976) On human body dynamics. Ann Biomed Eng 4:25-43

Huston RL, Passerello, CE, Harlow MW (1978) Dynamics of multirigid-body systems. J Appl Mech 45:889-894

Iberall T, Bingham G, Arbib MA (1986) Opposition space as a structuring concept for the analysis of skilled hand movements. In: Heuer H, Fromm C (eds.) Generation and modulation of action pattern.

Iberall T, MacKenzie CL (1990) Opposition space and human prehension. In: Venkataraman ST, Iberall T (eds.) Dextrous robot hands. Springer-Verlag, NY, pp 32-54

Ilić M, Vasiljević D, Popović D (1994) A programmable electronic stimulator for FES systems. IEEE Trans Rehabil Eng TRE-2:234-239

Illert M, Lundberg A, Padel Y, Tanaka R (1978) Integration in descending motor pathways controlling the forelimb in the cat. 5. Properties of and monosynaptic excitatory convergence on C3-C4 propriospinal neurons. Exp Brain Res 33:101-130

Illert M, Trauner M, Weller E, Wiedemann E (1986) Forearm muscles of man can reverse their function after tendon transfers: an electromyographic study. Neurosci Lett 67:129-134

Inman VT, Ralston HJ, Todd F (1981) Human Walking. Williams and Wilkins, Baltimore

Irby SE, Kaufman KR, Mathewson JW, Sutherland DH (1999a) Automatic control design for a dynamic knee-brace system. IEEE Trans Rehabil Eng TRE-7(2):135-139

Irby SE, Kaufman KR, Wirta RW, Sutherland DH (1999b) Optimization and application of a wrap-spring clutch to a dynamic knee-ankle-foot orthosis. IEEE Trans Rehabil Eng TRE- 7(2):130-134

Jackson JH (1932) Selected Writings of John Hughlings Jackson. In: Taylor HJ (ed.). Hodder and Stoughton, London

Jacobs PL, Nash MS, Klose KJ, Guest RS, Needham-Shropshire BM, Green BA (1997) Evaluation of a training program for persons with SCI paraplegia using the Parastep 1 ambulation system: part 2. Effects on physiological responses to peak arm ergometry. Arch Phys Med Rehabil 78(8):794-798

Jacobsen SC, Knutti DF, Johnson RT, Sears HH (1982) Development of the Utah artificial arm. IEEE Trans Biomed Eng BME-29:249-269

Jacobsen SC, Smith CC, Biggers KB, Iversen EK (1989) Behavior based design for robot effectors. In: Brady M (ed.) Robotics science. MIT Press, Cambridge, pp 505-539

Jacobson LS, Goodale MA (1991) Factors affecting higher-order movement planning: A kinematic analysis of human prehension. Exp Brain Res 86:199-208

Jaeger RJ (1986) Design and simulation of closed-loop electrical stimulation orthosis for restoration of quiet standing in paraplegia. J Biomech 19:825-835

Jaeger RJ, Yarkony GY, Smith R (1989) Standing the spinal cord injured patient by electrical stimulation: Refinement of a protocol for clinical use. IEEE Trans Biomed Eng BME-36:720-728

Jagacinski RJ, Repperger DW, Moran MS, Ward SL, Glass B (1980) Fitt's law and microstructure of rapid discrete movements. J Exp Psychol: Human Percept Perform 6:309-320

James K (1983) Improved knee joints for Above-Knee Amputees. Fragment, pp 56-57

James K, Stein RB, Rolf R, Tepavac D (1990) Active suspension above-knee prosthesis. In: Goh JC (ed.) 6th Int Conf Biomech Eng, pp 317-320

James K, Waldon V, Popović D, Stein R (1991) High power four channel stimulator for use in FES systems. Eng Found Conf: Motor Control III - Neuroprostheses, Banff, pp 25

James WV, Orr JF (1984) Upper limb weakness in children with Duchenne muscular dystrophy-a neglected problem. Prosthet Orthot Int 8(2):111-113

Jang JSR (1993) ANFIS: Adaptive-Network-based Fuzzy Inference Systems. IEEE Trans Sys Man Cybern SMC-23:665-685

Jaspers P, Petegem W van, Perre G van der, Peeraer L (1996) Design of an automatic step intention detection system for a hybrid gait orthosis. In: Proc 18th Ann Int IEEE Conf EMBS, Amsterdam, pp 457-458

Jeannerod M, Hecaen H (1979) Adaptation et restaurations des fonctions motrices. Simep, Villeurbanes

Jeannerod M (1981) Intersegmental coordination during reaching at natural visual objects. In: Long J, Baddeley A (eds.). Lawrence Erlbaum Associates, Hillsdale, NJ

Jeannerod M, Biguer B (1982) Visuomotor mechanisms in reaching within extrapersonal space. In: Ingle DJ, Goodale MA, Mansfield RJW (eds.) Analysis of visual behavior. MIT Press, Cambridge MA, pp 387-409

Jeannerod M (1984) The timing of natural prehension movements. J Motor Behav 16(3):235-254

Jeannerod M (1986) The formation of finger grip during prehension. A cortically mediated visuomotor pattern. Behav Brain Res 19(2):99-116

Jeannerod M (1988) The neural and behavioural organization of goal-directed movements. Clarendon Press, Oxford

Jeannerod M (1993) The hand and the object: the role of posterior parietal cortex in forming motor representations. J Physiol Pharmacol 72:535-541

Jeannerod M (1994) Object oriented action. In: Bennett KMB, Castiello U (eds.) Insights into the reach and grasp movement. Elsevier/North-Holland, Amsterdam, pp 3-15

Jeannerod M, Arbib M, Rizzolatti G, Sakata H (1995) Grasping objects: the cortical mechanisms of visuomotor transformation. Trends in Neurosci 18:12-19

Jefferson RJ, Whittle MW (1990) Performance of three walking orthoses for the paralysed : a case study using gait analysis. Prosthet Orthot Int 14:103-110

Jenmalm P, Goodwin AW, Johansson RS (1998) Control of grasp stability when humans lift objects with different surface curvatures. J Neurophysiol 79(4):1643-1652

Jennett B, Teasdale G (eds.) (1984) Management of Head Injuries. Davis FA, Philadelphia

Jenq CB, Coggeshall RE (1987) Permeable tubes increase the length of the gap that regenerating axons can span. Brain Res 408(1-2):239-242

Jensen W, Riso R, Sinkjær T (1998) Position Information in Whole Nerve Cuff Recordings of Muscle Afferents in a Rabbit Model of Normal and Paraplegic Standing. In: Proc of 20th Int Conf IEEE EMBS 5/6:2523-2526

Jezernik S, Sinkjaer T (1999) On statistical properties of whole nerve cuff recordings. IEEE Trans Biomed Eng BME-46(10):1240 -1245

Johansson RS, Vallbo AB (1979) Tactile sensibility in the human hand: relative and absolute densities of four types of mechanoreceptive units in glabroud skin. J Physiol (Lond) 286:283-300

Johansson RS, LaMotte RH (1983) Tactile detection thresholds for a single asperity on an otherwise smooth surface. Somatosens Motor Res 1:21-31

Johansson RS, Westling G (1987) Signals in tactile afferents from the fingers eliciting adaptive motor resposnes during precision grip. Exp Brain Res 66:141-154

Johansson RS, Westling G (1990) Tactile afferent signals in the control of precision grip. In: Jeannerod M (ed.) Attention and performance XIII. Lawrence Erlbaum Associates, Hillsdale NJ, pp 677-736

Johnson KO, Hsiao SS (1992) Tactual form and texture perception. Ann Rev Neurosci 15: 227-250

Johnson MW, Peckham PH, Bhadra N, Kilgore KL, Gazdik MM, Keith MW, Strojnik P (1999) Implantable transducer for two-degree of freedom joint angle sensing. IEEE Trans Rehabil Eng TRE-7(3):349-359

Jonić J, Popović D (1997) Rule-based controller for locomotion - use of radial basis function ANN. In: Proc of the Neurel '97, Belgrade, pp 49-52

Jonić S, Janković T, Gajić V, Popović DB (1999) Three machine learning techniques for automatic determination of rules to control locomotion. IEEE Trans Biomed Eng BME-46(3):300-310

Jonić S, Popović D, Struijk JJ, Sinkjær T (2000) Ballistic and near-ballistic walking assisted by FES, J Biomech (accepted)

Kalanović VD (1996) Total Energy Extraction from a class of Nonlinear systems via Feedback Error Learning. In: Proc IEEE SMC Conf, Lille, pp 231-234

Kalanović VD, Tseng WH (1996) Back Propagation in Feedback Error Learning. In: Proc Int Conf Neural, Parallel and Scientific Computations, 1: 239-242

Kalanović VD, Popović D, Skaug NT (2000) Feedback error learning neural network for above-knee prosthesis. IEEE Trans Rehabil Eng TRE-8(1):71-80

Kalaska JF, Caminiti R, Georgopoulos AP (1983) Cortical mechanisms related to the direction of two-dimensional arm movements. Relations in parietal area 5 and comparison with motor cortex. Exp Brain Res 51:247-260

Kalaska JF, Cohen DAD, Hyde ML, Prud'homme M (1989) A comparison of movement direction-related versus load direction-related activity in primate motor cortex, using a two-dimensional reaching task. J Neurosci 9:2080-2102

Kalaska JF, Crammond DJ (1992) Cerebral cortical mechanisms of reaching movements. Science 255:1517-1523

Kalaska JF, Scott SH, Cisek P, Sergio LE (1997) Cortical control of reaching movements. Curr Opin Neurobiol 7:849-859

Kallesøe JA, Hoffer JA, Strange K, Valenzuela I (1996) Implantable cuff having improved closure: United States Patent No 5, 487, 756, awarded January 30

Kandel ER, Schwartz JH, Jessell MJ (eds.) (1999) Principles of neural science, 4th edn. McGraw Hill, New York

Kane TR, Levinson DA (1985) Dynamics: Theoruy and Application. McGraw Hill, New York

Karu ZZ, Durfee WK, Barzilai AM (1995) Reducing muscle fatigue in FES applications by stimulating with N-let pulse trains. IEEE Trans Biomed Eng BME-42(8):809-817

Katz D (1989) The World of Touch. Erlaum, Hillsdale, NJ (originally published in 1925)

Kawato M, Furukawa K, Suzuki R (1987) A Hierarchical Neural-Network Model for Control and Learning of Voluntary Movement. Biol Cybern 57:169-185

Kawato M (1990) Feedback-Error-Learning Neural Network for Supervised Motor Learning. Advanced Neural Computers, pp 365-372

Kawato M (1996) Trajectory formation in arm movements: Minimization principles and procedures. In: Zelaznik N (ed) Advances in motor learning and control. Human Kinetics Publisher, Champaign, pp 225-259

Kearney RE, Stein RB, Parameswaran L (1994) Identification of intrinsic and reflex contributions to human ankle stiffness dynamics. IEEE Trans Biomed Eng BME-44:493-504

Keele SW, Posner MI (1968) Processing of visual feedback in rapid movements. J Exp Physiol 77:155-158

Keith RA, Granger CV, Hamilton BB, Sherwin FS (1987) The functional independence measure: a new tool for rehabilitation. Adv Clin Rehabil, pp 6-18

Keith MW, Peckham, PH, Thrope GB, Buckett JR, Stroh KC, Menger V (1988) Functional neuromuscular stimulation for the tetraplegic hand. Clin Orthop Rel Res 233:25-33

Kelih B, Rozman J, Stanič U, Kljajić M (1988) Dual channel implantable stimulator. In: Wallinga W, Boom HBK, de Vries J (eds.) Electrophysiological Kinesiology. Elsevier Science Publichers, pp 127-130

Keller T, Curt A, Popović RM, Dietz V, Signer A (1998) Grasping in High Lesioned Tetraplegic Subjects Using the EMG Controlled Neuroprosthesis. J Neurorehab 10:251-255

Kelly JP (1985) Reactions of neurons to injury. In: Kandel ER, Schwartz JH (eds.) Principals of neural science, 2nd edn. Elsevier, New York, pp 187-195

Kelso JAS, Southard DL, Goodman D (1979) On the nature of human interlimb coordination. Science 203:1029-1031

Kennedy PR (1989) The cone electrode: a long-term electrode that records from neurites grown onto its recording surface. J Neurosci Methods 29(3):181-193

Kennedy PR, Mirra SS, Bakay RA (1992) The cone electrode: ultrastructural studies following long-term recording in rat and monkey cortex. Neurosci Lett 142(1):89-94

Kernell D, Donselaar Y, Eerbeek O (1987a) Effects of physiological amounts of highand low-rate chronic stimulation on fast-twitch muscle of the cat hindlimb. II: endurance-related properties. J Neurophysiol 58:614-627

Kernell D, Eerbeek O, Verhey BA, Donselaar Y (1987b) Effects of physiological amounts of highand low-rate chronic stimulation on fasttwitch muscle of the cat hindlimb. I: speed force-related properties. J Neurophysiol 58:598-613

Kernell D, Eerbeek O (1989) Physiological effects of different patterns of chronic stimulation on muscle properties. In: Rose F, Bones R (eds.) Neuromuscular Stimulation. Demos Publications, New York, pp 193-200

Kettner RE, Marcario JK, Clark-Phelps MC (1996a) Control of remembered reaching sequences in monkey. I. Activity during movement in motor and premotor cortex. Exp Brain Res 112:335-346

Kettner RE, Marcario JK, Port NL (1996b) Control of remembered reaching sequences in monkey. II. Storage and preparation before movement in motor and premotor cortex. Exp Brain Res 112:347-358

Khang G (1988) Paraplegic standing controlled by finctional neuromuscular stimulation: computer model, control system design, and simulation studies. PhD thesis, Stanford University

Khang G, Zajac FE (1989a) Paraplegic standing controlled by functional electrical stimulation: part I - computer model and control-system design. IEEE Trans Biomed Eng BME-36:873-884

Khang G, Zajac FE (1989b) Paraplegic standing controlled by functional electrical stimulation. part II .- computer simulation studies. IEEE Trans Biomed Eng BME-36:885-893

Kilgore KL, Peckham PH, Thrope GB, Keith MW, Gallaher-Stone KA (1989) Synthesis of hand grasp using functional neuromuscular stimulation. IEEE Trans Biomed Eng 36(7):761-770

Kilgore KL, Peckham PH (1993a) Grasp synthesis for upper-extremity FNS, Part 1: Automated method for synthesising the stimulus map. Med Biol Eng Comp 31:607-614

Kilgore KL, Peckham PH (1993b) Grasp synthesis for upper-extremity FNS, Part 2: Evaluation of the influence of electrode recruitment properties. Med Biol Eng Comp 31:615-622

Kilgore KL, Peckham PH, Keith MW, Thrope GB, Wuolle KS, Bryden AM, Hart RT (1997) An implanted upper-extremity neuroprosthesis. Follow-up of five patients. J Bone Joint Surg Am 79:533-541

Kirkwood CA, Andrews BJ, Mowforth P (1989) Automatic detection of gait events: a case study using inductive learning techniques. J Biomed Eng 11:511-516

Kitazawa S, Kimura T, Ping-Bo Y (1998) Cerebellar complex spikes encode both destinations and errors in arm movements. Nature 392:494-497

Klatzky RL, Lederman SJ (1987) The intelligent hand. In: Bower GH (ed) The psychology of lerning and motivation. (vol 21) Academic Press, San Diego

Kljajič M, Aćimović R, Maležić M, Stanič U, Pangrsič B, Rozman J (1993) Long-term follow up of gait in hemiparetic patients using subcutaneous peroneal electrical stimulation. In: Proc Ljubljana FES Conf pp 49-52

Klose KJ, Jacobs PL, Broton JG, Guest RS, Needham-Shropshire BM, Lebwohl N, et al. (1997) Evaluation of a training program for persons with SCI paraplegia using the Parastep 1 ambulation system: part 1. Ambulation performance and anthropometric measures. Arch Phys Med Rehabil 78(8):789-793

Knaflitz M, Merletti R (1988) Suppression of stimulation artifacts from myoelectric-evoked potential recordings. IEEE Trans Biom Eng 35(9):758-763

Knutsson E (1985) Studies of gait in patients with spastic paresis. In: Delwaide PJ, Yang RR (eds.) Clinical neurophysiology in spasticity. Elsevier, Amsterdam, pp 175-183

Knuttson E, Richards C (1979) Different types of disturbed motor control in gait of hemiparetic patients. Brain 102:405-430

Ko WH (1986) Solid state physical transducers for biomedical research. IEEE Trans Biomed Eng BME-33(2):153-162

Kobetič R, Marsolais EB (1994) Synthesis of paraplegic gait with multichannel functional electrical stimulation. IEEE Trans Rehab Eng TRE-2:66-79

Kobetič R, Triolo RJ, Marsolais EB (1997) Muscle selection and walking performance of multichannel FES systems for ambulation in paraplegia. IEEE Trans Rehab Eng TRE-5:23-29

Kobetič R, Triolo RJ, Uhlir JP, Bieri C, Wibowo M, Polando G, et al. (1999) Implanted functional electrical stimulation system for mobility in paraplegia: a follow-up case report. IEEE Trans Rehab Eng TRE-7:390-398

Koganezawa E, Fujimoto H, Kato I (1987) Multifunctional Above-Knee Prosthesis for Stairs Walking. Pros Orth Int 11:139-145

Koozekanani SH, Barin K, McGhee RB, Chang HT (1983) A recursive free body approach to computer simulation of human postural dynamics. IEEE Trans Biomed Eng BME-30:787-792

Kostov A, Stein RB, Armstrong WW, Thomas M (1992) Evaluation of Adaptive Logic Networks for Control of Walking in Paralyzed Patients. In: Proc of the 14th Ann Int Conf IEEE EMBS, Paris, pp 1332-1334

Kostov A, Stein RB, Popović DB, Armstrong WW (1994) Improved Methods for Control of FES for Locomotion. In: Proc IFAC Symp Modeling Biomed Eng Galveston, Texas, pp 422-427

Kostov A (1995) Machine learning techniques for the control of FES-assisted locomotion after spinal cord injury. PhD thesis, Univ of Alberta, Edmonton

Kostov A, Andrews B, Popović D, Stein RB, Armstrong WW (1995) Machine learning in control of functional electrical stimulation (FES) for locomotion. IEEE Trans Biomed Eng BME-42:541-551

Kostov A, Hansen M, Haugland M, Sinkjær T (1999) Adaptive restriction rules provide functional and safe stimulation pattern for foot-drop correction. Artificial Organs 23(5): 443-446

Kralj A, Grobelink S (1973) Functional electrical stimulation - a new hope for paraplegic patients. Bull Prosth Res 20:7S

Kralj A, Bajd T, Turk R (1980) Electrical stimulation providing functional use of paraplegic patient muscles. Med Prog Technol 7:3-9

Kralj A, Bajd T, Turk T, Krajnik J, Benko H (1983) Gait restoration in paraplegic patients: a feasibility demonstration using multichannel surface electrode FES. J Rehab Res Developm 20:3-20

Kralj A, Bajd T, Turk R, Benko H (1987) Results of FES application to 71 SCI patients. In: Proc RESNA 10th Ann Conf Rehabil Techn, San Jose, pp 645- 647

Kralj A, Bajd T (1989) Functional Electrical Stimulation: Standing and walking after spinal Cord Injury. CRC Press, Boca Raton, Florida

Krarup C, Loeb GE (1987) Conduction studies in peripheral cat nerve using implanted electrodes: I. Methods and findings in control. Muscle and Nerve 11:922-932

Krarup C, Loeb GE, Pezeshkpour GH (1988) Conduction studies in peripheral cat nerve using implanted electrodes: II The effects of prolonged constriction on regeneration of crushed nerve fibers. Muscle and Nerve 11:933-944

Krarup C, Loeb GE, Pezeshkpour GH (1989) Conduction studies in peripheral cat nerve using implanted electrodes: III The effects of prolonged constriction on the distal nerve segment. Muscle and Nerve 12:915-928

Krebs HI, Hogan N, Aisen ML, Volpe BT (1998) Robot-aided neurorehabilitation. IEEE Trans Rehabil Eng 6(1):75-87

Kromer LF, Cornbrooks CJ (1985) Transplants of Schwann cell cultures promote axonal regeneration in the adult mammalian brain. Proc Natl Acad Sci USA 82(18):6330-6334

Kuhlengel KR, Bunge MB, Bunge RP, Burton H (1990) Implantation of cultured sensory neurons and Schwann cells into lesioned neonatal rat spinal cord. II. Implant characteristics and examination of corticospinal tract growth. J Comp Neurol 293(1):74-91

Kuhn RA (1950) Functional capacity of the isolated human spinal cord. Brain 73:1-51

Kuypers HG (1981) Anatomy of the descending pathways. In: Brook VB (ed.) Handbook of Physiology: The Nervous System. (vol II) American Physiol Soc Bethesda, pp 597-666

Kyberd PJ, Chappell PH (1994) The Southampton hand: an intelligent myoelectric prosthesis. J Rehabil Dev 31(4):326-334

Lackner J, DiZio P (1995) Rapid adaptation to Coriolis force perturbations of arm trajectory. J Neurophysiol 72:299-313

Lamoreaux L (1981) Exoskeleton goniometry. Bull Prosthet Res BPR-10-35 18:288

LaMotte RH, Whitehouse JM (1986) Tactile detection of a dot on a smooth surface: peripheral neural events. J Neurophysiol 56:1109-1128

LaMotte RH, Srinivasan MA (1991) Surface microgeometry: Tactile perception and neural encoding. In: Franzen O, Westman J (eds.) Information Processing in the Somatosensory System. Macmillan, London, pp 49-58

Lan N, Crago PE, Chizeck HJ (1991) Feedback control methods for task regulation by electrical stimulation of muscles. IEEE Trans Biomed Eng BME-38:1213-1223

Lan N, Crago PE (1994) Optimal control of antagonistic muscle stiffness during voluntary movements. Biol Cybern 71:123-135

Lan N, Feng H, Crago PE (1994) Neural network generation of muscle stimulation patterns for control of arm movements. IEEE Trans Rehabil Eng TRE-2:213-223

Landau W (1980) Spasticity: What is it? What is it not? In: Feldman R, Young R, Koella W (eds.) Spasticity: Disordered Motor Control. Year Book Med Publ, Chicago, pp 17-24

Larsen JO, Thomsen M, Haugland M, Sinkjær T (1998) Degeneration and regeneration in rabbit peripheral nerve with long-term nerve cuff electrode implant. A stereological study of myelinated and unmyelinated axons. Acta Neuropathol 96:365-378

Latash ML (1993) Control of Human Movement. Human Kinetics Publisher, Chicago

Latash ML (1996) How does our brain make its choices? In: Latash ML, Turvey MT (eds.) Dexterity and its Development. Elbaum, NJ, pp 277-304

Lee MY, Wong MK, Tang FT (1996) Clinical evaluation of a new biofeedback standing balance training device. J Med Eng Tech 20(2):60-66

Leeds EM, Klose KJ, Gang W, Serafini A, Green B (1990) Bone mineral density after bicycle ergometry training. Arch Phys Med Rehabil 71:207-209

Leffert RD, Meister M (1976) Patterns of neuromuscular activity following tendon transfer in the upper limb: a preliminary study. J Hand Surg 1A:183-189

Lehmann JF, de Lateur BJ, Warren CG, Simons BC, Guy AW (1969) Biomechanical evaluation of braces for paraplegics. Arch Phys Med Rehab 50:179-188

Lehmann JF, Warren CG, Hertling D, McGheen Simons BC, Dralle A (1976) Craig-Scott Orthosis : A biomechanical and functional evaluation. Arch Phys Med Rehab 57:438-442

Lemay MA, Crago PE, Katorgi M, Chapman GJ (1993) Automated tuning of a closed-loop hand grasp neuroprosthesis. IEEE Trans Biomed Eng BME-40:673-685

Lemay MA, Crago PE (1997) Closed loop stabilization in C4 and C5 tetraplegia. IEEE Trans Rehab Eng TRE-5:244-252

Lemay MA, Galagan JA, Hogan N, Bizzi E (1997) Vector summation of spinal force field primitives using multiple levels of co-stimulation (abstract). Neurosci 23:1300

Lemay MA, Grill WM (1999) Spinal force fields in the cat spinal cord (abstract). Soc for Neurosci 25:1396

Lenman JR, Tulley FM, Vrbova G, Dimitrijević MR, Towle JA (1989) Muscle fatigue in some neurological disorders. Muscle Nerve 12:938-942

Lestienne F, Soechting J, Berthoz A (1977) Postural readjustment induced by linear motion of visual scenes. Exp Brain Res 28:363-384

Lestienne F (1979) Effects of inertial loads and velocity on the braking process of voluntary limb movements. Exp Brain Res 35: 407-418

Levin O, Mizrahi J (1999) EMG and metabolite-based prediction of force in paralyzed quadriceps muscle under interrupted stimulation. IEEE Trans Rehabil Eng TRE-7(3):301-314

Levy M, Mizrahi J, Susak Z (1990) Recruitment, force and fatigue characteristics of quadriceps muscles of paraplegics, isometrically activated by surface FES. J Biomed Eng 12:150-156

Liberson WF, Holmquest HJ, Scott D, Dow A (1961) Functional electrotherapy: stimulation of the peroneal nerve synchronized with the swing phase of the gait in hemiplegic patients. Arch Phys Med Rehab 42:101-105

Lieber RL, Fridén JO, Hargens AR, Feringa ER (1986b) Long-term effects of spinal cord transection on fast and slow rat skeletal muscle. II. Morphometric properties. Exp Neurol 91(3): 435-448

Lieber RL, Johansson CB, Vahlsing HL, Hargens AR, Feringa ER (1986a) Long-term effects of spinal cord transection on fast and slow rat skeletal muscle. I. Contractile properties. Exp Neurol 91(3):423-434

Lima PU, Saridis GN (1999) Intelligent controllers as hierarchical stochastic automata. IEEE Trans Syst Man Cybern SMC(B)-29(2):151-63

Lin S, Si J, Schwartz AB (1997) Self-organization of firing activities in monkey's motor cortex: trajectory computation from spike signals. Neural Comput 9(3):607-621

Lindblom U (1981) Qunatitative testing of sensibility including pain. In: Stalberg E, Young RR (eds.) Clinical Neurophysiology, Neurology I. Butterworth, London, pp 168-190

Lippmann RP (1987) An introduction to computing with neural nets. IEEE ASSP Mag

Little JW (1986) Serial recording of reflexes after feline spinal cord transection. Exp Neurol 93:510-521

Lloyd DPC (1943) Conduction and synaptic transmission of the reflex response to stretch in spinal cats. J Neurophysiol 6:317-326

Loeb GE, Marks WB, Hoffer JA (1987) Cat hindlimb motoneurons during locomotion. IV. Participation in cutaneous reflexes. J Neurophysiol 57:563-573

Loeb GE, Peck RA (1996) Cuff electrodes for chronic stimulation and recording of peripheral nerve activity. J Neurosc Meth 64:95-103

Loeb GE, Brown LE, Cheng EJ (1999) A hierarchical foundation for models of sensorymotor control. Exp Brain Res 126(1):1-18

Long II C, Masciarelli CV (1963) An electrophysiologic splint for the hand. Arch Phys Med Rehab 44:499-503

Loomis ME (1985) Levels of contracting. J Psychosoc Nurs Ment Health Serv 23(3):9-14

Lovely RG, Gregor RJ, Roy RR (1986) Effects of training on the recovery of full-weight-bearing stepping in the spinal adult cat. Exp Neurol 92:421-435

Lowenthal M, Tobis JS (1957) Contractures in chronic neurologic disease. Arch Phys Med Rehabil 38:640-645

Luh JYS, Walker MW, Paul RP (1980) On line computational scheme for mechanical manipulators. Trans ASME J Dynam Syst Meas Contr 102:69-76

Lukert B (1982), Osteoporosis - a review and update. Arch Phys Med Rehabil 63:480-484

Lum PS, Burgar CG, Kenney DE, Van der Loos HF (1999) Quantification of force abnormalities during passive and active-assisted upper-limb reaching movements in post-stroke hemiparesis. IEEE Trans Biomed Eng BME-46(6):652-562

Lund S, Broberg C (1983) Effects of different head positions on postural sway in human induced by a reproducible vestibular error signal. Acta Physiol Scand 117:307-309

Lundborg G, Dahlin LB, Danielsen N, Gelberman RH, Longo FM, Powell HC, Varon S (1982) Nerve regeneration in silicone chambers: influence of gap length and of distal stump components. Exp Neurol 76(2):361-375

Lyles M, Munday J (1992) Report on the evaluation of the Vannini-Rizzoli Stabilizing Limb Orthosis. J Rehabil Res Dev 29(2):77-104

Maalej N, Zhu H, Webster JG, Thomkins WJ, Wertsch JJ, Bach-y-Rita P (1987) Pressure monitoring under insensate feet. In: Proc Ann Int Conf IEEE EMBS, pp 1823-1824

Maalej N, Webster JG (1988) A miniature electrooptical force transducer. IEEE Trans Biomed Eng BME-35(1):93-98

MacGregor J (1979) The objective measurement of physical performance with Long term Ambulatory Physiological Surveillance Equipment (LAPSE). In: Stott FD, Raftery EB, Goulding J (eds.) Proc of 3rd Int Symp Ambulatory Monitoring. Academic Press, London, pp 29-39

MacGregor J (1981) The evaluation of patient performance using long term ambulatory monitoring technique in the domiciliary environment. Physiother 67:30-33

MacKenzie CL, Iberall T (1994) The Grasping Hand. In: Stelmach GE, Vroon PA (eds.) Advances in Psychology Series 104. North-Holland

Mackinnon SE, Dellon AL (1990) Clinical nerve reconstruction with a bioabsorbable polyglycolic acid tube. Plast Reconstr Surg 85(3):419-424

Magnus R (1924) Der Körperstellung. Springer Verlag, Berlin

Maležić M, Trnkoczy A, Reberšek S, Aćimović R, Gros N, Strojnik P, Stanič U (1978) Advanced cutaneous stimulators for paretic patients' personal use. In: Proc 6th Int Symp on External Control of Human Extremities, Dubrovnik, pp 233-241

Maležič M, Stanič U, Kljajić M, Aćimović R, Krajnik J, Gros N, Stopar M (1984) Multichannel Electrical Stimulation of Gait in Motor disabled Patients. Orthopedics 7 (7):1187-1195

Maležić M, Bogataj U, Gros N, Decman I, Vrtačnik P, Kljajić M (1992) Application of a programmable dual-channel adaptive electrical stimulation system for the control and analysis of gait. J Rehabil Res and Dev 29(4):41-53

Malouin F, Bonneau C, Pichard L, Corriveau D (1997) Non-reflex mediated changes in plantar flexor muscles early after stroke. Acta Phys Med Rehabil 29(3):147-153

Mannard A, Stein RB (1973) Determination of the frequency response of isometric soleus muscle in the cat using random nerve stimulation. J Physiol 229:275-296

Mano N, Kanazawa I, Yamamoto K (1986) Complex spike activity of cerebellar Purkinje cells related to wrist movement in monkey. J Neurophysiol 56:137-158

Mano N, Kanazawa I, Yamamoto K (1989) Voluntary movements and complex-spike discharges of cerebellar Purkinje cells. Exp Brain Res 17:265-280

Mansour JM, Pereira JM (1987) Quantitative functional anatomy of the lower limb with application to human gait. J Biomech 20(1):51-58

Marks WB, Loeb GE (1976) Action currents, internodal potentials and extracellular records of myelinated mammalian nerve fibres derived from node potentials. J Biophys 16:655-668

Maroudas A (1975) Biophysical chemistry of cartilaginous tissues with special reference to solute and fluid transport. Bioarheology 12:233-248

Marshall RN, Jensen RK, Wood GA (1985) A general Newtonian simulation of an n-segment open chain model. J Biomech 18:359-367

Marsolais EB, Kobetič R (1983) Functional walking in paralyzed patients by means of electrical stimulation. Clin Orthop 175:30-36

Marsolais EB, Kobetič R (1987) Functional electrical stimulation for walking in paraplegics. J Bone Jt Surg 69:728-733

Marsolais EB, Edwards BG (1988) Energy costs of walking and standing with functional neuromuscular stimulation and long leg braces. Arch Phys Med Rehabil 69:243-249

Marsolais EB, Kobetič R, Jacobs J (1990) Comparison of FES treatment in the stroke and spinal cord injury patient. In: Popović D (ed.) Advances in External Control of Human Extremities X, Nauka, Belgrade, pp 213-218

Marteniuk RG, MacKenzie CL, Jeannerod M (1987) Constraints on human arm movement trajectories. Can J Psychol 41:365-378

Marteniuk RG, MacKenzie CL, Leavitt JL (1990) The inadequacies of a straight physical account of motor control. In: Whiting HTA, Meijer OG, van Wieringen PCW (eds.) The Natural-Physical Approach to Movement Control. Free Univ Press, Amsterdam, pp 95-115

Martin D, Schoenen J, Delree R, Rigo JM, Rogister B, Leprince R, Moonen G (1993) Syngeneic grafting of adult rat DRG-derived Schwann cells to the injured spinal cord. Brain Res Bull 30:507-514

Martin T, Stein RB, Hoepner PT, Reid DR (1992) The influence of functional electrical stimulation on the morphological metabolic properties of paralysed muscle. J Appl Physiol 72:1401-1406

Massion J (1992) Movement, posture and equilibrium: interaction and coordination. Prog Neurobiol 38:35-56

Massion J (1998) Postural control systems in developmental perspective. Neurosci Behav Rev 22:465-472

Matjačić Z, Bajd T (1998a) Arm-free paraplegic standing - part I: Control model synthesis and simulation. IEEE Trans Rehab Eng TRE-6:125-134

Matjačić Z, Bajd T (1998b) Arm-free paraplegic standing part II: Experimental results. IEEE Trans Rehab Eng TRE-6:135-150

Matjačić Z, Sinkjær T (1999) A mechanical apparatus for arm free therapeutical paraplegic standing. In: Veltink PH, de Vries TJA, Koopman HFJM, Hermens HJ (eds.) Proc Int Biomechatronics Workshop, Enshcede, pp 158-161

Matjačić Z, Voigt M, Popović D, Sinkjær T (2000) Functional postural responses after perturbations in multiple direction in a standing man revealed by net joint torque: a principle of decoupled control. J Biomech, submitted

Matthews BHC (1933) Nerve ending in mammalian muscle J Physiol (Lond) 78:1-53

Matthews PBA (1959) A study of certain factors influencing the stretch reflex of the decerebrate cat. J Physiol (Lond) 147:547-564

Maynard FM Jr, Bracken MB, Creasey G, Ditunno JF Jr, Donovan WH, Ducker TB, et al. (1997) International Standards for Neurological and Functional Classification of Spinal Cord Injury. Am Spinal Injury Association. Spinal Cord 35(5):266-274

McPherson (1991) How flexible are muscles synergies? In: Humphrey, Freund (eds.) Motor control. Concept and issues. John Wiley and Sons Ltd, Chichester

McComas AJ (1977) Neuromuscular Functional Disorders. Butterworth, London

McCreery DB, Agnew WF, Yuen TG, Bullara LA (1995) Relationship between stimulus amplitude, stimulus frequency and neural damage during electrical stimulation of sciatic nerve of cat. Med Biol Eng Comput 33(3):426-429

McFarland DJ, McCane LM, Wolpaw JR (1998) EEG-based communication and control: short-term role of feedback. IEEE Trans Rehabil Eng TRE-6(1):7-11

McGeer T (1993) Dynamics and control of bipedal locomotion. J Theory Biol 163:277-314

McGraw MB (1943) Neuro-muscular maturation of the infant. Columbia Univ Press, New York

McMahon T (1984) Muscles, Reflexes, and Locomotion. Princeton Univ Press, Princeton

McNeal DR, Reswick JB (1976) Control of skeletal muscle by electrical stimulation. Adv Biomed Eng 6:209-256

McNeal DR, Bowman B (1985) Selective activation of muscle using peripheral nerve electrodes, Med Biol Eng Comp 23(3)249-253

McNeal DR, Nakai RJ, Meadows P, Tu W (1989) Open-loop control of the freely-swinging paralyzed leg. IEEE Trans Biomed Eng BME-36:895-905

McNeal DR, Baker L (1988) Effects of joint angle, electrodes and waveform on electrical stimulation of the quadriceps and hamstrings. Ann Biomed Eng 16:299-310

Medri E, Tepavac D, Needham-Shropshire B, Popović DB (1994) The comprehensive system for gait analysis in handicapped persons. In: Proc Ann Int Conf IEEE EMBS, pp 1234-1235

Meek SG, Wood JE, Jacobsen SC (1990) Model based EMG control of upper extremity prostheses. In: Winters J, Woo SLH (eds.) Multiple muscle systems. Springer, New York, pp 360-376

Meek SG, Fetherston SJ (1992) Comparison of signal-to-noise ratio of myoelectric filters for prosthesis control. J Reh Res Dev 29(4):9-20

Meier JH, Rutten WLC, Boom HBK (1995) Force recruitment during electrical nerve stimulation with multipolar intrafascicular electrodes. Med Biol Eng Comp 33:409-417

Meier JH, Rutten WL, Boom HB (1998) Extracellular potentials from active myelinated fibers inside insulated and noninsulated peripheral nerve. IEEE Trans Biomed Eng BME-45(9):1146-1153

Mendell LM (1988) Physiological aspects of synaptic plasticity: the Ia-Motoneuron connection model. In: Waxman SG (ed.) Advances in Neurology. (Functional recovery in Neurological Disease, vol 47) Raven Press, New York, pp 337-360

Merkel KD, Miller NE, Westbrook PR, Merritt JL (1984) Energy expenditure of paraplegic patients standing and walking with two knee ankle foot orthoses. Arch Phys Med Rehabil 65:121-124

Merzenich MM, Kaas JH, Wall J, Sur M, Nelson RJ, Felleman DJ (1983) Progression of change following median nerve section in the cortical representation of the hand in areas 3b and I in adult owl and squirrel monkey. Neurosci 10(3):639-665

Micera S, Sabatini AM, Dario P (1999) Adaptive fuzzy control of electrically stimulated muscles for arm movements. Med Biol Eng Comput 37(6):680-685

Michie D, Chambers RA (1968) Boxes: an experiment in adaptive control. In: Dale E, Michie D (eds.) Machine Intelligence 2. Edinburgh Univ Press, Edinburgh, pp 137-152

Mihelj M, Matjačić Z, Bajd T (1999) Postural activity of contstrained subject in response to disturbance in sagittal plane. Technology and Health Care 7:437-442

Miller LJ, Peckham PH, Keith MW (1989) Elbow extension in the C5 quadriplegic using functional neuromuscular stimulation. IEEE Trans Biomed Eng BME-36:771-780

Miller NE, Merritt JL, Merkel KD, Westbrook PR (1984) Paraplegic energy expenditure during negotiation of architectural barriers. Arch Phys Med Rehabil 65:778-779

Milner TE, Dugas C, Picard N, Smith AM (1991) Cutaneous afferent activity in the median nerve during grasping in the primate. Brain Res 548:228-241

Milner-Brown HS, Stein RB (1975) The relation between the surface electromyogram and muscular force. J Physiol (London) 246:549

Minns RJ, Soden PD, Jackson DS (1973) The role of the fibrous components and ground substances in the mechanical properties of biological tissues: A preliminary investigation. J Biomech 6:153-165

Minzly J, Mizrahi J, Isakov E, Susak Z, Verbeke M (1993) A computer controlled portable stimulator for paraplegic patients. J Biomed Eng 15:333-338

Mirbagheri MM, Kearney RE, Barbeau H (1998) Stretch reflex behavior of spastic ankle under passive and active conditions. In: Proc Ann Int IEEE EMBS Conf, CD ROM

Mittelstaedt H (1983) A new solution to the problem of the subjective vertical. Naturwissenschaften 70:272-281

Miyamoto H, Kawato M, Setoyama T, Suzuki R (1988) Feedback-Error-Learning Neural Network for Trajectory Control of a Robotic Manipulator. Neur Networks 1:251-265

Mizrahi J, Levy M, Ring H, Isakov E, Liberson A (1994) EMG as an indicator of fatigue of isometrically FES-activated paralyzed muscles. IEEE Trans Rehab Eng TRE-2:57-65

Mizrahi J (1997) Fatigue in muscles activated by FES. CRC Crit Rev Phys Rehabil Med 9(2):93-129

Mizrahi J, Seelenfreund D, Isakov E, Susak Z (1997) Predicted and measured muscle forces after recoveries of differing durations following fatigue in functional electrical stimulation. Artif Organs 21(3):236-239

Moberg E (1975) Surgical treatment for absent single-hand grip and elbow extension in quadriplegia. J Bone Bone Surg 57A(2):196-206

Moberg E (1978) The upper limb in tetraplegia, a new approach to surgical rehabilitation. George Thieme, Stuttgart

Moberg E (1990) Surgical rehabilitation of the upper limb in tetraplegia. Paraplegia 28:330-334

Mochon S, McMahon T (1980) Ballistic walking. J Biomech 13(1):49-57

Mochon S, McMahon T (1981) Ballistic walking: an improved model. Math Biosci 52:241-260

Montero-Menei CN, Pouplard-Barthelaix A, Gumpel M, Baron-Van Evercooren A (1992) Pure Schwann cell suspension grafts promote regeneration of the lesioned septohippocampal cholinergic pathway. Brain Res 570:198-208

Moore P, Stallard JS (1991) A clinical review of adult paraplegic patients with complete lesions using the ORLAU ParaWalker. Paraplegia 29:191-196

Morasso P (1981) Spatial control of arm movements. Exp Brain Res 42:223-227

Morasso P (1983) Three dimensional arm trajectories. Biol Cybern 48:187-194

Morasso P, Sanguinetti V (1997) From Cortical Maps to the Control of Muscles. In: Stelmach GE, Vroon P (eds.) A Self-organization, computational maps, and motor control. Advan Psychol Ser, Elsevier, pp 547-592

Morita H, Petersen N, Christensen LOD, Sinkjær T, Nielsen J (1998) Sensitivity of H-reflexes and stretch reflexes to presynaptic inhibition in man. J Neurol Phys 80:610-620

Morrissey TK, Kleitman N, Bunge RP (1991) Isolation and functional characterization of Schwann cells derived from adult peripheral nerve. J Neurosci 11(8):2433-2442

Morse AS (ed.) (1996) Control Using Logic-Based Switching. (Lecture Notes in Computer Science, no 222) Springer Verlag, New York

Mortimer T (1981) Motor prosthesis. In: Brooks VB (ed.) Handbook of Physiology. (Sect 1, vol 11, part 1(5)) Am Physiol Soc, Bethesda, pp 155-187

Moskowitz E, Lightbody FEH, Freitag NS (1972) Long-term follow-up of post stroke patient. Arch Phys Med 53:167

Motlock WM (1992) Principles of orthotic management for child and adult paraplegia and clinical experience with the isocentric ROO. In: Proc 7th World Cong of the Int Soc for Prosth and Orthot, Chicago, pp 28

Motlock WM, Elliott J (1966) Fitting and training children with Swivel Walkers. Artificial Limbs Autumn pp 27-38

Mountcastle VB, Poggio GF, Werner G (1963) The relation of thalamic cell response to peripheral stimuli varied over an intensive continuum. J Neurophysiol 6:807-334

Mountcastle VB, LaMotte RH, Carli G (1972) Detection thresholds for stimuli in humans and monkeys: comparison with threshold events in mechanoreceptive afferent nerve fibers innervating the monkey hand. J Neurophysiol 35:122-136

Muilenburg L, Wilson AB Jr (1996) A manual for Above-Knee Amputees. Electronic version presented by Dankmeyer, Inc, URL: *http://www.oandop.com*

Mulder AJ, Boom, HBK, Hermens HJ, Zilvold G (1990) Artificial-reflex stimulation for FES-induced standing with minimum quadriceps force. Med Biol Eng Comp 28:483-488

Mulder AJ, Veltink PH, Boom HB (1992a) On/off control in FES-induced standing up: a model study and experiments. Med Biol Eng Comput 30(2):205-212

Mulder AJ, Veltink PH, Boom HB, Zilvold G (1992b) Low-level finite state control of knee joint in paraplegic standing. J Biomed Eng 14(1):3-8

Munih M, de N Donaldson N, Hunt KJ, Barr FM (1997) Feedback control of unsupported standing in paraplegia-part II: experimental results. IEEE Trans Rehabil Eng TRE-5:4 341-52

Murphy JT, Kwan HH, MacKay HH, Wong YC (1982) Precentral unit activity correlated with angular components of a compound arm movement. Brain Res 246:141-145

Murray MP, Drought AB, Kory RC (1964) Walking patterns of normal men. J Bone Jt Surg 46:335

Mushahwar VK, Horch KW (1997) Proposed specifications for a lumbar spinal cord electrode array for control of lower extremities in paraplegia. IEEE Trans Rehabil Eng TRE-5(3):237-243

Mushahwar VK, Horch KW (2000) Muscle recruitment through electrical stimulation of the lumbo-sacral spinal cord. IEEE Trans Rehab Eng TRE-8(1):22-28

Mussa-Ivaldi E, Hogan N, Bizzi E (1985) Neural, mechanical and geometric factors subserving arm posture in humans. J Neurosci 5:2732-2743

Mussa-Ivaldi FA (1988) Do neurons in the motor cortex encode movement direction? An alternative hypothesis. Neurosci Lett 91:106-111

Mussa-Ivaldi FA, Giszter SF, Bizzi E (1994) Linear combinations of primitives in vertebrate motor control. In: Proc Natl Acad Sci USA 91:7534-7538

Nachemson AL and JH Evans (1968) Some mechanical properties of the third human lumbar interlaminar ligament (ligamentum flavum). J Biomech 1:211-220

Nannini N, Horch K (1991) Muscle recruitment with intrafascicular electrodes. IEEE Trans Biomed Eng BME-38:769-778

Naples GG, Mortimer JT, Scheiner A, Sweeney JD (1988) A spiral nerve cuff electrode for peripheral nerve stimulation. IEEE Trans Biomed Eng BME-35(11):905-916

Narazaki H, Watanabe T, Yamamoto M (1996) Reorganizing Knowledge in Neural Networks: An Explanatory Mechanism for Neural Networks in Data Classification Problems. IEEE Trans Sys Man Cybern SMC-26:107-117

Nash MS, Jacobs PL, Montalvo BM, Klose KJ, Guest RS, Needham-Shropshire BM (1997) Evaluation of a training program for persons with SCI paraplegia using the Parastep 1 ambulation system: part 5. Lower extremity blood flow and hyperemic responses to occlusion are augmented by ambulation training. Arch Phys Med Rehabil 78:8 808-14

Nashner LM (1972) A vestibular posture control model. Kybernetik 10:106-110

Nashner LM, Black FO, Wall C (1982) III.Adaptation to altered support and visual conditions during stance: patients with vestibular deficits. J Neurosci 2:536-544

Nashner LM, Shupert CL, Horak FB, Black FO (1989) Organization of posture control: an analysis of sensory and mechanical constraints. Prog Brain Res 80:411-418

Nathan PW, Smith MC, Cook AW (1986) Sensory effects in man of lesions of the posterior columns and of some other afferent pathways. Brain 109 (Pt 5): 1003-1041

Nathan RH (1989) An FNS-based system for generating upper limb function in the C4 quadriplegic. Med Biol Eng Comp 27:549-556

Nathan RH, Ohry A (1990) Upper limb functions regained in quadriplegia: A hybrid computerized neuromuscular stimulation system. Arch Phys Med Rehabil 71:415-421

Nathan R (1997) Handmaster NMS - present technology and the next generation. In: Popović D (ed.) Proc 2nd Int Symp FES, Burnaby, pp 139-140

Needham-Shropshire BM, Broton JG, Klose KJ, Lebwohl N, Guest RS, Jacobs PL (1997) Evaluation of a training program for persons with SCI paraplegia using the Parastep 1 ambulation system: part 3. Lack of effect on bone mineral density. Arch Phys Med Rehabil 78(8):799-803

Nelson W (1983) Physical principles for economies of skilled movements. Biol Cybern 46:135-147

Nene AY, Patrick JH (1989) Energy cost of paraplegic locomotion with the ORLAU ParaWalker. Paraplegia 27:5-15

Nene AV, Jennings SJ (1992) Physiological cost index of paraplegic locomotion using the ORLAU ParaWalker. Paraplegia 30:246-252

Ng SK, Chizeck HJ (1997) Fuzzy model identification for classification of gait-events in paraplegics. IEEE Trans Fuzzy Systems TFS-5:536-544

Nguyen D, Widrow B (1990) Improving the learning speed of the 2-layer neural networks by choosing initial values of the adaptive weights. In: Proc Int Joint Conf Neural Networks 3:21-26

Nielsen J, Petersen, N, Crone C (1995) Changes in transmission across synapses of Ia afferents in spastic patients. Brain 118:995-1004

Nikias C, Petropulu A (1993) Higher-Order Spectra Analysis. Prentice Hall, pp 7-122

Nikolić ZM, Popović DB, Stein RB, Kenwell Z (1994) Instrumentation for ENG and EMG recordings in FES systems. IEEE Trans Biomed Eng BME-41:703-706

Nikolić Z, Popović DB (1996) Automatic detection of production rules for locomotion. J Autom Control (Univ of Belgrade) 6:81-94

Nikolić Z, Popović DB (1998) Automatic rule determination for finite state model of locomotion IEEE Trans Biomed Eng BME-45:1081-1085

Noback CR, Demarest RL (1981) The Human Nervous System: Basic Principles of Neurobiology, 3rd edn. McGraw-Hill, New York

Nordgren RE, Meckl PH (1993) An Analytical Comparison of a Neural Network and a Model-Based Adaptive Controller. IEEE Trans on Neural Networks NN-4:595-601

Normann RA, Maynard EM, Rousche PJ, Warren DJ (1999) A neural interface for a cortical vision prosthesis. Vision Res 39(15):2577-87

Nudo RJ, Plautz EJ, Miliken GW (1997) Adaptive plasticity in primate motor cortex as a consequence of behavioral experience and neuronal injury. Seminars in Neuroscience 9:13-23

Oğuztöreli MN, Popović D, Stein RB (1994) Optimal control for musculo-skeletal systems. J Aut Control (Univ Belgrade) 4:1-16

Ojemann JG, Silbergeld DL (1995) Cortical stimulation mapping of phantom limb rolandic cortex. J Neurosurg 82:641-644

Olson L, Cheng H, Zetterstrom RH, Solomin L, Jansson L, Gimenez-Llort L, et al. (1998) On CNS repair and protection strategies: novel approaches with implications for spinal cord injury and Parkinson's disease. Brain Res Rev 26(2-3):302-305

Onyshko S, Winter DA (1980) A mathematical model for the dynamics of human walking. J Biomech 13:361-368

Orin DE, McGhee RB, Vukobratovic M, Hartoch G (1979) Kinematic and kinetic analysis of open-chain linkages utilizing Newton-Euler methods. Math Biosci 43:107-130

Ostry DJ, Munhall KG (1994) Control of jaw orientation and position in mastication and speech. Neurophysiol 71(4):1528-45

Paillard J, Jordan P, Brouchon M (1981) Visual motion cues in prismatic adaptation: evidence for two separate and additive processes. Acta Psychol 48:253-270

Paillard J (1982) The contribution of peripheral and central vision to visually guided reaching. In: Ingle DJ, Goodale MA, Mansfield RJW (eds.) Visually Oriented Behavior. MIT Press, Cambridge, pp 367-385

Paillard F (1999) Gene transfer to neurons with Herpes simplex virus/adeno-associated virus hybrid vectors. Hum Gene Ther 10(15):2441-2443

Palmer CI, Marks WB, Bak MJ (1985) The responses of cat motor cortical units to electrical cutaneous stimulation during locomotion and during lifting, falling and landing. Exp Brain Res 58:102-116

Pandy MG, Berme N (1988) Synthesis of human walking: a planar model for single support. J Biomech 21(12):1053-1056

Park E, Meek SG (1995) Adaptive filtering of the electromyographic signal for prosthetic control and force estimation. IEEE Trans Biomed Eng BME-42(10):1048-1052

Patla AE, Calvert TW, Stein RB (1985) Model of a pattern generator for locomotion in mammals. Am J Physiol 248(4 Pt 2):R484-494

Patla AE (1986) Adaptation of postural response to voluntary arm raises during locomotion in humans. Neurosci Lett 68(3):334-338

Patla AE (1991) Adaptability of human gait: Implication for the control of locomotion. Elsevier

Patla AE, Prentice SD, Robinson C, Neufeld J (1991) Visual control of locomotion: strategies for changing direction and for going over obstacles. J Exp Psychol Hum Percept Perform 17(3):603-634

Paulignan Y, MacKenzie CL, Marteniuk RG, Jeannerod M (1991) Selective perturbation of visual input during prehension movements. I. The effects of changing object position. Exp Brain Res 83:502-512

Pearson KG, Duysens J (1976) Function of segmental reflexes in the control of stepping in cockroaches and cats. In: Herman PM, Grillner S, Stein PSG, Stuart DG (eds.) Neural Control of Locomotion. Plenum Press, New York, pp 519-537

Pearson KG (1995) Propriceptive regulation of locomotion. Curr Opin Neurobiol 5:789-791

Pearson KG, Gordon J (1999) Locomotion. In: Kandel ER, Schwartz JH, Jessell TM (eds.) Principles of Neuroscience, 4th edn. Mc Graw Hill, Ney York, pp 737-755

Peckham PH, Mortimer JT, Marsolais EB (1976a) Alteration in the force and fatigability of skeletal muscle in quadriplegic humans following exercise induced by chronic electrical stimulation. Clin Orthop 114:326-333

Peckham PH, Mortimer JT, Marsolais EB (1976b) Upper and lower motor neuron lesions in the upper extremity muscles of tetraplegics. Paraplegia 14:115-121

Peckham PH, Mortimer JT, Marsolais EB (1980a) Controlled prehension and release in the C5 quadriplegic elicited by functional electrical stimulation of the paralyzed forearm muscles. Annals Biomed Eng 8:369-388

Peckham PH, Marsolais EB, Mortimer JT (1980b) Restoration of the key grip and release in the C6 quadriplegic through functional electrical stimulation. J Hand Surg 5:464-469

Peckham PH (1987) Functional electrical stimulation: current status and future prospects of applications to the neuromuscular system in spinal cord injury. Paraplegia, Silver Jubilee Number 25:274-288

Peckham PH (1988) Functional electrical stimulation. In: Webster JG (ed.) Encyclopedia of medial devices and instrumentation. John Wiley, New York, pp 1341-1358

Peckham PH, Keith MW, Freehafer AA (1988) Restoration of functional control by electrical stimulation in the upper extremity of the quadriplegic patient. J Bone Joint Surg 70a:144-148

Peckham PH, Keith MW (1992) Motor Prosthesis for restoration of upper extremity function. In: Stein RB, Peckham PH, Popović DB (eds.) Neural Prostheses: Replacing motor function after disease or disability. Oxford Univ Press, New York, pp 162-190

Pederson DR, Brand RA, Cheng C, Arora JS (1987) Direct comparison of muscle force predictions using linear and nonlienar programming. J Biomech Eng 109:192-199

Perry J (1981) Generic terminology for the phases of gait. Bull Prosthet Res BPR-10-35, 18:279

Perry J (1992) Gait analysis: normal and pathological function. Slack Inc, Thorofare, NJ

Peterson DK, Chizeck HJ (1987) Linear quadratic control of a loaded agonist-antagonist muscle pair. IEEE Trans Biome Eng BME-34:788-796

Petrofsky JS, Phillips CA (1983a) Active physical therapy: a modern approach for rehabilitation of the disabled. J Neurol Orthop Surg 4:165-173

Petrofsky JS, Phillips CA (1983b) Computer controlled walking in the paralyzed individual. J Neurol Orthop Surg 4:153-164

Petrofsky JS, Phillips CA (1985) Closed-loop control of movement of skeletal muscle. CRC Crit Rev Bioeng 13:35-96

Pette D, Vrbova G (1992) Adaptation of mammalian skeletal muscle to chronic electrical stimulation. Rev Physiol Biochem Pharmacol 120:115-202

Philipson L, Childress DS, Strysik J (1981) Digital approaches to myoelectric control of prostheses. Bul Pros Res 10-36:3-11

Phillips CA, Petrofsky JS, Hendershot DM, Stafford D (1984) Functional electrical exercise - a comprehensive approach for physical conditioning of the spinal cord injured patients. Ortoped 7:1112-1114

Phillips CA (1989) Electrical muscle stimulation in combination with a reciprocating gait orthosis for ambulation by paraplegics. J Biomed Eng 11:338-344

Phillips GF, Andrews BJ, Chizeck HJ, Barnckle K (1988) Finite state control of paraplegic gait using a hybrid FNS orthosis. In: Proc 10th Ann Int IEEE Conf EMBS, pp 1671

Pinter MM, Dimitrijević MR (1999) Gait after spinal cord injury and the central pattern generator for locomotion. Spinal Cord 37(8):531-537

Pitas I, Milios E, Venetsanopoulos AN (1992) Minimum Entropy Approach to Rule Learning from Examples. IEEE Trans Sys Man Cybern SMC-22:621-635

Polit A, Bizzi E (1979) Characteristics of motor programs underlying arm movement in monkey. J Neurophysiol 42:183-194

Popović D, Tomović R, Gračanin F (1979) Neue aspekte für den Bau fon Orthesen für die unteren Extremitäten. Ortopädie Technik 6:94-97

Popović D (1981) Design of assistive systems for humans with paralysis of legs. PhD Thesis, Univ of Belgrade, Belgrade

Popović D, Schwirtlich L (1986) Gait restoration by active SFMO. In: Naletz A (ed.) Control Aspects in Biomedical Robotics, IFAC, pp 87-94

Popović D, Schwirtlich L (1987) Hybrid powered orthoses. In: Popović D (ed.) Advances in External Control of Human Extremities IX, pp 95-104, ETAN, Belgrade

Popović D, Schwirtlich L (1988) Belgrade active A/K prosthesis. In: de Vries J (ed.) Electrophysiological Kinesiology. Excerpta Medica, Amsterdam, Int Congress Series No 804, pp 337-343

Popović D, Tomović R, Schwirtlich L (1989) Hybrid assistive system: Neuroprosthesis for motion. IEEE Trans Biomed Eng BME-36(7):729-738

Popović D (1990) Dynamics of self - fitting modular orthoses. IEEE Trans Robot Autom TRA-6:200-207

Popović D, Schwirtlich L, Radosavljević S (1990a) Powered hybrid assistive system. In: Popović D (ed.) Advances in external control of human extremities X, Nauka, Belgrade, pp 191-200

Popović D, Stein RB, James K (1990b) Biological and artificial sensors for rehabilitation neuroscience. In: Proc 3rd III Int Forum on ASICT'90, Bannf, pp 79-88

Popović D (1991) Control of locomotion in handicapped humans. In: Antognetti P, Milutinović V (eds.) Neural networks concepts, applications and implementations. Prentice Hall, 2:144-154

Popović D, Gordon T, Rafuse V, Prochazka A (1991a) Properties of implanted electrodes for functional electrical stimulation Ann Biomed Eng 19:303-316

Popović D, Tomović R, Tepavac D, Schwirtlich L (1991b) Control aspects an active A/K prosthesis. Int J Man-Machine Studies 35:751-767

Popović D, Oğuztöreli MN, Stein RB (1991c) Optimal control for the active above-knee prosthesis. Ann Biomed Eng 19:131-150

Popović D, Watt J, Stein RB (1991d) Functional electrical stimulation in the rehabilition of the spinal cord injured child. In: Proc Int Conf the IEEE Eng in Biol and Med Soc, Orlando, 3:93

Popović D, Raspopović V (1992) Afferent signals in palmar digital nerves. Proc 4th Vienna Int Workshop on FES, Vienna, pp 105-108

Popović D (1993) Finite state model of locomotion for functional electrical stimulation systems. Prog Brain Res 97:397-407

Popović D, Schwirtlich L (1993) Design and evaluation of the self-fitting modular orthosis (SFMO). IEEE Trans Rehabil Eng TRE-1:165-174

Popović D, Stein RB, Jovanović KL, Rongching D, Kostov A, Armstrong WW (1993) Sensory nerve recording for closed-loop control to restore motor functions. IEEE Trans Biomed Eng BME-40:1024-1031

Popović D, Oğuztöreli MN, Stein RB (1995) Optimal control for an above-knee prosthesis with two degrees of freedom. J Biomech 28:89-98

Popović D, Stojanović A, Pjanović A, Radosavljević S, Vulović D, Jović S, Popović M (1997) Application of FES to restore standing and walking. Phys Ther (Belgrade) 3(9):3-11

Popović D, Popović M (1998a) Tuning of a nonanalytical hierarchical control system for reaching with FES. IEEE Trans Biomed Eng BME-45(2):203-212

Popović D, Popović M (1998b) Belgrade grasping system. J Electronics (Banja Luka, Bosnia) 2:21-28

Popović D, Popović M, Stojanović A, Radosavljević S, Pjanović A, Vulović D (1998) Clinical Evaluation of the Belgrade grasping system. In: Proc V Int Workshop on FES, Vienna, pp 247-250

Popović D, Stojanović A, Pjanović A, Radosavljević S, Popović M, Jović S, Vulović D (1999a) Clinical evaluation of the bionic glove. Arch Phys Med Rehabil 80(3):299-304

Popović D, Stein RB, Oğuztöreli N, Lebiedowska M, Jonić S (1999b) Optimal control of walking with functional electrical stimulation: A computer simulation study. IEEE Trans Rehab Eng TRE-7:69-79

Popović D, Popović M (2000a) Nonanalytical control for assisting reaching in humans with disability. In: Winters JM, Crago PE (eds.) Control of Posture and Movement: Neuro-musculo-skeletal interaction and organization principles, Springer Verlag, in print

Popović D, Popović M (2000b) Control for an elbow neuroprosthesis: cloning biological synergies. IEEE Med Biol Eng Mag, accepted

Popović D, Sinkjær T (2000) Controlling Functional Electrical Stimulation to restore walking. J Physiotherapy (Honk Kong), in print

Popović M, Popović D (1983) Cybernetic actuator for prosthesis/orthosis. In: Proc 27th Yugoslav Conf on ETAN, II:285-292

Popović M, Tepavac D (1992) A portable 8-channel gait kinematics recording unit. In: Proc Ann Int Conf IEEE EMBS 4:1646-1647

Popović M, Popović D, Tomović R (1993) Simplified Arm Control in Goal-directed Movements. In: Proc 12th Southern IEEE Conf on BME, pp 24-27

Popović M, Jovanović N, Schwirtlich L (1994) Identification of parameters for control of assistive systems. J Aut Control (Univ Belgrade) 4:31-45

Popović M, Popović D (1994) A new approach to reaching control for tetraplegic subjects. J Electromyog and Kinesiol 4:242-253

Popović M (1995) A new method to control arm movement in tetraplegic subjects. PhD Thesis, Univ of Belgrade, Belgrade

Popović M, Popović D (1995) Enhanced reaching by means of FES. In: Proc 5th Vienna Int Workshop on FES, Vienna, pp 347-350

Popović M, Popović D, Tomović R (1999) Control of reaching movements: cloning biological control. In: Gantchev N, Gantchev G (eds.) From basic motor control to functional recovery Academic Publ House M Drinov, Sofia, pp 310-316

Popović M, Popović D (2000) Synergistic control for en elbow neuroprosthesis. In: Proc 6th Int Conf IFESS, Aalborg, in print

Popović MR, Keller T, Nakazawa K, Pappas I, Dietz V, Morari M (1999) Stability zones in able-bodied subjects during quiet standing. In: Gantchev N, Gantchev G (eds.) From basic motor control to functional recovery, Academic Publ House M Drinov, Sofia, pp 165-176

Popović MR Keller T, Pappas I, Dietz V, Morari M (2000) ETHZ-ParaCare grasping and walking neuroprostheses. IEEE Med Biol Eng Mag, accepted

Powers RK, Marder-Meyer J, Rymer WZ (1988) Quantitative relations between hypertonia and stretch reflex threshold in spastic hemiparesis. Ann Neurol 23:115-124

Prablanc C, Echallier JF, Komilis E, Jeannerod M (1979a) Optimal response of eye and hand motor systems in pointing at visual target. I. Spatio-temporal characteristics of eye and hand movements and their relationships when varying the amount of visual information. Biol Cybern 35:113-124

Prablanc C, Echallier JF, Komilis E, Jeannerod M (1979b) Optimal response of eye and hand motor systems in pointing at visual target. II. Static and dynamic visual cues in the control of hand movements. Biol Cybern 35:183-187

Pratt CA, Fung J, Machperson M (1994) Stance control in the chronic spinal cat. J Neurophysiol 71:1981-1985

Prilutsky BI, Petrova LN, Raitsin LM (1996) Comparison of mechanical energy expenditure of joint moments and muscle forces during human movement. J Biomech 29:405-416

Prochazka A, Davis LA (1992) Clinical experience with reinforced, anchored intramuscular electrodes for functional neuromuscular stimulation. J Neurosci Methods 42(3):175-184

Prochazka A (1993) Comparison of natural and artificial control of movement. IEEE Trans Rehabil Eng TRE-1:7-17

Prochazka A, Gauthier M, Wieler M, Kenwell Z (1997) The Bionic glove: an electrical stimulator garment that provides controlled grasp and hand opening in quadriplegia. Arch Phys Med Rehabil 78:608-614

Qi H, Tyler DJ, Durand DM (1999) Neurofuzzy adaptive controlling of selective stimulation for FES: a case study. IEEE Trans Rehabil Eng TRE-7: 183-192

Quintern J, Minwegen P, Mauritz KH (1989) Control mechanisms for restoring posture and movements in paraplegics. Prog Brain Res 80: 489-502

Rabishong P, Tomović R, Turajlić S, Bell A, et al. (1975) The Active Modular Orthosis for Locomotion (AMOLL) project. In: Advances in External Control of Human Extremities VI, ETAN, pp 33 – 44

Rack PMH, Ross HF, Thilmann AF (1984) The ankle stretch reflexes in normal and spastic subjects. The response to sinusoidal movement. Brain 107:637-654

Raczka R, Braun R, Waters RL (1984) Posterior deltoid-to-triceps transfer in quadriplegia. Clin Orthop 187:163-167

Radcliffe CW (1980) Biomechanical Basis for the Design of Prosthetic Knee Mechanisms. In: Proc Rehab Eng Int Seminar REIS '80 (J Biomechanisms), Tokyo, pp 68 -88

Rafil M, Firosnia M, Golimbu C, Sokolow J (1982) Bilateral acetabular stress fractures in a paraplegic patient. Arch Phys Med Rehabil 63:240-246

Raisman G (1997) Use of Schwann cells to induce repair of adult CNS tracts. Rev Neurol (Paris) 153(8-9):521-525

Rakić M (1964) An automatic hand prosthesis. Med Electron Biol Eng 2:47-55

Rakić M (1989) Multifingered robot hand with selfadaptibility. Robotics& Comp-Integr Manufact 5(2/3):269-276

Rakić P (1995) Radial versus tangential migration of neuronal clones in the developing cerebral cortex [comment] Proc Natl Acad Sci 92(25):11323-11327

Rakoš M, Freudernschuss B, Girsch W, Hofer C, Kaus J, Meiners T, et al. (1998) EMG-controlled FES for treatment of the paralyzed upper extremity. In: Proc 6th Vienna Int Workshop FES, Vienna, pp 259-262

Rangoussi M, Carayannis G (1995) Adaptive Detection of Noisy Speech using Third-Order Statistics. Int J Adapt Contr and Sig Proc, Special Issue on HOS

Rao DH, Bitner D, Gupta MM (1994) Feedback-error learning scheme using recurrent neural networks for nonlinear dynamic systems. Neural Networks, IEEE World Cong Comput Intelligence 1:175-180

Reberšek S, Vodovnik L (1973) Proportionally controlled functional electrical stimulation of hand. Arch Phys Med Rehabil 54:378-382

Reier PJ, Houle JD (1988) The glial scar: its bearing on axonal elongation and transplantation approaches to CNS repair. Adv Neurol 47: 87-138

Reinkensmeyer DJ, Dewald JP, Rymer WZ (1999) Guidance-based quantification of arm impairment following brain injury: a pilot study. IEEE Trans Rehabil Eng TRE-7(1):1-11

Reiser T, Waters RL (1986) Long term follow-up of the Moberg key grip procedure. J Hand Surg 11A:724-728

Richardson RM, Issa VMK, Aguayo AJ (1984) Regeneration of long spinal axons in the rat. J Neurocytol 13:165-182

Ridley BR (1990) A New Continuous-Time Model for Current-Mode Control. In: Proc DCM 21th Ann IEEE Power Electronics Specialists Conf, pp 382-389

Riener R, Fuhr T (1998) Patient-driven control of FES-supported standing up: A simulation study. IEEE Trans Rehab Eng TRE-6:113-124

Riess JA, Abbas JJ (1999) Control of cyclic movements as muscles fatigue using functional neuromuscular stimulation. In: Proc Ann Int IEEE EMBS Conf 1:659

Riso RR (1998) Perspectives on the role of natural sensors for cognitive feedback in neuromotor prostheses. Automedica 16:329-353

Riso RR, Fahard K, Jensen W, Sinkjær T (2000) Nerve Cuff Recordings of Muscle Afferent Activity from Tibial and Peroneal Nerves in Rabbit During Passive Ankle Motion. IEEE Trans Rehab Eng (June)

Roberts AH (1976) Long-term prognosis of severe accidental head injury. In: Proc R Soc Med 69:137-140

Rose G, Henshaw JT (1973) Swivel Walkers for paraplegics : Considerations and problems in their design and application. Bull Prosth Res 10-20:62-74

Rose G (1979) The principles and practice of Hip Guidance Articulations. Prosth and Orth Int 3:37-43

Rosen JM, Padilla JA, Nguyen KD, Padilla MA, Sabelman EE, Pham HN (1990) Artificial nerve graft using collagen as an extracellular matrix for nerve repair compared with sutured autograft in a rat model. Ann Plast Surg 25(5):375-87

Rosman N, Spira E (1974) Paraplegic use of walking braces: A survey. Arch Phys Med Rehabil 55:310-314

Rousche PJ, Normann RA (1999) Chronic intracortical microstimulation (ICMS) of cat sensory cortex using the Utah Intracortical Electrode Array. IEEE Trans Rehabil Eng TRE-7(1):56-68

Roy RR, Acosta R Jr (1986) Fiber type fiber size changes in selected thigh muscles six months after low thoracic spinal cord transection in adult cats: exercise effects. Exp Neurol 92:675-685

Roy RR, Baldwin KM, Edgerton VR (1991) The plasticity of skeletal muscle: effects of neuromuscular activity. Exerc Sports Sci Rev 19:269-312

Rozman J, Aćimović-Janežič R, Tekavčič I, Kljajić M, Trlep M (1994) Implantable stimulator for selective stimulation of the common peroneal nerve: a preliminary report. Journal of Med Eng and Technol 18(2):47-53

Rubin BP, Dusart I, Schwab ME (1994) A monoclonal antibody (IN-1) which neutralizes neurite growth inhibitory proteins in the rat CNS recognizes antigens localized in CNS myelin. J Neurocytol 23(4):209-217

Rudel D, Bajd T, Reberšek S, Vodovnik L (1984) FES assisted manipulation in quadriplegic patients. In: Popović D (ed.) Advances in external control of human extremities VIII. ETAN, pp 273-282

Rumelhart DE, Hinton GE, Williams RJ (1986) Learning interval representation by error propagation. In: Parallel distributed processing. (chap 8) MIT Press, Cambridge, pp 318-361

Rushton DN (1990) Choice of nerves roots for multichannel leg controller implant. In: Popović D (ed.) Advances in External Control X, Nauka, pp 99-108

Rutkowski JL, Tennekoon GI, McGillicuddy JE (1992) Selective culture of mitotically active human Schwann cells from adult sural nerves. Ann Neurol 31(6):580-586

Rutten WL, van Wier HJ, Put JH (1991) Sensitivity and selectivity of intraneural stimulation using a silicon electrode array. IEEE Trans Biomed Eng 38(2):192-198

Sagi-Dolev AM, Prutchi D, Nathan RH (1995) Three-dimensional current density distribution under surface stimulation electrodes. Med Biol Eng Comp 33: 403-408

Sainburg RL, Poizner H, Ghez C (1993) Loss of proprioception produces deficits in interjoint coordination. J Neurophysiol 70(5):2136-2147

Salatian AW, Yi KY, Zheng YF (1997) Reinforcement learning for a biped robot to climb sloping surfaces. J Robot Systems 14:283-296

Salisbury JK, Craig JJ (1982) Articulated hand: force control and kinematic issues. Int J Robot Res 1(1):4-17

Salisbury JK (1985) Integrated language, sensing and control for robot hand. In: Proc Int Symp Intel Autom, pp 54-61

Salmons S, Vrbova G (1969) The influence of activity on some contractile characteristics of mammalian fast slow muscles. J Physiol (Lond) 201:535-549

Salmons S, Henriksson J (1981) The adaptive response of skeletal muscle to increased use. Muscle Nerve 4:94-105

Sanes JN, Suner S, Donoghue (1990) Dynamic organization of primary motor output to target muscles in adult rats. I. Long term pattern of reorganization following motor or mixed peripheral nerve lesions. Exp Brain Res 79:479-491

Sanger TD (1996) Probability density estimation for the interpretation of neural population codes. J Neurophysiol 76:2790-2793

Sargeant AJ, Kernel D (eds.) (1993) Neuromuscular fatigue. Elsevier, Amsterdam

Saxena S, Nikolić S, Popović D (1995) An EMG controlled FES system for grasping in tetraplegics. J Rehabil Res Dev 32:17-23

Scheiner A, Mortimer JT, Roessmann U (1990) Imbalanced biphasic electrical stimulation: muscle tissue damage. Ann Biomed Eng 18(4):407-425

Scheiner A, Stein RB, Ferencz D, Chizeck HJ (1993) Improved models for the lower leg in paraplegics. In: Proc IEEE Ann Conf EMBS, San Diego, pp 1151-1153

Schieber MH, Hibbard LS (1993) How somatotopic is the motor cortex hand area? Science 261(5120):489-492

Schlesinger G (1919) Der Mechanisce Aufbau der kunstlischen Glieder. In: Borchardt M (ed.) Ersatzglieder und Arbeitshilfen fur Kriegsbeshadigte und Unfallverletzte. Springer, Berlin, pp 21-600

Schwab ME, Caroni P (1988) Oligodendrocytes and CNS myelin are nonpermissive substrates for neurite growth and fibroblast spreading in vitro. J Neurosci 8(7):2381-2393

Schwartz AB, Kettner RE, Georgopoulos AP (1988) Primate motor cortex and free arm movements to visual targets in three-dimensional space. I. Relations between single cell discharge and direction of movement. J Neurosci 8(8):2913-2927

Schwartz AB, Adams JL (1995) A method for detecting the time course of correlation between single-unit activity and EMG during a behavioral task. J Neurosci Methods 58(1-2):127-141

Schweighofer N, Arbib MA, Kawato M (1998) Role of the cerebellum in reaching movements in humans. II. distributed inverse dynamics control. Eur J Neurosci 10:86-94

Schwirtlich L, Popović D (1984) Hybrid orthoses for deficient locomotion. In: Popović D (ed.) Advances in External Control of Human Extremities VIII, ETAN, pp 23-32

Scott BA (1971) Engineering principles and fabrication techniques for the Scott-Craig long brace for paraplegics. Orthot Prosthet 25:14-19

Scott SH, Loeb GE (1994) The computation of position sense from spindles in mono- and multiarticular muscles. Neurosci 14:7529-7540

Scott SH (1997) Comparison of onset time and magnitude of activity for proximal arm muscles and motor cortical cells prior to reaching movements. J Neurophysiol 77:1016-1022

Scott TRD, Peckham PH, Kilgore KL (1996) Tri-state myoelectric control of bilateral upper extremity neuroprosthesis for tetraplegic individuals. IEEE Trans Rehab Eng TRE-4:251-263

Scrutton DR (1971) A reciprocating brace with polyplanar hip hinges used on spina bifida children. Physiotherapy 57:61-66

Seif-Naragfhi AH, Winters JM (1990) Optimized strategies for scaling goal-directed movements. In: Winters JM, Woo SL-Y (eds.) Multiple muscle systems. Biomechanics and movement organization. Springer-Verlag, New York, pp 312-334

Sennels S, Biering-Soerensen F, Anderson OT, Hansen SD (1997) Functional neuromuscular stimulation control by surface electromyographic signals produced by volitional activation of the same muscle: adaptive removal of the muscle response from the recorded EMG-signal. IEEE Trans Rehab Eng TRE-5:195:206

Seow KC (1988) Capacitive sensors. In: Webster JG (ed.) Tactile sensors for robotics and medicine. John Wiley, New York

Sepulveda F, Wells DM, Vaughan CL (1993) A neural network representation of electromyography and joint dynamics in human gait. J Biomech 26:101-109

Sepulveda F, Granat MH, Cliquet A Jr (1997) Two artificial neural systems for generation of gait swing by means of neuromuscular electrical stimulation. Med Eng Phys 19(1):21-28

Sepulveda F, Granat MH, Cliquet A Jr (1998) Gait Restoration in a spinal cord injured subject via neuromuscular electrical stimulation controlled by an artificial neural network. Int J Artif Org 21:49-62

Sergio L, Ostry DJ (1995) Coordination of multiple muscles in two degree of freedom elbow movements. Exp Brain Res 105(123):137-145

Sethi IK, Sarvarayudu GPR (1992) Hierarchical classifier design using mutual information. IEEE Trans Pattern Anal Mac Intel AMC-4:441-445

Shadmehr R, Mussa-Ivaldi F, Bizzi E (1993) Postural force fields of the human arm and their role in generating multi-joint movements. J Neurosci 13:45-62

Shadmehr R, Mussa-Ivaldi FA (1994) Adaptive representation of dynamics during learning of motor task. J Neurosci 5:3208-3224

Sharma M, Marsolais EB, Polando G, Triolo RJ, Davis JA Jr, Bhadra N, Uhlir JP (1998) Implantation of a 16-channel functional electrical stimulation walking system. Clin Orthop 347:236-242

Sherrington CS (1900) The muscular sense. In: Scheifer EA (ed.) Text-book of Physiology. (vol 2) Pentland, Edinburgh, pp 1002-1025

Sherrington CS (1906) Integrative action of the nervous system. Yale Univ Press, New Haven

Sherrington CS (1910) Flexion-reflex of the limb, crossed extension-reflex, and reflex stepping and standing. J Physiol 40:28-121

Shik ML, Severin FV, Orlovsky GN (1966) Control of walking and running by means of electrical stimulation of the mid-brain. Biophysics 11:756-765

Shik ML, Orlovsky GN (1976) Neurophysiology of locomotor automatism. Physiol Rev 56:465-501

Shoenning HA, Anderegg L, Berkostrom D, Fonda M, Steinke B, Ulrich P (1965) Numerical scoring of self-cared status of patients. Arch Phys Med 46:689

Shue G, Crago PE, Chizeck HJ (1995) Muscle-joint models incorporating activation dynamics, moment-angle and moment-velocity properties. IEEE Trans Bimed Eng BME-42:212-223

Shue GH, Crago PE (1998) Muscle-tendon model with length history dependent activation-velocity coupling. Ann Biomed Eng 26:369-380

Shumway-Cook A, Anson D, Haller S (1988) Postural sway biofeedback: its effect on reestablishing stance stability in hemiplegic patients. Arch Phys Med Rehab 69:395-400

Simpson DC (1974) The choice of control system for multi-movement prosthesis: Extended physiological proprioception (e.p.p.). In: Herberts P, Kadefors R, Magnuson R, Peterse I (eds.) Control of upper-extremity prostheses and orthoses. (chap 15) Springfiled

Simpson JI, Wylie DR, De Zeeuv CI (1996) On climbing fibers and their consequences. Behav Brain Sci 19:384-389

Sinkjær T, Toft E, Andreassen S, Horneman BC (1988) Muscle stiffness in human ankle dorsiflexors: Intrinsic and reflex components. J Neurophysiol 60:1110-1121

Sinkjær T, Gantchev N, Arendt-Nielsen L (1992) Mechanical properties of human ankle extensors after muscle potentiation. J Electroenceph Clin Neurophysiol 85:412-418

Sinkjær T, Toft E, Larsen K, Andreassen S, Hansen HJ (1993) Non-reflex and reflex mediated ankle joint stiffness in multiple sclerosis patients with spasticity. Muscle and Nerve 16:69-76

Sinkjær T, Haugland MK, Haase J (1994) Natural neural sensing and artificial muscle control in man. Exp Brain Res 98:542-546

Sinkjær T, Magnussen I (1994) Passive, intrinsic, and reflex-mediated stiffness in the ankle extensors of hemiparetic patients. Brain 117:355-363

Sinkjær T, Andersen JB, Nielsen JF (1996a) Impaired stretch reflex and joint torque modulation during spastic gait. J Neurology 243:566-574

Sinkjær T, Andersen JB, Larsen B (1996b) Soleus stretch reflex modulation during gait in humans. J Neurophysiol 76:1112-1120

Sinkjaer T (1997) Muscle, reflex and central components in the control of the ankle joint in healthy and spastic man. Acta Neurol Scand Suppl 170:1-28

Sinkjær T, Haugland M, Struijk J, Riso R (1999) Long-term cuff electrode recordings from peripheral nerves in animals and humans. In: Windhorst U, Johansson H (eds.) Modern Techniques in Neuroscience. Springer-Verlag, pp 787-802

Sinkjær T (1999) Muscle stiffness in spastic patients. Advances in Rehabilitation 1(3):23-35

Sinkjær T, Andersen JB, Ladouceur M, Christensen LOD, Nielsen JB (2000) Major role for sensory feedback in soleus EMG activity in the stance phase of walking in man. J Physiol, 532(3)817-827

Skinner SR, Skinner HB, Wyait HP (1994) Gait analysis. In: Webster J (ed.) Encyclopedia of Biomedical Devices and Instrumentation. Wiley, pp 1353-1364

Smidt C (1984) Muscle Strength Testing: A System Based on Mechanics. Physical Therapy, Univ of Iowa, Iowa City

Smith BT, Peckham PH, Keith MW, Roscoe DD (1987) An externally powered, multichannel, implantable stimulator for versatile control of paralyzed muscle. IEEE Trans Biomed Eng BME-34(7):499-508

Smith BT, Betz RR, Mulcahey MJ, Triolo RJ (1994) Reliability of percutaneous intramuscular electrodes for upper extremity functional neuromuscular stimulation in adolescents with C5 tetraplegia. Arch Phys Med Rehabil 75(9):939-945

Smith BT, Mulcahey BJ, Betz RP (1996) Development of an upper extremity FES system for individuals with C4 tetraplegia. IEEE Trans Rehab Eng TRE-4:264-270

Smith BT, Tang Z, Johnson MW, Pourmehdi S, Gazdik MM, Buckett JR, Peckham PH (1998) An externally powered multichannel, implantable stimulator-telemeter for control of paralyzed muscles. IEEE Trans Biomed Eng BME-45:463-475

Soechting JF, Lacquaniti F (1981) Invariant characteristics of a pointing movement in man. J Neurosci 1:710-720

Soechting JF (1989) Elements of coordinated arm movements in three-dimensional space. In: Wallace SA (ed.) Perspectives on the Coordination of Movement. North-Holland, Amsterdam, pp 47-83

Soechting JF, Flanders M (1989) Errors in pointing are due to approximations in sensorymotor transformations. J Neurophys 62:595-608

Soechting JF, Flanders M (1992) Moving in three-dimensional space: frames of reference, vectors and coordinate systems. Annu Rev Neurosci 5:167-191

Soechting JF, Bueno CA, Herrmann U, Flanders M (1995) Moving effortlessly in three dimensions: does Donders law apply to arm movements? J Neurosci 15:6271-6280

Soechting JF, Flanders M (1995) Psychophysiological approaches to motor control. Curr Opin Neurobiol 5:742-748

Solandt DY, Magladery JW (1942) A comparison of effects of upper and lower motor neurone lesions on skeletal muscle. J Neurophysiol 5:373-380

Solomonow M, Eldred E, Lyman J, Foster J (1983) Control of muscle contractile force through indirect high-frequency stimulation. Am J Phys 62:71-82

Solomonow M, Baratta R, Hirokawa S, Rightor N, Walker W, Beaudette P, Shoji H, D'Ambrosia R (1989) The RGO Generation II: muscle stimulation powered orthosis as a practical walking system for thoracic paraplegics. Orthopedics 12(10):1309-1315

Solomonow M, Aguilar E, Reisin E, Baratta RV, Best R, Coetzee T, D'Ambrosia R (1997a) Reciprocating gait orthosis powered with electrical muscle stimulation (RGO II). Part I: Performance evaluation of 70 paraplegic patients. Orthopedics 20(4):315-24

Solomonow M, Reisin E, Aguilar E, Baratta RV, Best R, D'Ambrosia R (1997b) Reciprocating gait orthosis powered with electrical muscle stimulation (RGO II). Part II: Medical evaluation of 70 paraplegic patients. Orthopedics 20(5):411-418

Sperry RW (1947) Effect of crossing nerves to antagonistic limb muscles in the monkey. Arch Neurol Psychiatr 58: 452-473

Srinivasan MA, Whitehouse JM, LaMotte RH (1990) Tactile detection of slip: Surface microgeometry and peripheral neural codes. J Neurophysiol 63:1323-1332

Stallard J, Rose GK, Tait JH, Davies JB (1978) Assessment of orthosis by means of speed and heart rate. J Med Eng Technol 2:22-24

Stallard J, Rose GK (1980) Clinical decision making with the aid of ambulatory monitoring of heart rate. Prosth and Orth Intnl 4:91-96

Stanič U, Aćimović-Janežič R, Gros N, Trnkoczy A, Bajd T (1978) Multichannel electrical stimulation for correction of hemiplegic gait. Scand J Rehab Med 10:75-92

Stefanovska A, Vodovnik L, Gros N, Reberšek S, Aćimović-Janežič R (1989) FES and spasticity, IEEE Trans Bimed Eng BME-36(7):738-745

Stein RB, Charles D, Davis L, Jhamandas J, Mannard A, Nichols TR (1975) Principles underlying new methods for chronic neural recording. Canad J Neurol Sci 2:235-244

Stein RB, Nichols TR, Jhamandas J, Davis AL, Charles D (1977) Stable long-term recordings from cat peripheral nerves. Brain Res 128:21-38

Stein RB, Gordon T, Oguztöreli MN, Lee RG (1981) Classifying sensory patterns and their effects on locomotion and tremor. Can J Physiol Pharmacol 59:645-655

Stein RB (1982) What muscle variable(s) does nervous system control in limb movements? Exp Brain Sci 5:535-577

Stein RB, Capaday C (1988) The modulation of human reflexes during functional motor tasks. Trends Neurosci 11:328-332

Stein RB, Gordon T, Jefferson J, Sharfenberger A, Yang JF, de Zepetnek JT, Bélanger M (1992) Optimal stimulation of paralyzed muscle after human spinal cord injury. J Appl Physiol 72:1393-400

Stein RB, Bélanger M, Wheeler G, Wieler M, Popović D, Prochazka A, Davis L (1993) Electrical systems for improving locomotion after incomplete spinal cord injury: An assessment. Arch Phys Med Rehabil 74:954-959

Stein RB (1995) Presynaptic inhibition in humans. Prog Neurobiol 47:533-544

Stein RB, Zehr EP, Lebiedowska MK, Popović D, Scheiner A, Chizeck HJ (1996) Estimating mechanical parameters of leg segments in neurologically intact and humans with disabilites. IEEE Trans Rehabil Eng TRE-4:201-211

Stepanenko Y, Vukobratović M (1976) Dynamics of articulated open-chain active mechanisms. Math Biosci 28:137-170

Stichel CC, Lips K, Muller HW (1995) Transplantation of Schwann cell suspension promotes regeneration in the transected posteommissural fornix of adult rats. J Neurotrauma 12:375

Strain RE, Olson WH (1975) Selective damage of large diameter peripheral nerve fibers by compression: An application of Laplace's law. Exp Neurol 47:68-80

Strange KD, Hoffer JA (1999a) Restoration of use of paralyzed limb muscles using sensory nerve signals for state control of FES-assisted walking. IEEE Trans Rehab Eng TRE-7:289-300

Strange KD, Hoffer JA (1999b) Gait phase information provided by sensory nerve activity during walking: Applicability of state controller feedback for FES. IEEE Trans Biomed Eng BME-46:797-810

Strojnik P, Aćimović-Janežič R, Vavken E, Simić V, Stanič U (1987) Treatment of drop foot using an implantable peroneal underknee stimulator. Scand J Rehabil Med 19:37-43

Strojnik P, Whitmoyer D, Schulman J (1990) An implantable stimulator for all season. In: Popović D (ed.) Advances in External Control of Human Extremities X, Nauka, pp 335-344

Strojnik P, Schulman J, Loeb G, Troyk P (1993) Multichannel FES system with distributed microstimulators. In: Proc Ann Int Conf IEEE EMBS, pp 1352-1353

Sunderland S (1978) Nerves and Nerve Injuries, 2nd edn. Churchill-Livingstone, Edinburgh

Sutherland DH, Hagy JL (1972) Measurement of gait movements from motion picture film. J Bone Jt Surg 54:787

Suton RS (1988) Learning to predict by the methods of temporal differences. Machine Learning pp 9-44

Sweeney JD, Mortimer JT (1986) An asymmetric two electrode cuff for generation of unidirectionally propagated action potentials. IEEE Trans Biomed Eng BME-33:541-549

Sweeney JD, Ksienski DA, Mortimer JT (1990) A nerve cuff technique for selective excitation of peripheral nerve trunk regions. IEEE Trans Biomed Eng BME-37(7):706-715

Sweeney JD, Crawford NR, Brandon TA (1995) Neuromuscular stimulation selectivity of multiple-contact nerve cuff electrode arrays. Med Biol Eng Comp 33:418-425

Sweeney PC, Lyons GM (1999) Fuzzy Gait Event Detection in a Finite State Controlled FES Drop Foot Correction System. J Bone Joint Surg (BR) 81-B:93-93

Szabo RR, Szabo P, Pandya AS (1994) Neural Network as Robot Arm Manipulator Controller. In: Proc Southeast IEEE Creative Tech Transfer - A Global Affair, pp 139–141

Tai C, Booth AM, Robinson CJ, de Groat WC, Roppolo JR (2000) Multielectrode stimulation within the cat L6 spinal cord: influences of electrode combinations and stimulus interleave time on knee joint extension torque. IEEE Trans Rehab Eng 8(1):1-10

Taira M, Boline J, Smyrnis N, Georgopoulos AP, Ashe J (1996) On the relation between single cell activity in the motor cortex and the direction and magnitude of three-dimensional static isometric force. Exp Brain Res 109:367-376

Talbot YM, Darian-Smith I, Kornbuber HH, Mounteastle VB (1968) The sense of flutter-vibration: comparison of the human capacity with response patterns of mechanoreceptive afferents from the -monkey hand. J Neurophysiol 31:301-334

Tashman S, Zajac FE (1992) Functional electrical stimulation for lower extremities. In: Stein RB, Peckham PH, Popović D (eds.) Neural Prostheses: Replacing Motor Function after Disease or Disability. Oxford Univ Press, New York, pp 252-280

Tashman S, Zajac FE, Perkash I (1995) Modeling and simulation of paraplegic ambulation in a reciprocating gait orthosis. J Biomech Eng 117(3):300-308

Tator CH, Rowed DW, Schwartz ML (eds.) (1982) Sunnybrook cord injury scales for assessing neurological injury and neurological recovery in early management of acute spinal cord injury. Raven Press, New York

Taub E, Perrella PN, Miller EA, Barro G (1975a) Diminution of early environmental control through perinatal and prenatal somatosensory deafferentation. Biol Psych 10(6):609-626

Taub E, Goldberg IA, Taub P (1975b) Deafferentation in monkeys: pointing at a target without visual feedback. Exp Neurol 46(1):178-186

Taub E, Miller NE, Novack TA, Cook EW 3d, Fleming WC, Nepomuceno CS et al. (1993) Technique to improve chronic motor deficit after stroke. Arch Phys Med Rehabil 74(4):347-354

Taylor CL, Schwartz RJ (1955) The anatomy and mechanics of the human hand. Artif limbs 2:22-35

Taylor PN (ed.) (1997) The Univ of Limerick Drop Foot Stimulator. The Inst Phys Eng Med, York, England

Tello F (1911) La influencia del neurotrophismo en la regeneracion de los centros nerviosos. Trabajos del Laboratorio de Investigaciones Biologicas de la Universidad de Madrid 9:123-159

Tepavac D, Nikolić Z (1992) A portable 8-hannel surface EMG recording system. In: Proc Ann Int Conf IEEE EMBS 4:14333-14334

Tepavac D, Medri E (1998) Programmable functional electrical stimulator with EMG feedback. In: Proc 6th Vienna Int Workshop FES, Vienna, pp 267-270

Thelen E, Bradshaw G, Ward JA (1981) Spontaneous kicking in month-old infants: manifestation of a human central locomotor program. Behav Neurol Biol 32(1):45-53

Thelen E (1983) Learning to walk is still an "old" problem: A reply to Zelazo. J Motor Behav 15:139-161

Thilmann A, Fellows SJ, Ross HF (1991) Biomechanic changes at the ankle joint after stroke. J Neurol Neurosurg & Psychiatry 54:134-139

Thoma H, Holle J, Moritz E, Stöhr H (1978) Walking after paraplegia - A principle concept. In: Advances in External Control of Human Extremities VI, ETAN, pp 71-84

Thoma H, Frey M, Hole J, Kern H, Mayr W, Schwanda G, Stoehr H (1987) Functional neurostimulation to substitute locomotion in paraplegia patients. In: Andrade JD (ed.) Artificial Organs. VCH Publishers, pp 515-529

Thomas CK, Westling G (1995) Tactile unit properties after human cervical spinal cord injury. Brain 18(Pt 6):1547-1556

Thompson WN (1967) What the Social Security Disability Program means to you and your patient. N C Med J 28(7):273-276

Thomsen M, Struijk JJ, Sinkjær T (1996) Artifact reduction with monopolar nerve cuff recording electrodes. In: 18th Ann Int Conf of the IEEE Eng in Med and Biol Soc, Amsterdam

Thoroughman KA, Shadmehr R (1999) Electromyographic correlates of learning an internal model of reaching movements. J Neurosci 19(19):8573-8588

Thorsen R, Ferrarin M, Spadone R, Frigo C (1998) An approach using wrist extension as control of FES for restoration of hand function in tetraplegics. In: Proc 6th Vienna Workshop on Functional Electrostimulation

Thorsen R, Ferrarin M, Spadone R, Frigo C (1999) Functional control of the hand in tetraplegics based on residual synergistic EMG activity. Artif Organs 23(5):470-473

Thrope GB, Peckham PH, Crago PE (1985) A computer-controlled multichannel stimulation system for laboratory use in functional neuromuscular stimulation. IEEE Trans Biomed Eng BME-31:363-370

Toft E, Sinkjær T, Espersen GT (1989a) Quantification of stretch reflexes. Acta Neurol Scandinav 79:384-390

Toft E, Sinkjær T, Kålund S, Espersen GT (1989b) Biomechanical properties of the human ankle in relation to passive stretch. J Biomechanics 22:1129-1132

Toft E, Sinkjær T, Andreassen S, Larsen K (1991) Mechanical and electromyographic responses to stretch of the human ankle extensors. J Neurophysiol 60:1110-1121

Tomović R, Boni G (1962) An adaptive artificial hand. IRE Trans Autom Contr AC-7:3-10

Tomović R, Popović D, Stein R (1995) Nonanalytical methods for motor control. World Sci Publ, Singapore

Tomović R, McGhee RB (1968) A finite state approach to the synthesis of bioengineering control systems. IEEE Trans Human Factors Eng HFE-7:65-69

Tomović R, Vukobratović M, Vodovnik L (1973) Hybrid actuators for orthotic systems - Hybrid assistive system. In: Advances in External Control of Human Extremities, ETAN, pp 73-88

Tomović R, Popović D, Gračanin F (1978) A technology for self-fitting of orthoses. In: Advances in External Control of Human Extremities (ECHE) VI, ETAN, pp 1-12

Tomović R, Turajlić S, Popović D (1981) Active modular unit for lower limb assistive devices. In: Advances in External Control of Human Extremities (ECHE) VII, ETAN, pp 1-15

Tomović R, Turajlić S, Popović D, McGhee RB (1982) Bioengineering actuator with non-numerical control. In: Control Aspects in Orthotics and Prosthetics, IFAC Proc, Pergamon Press, pp 145-151

Tomović R (1984) Control of assistive systems by external reflex arcs. In: Popović D, (ed.) Advances in external control of human extremities X, Nauka, pp 1-8

Tomović R (1991) Skill-based expert systems. In: Tzafestas T (ed.) Intelligent Robotics Systems. Marcel Decker, New York, pp 109-136

Tomović R, Anastasijević R, Vučo J, Tepavac D (1991) The study of locomotion by finite state models. Biol Cybern 63:271-276

Tong KY, Granat MH (1998) Virtual artificial sensor technique for functional electrical stimulation. Med Eng Phys 20:458-468

Tong KY, Granat MH (1999) Gait control system for functional electrical stimulation using neural networks. Med Biol Eng Comp 37:35-41

Tower SS (1937) Function and structure in the chronically isolated lumbosacral spinal cord of the dog. J Comp Neurol 67:109-131

Townsend MA, Seireg AA (1973) Effects of model complexity and gait criteria on the synthesis of bipedal locomotion. IEEE Biomed Eng BME-20:433-444

Tresch MC, Bizzi E (1999) Responses to spinal microstimulation in the chronically spinalized rat and their relationship to spinal systems activated by low threshold cutaneous stimulation. Exp Brain Res 129:401-416

Triolo R, Nathan R, Handa Y, Keith M, Betz RR, Carroll S, Kantor C (1996) Challenges to clinical deployment of upper limb neuroprostheses. J Rehabil Res Dev 33(2):111-122

Trnkoczy A (1978) Functional electrical stimulation of extremities: Its basis, technology and role in rehabilitation. Automedica 2:59-100

Troyk PR, Jaeger RJ, Haklin M, Poyezdala J, Bajzek T (1986) Design and implementation of an implantable goniometer. IEEE Trans Biomed Eng BME-33(2):215-222

Tubiana R (1984) Architecture and functions of the hand. In: Tubiana R, Thomine JM, Mackin E (eds.) Examination of the hand and upper limb. Saunders, Philadelphia, pp 1-97

Turajlić S Drakulić (1981) Above-Knee Prosthesis with attitudinal control. In: Advances in External Control of Human Extremities VII, ETAN, pp 529-541

Tyler DJ, Durand DM (1996) Selective stimulation with a chronic slowly penetrating interfascicular nerve electrode. In: Proc 18th Ann Int IEEE EMBS, pp 1233-1234

Uno Y, Kawato M, Suzuki R (1989) Formation and control of optimal trajectory in human multijoint arm movement-minimum torque-change model. Biol Cybern 61:89-101

Upshaw B, Sinkjær T (1998) Digital signal processing algorithms for the detection of afferent nerve activity recorded from cuff electrodes. IEEE Trans Rehab Eng TRE-6:172-181

Vallbo ÅB, Johansson RS (1984) Properties of cutaneous mechanoreceptors in the human hand related to touch sensation. Human Neurobiology 3:3-14

Van Boven RW, Johnson KO (1994) A psychophysical study of the mechanisms of sensory nerve recovery following nerve injury in humans. Brain 117:149-167

Van der Spek JH, Velthuis WJR, Veltink PH, Vries de TJA (1996) Neurofuzzy control of FES assisted freely swinging leg of paraplegic subjects. In: Proc of the 18th IEEE Conf EMBS Amsterdam, pp 2334-2335

Vaughan CL, Davis BL, O'Connor JC (1992) Dynamics of human gait. Human Kinetic Publishers, Il

Vaughan TM, Miner LA, McFarland DJ, Wolpaw JR (1998) EEG-based communication: analysis of concurrent EMG activity. Electroencephalogr Clin Neurophysiol 107(6):428-433

Veltink PH, Koopman AFM, Mulder AJ (1990) Control of cyclical lower leg movements generated by FES. In: Popović D (ed.) Advances in External Control of Human Extremities X, Nauka, pp 81-90

Veltink PH, Chizeck HJ, Crago PE, El-Bialy A (1992) Nonlinear joint angle control for artificially stimulated muscle. IEEE Trans Biomed Eng BME-39:368-380

Veltink PH, Franken HM (1996) Detection of knee unlock during stance by accelerometry. IEEE Trans Rehabil Eng TRE-6:395-402

Veltink PH, de Vries TJA, Koopman HFJA, Hermens HJ (eds.) (1999) Estimating orientation with gyroscopes and accelerometers. Institute for Biomedical Technology, Univ of Twente, Enschede

Veraart C, Grill WM, Mortimer JT (1993) Selective control of muscle activation with a multipolar nerve cuff electrode. IEEE Trans Biomed Eng BME-40(7):640-653

Visintin M, Barbeau H (1989) The effects of body weight support on the locomotion pattern of spastic patients. Can J Neurol Sci 16: 315-325

Vodovnik L, Crochetiere WJ, Reswick JB (1967) Control of a skeletal joint by electrical stimulation of antagonists. Med Biol Eng 5:97-109

Vodovnik L, Bajd T, Kralj A, Gračanin F, Strojnik P (1981) Functional electrical stimulation for control of locomotor systems. CRC Crit Rev Bioeng 6:63-131

Volz RG, Lieb M, Benjamin J (1980) Biomechanics of the wrist. Clin Orthop 149:112-117

von Hofsten C (1979) Development of visually guided reaching. The approach phase J Mot Behav 5:150-178

von Hofsten C (1980) Predictive reaching for moving objects by human infants. J Exp Child Psychol 30:369-392

Vossius G, Mueschen U, Hollander HJ (1987) Multichannel stimulation of the lower extremities with surface electrodes. In: Popović D (ed.) Advances in External Control of Human Extremities IX, ETAN, pp 193-203

Vukobratović M (1974) Development of Active Anthropomorphic Exoskeleton. J Biol Eng 12:66-80

Vukobratović M (1975) Legged Locomotion, Robots and Anthropomorphic Mechanisms. Institute Mihajlo Pupin, Belgrade

Vukobratović M, Stokić D (1980) Significance of force-feedback in controlling artificial locomotion-manipulation systems. IEEE Trans Biomed Eng 27(12):705-713

Wachholder K, Altenburger H (1926) Beitrage zur Physiologie der willkurlichen Bewegung. X Mitteilung. Einzelbewegungen. Pflügers Arch Ges Physiol 214:642-661

Wagner EM, Catranis JG (1954) New Developments in Lower-Extremity prostheses, In Klopsteg PE, Wilson PD (eds.) Human Limbs and Their Substitutes. McGraw-Hill, New York, Reprinted 1968

Watanabe S, (1985) Pattern Recognition. Wiley Interscience, New York

Waters RJ, Moore K, Graboff S, Paris K (1985a) Brachioradialis to flexor pollicis longus tendon transfer for active lateral pinch in the tetraplegic. J Hand Surg 10A:385-391

Waters RJ, McNeal DR, Faloon W, Clifford B (1985b) Functional electrical stimulation of the peroneal nerve for hemiplegia. J Bone Jt Surg 67:792-793

Waters RL, Barnes G, Husserl T, Silver L, Liss R (1988a) Comparable energy expenditure after arthrodesis of the hip and ankle. J Bone Joint Surg (Am) 70(7):1032-1037

Waters RL, Lunsford BR, Perry J, Byrd R (1988b) Energy-speed relationship of walking: standard tables. J Orthop Res 6(2):215-222

Waters RL, Yakura JS, Adkins RH, Sie I (1992) Recovery following complete paraplegia. Arch Phys Med Rehabil 73(9):784-789

Waters RL, Adkins RH, Yakura JS, Vigil D (1994) Prediction of ambulatory performance based on motor scores derived from standards of the American Spinal Injury Association. Arch Phys Med Rehabil 75(7):756-760

Waters RL, Sie IH, Gellman H, Tognella M (1996) Functional hand surgery following tetraplegia. Arch Phys Med Rehabil 77(1):86-94

Weber EH (1846) Der Tastsinn und das Cemeingefiihl. In: Wagner R (ed.) Handwbrterbuch der Physiologic. (vol III, abt. 2) Vieweg, Braunschweig, pp 481-588

Webster JG (ed.) (1988) Tactile sensors for robotics and medicine. J Wiley and Sons, New York

Wernig A, Herrarra AA (1986) Sprouting and remodeling at the nerve-muscle junction. Prog Neurobiol 27:251-291

Wernig A, Müller S (1990) Improvement of locomotion by prolonged training in patients with severe spinal cord lesions. In: Wernig A (ed.) Proc Int Symp Motor-Neuronal plasticity, Bonn, pp 31

Wernig A, Müller S (1992) Laufband locomotion with body weight support improved walking in persons with severe spinal cord injuries. Paraplegia 30(4):229-238

Wernig A, Müller S, Nanassy A, Cagol E (1995) Laufband therapy based on rules of spinal locomotion is effective in spinal cord injured patients. Europ J Neurosci 7:823-829

West SP, Roy RR, Edgerton VR (1986) Fiber type and fiber size of cat ankle, knee, and hip extensors and flexors following low thoracic spinal cord transaction at an early age. Exp Neurol 91:174-182

Westling G, Johansson RS (1984) Factors influencing the force control during precision grip. Exp Brain Res 53:277-284

White BL, Castle P, Held R (1964) Observations on the development of visually directed reaching. Child Develop 35:349-369

Whittle MW (1989) Biomechanical Assessment. The comparative evaluation of the Hip Guidance Orthosis (HGO) and the Reciprocating Gait Orthosis (RGO). HEI No 192, NHS Procurement Directorate, Dept of Health, UM Govt, United Kingdom

Wieler M, Stein RB, Ladouceur M, Whittaker M, Smith AW, Naaman S, et al. (1999) Multicenter evaluation of electrical stimulation systems for walking. Arch Phys Med Rehabil 80(5):495-500

Wiener N (1948) Cybernetics. Wiley, New York

Wijman AC, Stroh KC, Van Doren CL, Thrope GB, Peckham PH, Keith MW (1990) Functional evaluation of quadriplegic patients using a hand neuroprosthesis. Arch Phys Med Rehabil 32:1053-1057

Wilberg R, Guay M (1985) Long-term memory for a single movement. In: Goodman D, Wilberg R, Franks I (eds.) Differing perspectives in motor learning, memory, and control. Nort-Holland/Elsevier, Amsterdam

Wilhere GF, Crago PE, Chizeck HJ (1985) Design and evaluation of a digital closed-loop controller for the regulation of muscle forces by recruitment modulation. IEEE Trans Biomed Eng BME-32:668-676

Wilkie DR (1950) Relation between force and velocity in human muscles. J Physiol 204:443-460

Willemsen ATM, Bloemhof F, Boom HBK (1990a) Automatic Stance-Swing Phase Detection from Accelerometer Data for Peroneal Nerve Stimulation. IEEE Trans Biomed Eng BME-37(12):1201-1208

Willemsen ATM, van Alste JA, Boom HBK (1990b) Real-time gait assessment utilizing a new way of accelerometry. J Biomechanics 23(8):859-863

Wilson VJ, Melvill Jones G (1979) Mammalian Vestibular Physiology. Plenum press, New York

Wilson VJ, Peterson BW (1981) Vestibulospinal and reticulospinal system. In: Brooks VB (ed.) Handbook of Physiology. The Nervous System, Motor Control. Am Physiol Soc, Bethseda, pp 667-702

Winchester PK, Carrollo JJ, Parekh RN, Lutz LM, Aston JW (1993) A comparison of paraplegic gait performance using two types of reciprocating gait orthoses. Prosthet Orthot Int 17:101-106

Wing AM, Turton A, Fraser C (1986) Grasp size and accuracy of approach in reaching. J Motor Behav 18(3):245-260

Wing AM, Allison S, Jenner JR (1993) Retaining and retraining balance after stroke. Bailliers' Clin Neurol 2:87-120

Winter DA (1990) Biomechanics and Control of Human Movement. J Wiley, New York

Winter DA (1991) The Biomechanics and Motor Control of Human Gait: Normal, Elderly and Pathological. Univ of Waterloo Press, Waterloo

Winter DA (1992) Foot trajectory in human gait: a precise and multifunctional motor control task. Phys Ther 72:45-56

Winter DA, Prince F, Frank JS, Powell C, Zabjek KF (1996) Unified theory regarding A/P and M/L balance in quiet stance. J Neuropsys 76:2334-2343

Winters JM, Stark L (1987) Muscle models: what is gained and what is lost by varying model complexity. Biol Cybern 55:403-420

Winters JM (1990) Hill-based muscle models: a systems engineering perspective, In: Winters JM, Woo SLY (eds.) Multiple Muscle Systems: Biomechanics and Movement Organization. Springer-Verlag, New York, pp 69-73

Wolf SL, Binder-MacLeod SA (1983) Electromyographic biofeedback applications to the hemiplegic patient. Changes in upper extremity neuromuscular and functional status. Phys Ther 63(9):1393-1403

Wolf SL, Lecraw DE, Barton LA, Jann BB (1989) Forced use of hemiplegic upper extremities to reverse the effect of learned nonuse among chronic stroke and head-injured patients. Exp Neurol 104(2):125-132

Wolpaw JR, Carp JS (1990) Memory traces in spinal cord. Trends Neurosci 13(14):137-142

Wolpaw JR, Ramoser H, McFarland DJ, Pfurtscheller G (1998) EEG-based communication: improved accuracy by response verification. IEEE Trans Rehabil Eng TRE-6(3):326-33

Wolpert D, Gahramani Z, Jordan M (1994) Perceptual distortion contributes to the curvature of human reaching movements. Exp Brain Res 98:153-156

Wolpert D, Gahramani Z, Jordan M (1995) Are arm trajectories planned in kinematic or dynamic coordinates? Exp Brain Res 103:460-470

Wood-Jones F (1920) The principles of anatomy as seen in the hand. Churchill, London

Woodwort RS (1899) The accuracy of voluntary movement. Psychol Review Monograph (Suppl.3)

Woollacott MH, Debu B, Mowatt M (1987) Neuromuscular control of posture in the infant and child: Is vision dominant? J Motor Behav 19:167-186

Wrathall JR, Rigamonti DD, Braford MR, Kao CC (1982) Reconstruction of the contused cat spinal cord by the delayed nerve graft technique and cultured peripheral nonneuronal cells. Acta Neuropathol (Berlin) 57:59-69

Xerri C (1998) Plasticité post lésionnelle des cartes corticales somatosensorielles: une revue. CR Acad Sci Paris 321:135-151

Xu XM, Guenard V, Kleitman N, Aebischer P, Bunge MB (1995) A combination of BDNF and NT-3 promotes supraspinal axonal regeneration into Schwann cell grafts in adult rat thoracic spinal cord. Exp Neurol 134:261-272

Yakolev P, Lecours A (1967) The myologenetic cycles of regional maturation of the brain. In: Minkowski A (ed.) Regional development of the brain in early life. Davis, Phuladelphia, pp 3-70

Yamaguchi GT (1990) Performing whole body simulations of gait with 3D dynamic musculoskeletal models. In: Winters JM, Woo SL-Y (eds.) Multiple Muscle Systems: Biomechanics and Movement Organization. Springer Verlag, New York, pp 663-679

Yamaguchi GT, Zajac FE (1990) Restoring Unassisted Natural Gait to Paraplegics Via Functional Neuromuscular Stimulation: A Computer Simulation Study. IEEE Trans Biomed Eng BME-37:886-902

Yang JF, Stein RB, Jharnandas J, Gordon T (1990) Motor unit numbers and contractile properties after spinal cord injury. Ann Neurol 28:496-502

Yang JF, Fung J, Edamura M, Blunt R, Stein RB, Barbeau H (1991) H-reflex modulation during walking in spastic paretic subjects. Can J Neurol Sci 18:443-452

Yoshida K, Horch K (1993) Selective stimulation of peripheral nerve fibers using dual intrafascicular electrodes. IEEE Trans Biomed Eng BME-40:492-494

Yoshida K, Horch K (1996) Closed - loop control of ankle position using muscle afferent feedback with functional neuromuscular stimulation. IEEE Trans Biomed Eng 43(2):167-176

Zaal FTJM, Bootsma RJ, van Wieringen PCW (1998) Coordination in prehension. Exp Brain Res 119:427-435

Zadeh LA (1965) Fuzzy sets. Inform and Control 8:338-352

Zahalak GI (1990) Modeling muscle mechanics (and energetics). In: Winters JM, Woo S L-Y, (eds.) Multiple Muscle Systems: Biomechanics and Movement Organization. Springer Verlag, New York, pp 1-23

Zahalak GI (1992) An overview of muscle modeling, In: Stein RB, Peckham HP, Popović D (eds.) Neural Prostheses: Replacing Motor function after disease or disability. Oxford Univ Press, New York, pp 17-57

Zajac FE (1989) Muscle and tendon properties: models, scaling, and application to biomechanics and motor control. CRC Crit Rev Biomed Eng 17:359-411

Zajac FE, Gordon ME (1989) Determining muscles's force and action in multi-articular movement. Exercise Sport Sci Rev 17:187-230

Zancolli EA (1975) Surgery for the quadriplegic hand with active, strong wrist extension preserved: A study of 97 cases. Clin Otrhop 1(12):101-113

Zatsiorsky VM, Aruin AS, Selujanow WN (1984) Biomechanik des menschlichen Bewegungsapparates. Sportverlag, Berlin

Zheng YF, Shen JS (1990) Gait Synthesis for the SD-2 biped robot to climb sloping surfaces. IEEE Trans Robot Automat RA-6:86-96

Zhou BH, Baratta R, Solomonow M (1987) Manipulation of muscle force with various firing rate and recruitment control strategy. IEEE Trans Biomed Eng BME-34:128-139

Zhou BH, Katz SR, Baratta RV, Solomonow M, D'ambrosia RD (1997) Evaluation of antagonist coactivation strategies elicited from electrically stimulated muscles under load-moving conditions. IEEE Trans Biomed Eng BME-44:620-628

Zhou L, Munih M, Haugland M, Perkins TA, Donaldson N (1998) An implantable telemeter for ENG signals. In: Proc 6th Vienna Int Workshop on FES, Vienna, pp 327-330

Zill SN (1985a) Plasticity and proprioception in insects. II. Modes of reflex action of the locust metathoracic femoral chordotonal organ. J Exp Biol 116:463-480

Zill SN (1985b) Plasticity and proprioception in insects. I. Responses and cellular properties of individual receptors of the locust metathoracic femoral chordotonal organ. J Exp Biol 116: 435-461

Zong-Ming Li, Latash ML, Zatsiorsky VM (1998) Force sharing among fingers as a model of the redundancy problem. Exp Brain Res 119:276-286

Abbreviations

2D - Two-dimensional
3D - Three-dimensional
A/P - Antero / Posterior
ADL - Activities of Daily Living
AFO - Ankle-Foot Orthosis
AKP - Above-Knee Prosthesis
ALN - Adaptive Logic Network
ANFIS - Adaptive Network based Fuzzy Inference System
ANN - Artificial Neural Network
ARGO - Advanced Reciprocating Gait Orthosis
ARMA - Autoregressive Moving Average
ASIA - American Spinal Cord Injury Association
CNS - Central Nervous System
CoG - Center of Gravity
CoM - Center of Mass
CoP - Center of Pressure
CPG - Central Pattern Generator
DARMA - Deterministic Autoregressive Moving Average
DoF - Degree of Freedom
DSP - Double Support Phase
EMG - Electromyography
FA - Fast Adapting
FEL - Feedback Error Learning
FES - Functional Electrical Stimulation
FET - Field Effect Transistor
FIM - Functional Independence Measure
FIS - Fuzzy Inference System
FLC - Fuzzy Logic Control
FNS - Functional Neuromuscular Stimulation
FRO - Floor Reaction Orthosis
FSR - Force Sensing Resistor
GRF - Ground Reaction Force

HGO - Hip-Guidance Orthosis
HKAFO - Hip-Knee-Ankle-Foot Orthosis
IC - Infrared Camera
IL - Inductive Learning
IPI – Inter-pulse Interval
KAFO - Knee-Ankle-Foot Orthosis
LEMS - Lower Extremity Muscle Score
LIFE - Longitudinal Intra-fascicular Electrode
M/L - Medio/lateral
M1 zone - Primary Motor Cortex
MES - Myoelectric Signal
MLP - Multilayer Perceptron
NFM - Neuro-Fuzzy Model
NMES - Neuromuscular Electrical Stimulation
NP - Neuroprosthesis
PCI - Physiological Cost Index
PG - Pattern Generator
PI - Proportional-Integral
PID - Proportional-Integral-Derivative
PRC - Production Rule Control
PS - Pattern Shaper
PW - Pulse Width (duration)
QIF - Quadriplegia Index of Function
RBC - Rule-Based Control
RBF - Radial Basis Function
RBI - Rectified Bin Integrated
RF - Radio Frequency
RGO - Reciprocating Gait Orthosis
SAI and SAII - Slowly Adapting I and II
SCI - Spinal Cord Injury
SFMO - Self-Fitting Modular Orthosis
SP - Stimulation Period (reciprocal of pulse frequency)
SSP - Single Support Phase
SVD - Singular Value Decomposition
VA - Veterans Administration

Index

A

actuator level, 334, 410
adaptive control, 332, 337, 339, 340, 342
adaptive logic network (ALN), 246, 247, 248, 269, 356
adaptive network fuzzy inference system (ANFIS), 364
ADP, 396
advanced reciprocating gait orthosis (ARGO), 276, 283, 361
afferent fibers, 5, 6, 7, 19, 21, 23, 25, 26, 29, 30, 72, 75, 76
amplifier, 162, 244, 245, 251, 269
amplitude modulation (AM), 213, 363, 364, 366, 381, 382
amputation, 147, 299, 300, 310, 311, 318, 319, 324
anatomic synergists, 110
ankle-foot orthosis (AFO), 271, 277, 278, 343, 346, 349, 350, 379
anterolateral system, 6, 7
aperture, 102, 126, 127, 260, 398
artificial hand, 126, 250, 314, 326
artificial neural network (ANN), 341, 356, 362, 363, 366, 378, 383, 384, 385, 405
ascending pathway, 15
ASIA, 148, 149, 150
assessment, 125, 147, 151, 16, 195, 198, 283, 394, 410, 411
ATP, 36, 37
atrophied muscle, 205
auditory feedback, 186, 187, 196, 198, 199, 271
augmented training, 198, 200
autoregressive moving average (ARMA), 338

B

back-propagation algorithm, 383
basal ganglia, 10, 12, 74, 75, 87, 93, 129, 130
BDNF, 172, 173
Belgrade grasping system, 255
Belgrade leg, 358
bioartificial graft, 179
BION, 230
Bionic glove, 258
biphasic, 208, 211, 213, 231, 266
body-powered prosthesis, 319, 320, 321
body schema, 80
brain interface, 298
brain stem, 4, 6, 8, 9, 10, 11, 12, 71, 73, 74, 75, 77, 78, 87, 93, 96, 126, 176, 187, 293,
Brown-Sequard Syndrome, 134

C

capacitive sensor, 237
cauda equina, 131, 133
cell body, 13, 16, 17, 33, 135, 136, 137, 138, 139, 140
cell column, 5
center of gravity (COG), 70, 81, 90, 169, 278, 316
center of mass (CoM), 81, 82, 83, 84, 98, 101, 160, 163, 165, 169, 194, 197, 199, 277, 279, 280, 281, 283, 323, 326, 330, 331, 369
center of pressure (CoP), 1, 163, 169, 171, 172, 187, 196, 197, 202, 205, 209, 215, 233, 238, 290, 318, 357, 410
central pattern generator (CPG), 71, 90, 94, 95, 96, 97, 99, 189, 341, 391
cerebral hemispheres, 4, 8, 12, 126
cerebro-vascular infarction, 125
clavicle, 60, 61
clonus, 133, 134, 190, 196, 295
cocontraction map, 262, 399
cognitive feedback, 243

command interface, 209, 232, 254, 256, 407, 408
common mode rejection ratio, 251, 404
complete injury, 149, 174
concentric, 17, 23, 43, 45, 154, 253
cone electrode, 253
constant current, 227, 394
contractile force, 32, 38, 40, 44, 69
control of posture, 81, 82, 88, 275, 319
control of walking, 163, 271, 381, 382
controlled brake orthosis, 281
coordinated stepping, 99
coordination level, 354, 391, 393, 413
coordinative synergies 110
corticospinal system, 14, 74
current regulated, 210, 272
cycle-to-cycle control, 373

D

DC/DC converter, 227
decision level, 354
decomposition, 245, 363, 398
degree of freedom (DoF), 116, 118, 185, 253, 302, 312, 314, 321, 322, 324, 334
denervated muscle, 140, 142, 143, 145, 203, 208
de-noising, 247
dermatomes, 25, 150
deterministic autoregressive moving average (DARMA), 337
development of reaching, 112
development of walking, 89
diencephalon, 4, 10, 11, 127
digit, 56, 67
digital closed-loop control, 336
discrete time model, 337
disuse atrophy, 142, 143, 144
dorsal column, 6, 7, 20
dorsal column, 78
dorsal horn, 5, 6, 7, 14
dorsal horn, 76, 77
drop-foot see foot-drop
dynamic knee brace system, 281
dynamic model, 320, 321, 322, 323, 331, 351, 373, 390
dynamic optimization, 323
dynamic testing 151
eccentric, 42, 43, 45, 47, 138, 154, 204
efferent fibers, 9, 19, 23, 25, 214

elastomer, 232, 234
electrically powered prosthesis, 321, 322
electro-cutaneous interface, 200
endurance, 45, 161, 193, 203, 204, 206, 322
energy efficiency, 171, 296, 374
epimysial electrode, 218, 219, 248, 260, 261
epimysium, 32, 33
equilibrium point hypothesis, 1 16, 117
equilibrium, 10, 33, 43, 77, 81, 82, 83, 85, 86, 87, 90, 93, 98, 111, 114, 115, 116, 117, 120, 122,125, 168, 197, 277, 341, 367,406
excitation, 9, 16, 17, 18, 36, 39, 159, 210, 211, 213, 214, 217, 223, 229, 261, 328
external moment model, 397
exteroceptive, 19, 20
extrafusal fibers, 29, 30

F

facilitation, 9, 202
fast-twitch muscle, 203
fatigue, 41, 46, 120, 121, 125, 142, 144, 145, 161, 171, 203, 206, 214, 250, 255, 259, 265, 274, 285, 289, 322, 329, 336, 338, 339, 342, 366, 367, 371, 372, 374, 375, 377, 383, 387, 394, 398, 400, 407
feature extraction, 23, 200
feedback error learning, 390, 395
feed-forward control, 339, 341, 342, 367, 391
femur, 50, 51
fibula, 56, 57
FIM, 148, 151, 201
firing rate, 105, 253, 274, 338, 340
floor reaction orthosis (FRO), 279
FNS, 209
foot-drop, 226, 244, 265, 266, 267, 268, 382
footswitch, 158, 159
force plate, 160
force sensing resistor, 346, 381
Frankel, 148, 150, 384
Freehand, 226, 238, 254, 260, 261, 262, 263, 273, 400, 401, 405
Fugl-Meyer, 148, 292
fused contraction, 208
fuzzy inference system (FIS), 364
fuzzy logic control (FLC), 369
fuzzy logic network, 362
fuzzy model identification, 385

fuzzy system identification, 382

G

glia, 174, 175
glial cells, 16, 138,139
Golgi, 15, 28, 30, 86, 95
graft, 173, 176, 177, 178, 179, 180, 183
gray matter, 5, 6, 77, 116, 138, 225
guidance channel, 175, 176, 177, 178
gyroscope, 275
gyrus, 12, 128, 157, 234, 237, 238, 396

H

hand-crafted rules, 357, 361
Handmaster, 226, 254, 256, 257, 260
harness, 33, 100, 193, 194, 196, 319, 320, 321, 322
hemiparesis, 129, 187, 195, 266
hemiparetic, 194, 195, 196, 197, 198, 294, 373
hemiplegia, 129, 223, 257, 266
hemiplegic, 202, 205, 207, 291, 293, 375
hemisection, 134
hierarchical control, 75
hierarchical structure, 1
hierarchical structure, 82, 355, 409, 410
high frequency stimulation, 203, 342
Hill macroscopic model, 327
hip-disarticulation, 299, 311
hip-guidance orthosis (HGO), 275
hip-knee-ankle-foot orthosis (HKAFO) 272
histological study, 241, 242
humerus, 61, 62, 63, 64, 312
hybrid assistive system, 284, 288, 357, 361, 374
hybrid control, 334, 351, 352, 374, 391, 410
hybrid hierarchical control, 354
hybrid prosthesis, 317, 322, 323

I

IL, 226,270, 365,366,377,378,383,411,412
impedance, 200, 206, 210, 216, 217, 219, 222, 228, 244, 251, 258, 402, 404
implantable NP, 262, 269
implantable stimulator, 229, 262, 268, 269, 274, 407
inductive learning, 356, 365, 377, 411

infarction, 126, 128, 129, 215
instrumented walkway, 158
intermittent stimulation, 204, 206
interpulse interval, 215, 228, 266, 331, 333, 336, 337, 338, 340, 402
intracortical electrode, 248
intrafascicular electrode, 223
intrafusal fibers, 29, 30
intramuscular electrode, 212, 213, 218, 219, 221, 251, 254, 255, 256, 260, 272, 332, 341, 396, 407, 408
intraneural electrode, 223, 224
intraspinal stimulation, 225
involuntary stepping, 99, 189, 190
IPI, 215, 227, 336
isokinetic, 152, 153, 342, 369
isometric testing, 151
isometric, 37, 42, 43, 45, 204, 205, 341, 342, 369, 372, 394, 400, 405
isotonic, 37, 42, 43, 44, 205
I-T (amplitude-duration curve), 213

J

jerk, 71, 120, 322

K

key grip, 180, 183,184
knee cage, 276, 278
knee joint 50
knee joint mechanism, 287
knee-ankle-foot orthosis (KAFO), 272, 278, 279, 281, 286, 288, 296, 297

L

λ-model, 112
labyrinth, 80
lateral column, 6, 7, 77
lateral grasp, 124, 232, 262, 397
level of recruitment, 213, 214, 215
ligament, 48, 49, 149, 173, 397
locomotor rhythm, 90, 94, 98, 99, 100
long-term implant, 232, 241, 242, 264
LSU RGO, 286

M

machine learning, 356, 377, 379, 406, 412
macroscopic model, 327, 328

magnetic stimulation, 186
manual muscle testing, 183
Markovian decision process, 368
maximum precision, 119
mechanoreceptors, 22, 24, 26, 86, 263, 264, 265
median nerve, 70
mediolateral, 154
medulla oblongata, 8
medulla, 6, 7, 8, 12, 14, 15, 20, 78, 87, 127
membrane, 17, 18, 22, 23, 34, 36, 56, 136, 141, 211, 372
microscopic model, 327, 328
midbrain, 4, 8, 9, 14, 77, 78, 127, 129
minimum acceleration, 1 19
minimum effort, 116
minimum jerk, 1 19, 120, 121
minimum time, 120, 391, 404
minimum torque, 119, 121
model parameter, 324, 330, 332, 333
modeling, 114, 250, 251, 290, 325, 319, 322, 323, 342, 351, 352, 355, 361
modular orthosis, 277
motion analysis system, 378
motor cortex, 3, 10, 11, 14, 71, 73, 74, 96, 103, 104, 106, 107, 109, 128, 129, 186, 253
motor equivalence, 111, 114
motor execution, 121, 122
motor learning, 8, 194
motor level, 131, 133, 148, 149, 150
motor pathway, 12, 13, 14, 73, 293
motor planning, 88, 104
motor program, 82, 97, 98, 99, 104, 189, 194, 258, 410
motor score, 133, 148, 149, 150, 292, 296
movement analysis, 154, 155, 157, 160
multi-channel device, 230
Multiple sclerosis, 134
multi-purpose standing frame, 198
muscle activity, 15, muscle activity, 154, 172
muscle atrophy, 142, 301
muscle endurance, 145, 203
muscle function, 172
muscle length, 143
muscle length, 30, 37, 43, 44, 70, 82, 115, 203, 219, 394
muscle loading, 202
muscle score, 296

muscle spindle, 15, 23, 28, 29, 30, 33, 86, 95, 109
myelinated fibers, 16, 140, 242
myoelectric control, 250, 259, 263, 317, 321, 326, 401
myofibril, 34, 35
myopathic, 140
myopathies, 139, 142

N

natural sensor, 238, 248, 250, 361, 401
nerve damage, 241
neural engineering, 409
neural network, 94, 106, 224, 250, 341, 362, 366, 377, 384, 385, 387, 388, 389, 390, 391
neural pathways, 14
neuro muscular junction, 36
neurofuzzy control, 387, 390
neuro-fuzzy model (NFM), 246
neurogenic, 139, 140
neurological level, 133, 148, 150
neuromuscular junction, 139
neuron theory, 172
neuropathies, 141
neuroregeneration, 171
neurorehabilitation, 125, 187, 192, 195, 196, 197, 198, 289
neurotrophin, 173, 177
NGF, 172, 173, 179
NMES, 209

O

occipital lobe, 12, 127
Odstock stimulator, 226
opposition, 47, 68, 70, 124, 125, 256, 260, 263, 314, 315, 398
optimization, 114, 119, 120, 121, 317, 322, 323, 331, 341, 348, 350, 35 3, 355, 367, 371, 398, 406
orthoses, 171, 184, 262, 275, 276, 277, 278, 283, 285, 286, 295, 297
output stage, 227, 228

P

pain threshold, 28, 205
palmar grasp, 124, 261, 263, 407

paraplegia, 99, 100, 146, 148, 132, 192, 209, 224, 295, 297, 346, 349, 350, 367
paraplegic, 193, 198, 199, 200, 202, 207, 226, 273, 278, 284, 285, 294, 295, 296, 297, 298, 326, 332, 339, 349, 350, 357, 361, 366, 367, 374, 375, 376, 377, 378, 385,386,387,391,394
Parastep I, 226
paretic limb, 196, 197, 202
parietal lobe, 6, 12, 13, 20, 127
Parkinson, 130
patella, 53, 277
pattern generator (PG), 340
pattern shaper (PS), 340, 342
pelvis, 49
perception, 6, 7, 15, 20, 21, 26, 27 79, 86, 102, 103, 108, 109, 127, 129, 131, 134, 135, 140, 141
percutaneous electrode, 219, 272, 357, 386, 406
peripheral input, 72, 99, 100, 146, 294, 295
peroneal nerve, 60, 223, 249, 266, 271, 286
perturbation, 88, 201, 318
phalangeal joints, 343
phasic input, 189, 341
Physiological Cost Index (PCI), 289
PID controller, 337
piezoelectric, 159, 160, 235
piezoresistive sensor, 234, 235
plantar arch, 59
plantar extension, 56, 271
plantar flexion, 57, 146
polycentric knee mechanism, 300
pons, 4, 8, 9, 15, 78, 87, 127
population code, 23
population vector, 105, 106, 107
post-tetanic, 42
potentiation, 42, 214, 292, 374, 377
powered orthosis, 277
powered treadmill, 194, 346
preamplifier, 243, 251
preferred direction, 105, 106, 253
preparatory prosthesis, 311
presynaptic terminal, 137
primary motor cortex, 12, 104, 105, 106
pronation, 64, 65,312, 313, 322, 403, 407
proprioceptive, 2, 7, 19, 20, 85, 87, 91, 128, 135, 197, 201, 272
propriospinal neuron, 6, 75, 76,77, 104, 177

pulse width (PW), 213, 217, 221, 230, 275, 329, 331, 332, 333, 334, 398, 403
Purkinje cells, 107
pylon, 307, 308, 309, 310, 311, 323, 324
QIF, 148, 151, 152

R

radial basis function, 363
radial deviation, 68, 69, 257
radial nerve, 63, 70, 358
radio frequency (RF), 230, 232, 269, 275
radius, 62, 63, 64, 65, 67, 184, 216
range of movement, 31, 50, 57, 275, 292, 295, 306, 343, 348, 402
Ranvier, 17, 45
RBC, 355, 356, 358, 362
RBF, 363, 366, 378, 380
reaching movement, 3, 84, 102, 104 106, 107, 108, 109, 118, 121, 122
reciprocating gait orthosis (RGO), 281, 283, 286, 297, 298, 327
recruitment order, 210, 214
reference based control, 323
refractory period, 18
regeneration, 16, 140, 142, 172, 173, 174, 175, 176, 177, 178, 179, 180, 208, 225
relaxation, 31, 37, 39, 40, 41, 46, 134, 141, 142
repetitive training, 194
resorbable nerve graft, 179
restorative neurology, 188
restriction rules, 379
reticular formation, 8, 9, 10, 11, 14, 15, 71, 78, 87, 88, 96
robot hand, 325
rubrospinal pathway, 14
rule-based control, 232, 248, 286, 355, 357, 361, 374, 378

S

sacral cord, 134
sarcolemma, 34, 36
sarcomere, 34, 35, 38, 44
sarcoplasm, 33, 36, 37
scapula, 61, 62, 63
Schwann cell, 17, 137, 172, 173, 174, 175, 176, 177, 178, 179, 180

sciatic nerve, 60, 178, 179, 180, 221, 222, 249, 338, 382
self-coiling cuff, 239
self-fitting modular orthosis (SFMO), 279, 284, 285, 288
sensory afferent, 26
sensory capacity, 22, 26
sensory pathway, 3, 6, 7, 13
sensory score, 148, 150
sensory threshold, 21
shank, 49
shoulder joint, 61, 62
size principle, 210
skeletal muscle, 1, 6, 19, 28, 29, 69, 137, 139
sliding filament, 328
slow-twitch muscle, 204
socket, 50, 60, 61, 67, 300, 301, 310, 311, 316, 321, 322
somatic sensory cortex, 12
spasm, 146, 147, 294, 295, 319
spasticity, 127, 143, 146, 165, 171, 184, 190, 196, 207, 225, 266, 289, 290, 293, 294, 298, 333
spatial discrimination, 22
stability, 57, 63, 159, 173, 194, 197, 199, 248, 266, 276, 278, 282, 285, 296, 299, 304, 305, 308, 336, 337, 351, 388, 390
standing biofeedback, 198
standing frame, 197, 198, 275, 277
standing frame, 369
stepping movement, 189, 193
stepping movement, 89, 96, 99
stepping, 89, 95, 96, 99, 100, 189, 190, 192, 193, 194, 273
stiffness, 47, 48, 70, 81, 83, 103, 116, 120, 122, 146, 198, 199, 253, 290, 291, 292, 293, 294, 324, 332, 335, 339, 341, 367, 369, 370, 398, 399, 406, 407
stimulation period (SP), 331
stimulation regimen, 205
stimulus intensity, 21, 22, 23, 40, 371
strain gauge, 157, 234, 337, 378
strengthening, 60, 205, 206
stroke, 125, 126, 127
structural units, 110
sulcus, 12, 63
sural nerve, 245, 246, 269
switched systems, 353
switching curve controller, 368

Swivel walker, 283
synapse, 6, 13, 14
synaptic relay, 13
synergistic control, 113, 260, 398, 410
synergy, 47, 83, 88, 104, 111, 113, 123, 196, 409, 411, 412, 413
syringomyelia, 132, 135

T

tectospinal pathway, 15
tectum, 9, 14, 15, 77
telemetry, 161, 231, 274
temporal lobe, 12
temporal summation, 214, 215, 337, 372
tendon transfer, 180, 183, 185, 186, 260, 406, 408
tetanus, 37, 41, 42, 205, 215
tetraplegia, 152, 180, 183, 184, 192, 209, 224, 406, 407
thigh, 49
three-factor model, 328
tibia, 53
tibial nerve, 60
toe, 47, 59
transhumeral prosthesis, 312, 403, 409
transplantation, 175, 176, 177
transtibial prosthesis, 310, 324
treadmill walking, 93, 191, 192, 194, 196
triphasic pattern, 1 17
trophic factor, 139, 172, 180
twitch, 29, 37, 39, 40, 42, 203, 205, 214, 215, 292

U

ulna, 62, 63
ulnar deviation, 47, 68, 69, 257, 312
ulnar nerve, 70, 171
unmyelinated fibers, 16, 19, 242

V

velocity of conduction, 141
velocity of shortening, 37, 329, 393, 394
ventral column, 6, 77
ventral horn, 5, 6, 29, 33
ventral spinocerebral tract, 15
vestibular receptor, 86
vestibular system, 9

vestibulospinal pathway, 14, 15
vibrotactile feedback, 199
visual guidance, 97, 107, 108
volar flexion, 68, 256, 312
voltage regulated, 210

W

Wallerian degeneration, 137, 138
wavelet, 247, 356

weight support, 93, 193, 194, 275
white matter, 5, 6, 76, 78, 127, 138
wireless, 155, 162, 163, 227, 229, 230, 271, 410
wrist joint, 67, 68

Z

Z-domain, 336